Coronary Arteriography and Angioplasty

Coronary Arteriography
and Angioplasty

Spencer B. King III, M.D.
Professor of Medicine (Cardiology)
Professor of Radiology
Emory University School of Medicine
Director, Cardiovascular Laboratory
Emory Hospital
Atlanta

John S. Douglas, Jr., M.D.
Associate Professor of Medicine (Cardiology)
Assistant Professor of Radiology
Emory University School of Medicine
Atlanta

McGraw-Hill Book Company

New York St. Louis San Francisco Auckland Bogotá Guatemala Hamburg
Johannesburg Lisbon London Madrid Mexico Montreal New Delhi Panama
Paris San Juan São Paulo Singapore Sydney Tokyo Toronto

NOTICE

Medicine is an ever-changing science. As new research and clinical experience broaden our knowledge, changes in treatment and drug therapy are required. The editors and the publisher of this work have checked with sources believed to be reliable in their efforts to provide drug dosage schedules that are complete and in accord with the standards accepted at the time of publication. However, readers are advised to check the product information sheet included in the package of each drug they plan to administer to be certain that the information contained in these schedules is accurate and that changes have not been made in the recommended dose or in the contraindications for administration. This recommendation is of particular importance in connection with new or infrequently used drugs.

CORONARY ARTERIOGRAPHY

1234567890HALHAL8987654

ISBN 0-07-034616-X

This book was set in Times Roman by General Graphic Services, Inc.; the editors were Beth Ann Kaufman and Steven Tenney; the production supervisor was Avé McCracken. Halliday Lithograph Corporation was printer and binder.

Library of Congress Cataloging in Publication Data

Main entry under title:

Coronary arteriography and angioplasty.

Includes index.
1. Angiocardiography. 2. Coronary arteries—Radiography. 3. Transluminal angioplasty. I. King, Spencer B. III, date. II. Douglas, John S., Jr., date.
[DNLM: 1. Angiography—methods. 2. Coronary Vessels—radiography. 3. Angioplasty, Transluminal. 4. Coronary Disease—Therapy. WG 300 K54c]
RC683.5.A5C67 1985 616.1′2307572 84-12599
ISBN 0-07-034616-X

Dedicated to our wives, Gail and June

Contents

List of Contributors

RUSSELL E. AIKEN, M.S.
Phillips Medical Systems Division
Atlanta

JAMES M. BRADFORD, Ph.D
Senior Associate
Emory University School of Medicine
Atlanta

JAMES C. CAMPBELL, M.D.
Fellow in Medicine (Cardiology)
Emory University School of Medicine
Atlanta

JOHN S. DOUGLAS, Jr., M.D.
Associate Professor of Medicine (Cardiology)
Assistant Professor of Radiology
Emory University School of Medicine
Atlanta

ROBERT H. FRANCH, M.D.
Professor of Medicine (Cardiology)
Emory University School of Medicine
Atlanta

ANDREAS R. GRUENTZIG, M.D.
Professor of Medicine (Cardiology) and Radiology
Director, Interventional Cardiovascular Medicine
Emory University School of Medicine
Atlanta

FREDERICK A. HEUPLER, Jr., M.D.
Division of Cardiology
The Cleveland Clinic Foundation
Cleveland

J. WILLIS HURST, M.D.
Candler Professor of Medicine (Cardiology)
Chairman, Department of Medicine
Chief of Medicine
Emory University School of Medicine
Atlanta

EILEEN JUDKINS, R.N., N.P.
Loma Linda University School of Medicine
Loma Linda, California

MELVIN P. JUDKINS, M.D.
Professor of Radiology
Loma Linda University School of Medicine
Loma Linda, California

SPENCER B. KING III, M.D.
Professor of Medicine (Cardiology)
Professor of Radiology
Emory University School of Medicine
Director, Cardiovascular Laboratory
Emory Hospital
Atlanta

DOUGLAS C. MORRIS, M.D.
Associate Professor of Medicine
Emory University School of Medicine
Atlanta

PERRY SPRAWLS, Ph.D.
Professor and Director
Division of Radiological Sciences and Education
Department of Radiology
Emory University School of Medicine
Atlanta

WILLIAM H. WILLIS, Jr., M.D.
Professor of Medicine
Loma Linda University School of Medicine
Director, Cardiovascular Laboratories
Loma Linda Medical Group
Loma Linda, California

Preface

Coronary atherosclerosis remains the foremost cause of death in industrial societies; in developing societies its incidence—almost universally—is rising. As a diagnostic technique, coronary arteriography has proven critical in the identification and assessment of patients with coronary atherosclerosis. It has also provided the basis for the development of all revascularization procedures, and holds promise for the discovery of new interventions for alleviating obstructive coronary disease and evaluating methods of retarding atherosclerosis.

This book examines in depth the three leading techniques of coronary arteriography—the Sones, the Judkins, and the multipurpose—as well as the percutaneous technique for transluminal coronary angioplasty. The descriptions are of unprecedented detail, derived from performing thousands of procedures, and richly illustrated. They provide tips on the performance of coronary arteriography which will interest even the most experienced arteriographers. The authors analyze the many developments that have occurred in coronary arteriography in recent years, with special attention devoted to new imaging techniques and the use of hemiaxial views. Their extensive experience with coronary angioplasty informs the book throughout.

The book also features thorough discussions of normal and abnormal coronary anatomy; the pathoanatomy of coronary artery disease; the interpretation of coronary angiograms (interrelating coronary anatomy with functions of the left ventricle); management of the patient before, during, and after coronary arteriography, including possible complications; and selecting patients for coronary bypass surgery and percutaneous transluminal angioplasty.

We have written especially for cardiologists, fellows and residents in cardiology, practicing angiographers, and radiologists with an interest in cardiology—for all, in fact, concerned with clinical problems that relate to the coronary arteries. The wealth of basic information presented here nevertheless makes this text accessible to students coming to the techniques for the first time. Finally, we believe the book will be an invaluable resource for those surgeons and physicians faced with the difficult task of selecting treatment modalities for patients with coronary atherosclerotic heart disease.

No textbook can substitute for supervised, hands-on experience with the arteriographic procedure, but this volume will provide an excellent starting point for those learning coronary arteriography and a reliable road map for the proficient angiographer perfecting additional techniques.

We wish to thank Libby Adams and Dottie Miller for typing the manuscript.

Spencer B. King III
John S. Douglas, Jr.

Chapter 1

History of Cardiac Catheterization

J. Willis Hurst, M.D.

I have selected six major benchmarks that tell the story of cardiac catheterization. Many benchmarks could be discussed, because many important contributions have been made, but the six chosen are so important that the spotlight must be placed on them.

The reader already knows, or can quickly perceive, the scientific value of the events themselves but may not "know" the individuals involved in the events. Accordingly, I wish to present an account of the events as described by some of the individuals who were involved in them. In this way the reader should feel closer to the men and women involved in the creation of the events as well as to the events themselves.

BENCHMARK 1: THE BIRTH OF CARDIAC CATHETERIZATION

Cardiac catheterization began with Werner Forssmann in 1929.[1] He was searching for a method of injecting drugs directly into the right atrium in order to treat certain serious medical conditions. Such a procedure may have been performed by others earlier, but Forssmann's name is deeply etched near this benchmark.[2] Dr. James V. Warren wrote a delightful essay entitled "Fifty Years of Invasive Cardiology: Werner Forssmann (1904–1979)" and the reader is referred to this document for additional information.[3] Forssmann performed the procedure in a small hospital in Eberswald, Germany, and wrote the following account of the event in his autobiography.*[4]

> I decided to override Schneider's prohibition and go ahead with the experiment on my own heart, secretly and quickly. But I needed an assistant, the surgical

* This quotation is reprinted with the permission of Droste Verlag GmbH. Originally published in German copyright © 1972 by Droste Verlag GmbH, Düsseldorf. English version copyright © 1974 by Saint Martin's Press.

nurse. I had to win her over or I would have no access to the necessary sterile instruments.

I let a few days go by and then started to prowl around Nurse Gerda Ditzen like a sweet-toothed cat around the cream jug. I knew I'd be able to carry out my black deed only during afternoon siesta while everyone in the hospital was dozing, so I made a point of dawdling in the canteen after lunch, hoping to meet Nurse Gerda as she left the nurses' dining room. We often lent each other books, so it was easy to find something to gossip about; and she'd invite me back to her little office next to the operating room for a cup of coffee. . . . When, about a fortnight after my conversation with Schneider, she said with a sigh, "What a pity we can't do the experiment together!" I decided the time had come.

The following afternoon the good lady was sitting in her cubicle when I breezed in, whistling cheerfully. "Nurse Gerda, I want you to give me a set of instruments for a venesection under local anesthesia, and a uretheral catheter."

She started up suspiciously. "But no one in the ward's scheduled for a venesection. You're not planning to do that experiment of yours against boss's orders are you?"

"Nurse Gerda, you need to know nothing about what I'm going to do. But supposing I were to do the experiment—it'd be quite safe."

She eyed me closely. "Are you absolutely sure there's no danger?"

"Absolutely."

"All right then, do it to me. I put myself in your hands."

"Well, why not? You'll be the first person in history to undergo such an experiment."

Of course, I had no intention of going through with this, but it was the only way to get the instruments. She got everything ready in the little operating room, then sat down and held out her left arm. When I suggested she lie down on the operating table she flatly refused at first. But I reminded her how, as she knew from her own experience, patients sometimes collapse from even the smallest dose of novocaine, and so I preferred her to be lying down for the anesthetic. She gave in, and with the speed of light I strapped her legs down so tightly that she couldn't reach the buckle; I then tied down her hand. Amazingly enough she accepted my explanation that I had to take all these precautions against her falling off the table since I had no one to assist me. I'd pushed the instrument tray behind her head so she couldn't see what I was doing. In the twinkling of an eye I had anesthetized my left elbow. Now I went back to her and began to iodize her elbow ceremoniously, and then to lay a sterile cloth over it, all very slowly and deliberately in order to kill time. When my anesthetic began to take effect I quickly made an incision in my skin, inserted a Dechamps aneurysm needle under the vein, opened it and pushed the catheter about a foot inside. I packed it with gauze and laid a sterile split over it. Then I released Nurse Gerda's right hand and loosened the straps around her knees.

"There we are, it's ready now. Please call the x-ray nurse."

Only then did she realize what had happened. She started to yell at me for having deceived her. It wasn't far to the x-ray room, but we had to go down into the basement, and by the time we arrived Nurse Eva was waiting for us. Upon my instruction she placed me behind the fluoroscope screen.

News spread like wildfire in a hospital. Suddenly Romeis burst in, half asleep and his hair all tousled: "You idiot, what the hell are you doing?" He was so desperate he almost tried to pull the catheter out of my arm. I had to give him a few kicks in the shin to calm him down.

BENCHMARK 2: THE DEVELOPMENT OF CATHETERIZATION OF THE RIGHT SIDE OF THE HEART

Klein, working in Prague, used cardiac catheterization in human subjects to obtain blood samples in order to determine the cardiac output in human beings.[5]

Cournand, Richards, et al., working at Bellevue Hospital in New York, used catheterization of the right side of the heart to make physiological observations.[2] I recall hearing a presentation by Cournand when I was a senior medical student. I could not believe what I saw—a catheter threaded through the heart and into the left branch of the pulmonary artery! He deserves the credit for stimulating others in the United States to pick up their catheters, think, and work.[6–8] Baldwin, Dexter, and Bing were also great pioneers.[15]

BENCHMARK 3: THE USE OF CATHETERIZATION OF THE RIGHT SIDE OF THE HEART FOR DIAGNOSTIC PURPOSES

James Warren, working with Emmett Brannon and Heinz Weens in Eugene Stead's laboratory in the Department of Medicine of Emory University School of Medicine, was among the first to use cardiac catheterization for *diagnostic purposes*. Their article describing the diagnosis of atrial septal defect was published in 1945.[9]

Dr. Warren writes the following account of their early experiences using cardiac catheterization:

> I have been asked to tell the story of the first use of the cardiac catheter as a diagnostic tool in heart disease. The catheter had been used previously as a physiologic monitor, but the report from Emory University in 1945 was the first where it was used to diagnose a form of heart disease, in this instance atrial septal defect.[9]
>
> Of course the whole thing started in 1929 with Forssmann in Germany.[1] He had many ideas about the use of the catheter both diagnostic and therapeutic. His studies on patients were limited and did not lead us far beyond the fact that a human being could have his heart catheterized with little danger. There were several scattered reports in the following years, but I believe the real impact of the catheter in clinical medicine came with the shock studies that were being conducted in New York during World War II by Cournand, Richards, and their group at Bellevue Hospital.[6–8] They used the cardiac catheter as a device for physiologic observations. From blood samples they calculated the cardiac output by the Fick principle and gradually explored the various chambers of the right side of the heart. The earlier reports however deal with blood sampled only from the right atrium.
>
> This all took place during World War II. A major focus of medical research at that time related to the medical needs of the armed forces. An agency, the Office of Scientific Research and Development (OSRD), was set up in Washington as a funding mechanism for supporting this research. It was under an OSRD contract that the studies at Bellevue were undertaken. Lower Manhattan provided many casualties that simulated those on the battlefield. The program was based in the emergency room in Bellevue Hospital. Although highly commendable, this program was not large enough and efforts were made to establish another focus of studies on shock. As a result of this, Dr. Alfred Blalock, Professor of Surgery at Johns Hopkins, and a group of distinguished physicians visited Dr. Eugene A. Stead, Jr., Professor and Chairman of the Department of Medicine at Emory University with offices in Grady Hospital. Their mission was simple. They wished to establish a shock unit at Grady because its emergency room also had a considerable amount of trauma. If my memory serves me correctly, at that time there were over 300 patients with hemopneumothorax admitted per year. I was particularly enthusiastic about the problem and volunteered to go to New York to see the Bellevue operation for myself.
>
> My visit added to my enthusiasm and within literally a few days Dr. Stead also visited Bellevue and within a month I suddenly found myself listed as a special resident in pulmonary diseases at Bellevue so that I might be present for the shock studies day and night. After a period of training in the techniques there, I returned to Atlanta, assembled the necessary equipment and we were in business by mid 1943. We did indeed carry out studies on shock victims, but also found it wise to develop certain normal standards such as the cardiac output by the Fick principle, the effect of tilting, and the effect of anxiety.[10] The British medical journal, *Lancet,* in an editorial at this time noted that there were three major centers for this kind of clinical study, New York, London, and Atlanta. The shock work, however, didn't take all of our time. We spent long hours in the emergency room waiting for appropriate patients. This time was not wasted. Dr. Stead and I worked on some new theories about congestive heart failure which were published in 1945.[11]
>
> We further explored the catheter technique in new directions. We also found that the catheter could be placed in the hepatic veins draining the liver[12] and the renal veins draining the kidney.[13] The latter provided the final proof that the postulates of the clearance technique were true in man. The hepatic study produced an interesting byproduct in that patients with bacterial endocarditis were studied. It was shown that the liver was a highly efficient filter for bacteria under these circumstances.[14]
>
> In some way, the most exciting was the conceptualization that if an atrial septal defect was present, left to right shunting of blood through the defect could be detected by appropriate sampling of blood. The

presence of highly oxygenated blood, which had been through the pulmonary circulation, in the right atrium gave evidence of shunting even if the catheter did not go through the septal defect. One could then make a positive diagnosis. The first patient to be identified was studied in March of 1944. He was a 44-year-old male who had experienced dyspnea on exertion for nine years and occasional attacks of paroxysmal nocturnal dyspnea and othopnea for the past three years. His heart was enlarged, the rhythm was regular, and he had a low-pitched soft systolic murmur heard over the III and IV intercostal spaces. The pulmonary second sound was greater than the aortic second sound. No diastolic murmur was heard. X-ray examination confirmed the enlargement of the cardiac silhouette. The aortic knob was slightly shortened. The major branches of the pulmonary artery revealed only slight accentuation and did not show any unusual pulsation. There was no enlargement of the left atrium observed and the electrocardiogram showed only right axis deviation. A diagnosis of atrial septal defect was suggested, but was far from certain. Cardiac catheterization was carried out. The most exciting moment was when it could be seen after the catheter had been advanced into the right atrium in a usual way, but then passed into the left atrium and then headward into what we presume was pulmonary vein. Blood samples studied for oxygen content showed the classic and expected configuration. The difference in color was apparent to the naked eye. There had been some discussion of what the factors were that caused flow from the left atrium into the right. It had been suggested that pressure gradients related to posture might influence shunting. To test that theory, the patient was tilted in a head down position and the arterial blood oxygen saturation monitored. If shunting were to be reversed with flow from the right to the left, then oxygen saturation from the femoral artery would fall. This did not take place.

During the next year, an interesting opportunity came up through a referral from Dr. J. C. Massee.[9] He had a patient, a 39-year-old male, who had been seen in another institution and large mediastinal masses detected. It was felt that this might be Hodgkin's disease and radiation was attempted but without effect. Dr. Massee properly suspected that the masses might be vascular rather than neoplastic and referred the patient to us for catheter studies. It was a great pleasure to be able to give him a definitive answer. The masses were indeed large segments of the pulmonary artery. In this case, it was complicated by pulmonary arterial disease and pulmonary hypertension.

These, to the best of my knowledge, were the first patients studied with the catheter to diagnose congenital heart disease. In Dr. Cournand's book on catheter studies in congenital heart disease,[15] he has a chronologic list of papers in the literature on the topic. Chronologically the Atlanta paper heads the list.

BENCHMARK 4: THE DEVELOPMENT OF CATHETERIZATION OF THE LEFT SIDE OF THE HEART

The creation of contrast media and special recording equipment led to the development of cardiac angiography. The right side of the heart and pulmonary arteries were visualized without difficulty.

The invasion of the left side of the heart was more difficult. Accordingly, pressure records, blood oxygen determinations, and angiography of the left side of the heart came a bit later. Zimmerman, Scott, and Becker led the way and developed the technique which enabled them to study the aortic valve and left ventricle.[16] Dr. Henry Zimmerman writes the following account of the first catheterization in which the cardiac catheter passed from the aorta into the left ventricle:

> In 1947 with the encouragement of my chief, Roy W. Scott, M.D., I built the first cardiac laboratory in the midwest at Cleveland City Hospital and performed the first right-sided heart catheterization in the area.
>
> Almost immediately we not only used the catheter as a diagnostic tool but began to use it as a research tool, using it to study the pulmonary circulation under a variety of conditions.
>
> During this period we worked in almost total darkness and adapted our rod vision with red glasses for 20–30 minutes so that we could see. At this time we also perfected a method for electrical recording of pressures and other physiological data.
>
> We had a fair idea what was occurring on the right side of the heart but could only guess what might be occurring on the left side of the heart. Claude Beck, M.D., and I were discussing some cardiac problems

dealing with the left side lesions and I mentioned the possibility of catheterizing the left side of the heart. With one of his residents assisting, we did a number of dogs, placing the catheter retrograde through an artery in the leg into the left ventricle. Then after several in depth conferences my chief gave the go ahead to attempt to place a catheter into the left ventricle of man.

Now 35 years later the exact details are a bit hazy. Even our nurse, Heckman, who was my right hand and who spent 25 years in the cardiac catheterization laboratory, cannot clearly remember the events. The case is on microfilm. No one knows exactly where it is among thousands of reels in the record library.

As I recall the events we selected a male with a large heart due to aortic insufficiency. I decided that it would be best to have a surgeon on hand to aid in the isolation of and repair of the ulnar artery. Somehow the whole medical service knew of the event and several fellows including the chief dropped in to see the procedure. We started the procedure around 8 A.M. and by 10 A.M. we completed the first left side heart catheterization.

The ulnar artery was isolated in the antecubital space. The catheter was anointed with olive oil and filled with heparin. The artery was isolated by tapes and opened by a longitudinal incision. The catheter was inserted and passed rather easily, retrograde, into the aortic arch using almost constant fluoroscopy. The catheter was passed down the aorta and the aortic valve was passed rather easily. With the catheter in the left ventricle there were some premature contractions and occasional short runs of tachycardia which disappeared on moving the catheter tip. Pressures were recorded above and below the valve in the tip of the left ventricle as well as a pull back across the aortic valve. The catheter was removed and the radial artery was repaired. (We were hesitant at the time to use the brachial artery.) The radial and ulnar pulses were present, and with a sigh of relief the first catheterization of the left heart in man was completed.

On analysis of the tracing, we were much interested to learn that although the patient had wide open aortic insufficiency, the end-diastolic pressure in the ventricle was within normal range. Rather quickly we used the method to study patients with consecutive failure and to take electrical potentials from the cavity of the left ventricle. Soon we routinely had catheters in both sides of the heart simultaneously.

BENCHMARK 5: CORONARY ARTERIOGRAPHY ARRIVES

Baltaxe, Amplatz, and Levin have written an excellent article on the history of coronary angiography.[17] Many investigators worked to develop a technique to visualize the coronary arteries in animals and humans.[18–31] Finally Mason Sones developed *selective* coronary arteriography. The date was 1958, and the place was the Cleveland Clinic. This event changed the medical profession's entire approach to the diagnosis and treatment of coronary artery disease.

Mason Sones writes the following account of the first selective coronary arteriogram:

> In 1958 we initiated a program to study the possibility of opacifying the coronary arteries in an effort to provide an improved basic standard of diagnosis for patients with coronary atherosclerosis. Using a 5 inch image amplifier we noted incidental opacification of the coronary artery tree during the performance of left ventriculograms and aortograms on infants and small children. In a series of studies performed on dogs we learned that we could get satisfactory opacification about 80 percent of the time if we injected 20–30 cc of contrast agent directly into the coronary sinus adjacent to the coronary orifices. We "reasoned" that if we could see the small coronary vessels of infants with a 5 inch amplifier we should be able to accomplish the same thing with a larger image amplifier in adult patients. For this reason we purchased an 11 inch image amplifier and built an entirely new laboratory around it. This amplifier was six feet long, weighed over 600 pounds, and could not be moved vertically with the input phosphor facing downward because it used a metal casing that we soldered together in the final stage of its construction. If you turned it face downward the input phosphor would be destroyed by flecks of solder inside the casing. We therefore had to mount it beneath the table top facing upwards in a hole about five feet deep beneath the table. The additional severe limitation of this piece of apparatus was it only amplified light about 95 times. It was equipped with an optical system that permitted the operator standing in the hole beneath the table to see the image by looking up through the patient using an x-ray tube mounted above the table. The image

could only be seen however during actual cine runs because the image was imperceptible with x-ray doses administered at conventional fluoroscopic levels.

Using this extremely cumbersome equipment in 1959 we embarked on a series of studies in adult patients with congenital or acquired valve lesions. In practice this required that one physician manipulate the catheter above the table top using a 5 inch image amplifier to position the catheter in the heart chambers or great vessels. When the catheter was properly positioned for an injection of contrast media the physician climbed down into the hole while an associate controlled the mechanical injector above the table. On one such occasion in 1959 we performed a left ventriculogram in a patient with acquired valve disease. I was working in the hole beneath the table in order to observe the image amplifier screen during injection. I asked my associate to withdraw the catheter tip across the aortic valve to the ascending aorta so that we could complete the procedure by performing an aortogram with the catheter tip in the ascending aorta. My associate complied and we relied on the pressure change from the left ventricle to the ascending aorta without sliding the table top back under the five inch amplifier to confirm the exact location of the tip. I didn't think this was necessary because I was quite certain that the catheter tip lay in the ascending aorta just above the aortic valve.

My associate, Dr. Royston Lewis, made an injection of 40 cc of 90 percent Hypaque through the catheter. About one second before the injection was initiated, I hit the switch to initiate a cine run. When the injection began I was horrified to see the right coronary artery become heavily opacified and realized the catheter tip was actually inside the orifice of the dominant right coronary artery. I shouted, "Pull it out." Our combined reaction times to accomplish withdrawal of the catheter consumed from 3–4 seconds which meant that approximately 30 cc of 90 percent Hypaque had been delivered into the right coronary artery. I was of course horrified because I was certain that the patient would develop ventricular fibrillation. At that time we did not have direct current defibrillators and knew nothing about the application of closed chest cardiac massage. I climbed out of the hole and ran around the table looking for a scapel to open his chest in order to defibrillate him by direct application of the paddles of an alternating current defibrillator. I looked at the oscilloscope tracing of his electrocardiogram and it was evident that he was in asystole rather than ventricular fibrillation. I knew that an explosive cough could produce a very effective pressure pulse in the aorta and hoped this might push the contrast media through his myocardial capillary bed. Fortunately, he was still conscious and responded to my demand that he cough repeatedly. After three or four explosive coughs his heart began to beat again with initially a sinus bradycardia which accelerated to a sinus tachycardia within 15–20 seconds. He then made a perfectly uneventful recovery with no neurological deficit or other sequelae.

Initially, I could feel only unbelievable relief and gratitude that we had been fortunate enough to avert a grievous disaster. During the ensuing days I began to think that this accident might point the way for the development of a technique which was exactly what we had been seeking. If a human could tolerate such a massive injection of contrast media directly into a coronary artery it might be possible to accomplish this type of an opacification with small doses of more dilute contrast agent. With considerable fear and trepidation we embarked on a program to accomplish this objective. Its success has led to a very significant improvement in the life expectancy and functional capacity of hundreds of thousands of patients with coronary artery disease through appropriate surgical intervention.

BENCHMARK 6: THE BIRTH OF PERCUTANEOUS TRANSLUMINAL CORONARY ANGIOPLASTY

Andreas Gruentzig was the first person to work inside a human coronary artery. He developed transluminal percutaneous coronary angioplasty, and this in turn is certain to lead to other therapeutic measures. He developed the technique at the University Hospital in Zurich, Switzerland. Seven years of work preceded the first coronary dilatation, which took place on September 16, 1977. Now Andreas Gruentzig and his colleagues, Spencer King, John Douglas, and Douglas Morris in the Departments of Medicine and Radiology of Emory University School of Medicine, have performed more than 3000 coronary angioplasties with only three deaths.

Gruentzig prepared the following account of the first coronary angioplasty:

This description is not a report about an accidental and, therefore, surprising event but rather about one which was planned for months.

After working seven years to develop peripheral arterial dilatation, using animal experiments, post-mortem examinations and interoperative dilatations, we were ready to use the technique for coronary artery dilatation in man. We waited for the first patient to come to be an ideal candidate for the procedure.

It happened in September 1977 that we did coronary angiography on a 37-year-old insurance salesman with severe and exercise induced angina pectoris. The coronary angiography revealed single vessel disease with a proximal stenosis in the left anterior descending artery located immediately before the take-off of a large diagonal branch. The patient was informed about the availability of balloon angioplasty in his case. The idea of preventing coronary bypass surgery was appealing to him inspite of the fact that he was informed of his being the first patient ever treated with this technique. He enthusiastically gave his consent and the catheterization laboratory at the University Hospital in Zurich, Switzerland was set up for the procedure on September 16, 1977.

Early in the afternoon at a time when the anesthesiologist and the cardiac surgeon were available and no cardiac procedure was underway in the operating room, the patient came into our catheterization laboratory and was catheterized in the usual fashion using the Seldinger approach from the right groin and a Judkins-type guiding catheter. The chief of cardiology, the cardiac surgeon, anesthesiologist, cardiology and radiology fellows were in the recording booth to observe the procedure. The guiding catheter was placed in the left coronary orifice and the dilatation catheter was inserted. Both catheters were connected to the pressure lines. The left femoral artery was also punctured and a sheath was placed. This was done to have arterial blood available to pump in via a roller pump through the main lumen of the dilatation catheter into the coronary artery to perfuse the myocardium during balloon inflation. This had been shown to be effective for the prevention of acute ischemia during coronary experiments in dogs. We set the same system up for the patient because at that time we did not know how one would react to the sudden interruption of blood flow through the coronary artery when the balloon is inflated. I had planned to start the roller pump as soon as the patient would need it.

After all these lines were installed and tested, the stage was set. The dilatation catheter was advanced to the stenosis with no difficulty. The stenosis was severe but the catheter slipped through it without resistance. The catheter wedged the stenosis so that there was no antegrade flow and the distal coronary pressure was very low. To the surprise of all of us, no ST-elevation, ventricular fibrillation or even extrasystole occurred and the patient had no chest pain. At this moment, I decided not to start the coronary perfusion with the roller pump.

After the first balloon deflation, the distal coronary pressure rose nicely. Encouraged by this positive response, I inflated the balloon a second time to relieve the residual gradient. Again, the patient had no chest pain. After balloon deflation, the distal coronary blood pressure normalized as compared to the aortic pressure indicating a good relief of stenosis according to our prior experience in peripheral arterial dilatation. I pulled the dilatation catheter back and tested the anatomic result with distal dye injection using the main lumen of the dilatation catheter. My colleagues shouted from the booth that they also saw a narrowing in the proximal part of the diagonal artery and I should do dilatation there as well. Seduced from their enthusiasm, I recrossed the stenosis again and went into the diagonal branch and repeated balloon inflation. Afterwards, I realized that there was no real stenosis in this artery and the balloon inflation was unnecessary. Fortunately, no complication occurred. I removed the catheters and the immediate control angiography in several oblique projections revealed a marked reduction of the LAD-stenosis. There was no peripheral spasm or embolization. We, therefore, declared success.

Everyone was surprised about the ease of the procedure and I started to realize that my dreams had come true. The only rain on my parade came when we found on the EKG that the patient had developed a right bundle branch block. However, this cloud was lifted when four hours later the EKG normalized. Then we were ready to celebrate the occasion.

A few hours after the procedure, the patient phoned a newspaper, without my knowledge, and wanted to release his story. The reporter came to him but also asked me for further details and I begged him not to destroy me and the method by early advertisement of a procedure which had not proven to be effective at that point in time. I asked him to wait until more experience would have been accumulated.

After a heated discussion in my office, we came to a ''gentlemen's agreement'' to hold the story until more patients have been treated and until the first publication would have appeared in a medical journal. Fortunately, the press cooperated and kept the story secret until February 1978 when the first five cases were published in the *Lancet*.[32] Then the press took over and the story was given in all aspects and colors. By the way, the patient also had success otherwise, because he has now been symptom-free for five years.

SUMMARY

I have presented six benchmarks related to the development of cardiac catheterization.

The first benchmark was created by Forssmann, who, along with nurse Gerda, and despite his chief, did the first cardiac catheterization. He showed the world it *could be done* without complications.

The second benchmark belongs to Klein, Cournand, Richards, and others who used Forssmann's technique to study the *physiology* of the circulation in human beings. They, in turn, stimulated others to think and work. The best modern example of the use of the catheter to obtain useful physiological measurements is the work of Swan and Ganz.

The third benchmark belongs to Warren and others who used the technique to *diagnose* heart disease. This led to modern surgery for congenital and acquired heart disease.

The fourth benchmark is that of Zimmerman, Scott, and Becker, who pioneered the catheterization of the left side of the heart.

The fifth benchmark belongs to Mason Sones, who developed selective coronary arteriography. Others had visualized the coronary arteries, but modern diagnostic and therapeutic work on coronary disease would not be possible had Sones not developed selective coronary arteriography. Melvin Judkins and others modified the procedure leading to its broad application.

The sixth benchmark belongs to Andreas Gruentzig, who developed percutaneous transluminal coronary angioplasty and showed the world that one can use catheters to work inside the coronary artery.

The seventh benchmark will come in cardiac catheterization. The person performing the procedure will be named ——— and he or she will ———. The date of the procedure will be ——— and the location where the procedure will be done will be ———. In all likelihood the person who creates benchmark 7 will be an interesting and creative individual who will also have an interesting story to tell.

ACKNOWLEDGMENTS

I wish to thank my friends Jim Warren, Henry Zimmerman, Mason Sones, and Andreas Gruentzig for supplying me with their own accounts of their enormous contributions.

REFERENCES

1 Forssmann W: The catheterization of the right side of the heart. Klin Wochenschr, 8:2085, 1929.
2 Cournand A: Cardiac catheterization: Development of the technique, its contributions to experimental medicine, and its initial applications in man. Acta Med Scand [Suppl], 579:7, 1975.
3 Warren JV: Fifty years of invasive cardiology: Werner Forssmann (1904–1979). Am J Med, 69:10, 1980.
4 Forssmann W: *Experiments on Myself. Memoirs of a Surgeon in Germany*. Saint Martin's Press, New York, 1974, pp 84–85.
5 Klein O: Determining human cardiac output (minute volume) using Fick's principle (extraction of mixed venous blood by cardiac catheterization). Med Wochenschr, 77:1311, 1930.
6 Cournand A, Ranges HA: Catheterization of the right auricle in man. Proc Soc Exp Biol Med, 46:462, 1941.
7 Cournand A, Lauson HD, Bloomfield RA, Breed ES, Baldwin E deF: Recording of right heart pressures in man. Proc Soc Exp Biol Med, 55:34, 1944.

8 Cournand A, Riley RL, Bradley SE, et al: Studies of the circulation in clinical shock. Surgery, 13:964, 1943.

9 Brannon ES, Weens HS, Warren JW: Atrial septal defect: Study of hemodynamics by the technique of right heart catheterization. Am J Med Sci, 210:480, 1945.

10 Stead EA, Warren JV, Merrill AJ, Brannon ES: The cardiac output in male subjects as measured by the technique of right atrial catheterization: Normal values with observations on the effect of anxiety and tilting. J Clin Invest, 24(3):326, 1945.

11 Warren JV, Stead EA: Fluid dynamics in chronic congestive heart failure: An interpretation of the mechanisms producing the edema, increased plasma volume and elevated venous pressure in certain patients with prolonged congestive failure. Arch Intern Med, 73:138, 1944.

12 Warren JW, Brannon ES: A method of obtaining blood samples directly from the hepatic vein in man. Proc Soc Exp Biol Med, 55:144, 1944.

13 Warren JV, Brannon ES, Merrill AJ: A method of obtaining renal venous blood in unanesthetized persons with observations on the extraction of oxygen and sodium para-amino hippurate. Science, 100:108, 1944.

14 Beeson PB, Brannon ES, Warren JV: Observations on the sites of removal of bacteria from the blood in patients with bacterial endocarditis. J Exp Med, 81:9, 1945.

15 Cournand A, Baldwin JS, Himmelstein A: Cardiac catheterization in congenital heart disease, in *A Clinical and Physiological Study in Infants and Children*. Commonwealth Fund, New York, 1949.

16 Zimmerman HA, Scott RW, Becker NO: Catheterization of the left side of the heart in man. Circulation, 1:357, 1950.

17 Baltaxe HA, Amplatz K, Levin DC: *Coronary Angiography*. Charles C Thomas, Springfield, Ill, 1976.

18 Moniz E, DeCarvalho L, Lima A: Angiopneumographie. Presse Méd, 39:996, 1931.

19 Reboul H, Racine M: La ventriculographie cardiaque expérimentale. Presse Med, 1:763, 1933.

20 Radner S: An attempt at the roentgenologic visualization of the coronary blood vessels in man. Acta Radiol, 26:497, 1945.

21 DiGuglielmo L, Guttaduro M: Roentgenologic study of coronary arteries in living. Acta Radiol [Suppl] (Stockh), 97, December 1952.

22 DiGuglielmo L, Guttaduro M: Visualization of arteries in living: Review of 413 observations. Radiol Med, 40:945, 1954.

23 Dotter CT, Frische LH: Visualization of the coronary circulation by occlusion aortography: A practical method. Radiology, 76:502, 1958.

24 Arnulf G, Chacornac R: Communication to La Société de Chirurgie de Lyon, November 14, 1957, in Arnulf G: L'arteriographie méthodique des artères coronaires grâce à l'utilisation de l'acetylcholine: Données expérimentales et cliniques. Bull Acad Natl Med (Paris), 25–26:661, 1958.

25 Richards LS, Thal AP: Phasic dye injection control system for coronary arteriography in the human. Surg Gynecol Obstet, 107:739, 1958.

26 Bellman S, Frank HA, Lambert PB, Littman D, Williams JA: Coronary arteriography: I. Differential opacification of the aortic stream catheters of special design—experimental development. N Engl J Med, 262:325, 1960.

27 Nordenstrom B: Contrast examination of the cardiovascular system during increased intrabronchial pressure. Acta Radiol [Suppl] (Stockh), 200:110, 1960.

28 Bilgutay AM, Gannon P, Sterns LP, Ferlic R, Lillehei CW: Coronary arteriography: New method under induced hypotension by pacing—experimental and clinical application. Arch Surg, 89(no. 5):899, 1964.

29 Sones FM Jr: Coronary arteriography. Read before the Eighth Annual Convention of the American College of Cardiology, Philadelphia, 1959.

30 Sones FM Jr, et al: Cine coronary arteriography, in Abstracts of the 32nd Scientific Session of the American Heart Association, Circulation, 20:773, October 1959.

31 Ricketts HJ, Abrams HL: Percutaneous selective coronary cine arteriography. JAMA, 181:620, 1962.

32 Gruentzig AR: Transluminal dilatation of coronary-artery stenoses. Lancet, 1:263, 1978 (Letters to the Editor).

Chapter 2

Normal Coronary Anatomy

Spencer B. King III, M.D.
John S. Douglas, Jr., M.D.

The anatomy of the coronary arteries was described by Vieussens over 350 years ago.[1]

The understanding of the relationship of coronary artery obstructive disease to angina pectoris and myocardial ischemia established by Edward Jenner in 1799[2] and Allan Burns in 1809[3] brought little interest from others concerning the anatomy of the coronary arteries. Only at the time of the contributions of Sir James McKenzie[4] in the twentieth century did coronary anatomy become of more than academic interest. The development of selective coronary arteriography in 1958 by Mason Sones[5] and the introduction of coronary bypass surgery in 1968 by René Favaloro[6] and Dudley Johnson[7] have done more to further the interest in coronary anatomy than all previous events. Careful postmortem studies utilizing injection techniques have provided the most definitive description of normal coronary anatomy.[8,9] The necessity for a clear understanding of the coronary anatomy for the purposes of myocardial revascularization is obvious. It is now necessary for all cardiologists and internists to have an appreciation of the anatomic distribution of the coronary arteries in order to make intelligent decisions regarding management of their patients with coronary artery disease.

Left Coronary Artery

The left coronary artery arises as a main trunk from the center of the upper portion of the left coronary sinus. This orifice therefore lies directly between the posterior portion of the pulmonary artery and the anterior portion of the left atrial appendage (Fig. 2-1). The left main artery courses in the epicardial fat for distances varying from less than 1 mm to several centimeters. This vessel then divides into the anterior descending artery and the circumflex artery. Frequently there is a third branch arising in

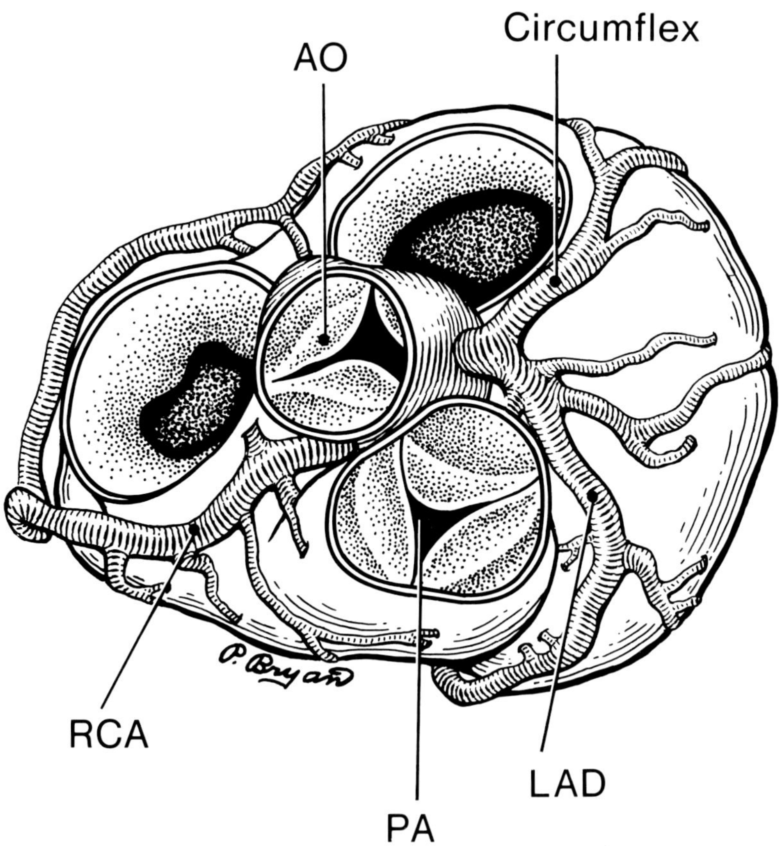

Figure 2-1 Superior view of the heart. The left coronary artery arises from the left coronary sinus and divides into the anterior descending and circumflex arteries. The anterior descending courses anterior around the pulmonary artery to reach the anterior interventricular groove. The circumflex travels under the atrial appendage in the left atrioventricular groove. The right coronary artery arises from the right coronary sinus and travels in epicardial fat to reach the right atrioventricular groove. AO = aorta, LAD = left anterior descending artery, PA = pulmonary artery, RCA = right coronary artery.

the crotch between the anterior descending and circumflex called the intermediate or diagonal branch. The anterior descending artery courses as a continuation of the left main around the pulmonary artery to reach the anterior interventricular sulcus in which it travels to and around the left ventricular apex. The circumflex artery turns posterior to travel in the atrioventricular groove.

Left Anterior Descending Artery

When the heart is viewed frontally, the anterior descending artery is seen as it curves around and emerges from behind the pulmonary artery (Fig. 2-2). This vessel in combination with the left main artery forms a curve that resembles a reverse S-shape. The tight upper curve brings the anterior descending around the pulmonary artery in order to reach the uppermost portions of the interventricular septum, and the lower portion curves in the opposite direction as it follows the interventricular septum towards the apex and around it. Major branches arising from the anterior descending artery are those that penetrate the interventricular septum and those that travel on the left ventricular free wall. Small, rather insignificant branches occasionally distribute to the right ventricular surface. The uppermost artery to course over the right ventricle is the branch which forms a loop with a similar branch coming to meet it from the right coronary artery. This potential anastomotic branch was first described by Vieussens.[10]

Septal Perforating Branches

The perforating branches in the upper septum arise at almost a right angle from the anterior descending

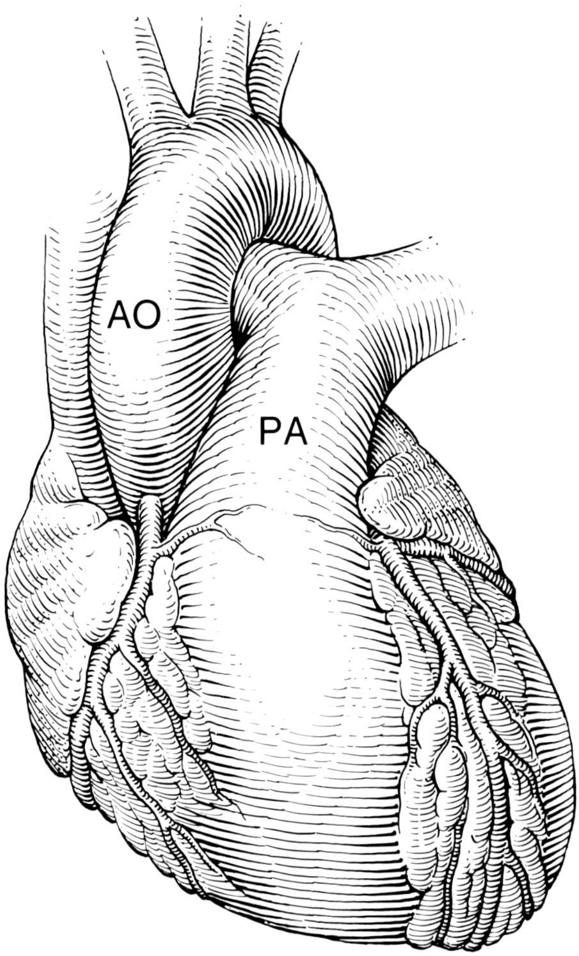

Figure 2-2 Anterior view of the heart. Note the left anterior descending coronary artery emerging from behind the pulmonary artery and under the left atrial appendage to travel in the interventricular groove. Epicardial fat has been removed to show the course of the right coronary artery arising anterior and rightward from the aorta to travel in the right atrioventricular groove. AO = aorta, PA = pulmonary artery.

artery and penetrate deep through the interventricular septum (Fig. 2-3). The first branch of this group is usually the largest and supplies the basal portion of septal myocardium. These septal perforating vessels become progressively smaller and may assume more acute angles at their origin from the anterior descending as the vessel approaches the apex. In some hearts there are many septal perforating vessels, while in others two or three major trunks take off from the anterior descending artery and then branch into many secondary and tertiary septal branches.

Diagonal Branches

The arteries that run over the left ventricular surface arise at acute angles from the left anterior descending artery (LAD) and are called the diagonal branches. These arteries vary from two to six in number. The larger diagonal branches arise from the upper portion of the anterior descending artery, and they become progressively smaller as the LAD approaches the apex. They run parallel to one another and also parallel to the intermediate branch arising from the left main artery when that artery

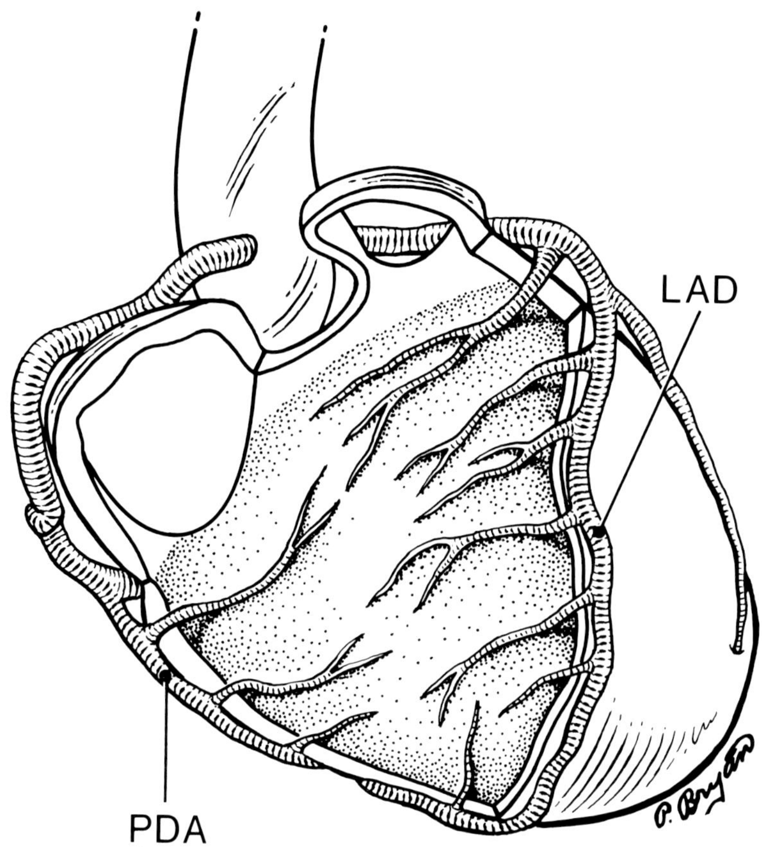

Figure 2-3 Right anterior oblique view of the heart with the right ventricle removed showing the circulation to the interventricular septum. Note the septal vessels originating at near 90° from the anterior descending to travel into the interventricular septum and the branches from the posterior descending travelling to meet them in the posterior interventricular septum. Notice that approximately two-thirds of the interventricular septum is supplied by the perforating branches of the anterior descending artery in this example. LAD = left anterior descending artery, PDA = posterior descending artery.

is present (Fig. 2-4). Occasionally a large diagonal branch will be equal in size to the anterior descending artery itself or even larger. Contrary to the traditional belief that septal perforating branches always arise from the anterior descending, they rarely may arise from the most proximal portion of the first diagonal branch.

Since the anterior descending artery gives rise to many progressively smaller septal perforating and diagonal branches, the parent vessel throughout its course is reduced in lumen diameter as it nears the apex. This gradual reduction in size of the trunk artery can be likened to a fir tree which gives off branches as it nears its apex. The major determining factor of the size of any coronary artery is the amount of blood flow it must carry and that in turn is determined by the amount of myocardium served. With each departing septal and diagonal branch, the blood flow demanded of the artery just beyond the point is reduced, and therefore the size of the artery is also progressively reduced. The anterior descending most often courses around the apex and up the posterior interventricular groove where it supplies some septal perforating branches to the posterior apical portion of the interventricular septum (Fig. 2-3).

The Left Circumflex Artery

The left circumflex artery arises from the left main artery at its bifurcation and travels posteriorly under the left atrial appendage to reach the left atrioventricular groove. The takeoff of this artery is frequently at right angles to the left main artery, although the angle may be more or less acute in some patients and may, when combined with the LAD and left main arteries, form an inverted "Y"

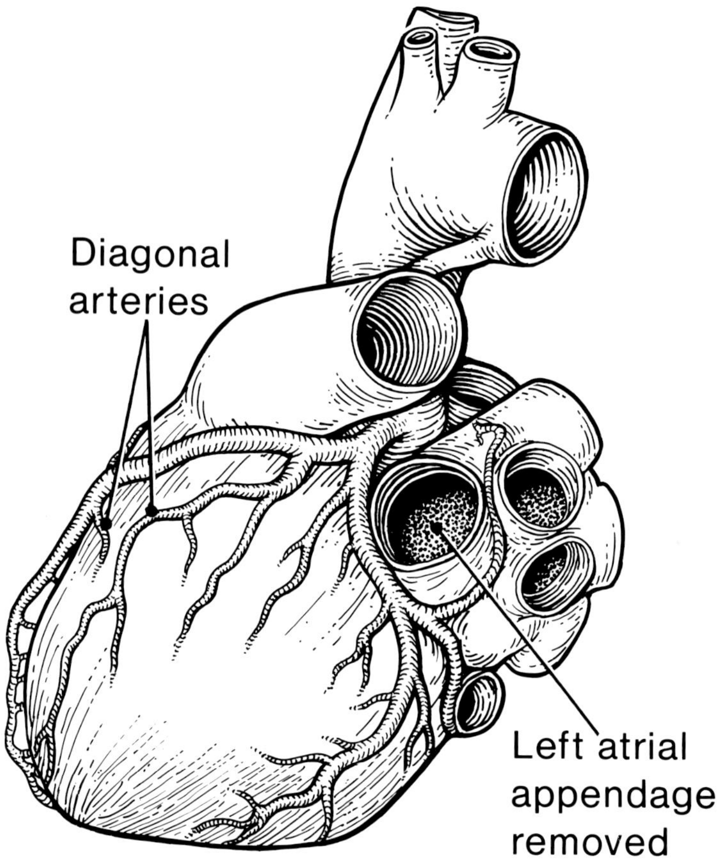

Figure 2-4 Left anterior oblique view of the heart with the left atrial appendage removed. The diagonal branches originate from the anterior descending artery and travel in a direction parallel to the marginal branches, which originate from the circumflex artery.

(Fig. 2-5). As the artery emerges from under the left atrial appendage, it reaches the obtuse margin of the heart and sends from one to four branches parallel to the intermediate branch and the diagonal branches of the LAD coursing over the obtuse margin of the heart toward the apex (Fig. 2-6).

Anatomic variation is quite common here, but there is at least one major branch over the left margin. When a single large branch is present, early secondary and tertiary branching of the vessel is extensive. Commonly two or three vessels are present. In these cases the vessels are of more or less equal size, and their secondary branching is less extensive. The nomenclature of these obtuse marginal branches depends on their origin from the circumflex rather than the course they take over the obtuse margin of the heart.

Diagonal branches and the intermediate branch also may course over portions of the obtuse margin (Fig. 2-5). If several obtuse marginal branches exist, then a parent vessel continues to run in the atrioventricular groove toward the posterior portion of the heart. In about 10 percent of hearts, the circumflex artery reaches the posterior interventricular sulcus and crosses it, then turns toward the apex and runs in the posterior interventricular groove as the posterior descending branch. In somewhat less than half of human hearts, the sinus node branch arises from the circumflex trunk and courses over the atrial surface to reach the right atrial superior vena cava junction, where it encircles the superior vena cava and penetrates the sinus node (Fig. 2-4). Another branch, the left atrial circumflex, may travel parallel to the atrioventricular groove above

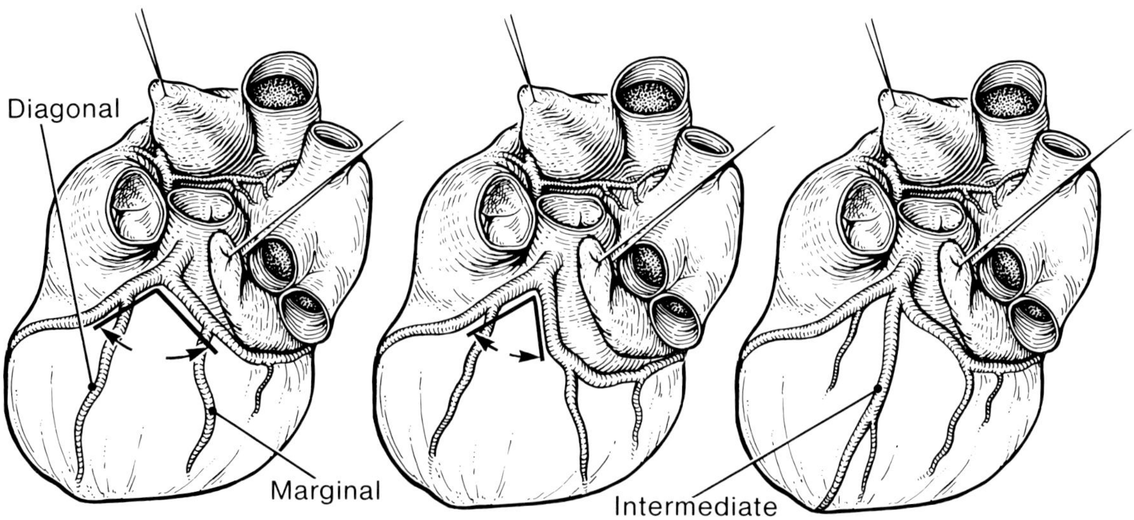

Figure 2-5 Left anterior oblique and superior view of the heart illustrating the variations in the left main bifurcation. (*a*) A wide angle is subtended by the anterior descending and circumflex arteries. (*b*) The angle formed by the anterior descending and circumflex arteries is narrow. (*c*) The left main terminates in a trifurcation forming the anterior descending, the intermediate branch, and the circumflex artery.

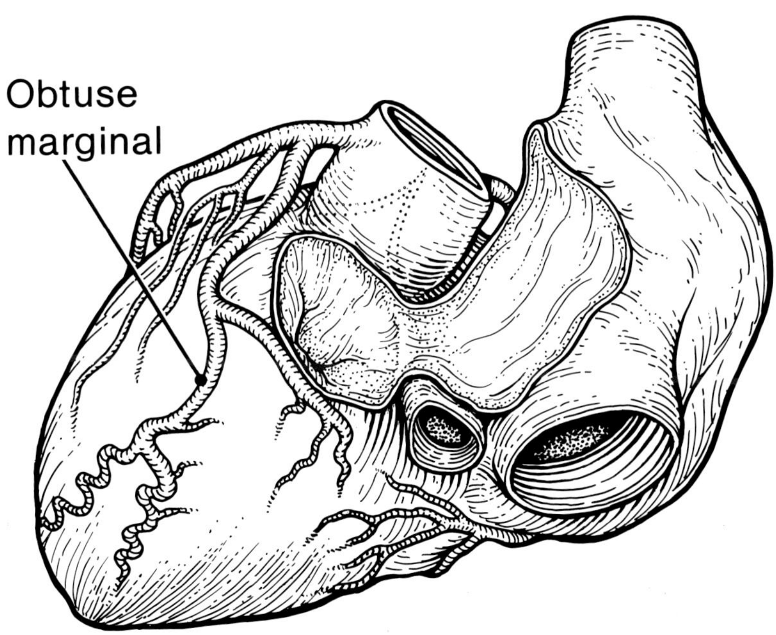

Figure 2-6 Left lateral view of the heart with the left atrium removed showing the course of the circumflex artery and its marginal branches over the lateral surface of the left ventricle.

the parent circumflex artery and circle the left atrium giving rise to most of the atrial blood supply. Although the origin of the sinus node branch from the circumflex artery is usually from its proximal portion, the location of its orifice may vary widely and may even arise several centimeters from the origin of the circumflex.

Obtuse Marginal Branches

In most cases, the first obtuse marginal branch arising from the circumflex artery is very large, and therefore the parent circumflex vessel in the atrioventricular groove is reduced in size dramatically at that branch point. Branch points at the origin of the marginal branches form acute angles pointing back against the direction of flow. The main circumflex artery usually gives rise to two to three marginal branches of more or less equal size. If the circumflex does not supply the posterior descending branch, then it is rapidly attenuated after the takeoff of the last marginal branch.

In those hearts in which the circumflex artery reaches the posterior interventricular groove, crosses it, and forms the posterior descending artery, this crossing is accomplished by a U-shaped turn into the myocardium at the junction of the interatrial and interventricular grooves. From this U-turn arises the artery to the atrioventricular (AV) node. This small artery travels superiorly, piercing the uppermost portion of the interventricular septum to reach the AV node.

Right Coronary Artery

The right coronary artery arises from the middle of the right coronary sinus in a variable distribution from low near the valve to high near the sinotubular ridge. It courses in the epicardial fat into the right atrioventricular sulcus. In the vast majority of hearts, the right coronary artery travels as a large conduit vessel in the atrioventricular sulcus toward the posterior interventricular groove (Fig. 2-7). There are characteristically few major branches arising from the right coronary artery throughout its course prior to reaching the posterior portion of the heart; therefore, its diameter remains unchanged to that point.

The first branch is the conus artery, which arises from the very proximal portion of the right coronary artery or, in almost half of human hearts, from a separate orifice located 1 to 2 mm anterior to the right coronary orifice. That vessel courses around the conus of the right ventricle near the level of the pulmonary valve. The sinus node artery originates from the proximal right coronary in just over 50 percent of human hearts. It arises from the superior right side of the artery and travels in the opposite direction from the conus branch, coursing directly to the right atrium where it pierces the sinoatrial node and encircles the superior vena cava. Subsequent branches of the right coronary artery take off at almost right angles and either perfuse the anterior portion of the right ventricle or turn backward to perfuse the right atrium. These vessels are seldom of clinical significance. There is usually a larger branch at the acute margin of the heart which travels toward the apex and in some cases reaches the apex, supplying that portion of the interventricular septum.

The conduit portion of the right coronary continues in its long course around the right atrioventricular groove until it nears the crux of the heart. There it usually bifurcates into two large branches, one turning down toward the apex in the interventricular groove as the posterior descending branch while the other dips intramyocardial at the crux of the heart to form a U-shape and emerge to the left of the atrioventricular groove, where it gives one to two branches to the posterior portion of the left ventricle running toward the apex parallel to the obtuse marginal branches of the circumflex artery. In some hearts, these left ventricular branches are as large as the posterior descending branch itself.

Reciprocal Relationship Between the Circumflex and Right Coronary Arteries

The posterior portion of the heart is variously supplied by the right coronary artery (RCA) and the circumflex coronary artery. In approximately 90 percent of hearts, the right coronary artery crosses the posterior interventricular groove and supplies the posterior descending branch as well as branches

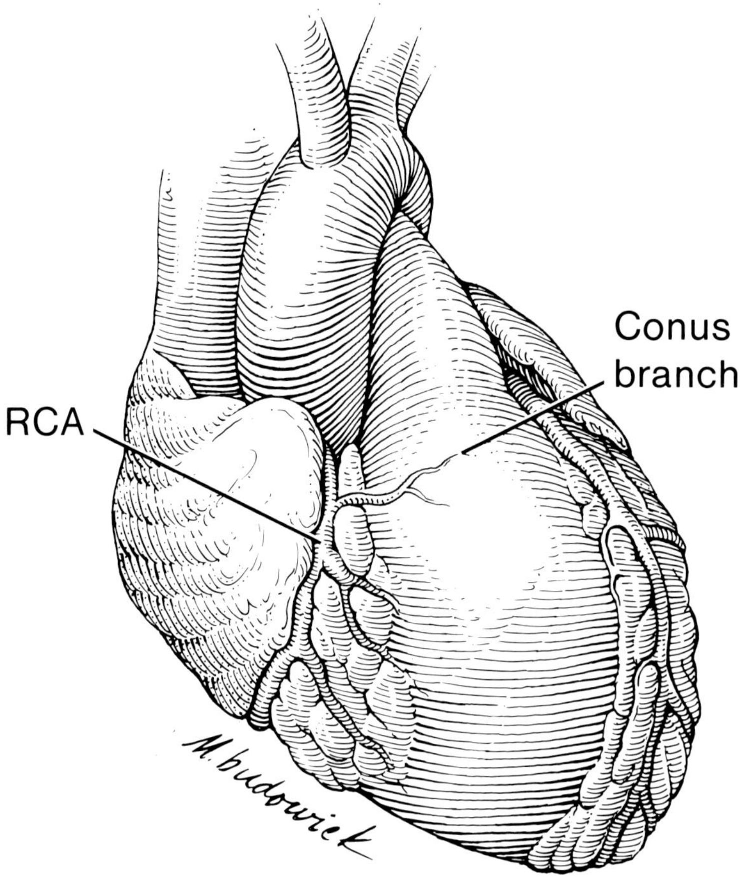

Figure 2-7 Right lateral view of the heart showing the right atrial and right ventricular branches as they travel in the atrioventricular groove. RCA = right coronary artery.

to the left ventricle (Fig. 2-8). In 10 percent of hearts, the circumflex coronary artery crosses the interventricular groove and supplies branches to the posterior right ventricular surface (Fig. 2-9). Occasionally posterior descending arteries are supplied from both the RCA and the circumflex. As previously indicated, the acute marginal artery may reach the posterior interventricular sulcus in its midportion and run in it toward the apex supplying posterior septal perforating arteries. In this case, the posterior descending artery is short, ending before the point of arrival of the acute marginal artery in the posterior interventricular sulcus, and therefore supplies posterior septal perforating vessels only to the atrial half of the interventricular septum.

Classically, the artery that crosses the crux of the heart and supplies the posterior descending branch has been called the dominant coronary artery. This is a misnomer since the left coronary artery almost always is the dominant artery in supplying the majority of the left ventricular myocardium. A more descriptive term for the artery which crosses the crux and supplies the posterior interventricular groove is "dominant posterior artery."

DISTRIBUTION OF THE CORONARY ARTERIES TO SPECIFIC REGIONS OF THE LEFT VENTRICULAR MYOCARDIUM

The coronary arteries are distributed so as to bring adequate blood supply to all areas of the left ventricular myocardium. Despite numerous variations, this rule is always met in healthy hearts. An analysis of the total distribution of the coronary arteries in the heart will show that no areas are left devoid

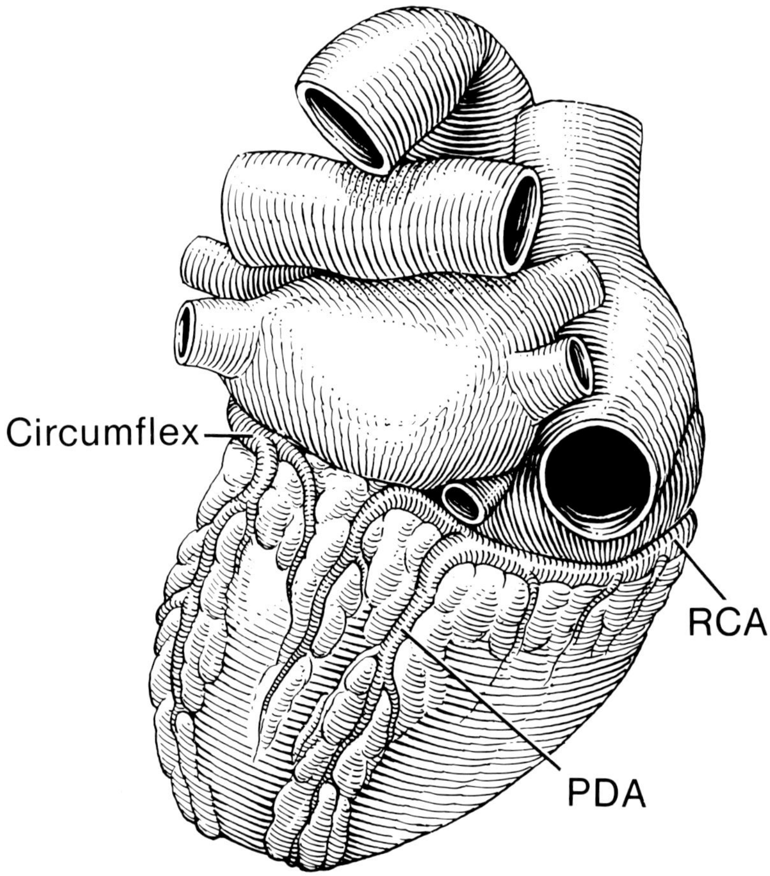

Figure 2-8 Posterior view of the heart. The posterior descending artery is a continuation of the right coronary artery turning to travel in the interventricular groove. PDA = posterior descending artery, RCA = right coronary artery.

of blood supply. The left anterior descending coronary artery usually supplies approximately 50 percent of the left ventricular myocardial mass if its diagonal branches are included. This is a fairly consistent finding. The circumflex artery, when it is of average size, supplies about 25 percent of the left ventricular myocardium, while the right coronary artery of approximately equal size will supply the other 25 percent. As previously mentioned, there is a reciprocal relationship between the right and circumflex arteries in which it is possible for one or the other artery to supply the remaining 50 percent of the left ventricular myocardium while the other vessel supplies essentially none. New techniques of digital subtraction provide direct visualization of the myocardium perfused by each artery (Fig. 2-10).

Interventricular Septum

The anterior descending coronary artery consistently supplies the major portion of the interventricular septum. This supply includes the anterior two-thirds to three-quarters of the upper portion of the interventricular septum and essentially the full thickness of the apical portion. The remaining posterior one-quarter to one-third of the upper interventricular septum is supplied by posterior perforating branches of the posterior descending coronary artery which arise either from the right or the circumflex branch.

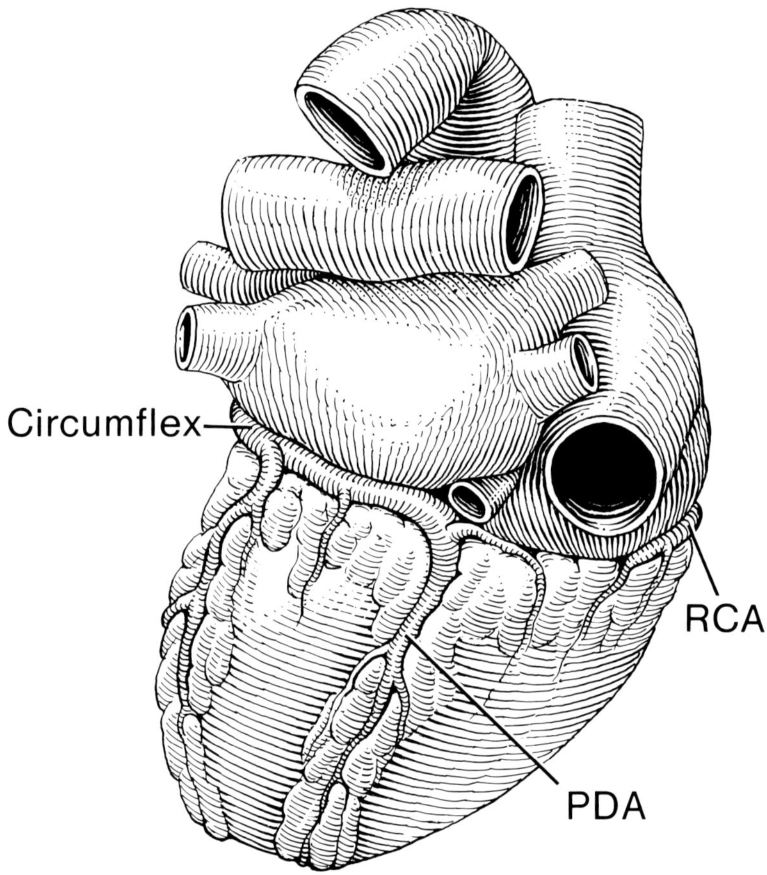

Figure 2-9 Posterior view of the heart. The circumflex artery supplies the posterior descending artery as it turns to travel in the interventricular groove. PDA = posterior descending artery, RCA = right coronary artery.

The Left Ventricular Free Wall

The anterior free wall of the left ventricle is supplied by the diagonal branches of the anterior descending artery for varying distances lateral to the anterior interventricular groove. When there are few diagonal branches and these are short and close to the LAD, then there are always large marginal branches of the circumflex which run quite anterior and pick up the blood supply at that point. If a large intermediate branch exists, then the diagonal branches are reciprocally smaller and fewer in number and supply an area close to the LAD while the intermediate branch supplies the next more lateral segment of the free wall, and then the circumflex marginal branches pick up the supply as one approaches the posterior lateral portion of the left ventricular free wall.

Papillary Muscles

The left ventricular papillary muscles both lie on the free wall and are supplied by the overlying epicardial arteries. The anterolateral papillary muscle is supplied by the diagonal branches of the anterior descending artery, and the posterior medial papillary muscle by the circumflex marginal branches which overlie it[11] (Fig. 2-11), or, in the case of the posterior dominant right coronary artery, it is supplied by the left ventricular branches of that

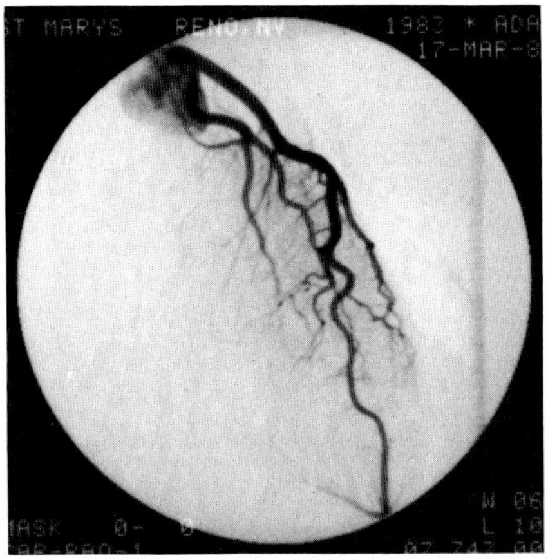

A

Figure 2-10 Digital subtraction study of an injection of the anterior descending artery in the right anterior oblique view. (*a*) Arterial phase of filling of the anterior descending artery. (*b*) Late arterial phase with capillary filling. (*c*) Capillary phase illustrating the mass of myocardium served by the anterior descending coronary artery. (*d*) Digital subtraction image of left anterior descending injection showing collateral filling of the posterior descending artery. (*e*) Capillary phase showing the entire left ventricular myocardium filled from this left coronary artery injection when the right coronary artery is occluded.

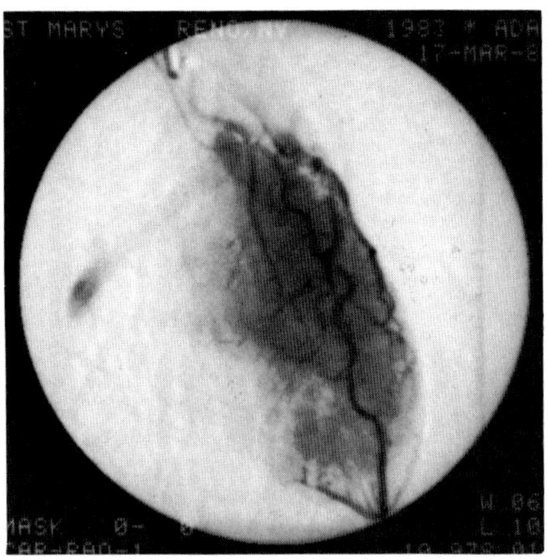

B

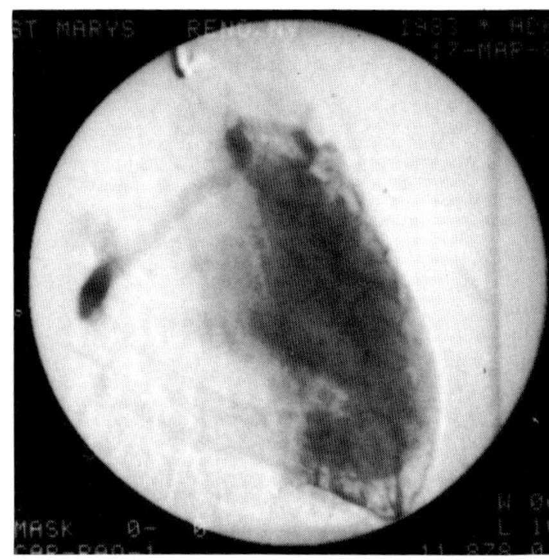

C

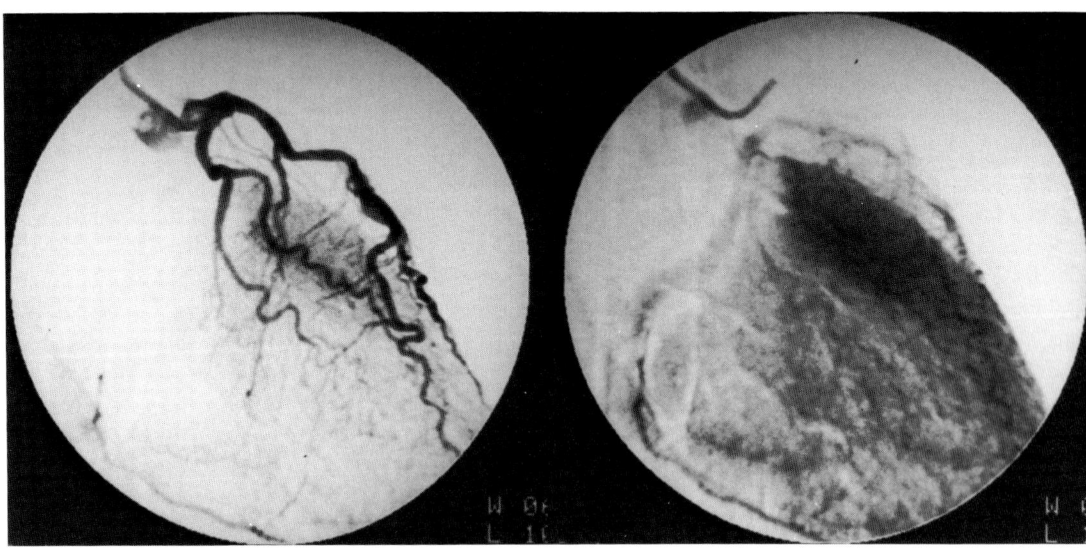

D

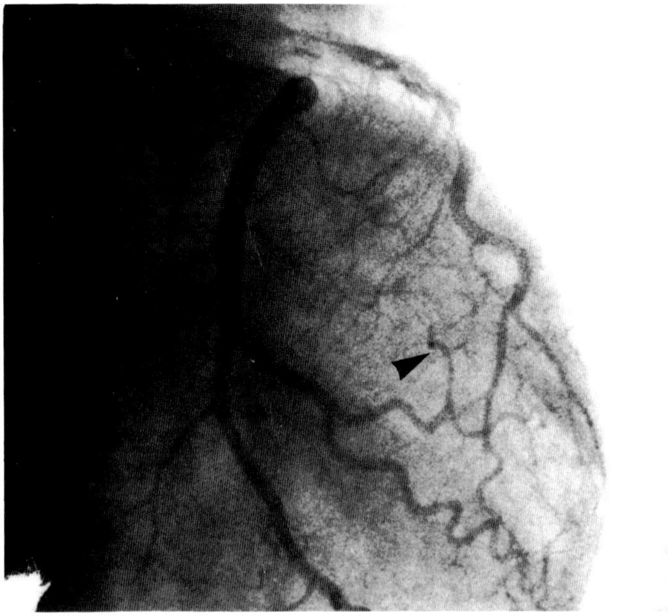

A

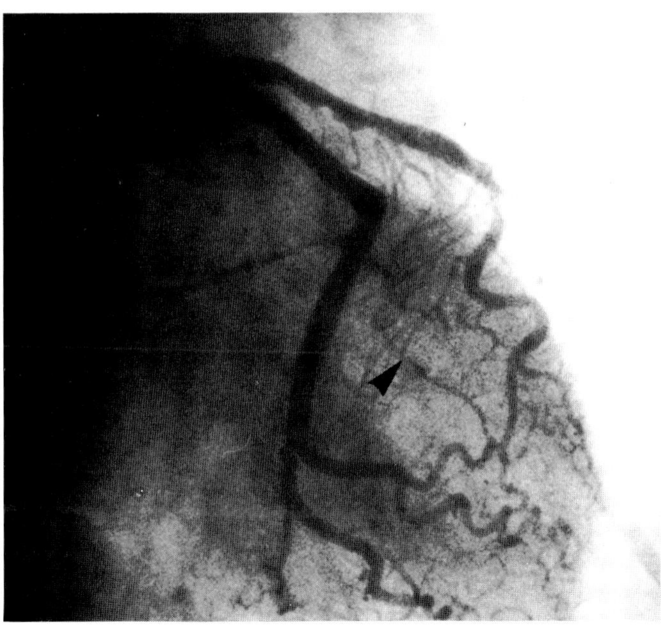

B

Figure 2-11 Right anterior oblique view of left coronary artery. (*a*) Arrow points to the artery to papillary muscle arising from obtuse marginal branch as viewed in diastole. (*b*) Arrow points to the artery to papillary muscle as viewed in systole. Note the stretching out, or extension, of the artery in the papillary muscle toward the mitral annulus which occurred during systole in this patient with mitral valve prolapse (this artery is seldom seen angiographically except in examples of mitral valve prolapse).

vessel. There may commonly be a dual supply to the posterior papillary muscle from the terminal branches of the right coronary artery and the posterolateral branches of the circumflex.

The Sinus Node

The sinus node, located at the junction of the superior vena cava and the right atrium, is supplied in slightly over one-half of hearts from a proximal branch of the right coronary artery which courses into its substance and circles the superior vena cava. In slightly less than 50 percent of human hearts, the sinus node artery arises from the circumflex artery and passes directly to the superior vena cava, where it again circles that structure, supplying the sinus node.

James has pointed out that the origin of the sinus node artery is usually very proximal in the circumflex branch, and occlusions that involve that sinus node artery might threaten the left main coronary.[12] That location is common indeed; however, we have observed many hearts in which the sinus node artery arises some distance from the left main artery, including the mid to even distal portions of the circumflex artery.

The Atrioventricular Node

The atrioventricular (AV) node is supplied by a single cranially directed artery that arises from the vessel that crosses the crux of the heart forming the U-turn at that point. This is the right coronary artery in 90 percent of cases and the circumflex in the remaining 10 percent.[13] There may be a dual blood supply coming to this area from the anterior circulation with a small branch, Kugel's artery, arising from the LAD or the circumflex branch and coursing through the upper interatrial septum.

Right Ventricle

The right ventricular blood supply has been largely ignored and certainly does not carry the same significance as the blood supply to the left ventricle. There is increasing awareness, however, of right ventricular infarction which, when it occurs, is almost always associated with left ventricular infarction. The anterior portion of the right ventricle adjacent to the interventricular septum is supplied by branches of the anterior descending coronary artery and may be involved in anterior myocardial infarctions. The posterior portion of the right ventricle is supplied by the distal right coronary artery and acute marginal branches in 90 percent of hearts. In 10 percent of the cases, the circumflex artery crosses the crux and supplies a portion of the right ventricular myocardium in that area. Posterior myocardial infarctions frequently involve the right ventricular posterior surface.[14]

CORONARY ARTERIAL ANATOMY AS VIEWED ON CORONARY ANGIOGRAMS

It is important to gain an appreciation for the distribution of the coronary arteries in space as three-dimensional objects from the two-dimensional shadows cast on an image intensifier tube. To facilitate this spatial orientation, a model is helpful (Fig. 2-12). A wire circle is constructed to which an elliptical loop is added at right angles. The circle represents a combination of the C-curve created by the right coronary artery travelling in the right atrioventricular groove joining with the reverse C-curve formed by the circumflex artery travelling in the left atrioventricular groove. The elliptical loop arising from the circle represents the anterior descending artery on the superior aspect and the posterior descending artery below as they run in the anterior and inferior interventricular grooves to meet near the cardiac apex. This stylized model of the coronary circulation is held in front of a projected light source, casting a shadow on a screen or wall. Rotation of the object will cast shadows which illustrate different images created when the coronary arteries are viewed in various positions. By viewing the shadow from the side as the coronary arteries are viewed in the right anterior oblique projection, the loop is seen on its side, and the circle appears as a straight line with the two shadows of the right and circumflex arteries overlapping (Fig. 2-12*a*). Viewed from the apex of the loop, the circle is seen en face and the loop representing the

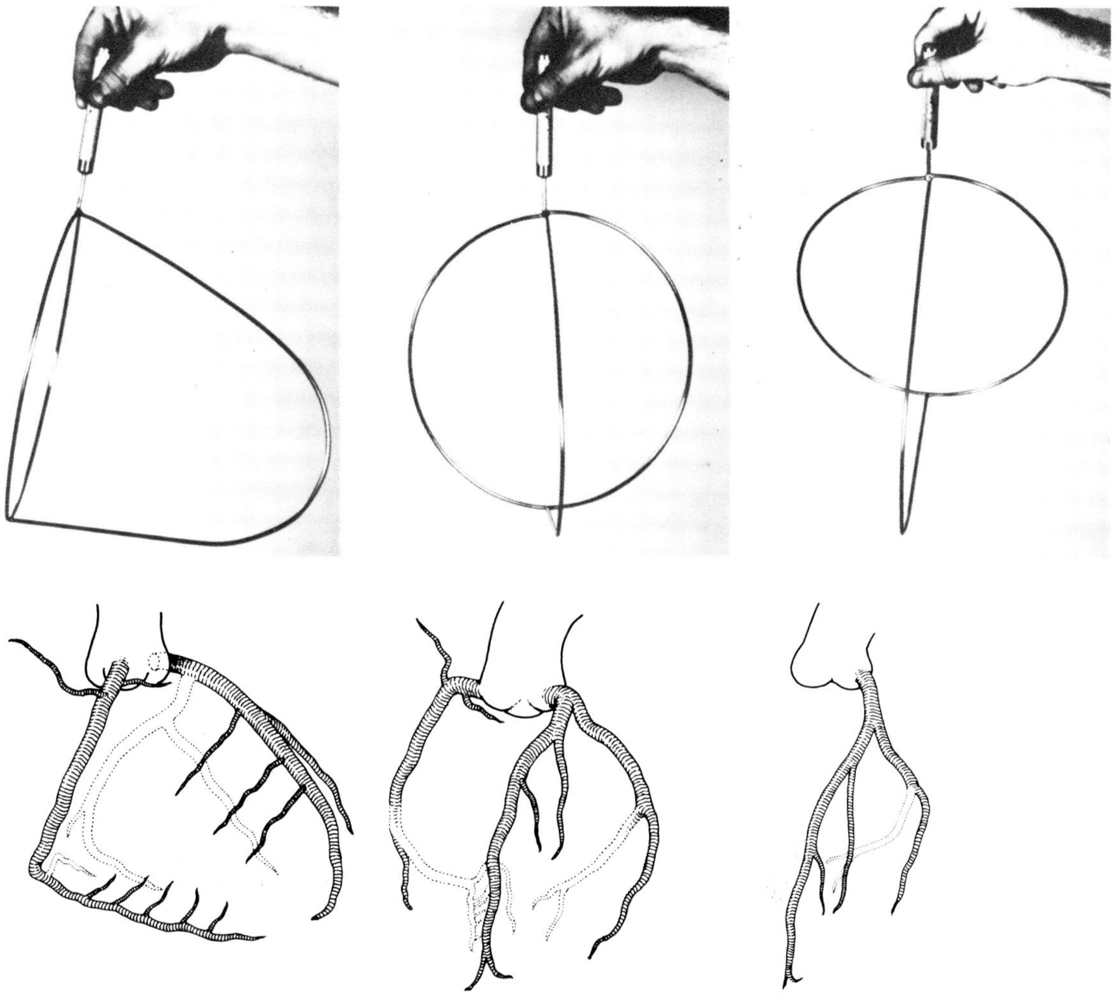

A B C

Figure 2-12 Demonstration of the spatial appearance of the coronary anatomy using a wire teaching model. (*a*) Right anterior oblique view of the model and the corresponding circulation. (*b*) Left anterior oblique view. (*c*) Left anterior oblique view with cranial angulation of the overtable image intensifier. *(From Franch RH, King SB III, Douglas JS: Techniques of cardiac catheterization including coronary arteriography, in Hurst JW (ed):* The Heart (5th ed). *McGraw-Hill, New York, p 1866. With permission of the authors.)*

LAD and posterior descending appear as straight lines facing the observer (Fig. 2-12*b*). By adding wires to the anterior descending artery running diagonally and to the circumflex artery also running diagonally and parallel to the anterior descending branches, diagonal and circumflex marginal arteries can be simulated. Further manipulations of this model can easily demonstrate those views which will be most successful in casting shadows of the coronary arteries free of overlap or significant foreshortening (Fig. 12-12*c*).

Nomenclature of Views

A brief review of the nomenclature of the views is needed. Each view is named for the position of the image intensifier and not for the direction of the x-ray beam. One may think of each view as though one were looking at the heart from the position of the image intensifier. Therefore, *frontal* means that the image tube is directly over the sternum. *Left* or *right lateral* refers to the image tube on that side with the x-ray beam perpendicular to the frontal view. *Right anterior oblique* places the image tube over the right side of the chest looking obliquely at the heart, while *left anterior oblique* places the image tube over the left side of the chest. *Cranial angulation* refers to the location of the image tube in a direction toward the head and *caudal* toward the feet. *Cranial* and *caudal* are not used to indicate the direction of the x-ray beam but the view one would obtain by observing the heart with one's eye at the position of the image intensifier.

The Left Coronary Artery

The left coronary orifice is located in the middle of the upper portion of the left coronary sinus. The left main artery travels leftward and slightly posterior for lengths varying from 1 to 25 to 30 mm before dividing into two or three branches. Occasionally the left main artery is absent, with the anterior descending artery and circumflex branch arising from separate orifices or from a common orifice but with no left main identifiable. A frontal projection will usually show the left coronary orifice and the left main segment to best advantage (Fig. 2-13). This will cast the shadow of the left main artery directly over the spine, but adequate x-ray penetration is possible with modern x-ray equipment. This view will not identify the portion of the left main artery that bifurcates. For that view, the left anterior oblique projection with steep cranial angulation will give an additional view of the left main artery and show the area of the bifurcation (Fig. 2-14). If the left main travels in a horizontal or slightly vertical direction, then foreshortening may limit the value of the left anterior oblique cranial view for left main visualization. Further discussion of the value of cranial and caudal angle views will be forthcoming in Chap. 9.

As the left main coronary curves around the pulmonary artery, it continues in the anterior interventricular sulcus as the anterior descending branch. The circumflex artery arises at the bifurcation, sometimes inscribing an acute angle with the anterior descending artery and at other times taking off the left main at almost a 90° angle. When the

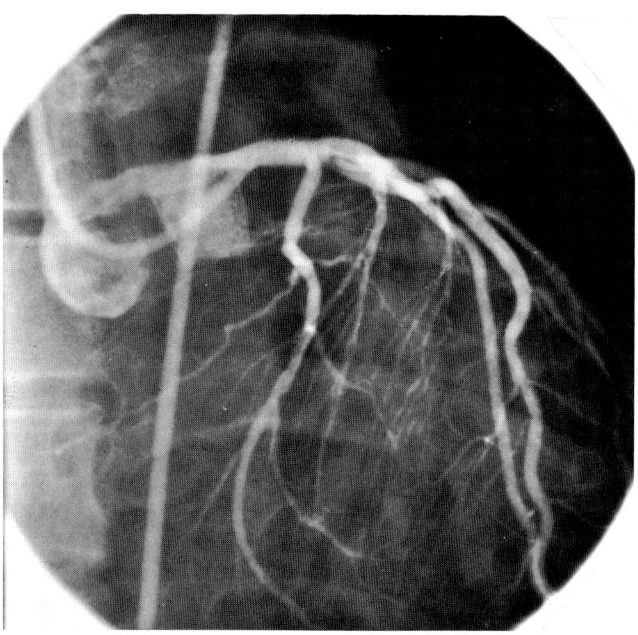

Figure 2-13 Frontal view of the left coronary artery showing the left main segment to include its orifice. Note backflow of contrast medium into the aortic sinus.

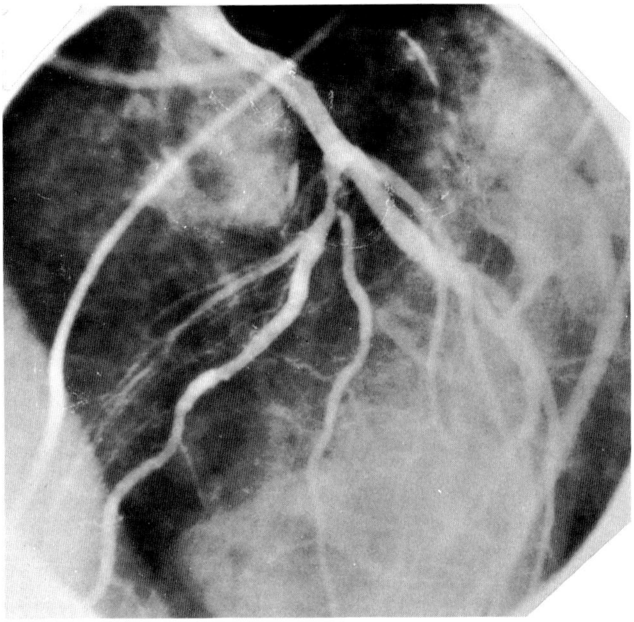

Figure 2-14 Left anterior oblique cranial view showing the bifurcation of the left coronary artery into the anterior descending and circumflex arteries.

third branch (the intermediate branch) arises between the anterior descending and circumflex arteries forming a trifurcation of the left main, then this branch point can best be visualized in the left anterior oblique view with significant cranial angulation. All frontal and right anterior oblique views will overlap this bifurcation point and obscure the origin of these three vessels. Occasionally in very horizontal hearts, a caudal angulation of the left anterior oblique view will "look up under the left main artery" providing a good view of the division of the left main into its more distal branches (Fig. 2-15).

Anterior Descending Artery

The anterior descending artery continues to sweep in a gentle curve into the interventricular groove travelling toward the left ventricular apex. When viewed in the right anterior oblique projection, the septal perforating branches can be seen travelling deep into the muscular septum (Fig. 2-16). The straight lateral view also gives an excellent image of the septal perforating branches as they take off at right angles from the anterior descending branch. In the left anterior oblique views, the septal vessels overlap with the LAD, and very little estimation of them can be made. These septal vessels differ from the epicardial vessels in that they are straighter and move little with cardiac action, in contrast to the buckling of the epicardial arteries during systole.

In the 30° right anterior oblique view, the anterior descending artery is seen travelling inside the border of the heart by 1 to 2 cm (Fig. 2-16). As it reaches the cardiac apex, the most common circumstance is for the anterior descending to continue around the apex and proceed for a short distance up the inferior surface of the heart. Occasionally the anterior descending may stop short of the apex in conjunction with a very long posterior descending branch of the right coronary artery which circles the apex and extends up the anterior portion of the ventricular groove.

Diagonal Branches

Diagonal arteries that originate from the anterior descending course over the anterior left ventricular free wall and appear on the lateral border of the

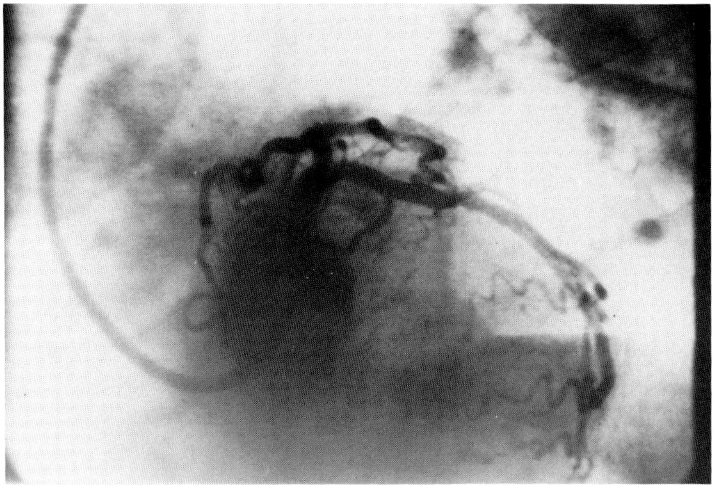

Figure 2-15 Left anterior oblique caudal view of the left coronary artery showing the separation of the proximal portion of the branch vessels of the left main.

heart as the heart is viewed in the right anterior oblique projection. This shadow of the diagonal branch on the anterolateral tangent of the heart distinguishes it from the anterior descending, which travels inside that border toward the left ventricular apex. In the right anterior oblique view, the LAD and diagonal branches often overlap in their proximal portions, making any examination of them difficult (Fig. 2-16). When viewed in a left anterior oblique projection, the diagonal branches can be seen clearly separated from the anterior descending artery. Addition of cranial angulation to the left anterior oblique view will further enhance the ability to separate the origin of the diagonal branches and the course of these vessels as they extend over the anterior left ventricular free wall (Fig. 2-17).

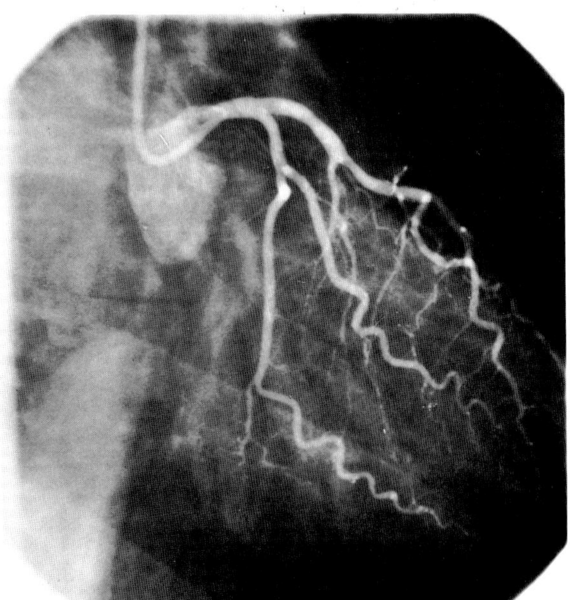

Figure 2-16 Right anterior oblique view of left coronary artery. Note large septal perforator and smaller perforating vessels extending down the length of the anterior descending artery.

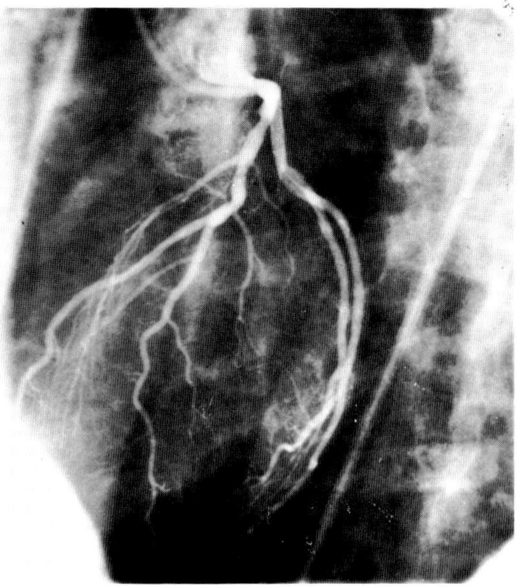

Figure 2-17 Left anterior oblique cranial view of left coronary artery showing takeoff of diagonal branch.

Circumflex Artery

Although the bifurcation of the left main artery is frequently thought of as a straight continuation of the LAD and a right angle takeoff of the circumflex, the angles subtended by these two arteries vary from 30° to 180°.[8,15] When this angle is very wide, the right anterior oblique view gives good visualization of the proximal circumflex artery, but when the angle is narrow, there is great overlap with the LAD in the right anterior oblique view. The left anterior oblique view with cranial angulation remains an excellent view for the proximal portion of the circumflex artery in those cases with a narrow angle. The addition of caudal angulation to the right anterior oblique view will improve visualization of the proximal circumflex artery without overlap. In the right anterior oblique view, the circumflex artery travels away from the image intensifier as it courses in the atrioventricular groove. One must realize this potential for foreshortening in the right anterior oblique view and recognize that this is not an optimal view for the atrioventricular groove portion of the circumflex artery. As the circumflex gives rise to marginal branches, however, they travel in a direction perpendicular to the x-ray beam, and therefore are well-visualized in all the right anterior oblique views (Fig. 2-18). The left anterior oblique view gives an excellent projection of the atrioventricular groove portion of the circumflex artery; however, the takeoffs of the marginal branches are usually obscured in this view. When the circumflex artery forms the dominant posterior circulation, the bifurcation of the posterior descending and right ventricular branches is equally obscured in the left anterior oblique view, since these vessels are coming directly toward the image intensifier and are grossly foreshortened. Addition of cranial angulation to the left anterior oblique views enhances the ability to see these posterior vessels. The posterior descending artery arising from the circumflex is best seen in the right anterior oblique projection, on its side. The discussion of these special views will be discussed in detail in Chap. 9.

Right Coronary Artery

The right coronary orifice is located in the right coronary sinus from the lower portion to high near the sinotubular ridge. Its takeoff is anterior and 30° to 40° to the right of the sagittal plane. The proximal portion of the artery travels in the epicardial

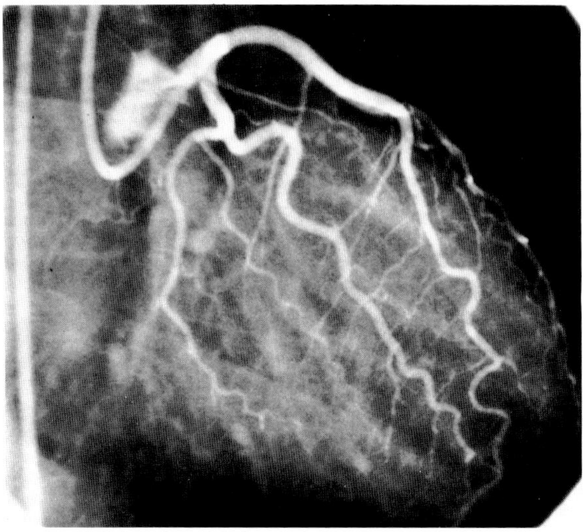

Figure 2-18 Right anterior oblique caudal view of left coronary artery showing the marginal branches of the circumflex coronary to best advantage.

fat in a more or less anterior direction, then curves posteriorly into the atrioventricular groove on the right side. The proximal part of the right coronary artery varies greatly and may travel from an almost caudal direction, through a wide range of orientations, to an almost cranial direction (Fig. 2-19).

After a short distance, however, the vessel does turn in a direction posterior and caudal to travel in the right atrioventricular groove. It proceeds as a long conduit vessel changing little in diameter to reach the posterior portion of the heart. The first branch, the conus artery, frequently arises either as a separate orifice or from the very proximal portion of the right coronary artery, and because of that location is frequently not opacified by the selective right coronary injection. The conus artery courses medially around the pulmonary outflow tract at the level of the pulmonary valve. Several other small right ventricular branches arise at right angles from the right coronary artery and travel in a tortuous fashion over the right ventricular free wall. In 55 percent of cases, the sinus node artery originates from the proximal portion of the right coronary artery and travels atrially to reach the sinus node. At the acute margin of the heart, there is usually a larger right ventricular branch which travels along the acute margin toward the apex of the heart. Occasionally this branch supplies a significant portion of the interventricular septum in its posterior apical aspect.

The C-shape of the right coronary artery seen en face can best be appreciated in the left anterior oblique view (Fig. 2-19). This usually gives an excellent view of the right coronary artery throughout its length until the posterior ventricular branches are reached. The posterior descending artery travelling on the inferior surface of the heart will be directed toward the image intensifier in the left anterior oblique views and therefore will be greatly foreshortened. Addition of cranial angulation in this view will improve visualization of that posterior descending artery considerably (Fig. 2-20). Right anterior oblique views will display the posterior descending artery perpendicular to the x-ray beam and will give excellent visualization of the vessel throughout its length. When there is a large left ventricular branch of the right coronary artery, that vessel may be superimposed on the posterior descending in the right anterior oblique view. The addition of cranial angulation in the right anterior oblique view may separate these vessels. However, cranial angulation in the left anterior oblique view will best separate the origin of the posterior descending branch and the left ventricular branch. The AV node artery consistently travels in a cranial direction from the U-turn of the right coronary ar-

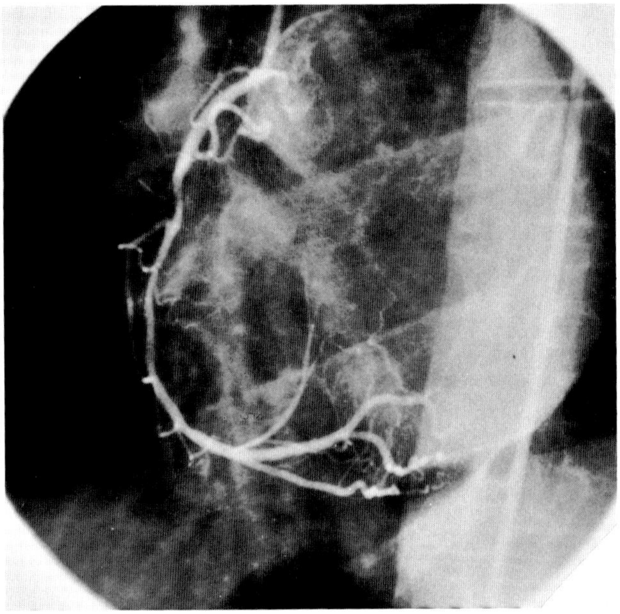

A

Figure 2-19 (a) Left anterior oblique view of right coronary artery showing caudal orientation of the proximal segment. (b) Left anterior oblique view of right coronary artery showing cranial orientation of proximal segment.

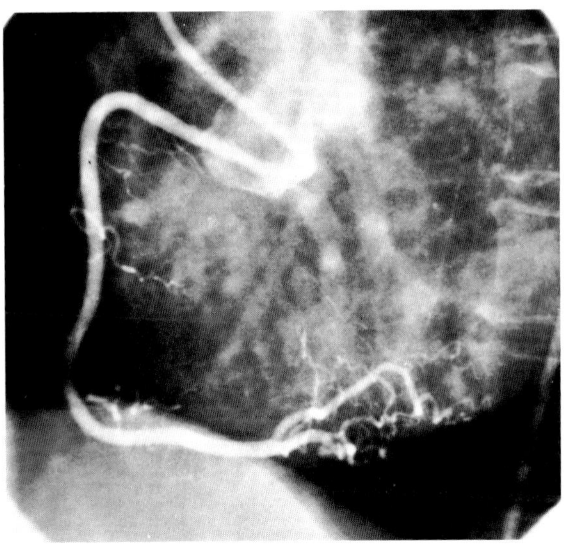

B

tery at the crux. This artery can be identified radiographically as a single branch directed cranially and terminating in a T-configuration created by two short lateral branches.

When the left circumflex artery is the dominant posterior artery, the right coronary usually bifurcates early into one branch travelling in the atrioventricular groove and another right ventricular branch of almost equal size. The smooth tapering of these vessels and the small diameter of the prox-

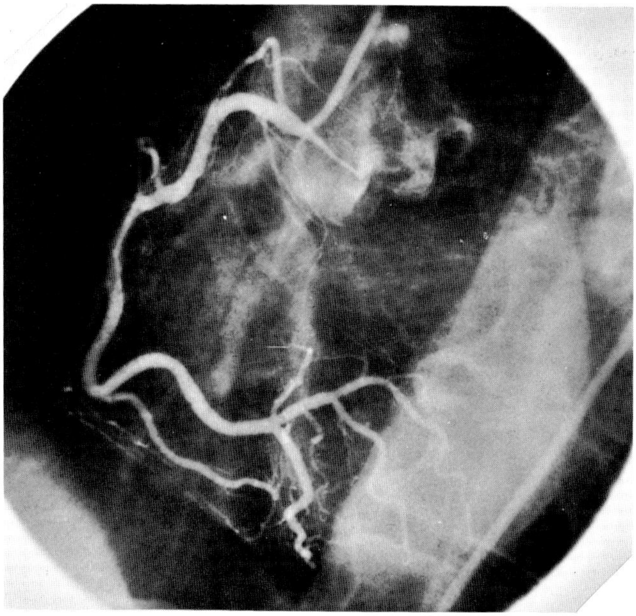

A

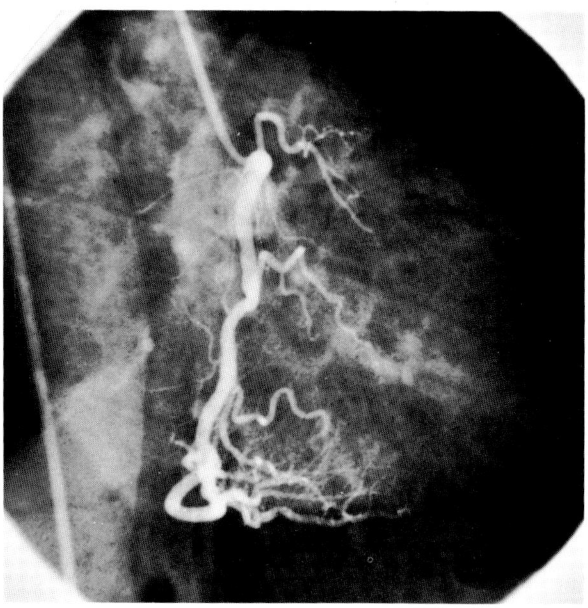

B

Figure 2-20 (*a*) Left anterior oblique cranial view of right coronary artery showing the origin of the posterior descending artery and the atrioventricular node artery travelling in the opposite direction. (*b*) Right anterior oblique view of right coronary artery showing the distal posterior descending artery without foreshortening.

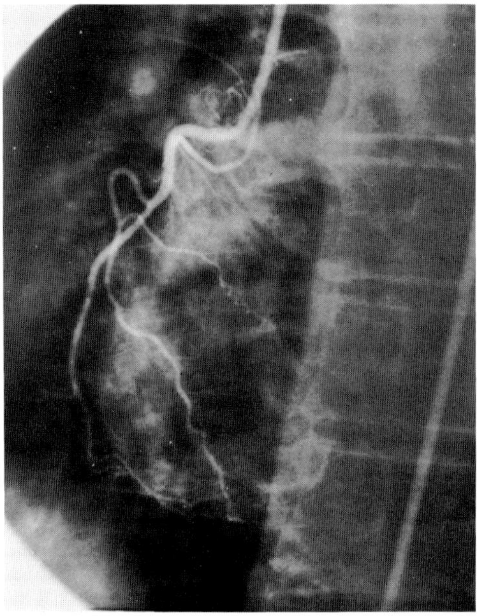

Figure 2-21 Left anterior oblique view of nondominant right coronary artery.

imal portion of the right coronary artery combined with the large posterior circulation of the circumflex artery identify this as a nondominant right coronary rather than a totally occluded right coronary artery (Fig. 2-21).

One overriding consideration in the evaluation of the radiographic anatomy of the coronary circulation is the realization that the anatomy may be quite variable; however, all segments of the left ventricular myocardium are perfused adequately in the healthy heart. It is therefore necessary to integrate the surface coronary anatomy as seen in both the left coronary artery injections and the right coronary artery injections in order to form a spacial appreciation of the distribution of these vessels over the epicardial surface of the heart to ensure that all areas are served by adequate coronary circulation. If gaps are seen or areas are devoid of coronary circulation, then the possibility exists that occlusion of an artery is present or an anomalous origin of a coronary artery exists and that vessels have not yet been opacified.

REFERENCES

1. Vieussens R: *Traité Nouveau de la Structure et Causes du Movements Natural du Coeur*. Toulouse, France, 1715.
2. Willius FA, Dry DJ: *A History of the Heart and Circulation*. Saunders, Philadelphia, 1948, p 95.
3. Ibid, p 110.
4. Ibid, p 234.
5. Sones FM Jr, Farra EK: Cine coronary Arteriography. Mod Concepts Cardiovasc Dis, 31:735, 1962.
6. Favaloro RG: Saphenous vein graft in the surgical treatment of coronary artery disease: Operative technique. J Thorac Cardiovasc Surg, 58:178, 1969.
7. Johnson WD, Flemma RJ, Lepley T Jr, et al: Extended treatment of severe coronary artery disease: A total surgical approach Ann Surg 170:460, 1969.
8. James TN: *Anatomy of the Coronary Arteries*. Hoeber Medical Division, Harper & Row, New York, 1961.
9. McAlpine WA: *Heart and Coronary Arteries*. Springer-Verlag, New York, 1975.
10. Vieussens R: *Nouvelles de Couvertes Sur le Coeur*. Paris, France, 1706.

11 Cobbs BW Jr, King SB III: Ventricular buckling: A factor in the abnormal ventriculogram and peculiar hemodynamics associated with mitral valve prolapse. Am Heart J, 93:741–758, 1977.

12 James TN: Myocardial infarction and atrial arrhythmias. Circulation, 24:761, 1961.

13 James TN: The coronary circulation and conduction system in acute myocardial infarction. Prog Cardiovasc Dis, 10:410, 1968.

14 Chou T, Van der Bel-Kahn J, Allan J, Brockmeier L, Fowler NO: Electrocardiographic diagnosis of right ventricular infarction. Am J Med, 70(6):1175, 1981.

15 King SB III, Douglas JS Jr, Morris DC: New angiographic views for coronary arteriography, in Hurst JW (ed): *Update IV: The Heart*. McGraw-Hill, New York, 1981.

Chapter 3

Coronary Artery Anomalies

John S. Douglas, Jr., M.D.
Robert H. Franch, M.D.
Spencer B. King III, M.D.

This chapter deals with anomalies of coronary artery origin, distribution, or structure, which may be encountered in performing and interpreting coronary arteriograms. Coronary anomalies (Table 3-1) are reported to occur in roughly 1 percent of the population catheterized, and this is consistent with our experiences. Coronary anomalies are frequently incidental findings, in which anatomy is altered but physiology is normal; that is, coronary blood flow is normal. However, certain anomalies are associated with myocardial ischemia or infarction, heart failure, and sudden death. In some of these cases, modern cardiac surgical techniques may relieve patients' symptoms and offer improved longevity.

Anomalies cause technical problems in coronary arteriography due to unusual positions of coronary artery ostia. Failure to cannulate and opacify an anomalous coronary artery may lead to the false conclusion that the missing artery is occluded. Anomalies of the coronary arteries may increase the risk of coronary arterial insult during cardiac surgery, serve as a site for development of endocarditis or thrombus formation, and in the case of coronary arterial venous fistulas, produce striking murmurs and significant left-to-right heart shunts.

An understanding of these anomalies is essential to those performing coronary arteriograms in order that a safe, complete initial study may be carried out even when the anomaly is encountered unexpectedly for the first time. This point is emphasized by reports that almost 40 percent of patients with coronary anomalies have required a second angiographic procedure to elucidate the anomaly clearly.[1]

Table 3-1 Anomalies of the Coronary Arteries

- **I** Anomalous origin from the aorta
  - **A** High aortic origin
  - **B** Origin from the contralateral sinus of Valsalva or coronary artery
    - **1** Circumflex coronary artery from right sinus of Valsalva or right coronary artery
    - **2** LAD from right sinus of Valsalva or right coronary artery
    - **3** Left coronary artery from right sinus of Valsalva
    - **4** Right coronary artery from left sinus of Valsalva
  - **C** Single coronary artery
- **II** Anomalous origin from the pulmonary artery
- **III** Coronary arteriovenous fistulas
- **IV** Coronary artery atresia or hypoplasia
- **V** Coronary artery aneurysms
- **VI** Variation in patients with congenital heart disease
  - **A** Tetralogy of Fallot
  - **B** Transposition of the great arteries
  - **C** Pulmonary atresia with intact ventricular septum
  - **D** Univentricular heart, including tricuspid atresia
  - **E** Congenitally corrected transposition of the great arteries
  - **F** Truncus arteriosus
  - **G** Double-outlet right ventricle
  - **H** Bicuspid aortic valve
  - **I** Supravalvular aortic stenosis and coarctation of the aorta
  - **J** Supravalvular mitral stenosis
  - **K** Superior-inferior heart (crisscross pattern)
  - **L** Situs inversus

ANOMALOUS ORIGIN FROM THE AORTA

High Aortic Origin

There is considerable variation in the location of the coronary ostia. Vlodaver[2] reported that both coronary ostia arose above the sinotubular junction in 6 percent of unselected adult hearts. Ogden[3] considered unusually high origin of the coronary ostia (more than a centimeter or so above the sinotubular ridge) to be a minor coronary anomaly. In our hands and others', [4] high origin of the coronary arteries has presented no major technical problems in performing coronary arteriography unless the right coronary artery is anomalously located high over the left coronary sinus. In this case selective intubation of the coronary artery may be extremely difficult[5] (see "Right Coronary Artery from the Left Sinus of Valsalva"). Use of a left Amplatz catheter may facilitate selective catheterization.

Origin from Contralateral Sinus of Valsalva

Circumflex from the Right Sinus of Valsalva Origin of the circumflex coronary artery from the right sinus of Valsalva or right coronary artery is the most common anomaly encountered by the coronary angiographer (Fig. 3-1). It was first described by Antopol and Kugel in 1933.[6] The incidence of this anomaly during routine coronary arteriography was reported by Donaldson et al. to be 0.3 percent,[7] by Kimbiris et al. to be 0.37 percent,[8] by Chaitman et al. to be 0.45 percent,[9] and

Figure 3-1 Artist's sketch of the circumflex coronary artery arising anomalously from the right sinus of Valsalva. AO = aorta, PA = pulmonary artery.

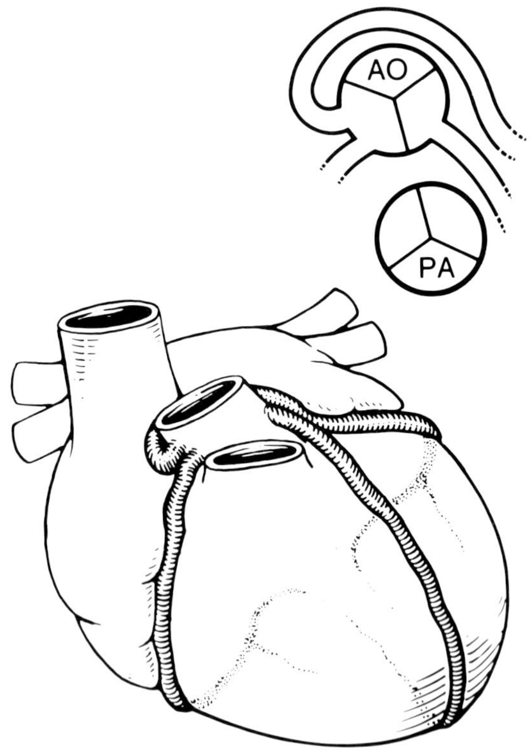

by Page et al. to be 0.67 percent.[10] In our last 5000 patients, this anomaly was observed in 18 patients (0.4 percent). This coronary anomaly is benign, and its clinical importance lies in the recognition of its presence so that complete evaluation of the coronary arterial tree can be carried out.

The anomalous circumflex artery invariably arises in the right sinus of Valsalva just posterior (and usually inferior) to the right coronary artery itself. It passes posterior to the aortic root, entering the left atrioventricular groove, and subsequently distributes branches to the posterior lateral left ventricle. The anomalous circumflex artery is commonly rather small.

Aberrant origin of the circumflex is suspected when injection of the left coronary artery fills only the left anterior descending coronary artery, with an apparent avascular area in the posterior lateral left ventricular myocardium (Fig. 3-2). Page et al.[10] called this angiographic appearance a sign of nonperfused myocardium. It is more common for the circumflex coronary artery to originate from the right sinus of Valsalva than from a separate orifice in the left coronary sinus, which is the other possibility that must be considered. Page et al. also called attention to the ''aortic root sign'' as a clue to the recognition of an anomalous circumflex artery from the right sinus of Valsalva. This aortic root sign is the visualization of the opacified anomalous coronary artery behind the aortic root during left ventriculography in the right anterior oblique (RAO) projection. Selective catheterization of the anomalous circumflex artery can usually be accomplished with a Judkins right coronary catheter or with a multipurpose catheter. Although generally considered a benign anomaly, at least one sudden death has been reported: a 20-year-old male with this anomaly.[11] The presence of this anomaly may be a complicating factor in mitral valve surgery[12] and in aortic valve surgery when coronary artery perfusion is attempted.

Left Anterior Descending Artery from Right Sinus of Valsalva Origin of the left anterior descending (LAD) coronary artery from the right sinus of Valsalva or right coronary artery is a rare anomaly (Fig. 3-3). It was reported to occur during routine coronary arteriography in 0.03 percent of patients by Kimbiris,[8] in 0.04 percent by Donaldson,[7] and 0.2 percent by Engel,[3] and was not seen at all by Levin.[13] Some of the variation in reported frequency of this anomaly may be due to difficulty in determining whether the LAD originates in the right sinus of Valsalva as a separate orifice or from a common trunk, in which case it may be classified as a single coronary artery anomaly. The anomalous LAD arises anteriorly in the right sinus of Valsalva or from the right coronary artery and passes either between the aorta and pulmonary artery or anterior to the pulmonary artery to reach the anterior interventricular groove.

Anomalous origin of the LAD from the right sinus of Valsalva is one of the anatomic variations that must be considered when injection of contrast medium in the left sinus of Valsalva reveals only a circumflex coronary artery. It is helpful to remember, however, that separate orifice of the LAD and circumflex in the left sinus of Valsalva is more common than anomalous origin of the LAD from the right sinus of Valsalva. Anomalous septal perforating branches arising from the right sinus of Valsalva are seen with approximately the same frequency as LAD originating from the same site.[3,8]

Origin of the LAD or septal perforating branch from the right sinus of Valsalva has been considered a benign anomaly. This is in contrast with the origin of the left main coronary artery from the right sinus of Valsalva (see below). Anomalous origin of the LAD from the right sinus of Valsalva is the most common coronary anomaly seen in tetralogy of Fallot (see Figs. 3-28 and 3-29), where it occurs in over 2 percent of patients.[14] Inadvertent transection of the anomalous LAD is a known complication of complete repair of tetralogy of Fallot, which is usually, but not invariably, fatal.[15] The increased frequency of anomalous LAD from the right coronary sinus and other anomalies in complex congenital heart disease has lead most cardiologists and surgeons to advocate routine preoperative coronary arteriography in these patients.[14]

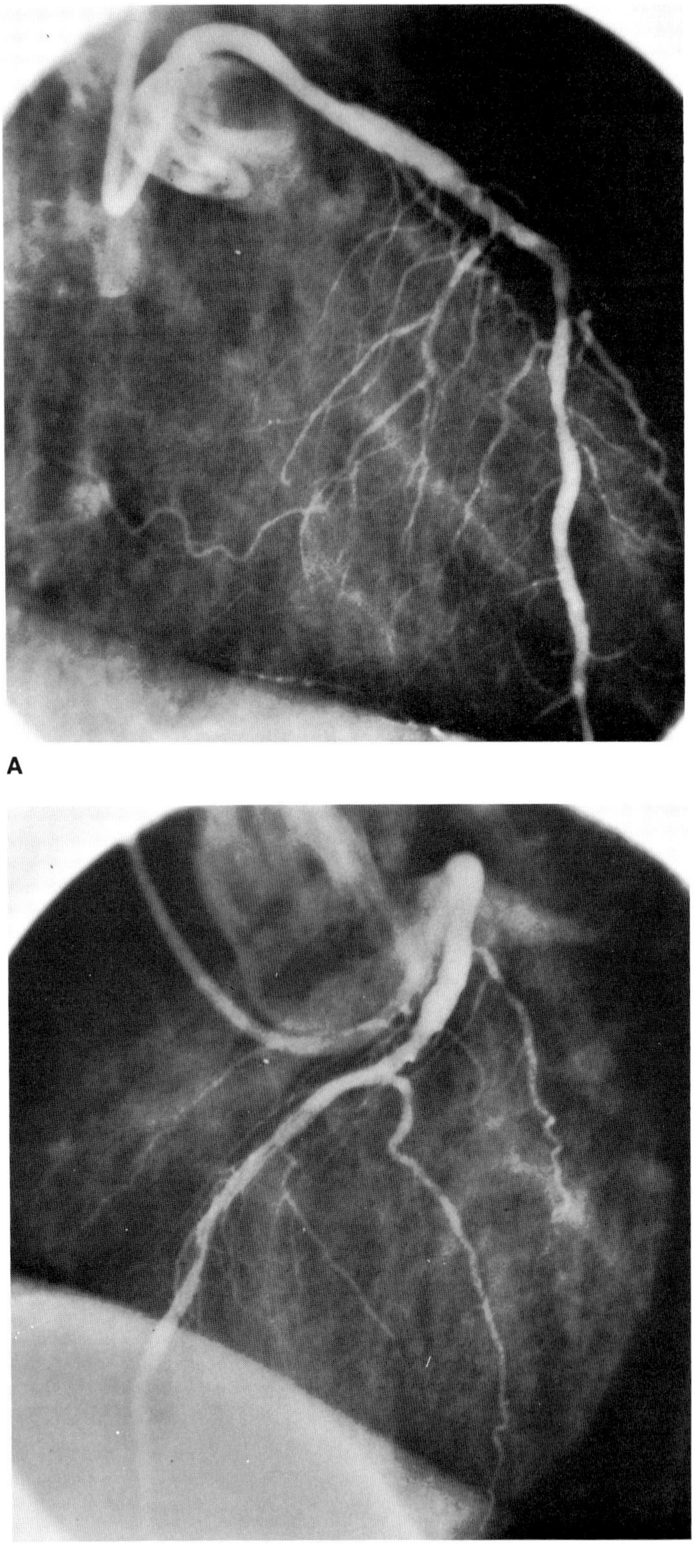

A

B

Figure 3-2 Coronary arteriogram showing injection of the left coronary artery arising from the left sinus of Valsalva in right anterior oblique (*a*) and left anterior oblique (*b*) projections. Note the absence of the circumflex coronary artery. The circumflex arises anomalously from the right sinus of Valsalva as shown in left anterior oblique (*c*) and right anterior oblique (*d*) projections and passes posterior to the aorta to reach the lateral wall of the left ventricle.

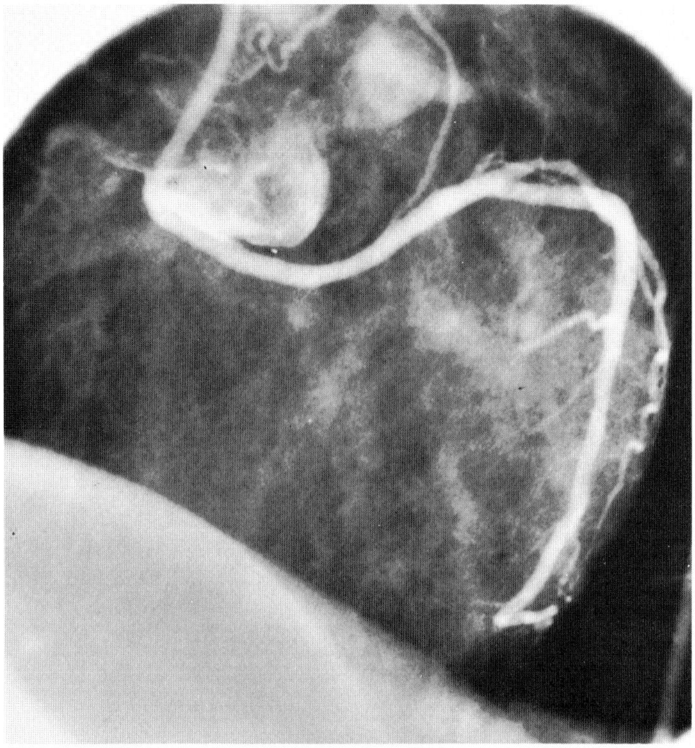

C

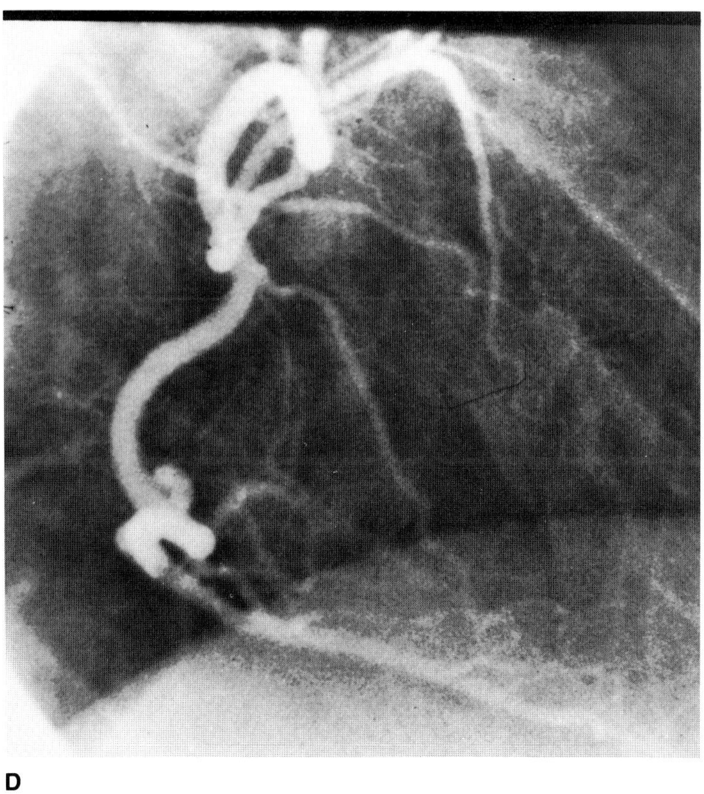

D

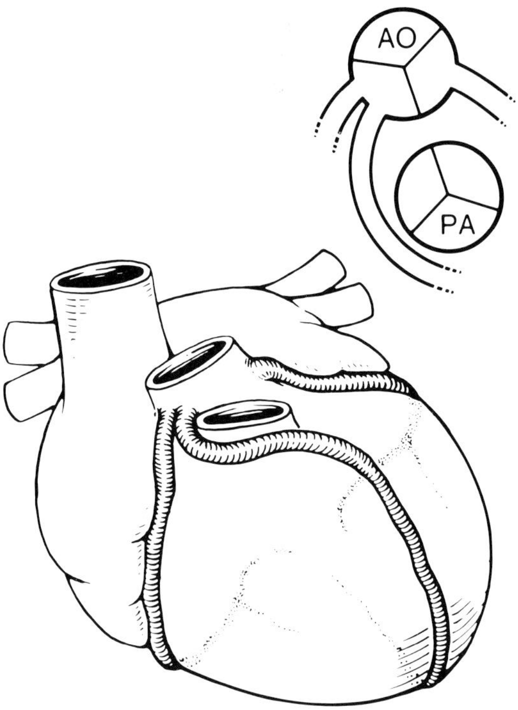

Figure 3-3 Artist's sketch of the left anterior descending coronary artery arising from the right sinus of Valsalva and passing anterior to the pulmonary artery to reach the anterior interventricular groove. The anomalous left anterior descending may also pass between the great vessels. AO = aorta, PA = pulmonary artery.

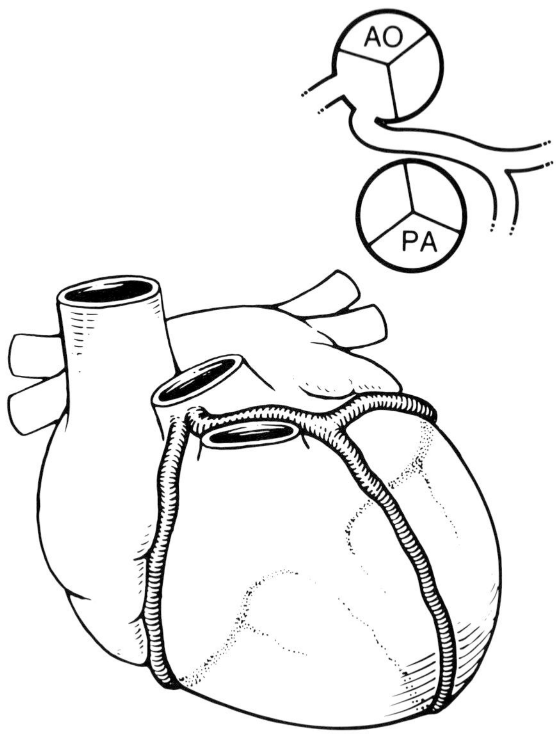

Figure 3-4 Artist's sketch showing the left main coronary artery originating in the right sinus of Valsalva and passing between the aorta and pulmonary artery. In some patients, the anomalous left coronary artery is incorporated into the anterior wall of the aorta, where compression may occur. AO = aorta, PA = pulmonary artery.

Left Main Coronary Artery from Right Sinus of Valsalva Origin of the left main coronary artery from the right sinus of Valsalva is a rare anomaly which has been associated with sudden death (Figs. 3-4 and 3-5). The frequency of this anomaly during routine coronary arteriography is reported to be 0.04 percent by Kimbiris,[8] 0.02 percent by Moodie,[16] 0.02 percent by Engel,[5] and 0.04 percent by Donaldson.[7] We have observed six such cases in the last 5000 coronary arteriograms for an incidence of 0.12 percent. In a majority of cases, the anomalous left main coronary artery arises just anterior to the right coronary artery in the right sinus of Valsalva and passes between the right ventricular outflow tract and aorta, after which it bifurcates into the left anterior descending and circumflex branches. The anomalous artery may tunnel on an intramyocardial course within the interventricular septum to reach the anterior interventricular groove, where it bifurcates into the major branches. Rarely, the left main coronary may pass anterior to the pulmonary artery, as observed in two of our last six patients with this anomaly, or posterior to the aorta.[8,13]

Significant cardiac morbidity with this anomaly was first reported in 1964, when Cohen[17] observed fatal myocardial infarction in an 11-year-old boy who was otherwise healthy. Benson reported sudden death in a 56-year-old male with this anomaly and collected five cases from the literature, noting that four were teenage males who died following exercise.[18] Cheitlin[19] reviewed the Armed Forces Institute of Pathology experience, finding 19 cases

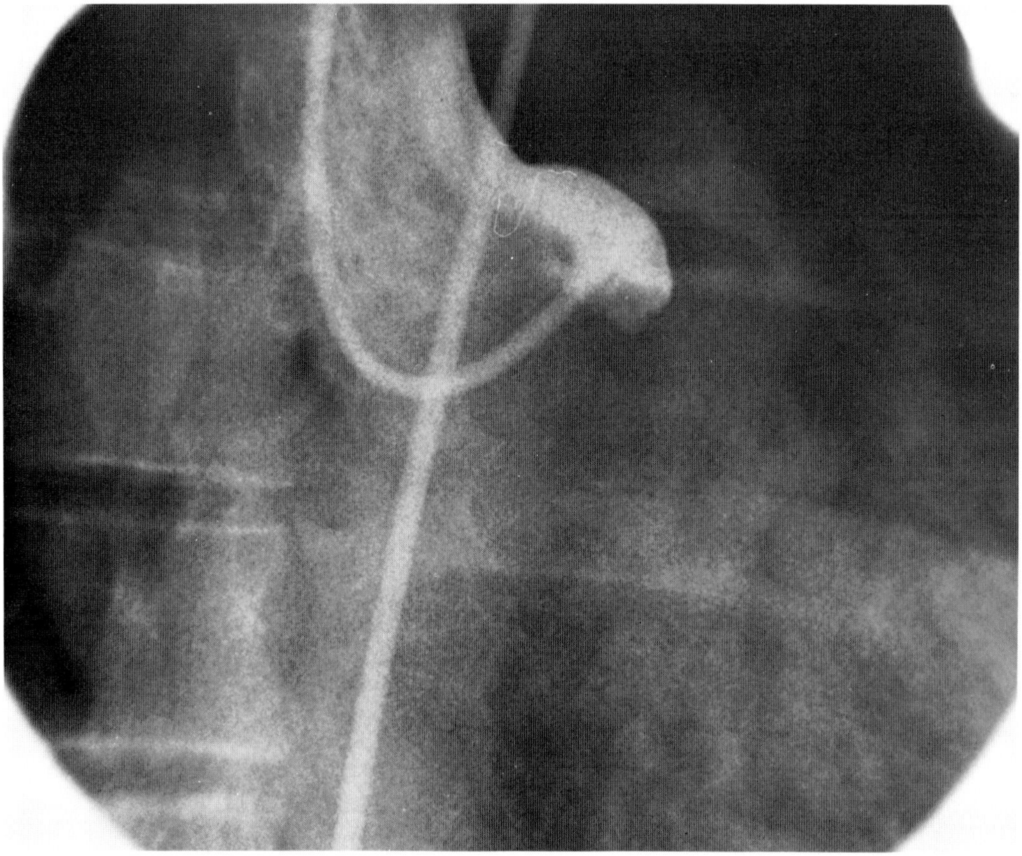

A

Figure 3-5 Coronary arteriogram in a 60-year-old female with anomalous left coronary artery arising from the right sinus of Valsalva and passing between the aorta and pulmonary artery. Injection of contrast medium in the left aortic sinus revealed no coronary artery (*a*), but selective left coronary injections in the left anterior oblique (*b*), right anterior oblique (*c*), and right anterior oblique cranial projection (*d*) demonstrate the site of origin of the left coronary artery in the right sinus of Valsalva. The anterior concavity of the initial portion of the left coronary artery in the right anterior oblique view is produced by the pulmonary artery, around and behind which the left coronary artery passes.

of left main coronary artery originating from the right sinus of Valsalva of which 7 (36 percent) died suddenly during or immediately following exercise with no other apparent cause of death detectable at autopsy. In all of these patients, the left main coronary artery passed between the aorta and the right ventricular infundibulum, and it was suggested that the mechanism of sudden death in these cases was related to compromise of the ostium of the left main artery, which arose tangentially from the anterior aspect of the right coronary sinus, or compression of the left main artery between the great vessels (Fig. 3-6). In addition, stretching and compression may occur in those arteries whose initial course is actually within the wall of the aorta, these effects being greatest during exercise (Fig. 3-7). Chaitman et al.[19a] noted that cardiac morbidity was not confined to those patients in whom the anomalous left main artery passed between the aorta and the right ventricular infundibulum. Myocardial infarction was reported in patients in whom the left main artery arose from the right sinus of Valsalva

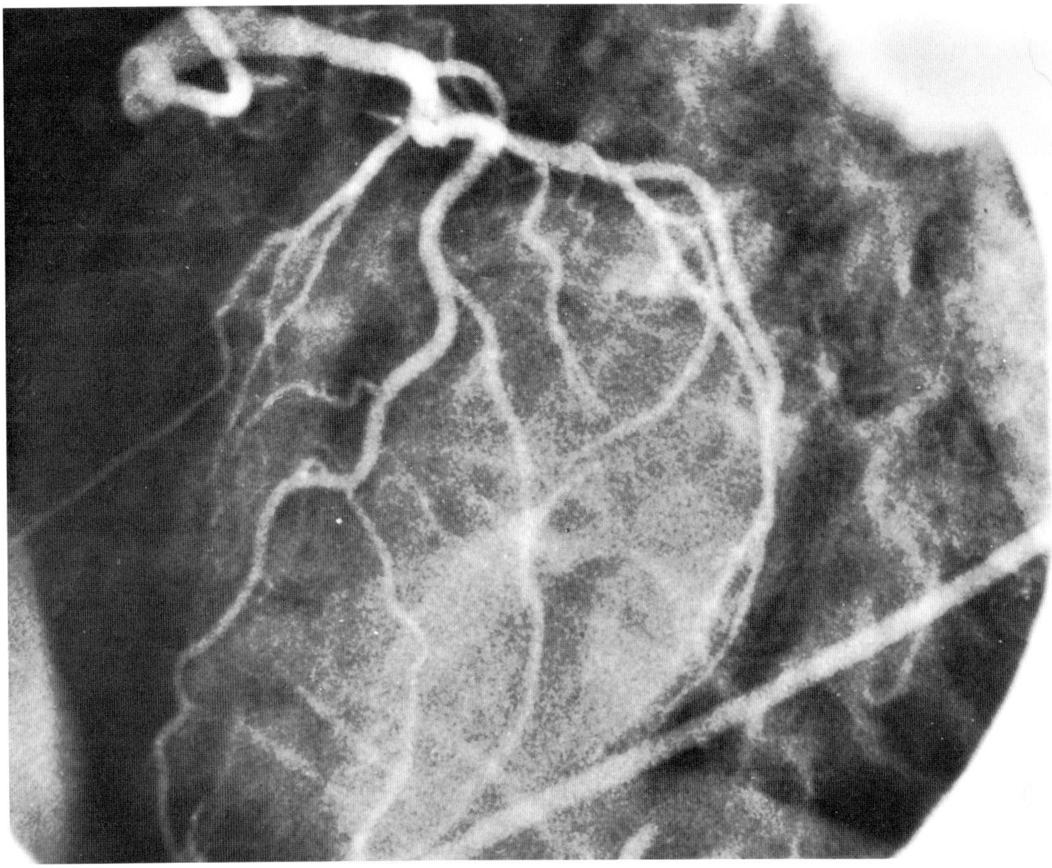

B *(Figure 3-5, continued)*

and passed either posterior to the aorta or anterior to the pulmonary artery.

In our experience, angiographic recognition of this anomaly is not difficult. Some difficulty has been noted in determining whether the anomalous artery passed anterior or posterior to the right ventricular infundibulum. Moodie[16] simultaneously injected contrast medium into the right ventricle and the anomalous artery to clarify this anatomic relationship, and Liberthson[20] found placement of a catheter in the pulmonary artery to be helpful.

Management of patients with this anomaly is not standardized. In older patients who are asymptomatic, free of ischemic signs and symptoms, and in whom the orifice of the anomalous artery is uncompromised, a conservative approach may be advocated. Highly stressful exercise is to be avoided. In a very small number of symptomatic and mostly younger patients, surgical revascularization has been carried out.[15–16a] Use of thallium-201 myocardial perfusion scintigraphy and/or technetium blood pool left ventriculography during stress may be helpful in evaluating the functional significance of this anomaly. Usually conventional aortocoronary bypass is performed with saphenous vein or internal mammary artery grafting; however, Yacoub et al. advocate a primary repair in which normal anatomic positioning of the left ostium is achieved (Fig. 3-8).[1,16a]

Right Coronary Artery from Left Sinus of Valsalva Origin of the right coronary artery from the left sinus of Valsalva is an uncommon anomaly which is difficult to demonstrate angiographically

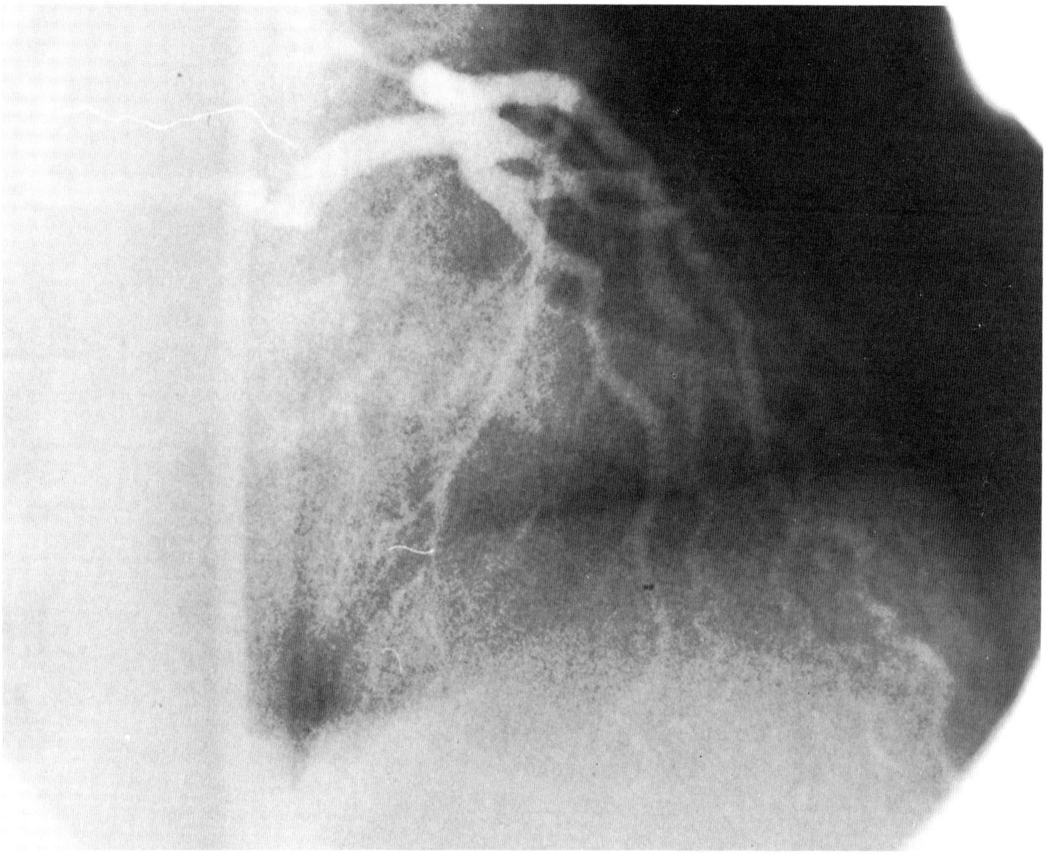

C *(Figure 3-5, continued)*

(Fig. 3-9). It has only recently been associated with significant cardiac morbidity. This anomaly was recognized in 0.02 percent of coronary arteriograms performed by Donaldson et al.,[7] 0.04 percent of studies by Engel,[3] 0.17 percent by Kimbiris,[8] and 0.16 percent by Chaitman.[9] The anomalous right coronary artery arises anterior to the left main coronary artery in the left sinus of Valsalva (Figs. 3-10 and 3-11) and almost invariably passes between the aorta and pulmonary artery to reach the right atrioventricular groove. This anomaly must be considered when the right coronary artery is not found in the right sinus of Valsalva. Commonly, injections in the left main coronary artery fail to opacify the anomalous vessel, which must be searched for specifically. In our experience, both right and left Judkins catheters and multipurpose catheters may fail to reach the anomalous vessel, and others report difficulty in selectively catheterizing this artery.[3,5] Amplatz-type left coronary artery catheters have been the most successful catheter in our experience.

Until recently, aberrant origin of the right coronary artery was considered to be a benign condition. Thompson[21] reported two patients with typical angina pectoris and Liberthson[20] had two patients with hypoplasia of the proximal portion of the anomalous right coronary artery. Cheitlin[19] and Benge[5] reported young adult males with inferior myocardial infarctions in the distribution of nonatheromatous aberrant right coronary arteries. Roberts[22] reported necropsy findings in 10 patients in whom the right coronary artery arose from the left aortic sinus. Three of these patients died sud-

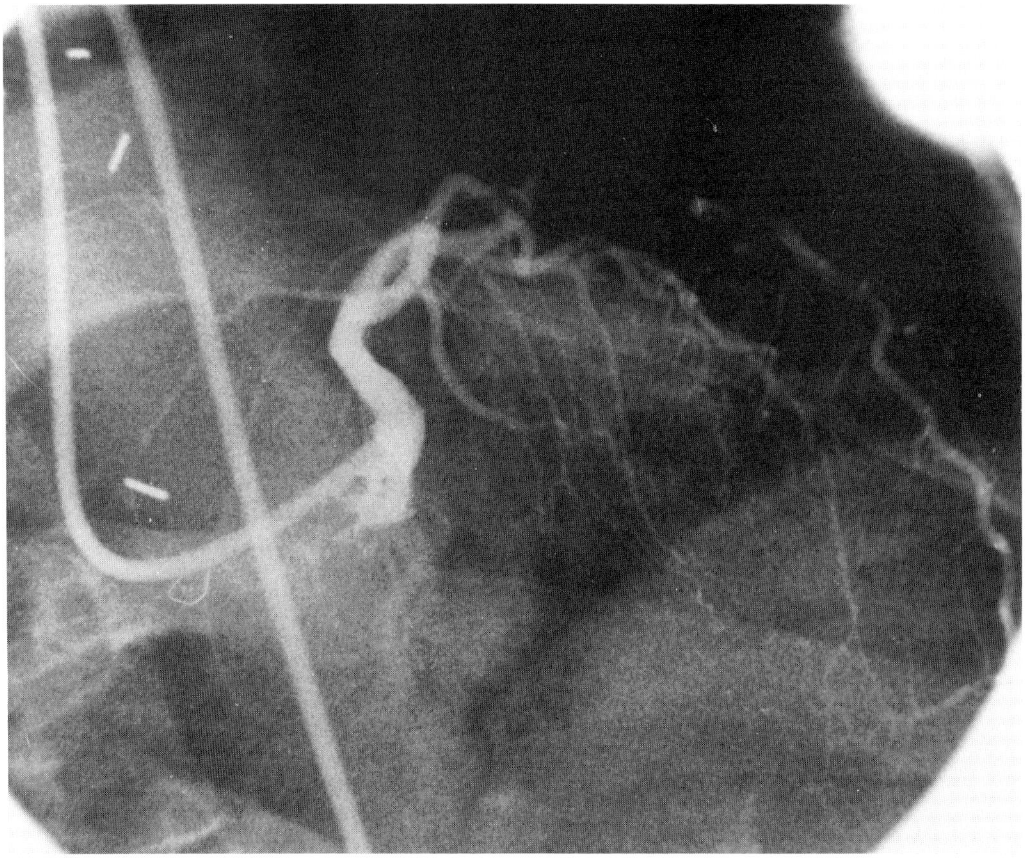

D (Figure 3-5, continued)

denly during physical exertion, and death was attributed to the anomaly. In all 10 patients the ostium of the right coronary artery was slitlike, with the largest diameter oriented in a superior-inferior axis (Fig. 3-11). In contrast, the left main orifice was round, or nearly so. Grossly visible ventricular scars were present in two of the three patients who died suddenly. It was suggested that coronary blood flow might be limited by an alteration of the slitlike ostial lumen during exercise (Fig. 3-12). When dilatation of the aorta occurred during exercise, the slitlike ostia could become more narrow. Recently the use of coronary bypass surgery for treatment of this anomaly has been reported.[22a] Doppler flow studies at the time of surgery indicated that coronary reserve, as assessed by reactive hyperemia after transient occlusion, was decreased by almost 50 percent.

Single Coronary Artery The origin of both coronary arteries from a single ostium is an infrequent anomaly which was, according to Ogden,[23] first reported in 1841 (Fig. 3-13). Sharbaugh[24] estimated that single coronary artery occurs in 0.04 percent of the population and that in 41 percent there is an associated cardiac anomaly, commonly transposition of the great vessels. Lipton[25] reported that single coronary artery occurs as an isolated anomaly in 0.02 percent of the general population but found 10 cases during the performance of 4382 coronary arteriograms, for an incidence of 0.2 per-

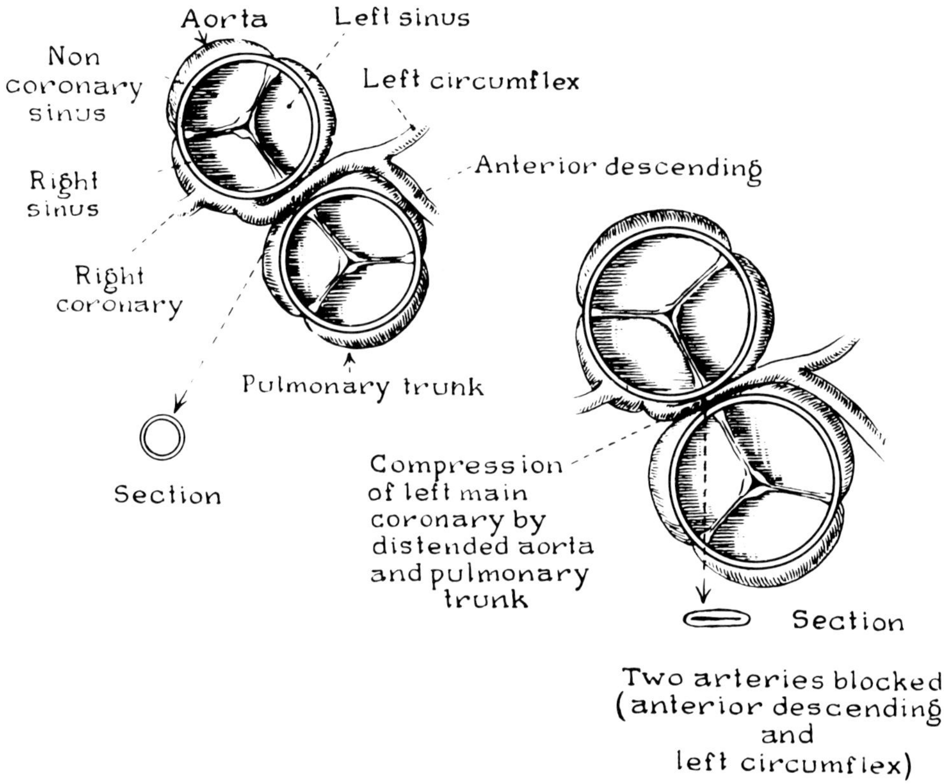

Figure 3-6 Artist's sketch of the relationships of the great vessels to the anomalous left coronary artery arising from the right sinus of Valsalva showing possible compression of the coronary artery during exercise. *(From Roberts WC, Siegel RJ, Zipes DP: Origin of the right coronary artery from the left sinus of Valsalva and its functional consequences: Analysis of 10 necropsy patients, Am J Cardiol, 49:863, 1982, with permission of the authors and publisher.)*

cent. Engle[3] found no cases in 4250 coronary arteriograms, and Kimbiris[8] observed one case during 7000 coronary arteriograms. We observed five patients with single coronary artery during the past 5000 coronary arteriograms at Emory University Hospital (Fig. 3-14). The occurrence rates of single left and right coronary arteries are reported to be approximately equal.[24] There are numerous varieties of this anomaly. An adaptation from a classification by Smith[26] and Lipton [25] is shown in Fig. 3-13. The anomaly is designated as an R or L pattern, depending on whether it is a single right (R) or left (L) coronary artery, and then further classified according to the distribution of the branches.

The clinical significance of the isolated single coronary artery anomaly depends on the adequacy of its orifice and on whether there is any acute angulation or compromise of the major branches as they traverse the base of the heart passing between or around the great vessels. In some cases an aortic intramural course of a portion of the left coronary artery has been established,[1,16a] Compromise of the ostium or compression of proximal vessels poses the risk of global myocardial ischemia. Angina pectoris, myocardial infarction, and sudden death are known complications of single coronary artery.[2,9,19,21,23–27] Sharbaugh reported that 15 percent of patients with single coronary artery as an isolated anomaly develop severe cardiac

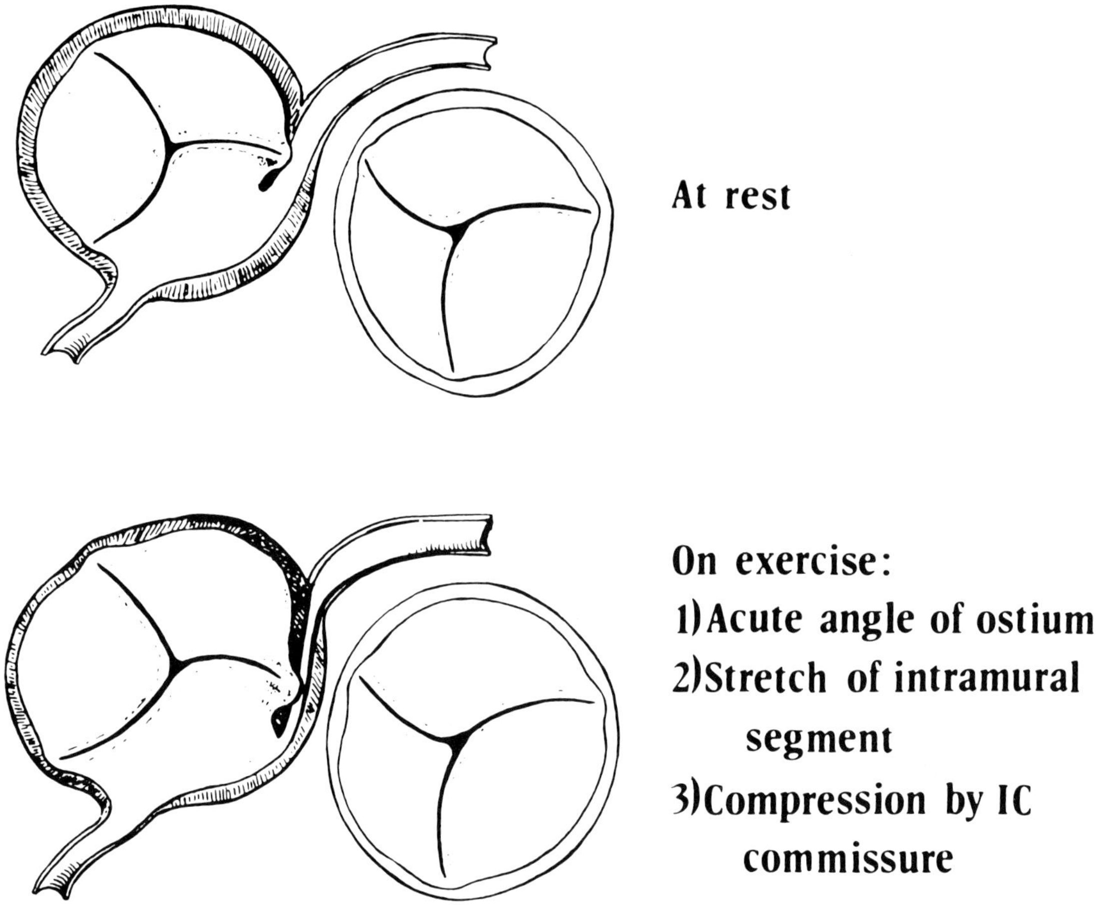

Figure 3-7 Artist's sketch showing compression and stretching of the proximal left coronary artery as it passes within the anterior aortic wall from its origin in the right aortic sinus. IC = commissure between right and left coronary cusps. *(From Mustafa I, Gula G, Radley-Smith R, Durrer S, Yacoub M: Anomalous origin of the left coronary artery from the anterior aortic sinus: A potential cause of sudden death. Anatomic characterization and surgical treatment, J Thorac Cardiovasc Surg, 82:297, 1981, with permission of the authors and publisher.)*

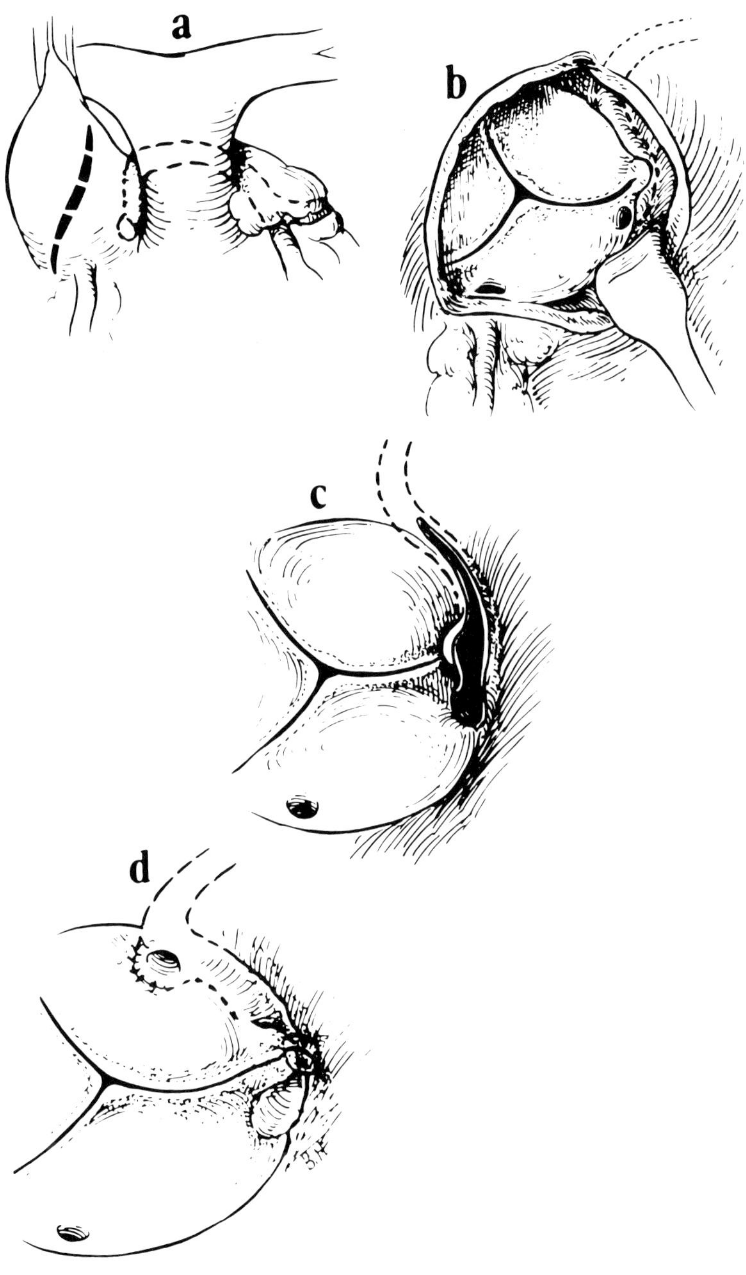

Figure 3-8 Diagram showing the anatomy of the anomalous left coronary artery arising from the right sinus of Valsalva (*a*) and a technique used for anatomic correction (*b–d*) in a 12-year-old boy. *(From Mustafa I, Gula G, Radley-Smith R, Durrer S, Yacoub M: Anomalous origin of the left coronary artery from the anterior aortic sinus: A potential cause of sudden death. Anatomic characterization and surgical treatment, J Thorac Cardiovasc Surg, 82:297, 1981, with permission of the author and publisher.)*

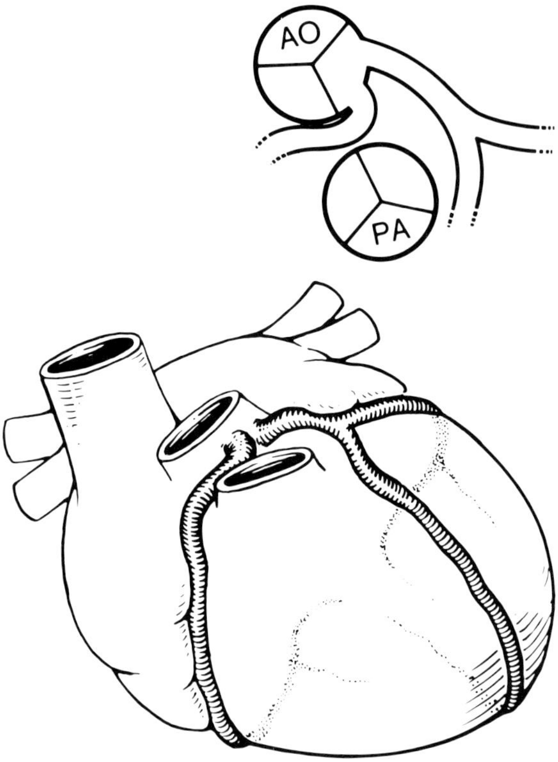

Figure 3-9 Artist's sketch showing anomalous origin of the right coronary artery from the left sinus of Valsalva. Selective catheterization of this anomalous coronary artery is usually difficult. The orifice may be slitlike and lead to cardiac morbidity. AO = aorta, PA = pulmonary artery.

problems before age 40.[24] Angina pectoris has been reported to occur due to hypoplasia, acute angulation of an artery, or atherosclerosis of the proximal vessel.[28] Congestive heart failure and death have been reported to occur in over a dozen patients with single coronary artery and no atherosclerosis.[25] Sudden death in seven young patients was reviewed by Sharbaugh.[26] The mechanism of death is uncertain, but is believed to be on an ischemic basis.

Little attention has been given to treatment modalities in this condition. Yacoub et al.[16a] reported surgical correction in a 54-year-old male of a single right coronary artery in which the left coronary artery arose from the proximal right coronary and passed between the aorta and pulmonary artery (type RII-B). At surgery, the left coronary appeared to be compressed as it ran in close proximity to the anterior aortic wall, and correction involved moving the left coronary orifice to the left sinus of Valsalva, as in Fig. 3-8.

In the absence of clear-cut guidelines for management, therapeutic decisions must hinge on factors such as the degree of apparent compromise caused by the anomaly, presence of ischemia as assessed by symptoms and testing (with stress thallium-201 myocardial perfusion imaging and other methods), and by an estimate of the feasibility and risk of surgical correction. None of our adult patients with this anomaly have required surgery for this problem alone.

ANOMALOUS ORIGIN OF THE LEFT CORONARY ARTERY FROM THE PULMONARY ARTERY

In 1 in 300,000 live births and in 0.24 percent of a population with known congenital heart disease the left coronary artery arises anomalously from the posterior aspect of the main pulmonary artery (Fig. 3-15).[29] The right coronary artery arises normally from the right aortic sinus. In utero the left

Figure 3-10 View of aortic valve and proximal right (RCA) and left main (LM) coronary arteries from above with origin of the right coronary artery from the left aortic sinus. L = left, P = posterior, R = right sinus of Valsalva, respectively. *(From Roberts WC, Siegel RJ, Zipes DP: Origin of the right coronary artery from the left sinus of Valsalva and its functional consequences: Analysis of 10 necropsy patients, Am J Cardiol, 49:863, 1982, with permission of authors and publisher.)*

Figure 3-11 Opened aorta showing the round ostium of the left main (LCA) and slitlike ostium of the right coronary artery (RCA). L = left, P = posterior, R = right sinus of Valsalva, respectively. *(From Roberts WC, Siegel RJ, Zipes DP: Origin of the left sinus of Valsalva and its functional consequences: Analysis of 10 necropsy patients, Am J Cardiol, 49:863, 1982, with permission of authors and publisher.)*

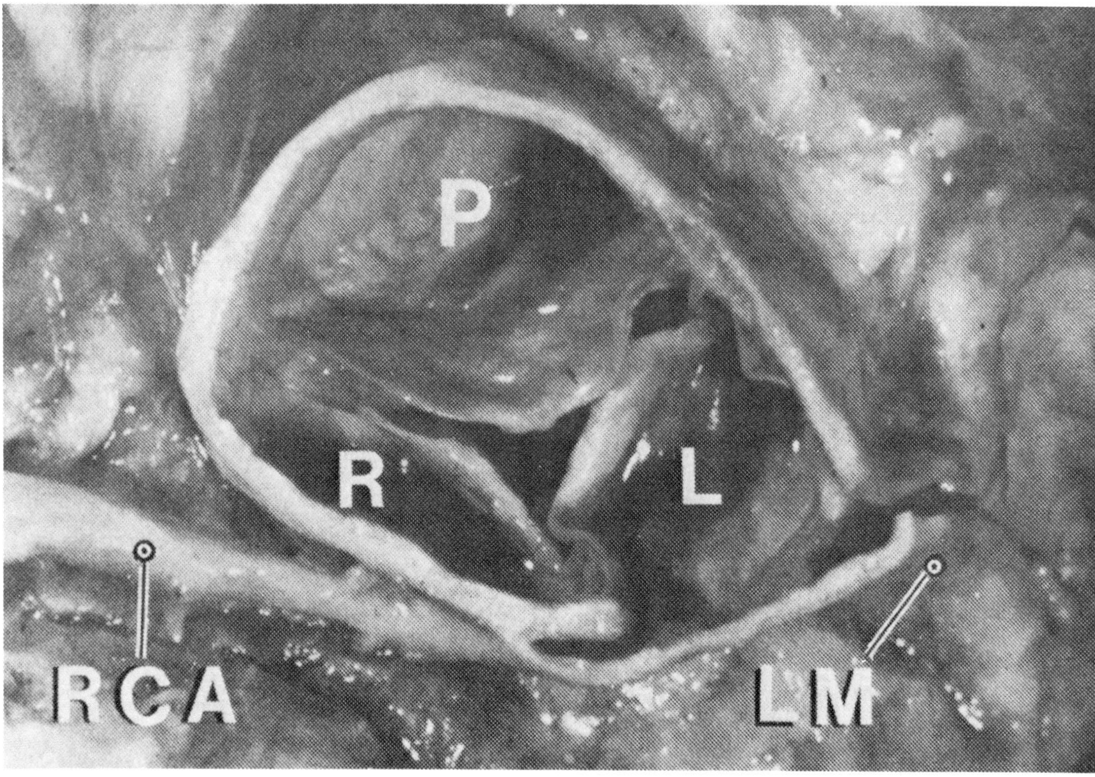

Figure 3-10

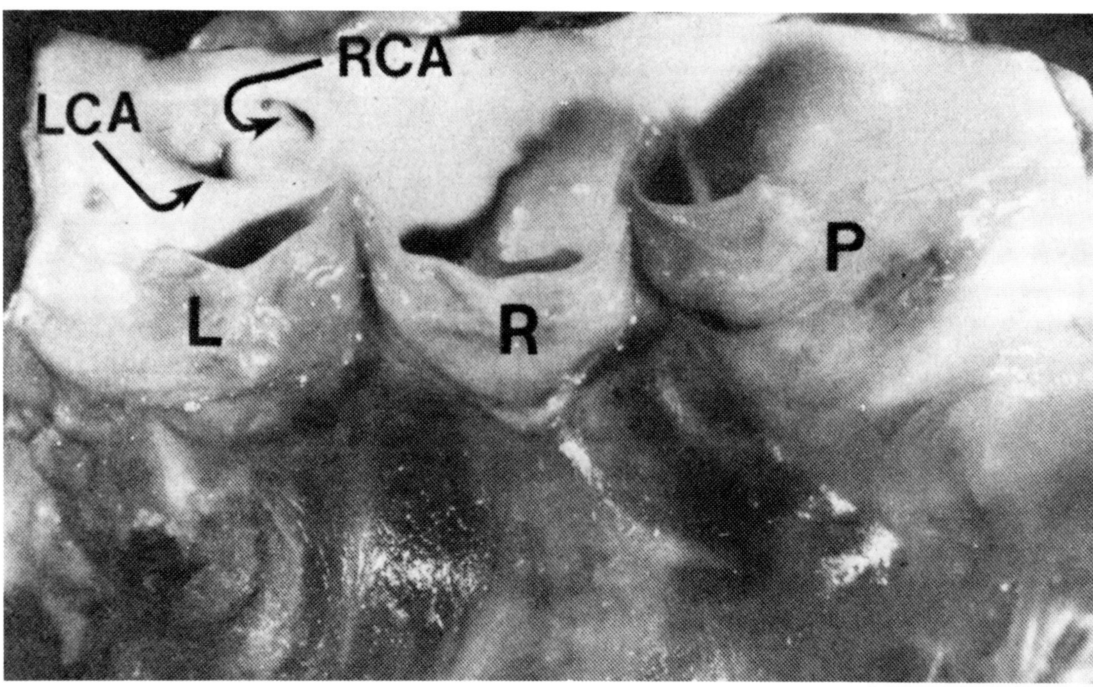

Figure 3-11

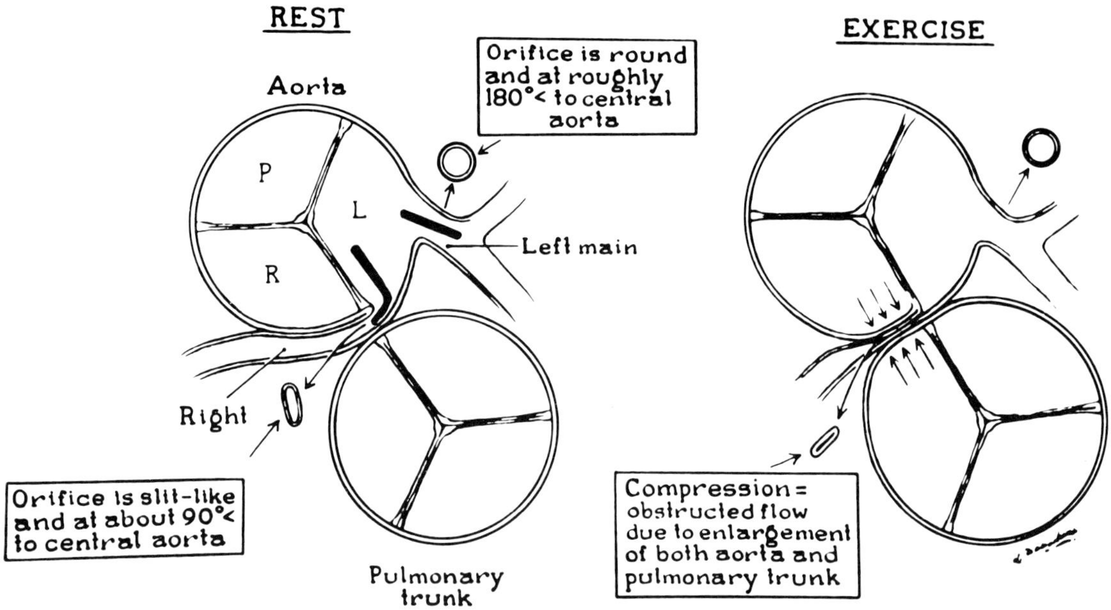

Figure 3-12 Diagrams showing possible mechanism by which origin of the right coronary artery from the left aortic sinus causes cardiac dysfunction. L = left, P = posterior, R = right sinus of Valsalva, respectively. *(From Roberts WC, Siegel TJ, Zipes DP: Origin of the left sinus of Valsalva and its functional consequences: Analysis of 10 necropsy patients, Am J Cardiol, 49:863, 1982, with permission of authors and publisher.)*

ventricular myocardium is well perfused via the anomalous left coronary artery, but as pulmonary artery pressure falls in the neonatal period, the decrease in perfusion pressure results in left ventricular ischemia. If the right coronary artery is dominant with prominent left ventricular (LV) branches, the posterior and lateral wall of the left ventricle is protected. In the absence of significant intercoronary artery collaterals between the high-pressure right coronary artery system and the low-pressure left coronary artery system, ischemia and a major myocardial infarction occurs; in the presence of excellent collaterals, the myocardium of the left ventricle may be spared or may suffer nontransmural injury. Neither the decreased oxygen saturation of blood in the anomalous left coronary artery arising from the main pulmonary artery nor the normal fall in total hemoglobin in the maturing infant nor the fall in percent hemoglobin A in the first 3 months of infancy plays a significant role in the ischemic process in the left ventricle.

In the postmortem examination of the infant heart there is extensive anterolateral and septal transmural myocardial infarction. The left ventricle is dilated and thin-walled in the region of distribution of the left coronary artery but hypertrophied in the zone of right coronary artery supply. Extensive endocardial fibrosis may occur, as well as progressive patchy replacement fibrosis and calcification of the anterior wall. The papillary muscles may be scarred, explaining known antemortem mitral valve regurgitation. In the operating room pallor and feeble paradoxical pulsations of the anteroapical wall of the left ventricle are described. The anomalous left coronary artery has a veinlike wall. There are usually no associated cardiac anomalies.[30] Six cases have been reported with congenital ventricular septal defect; less commonly reported are tetralogy of Fallot, common atrioventricular canal plus coarctation of the aorta plus aortic stenosis, and patent ductus arteriosus plus valvular pulmonic stenosis.[31,32]

Clinical Picture

The majority (over 80 percent) of these infants die in the first few months of life. They do well at birth and in the first month of life, but symptoms tend to begin in the second and third months and include respiratory distress secondary to left ventricular failure, episodes of angina with episodic pallor, irritability, and cold sweating and dyspnea.[33]

An occasional infant may have symptoms of left ventricular failure early with gradual improvement and be relatively symptom-free by age 3 or 4 years.[34] This is presumably related in part to improved collateral circulation. A surviving small minority may reach adolescence and adulthood with no symptoms or with complaints of exertional chest pain or palpitations.[35,36] Sudden death in the mid-30s has been reported. Adult patients with anomalous left coronary artery from the pulmonary artery may present for the first time as follows: (1) a 49-year-old female developed atrial arrhythmias and premature ventricular contractions; (2) a 16-year-old male presented with a murmur and palpitations; (3) a 46-year-old asymptomatic female had a normal chest x-ray but abnormal exercise tolerance test; (4) a 40-year-old female with a history of having a murmur noted at 5 years of age had a 3-year history of angina; (5) a 42-year-old mother of three children had angina for 1 year; (6) a 60-year-old female was autopsied after she died in an accident. In these adults the left ventricular muscle is viable but hypoperfused, and benefit would seem to result from restoring a two–coronary artery circulation.[37]

On physical exam an anterolateral precordial bulge may be felt with a displaced, sustained, or paradoxical apical left ventricular impulse. A soft continuous murmur louder in diastole reflects the presence of good collateral flow and sizable shunting

Figure 3-13 Classification of types of isolated single coronary artery patterns adapted from Smith[26] and Lipton.[25] In group I (*a,b*) the initial portion of the single coronary artery follows the path of a normal right (R) or left (L) coronary artery, but the artery continues posteriorly in the atrioventricular groove to reach regions of the heart usually supplied from the contralateral coronary sinus. In group II (*c–h*) the single coronary artery arises in either the left or right coronary sinus, and a single large coronary trunk traverses the base of the heart either anterior to the pulmonary artery (A), between the great vessels (B), or posterior to the aorta (P). In group III (*i,j*) the single coronary artery arises in the right sinus of Valsalva and trifurcates, with passage of the circumflex coronary artery posterior to the aorta and the left anterior descending either between the great vessels or anterior to the pulmonary artery.

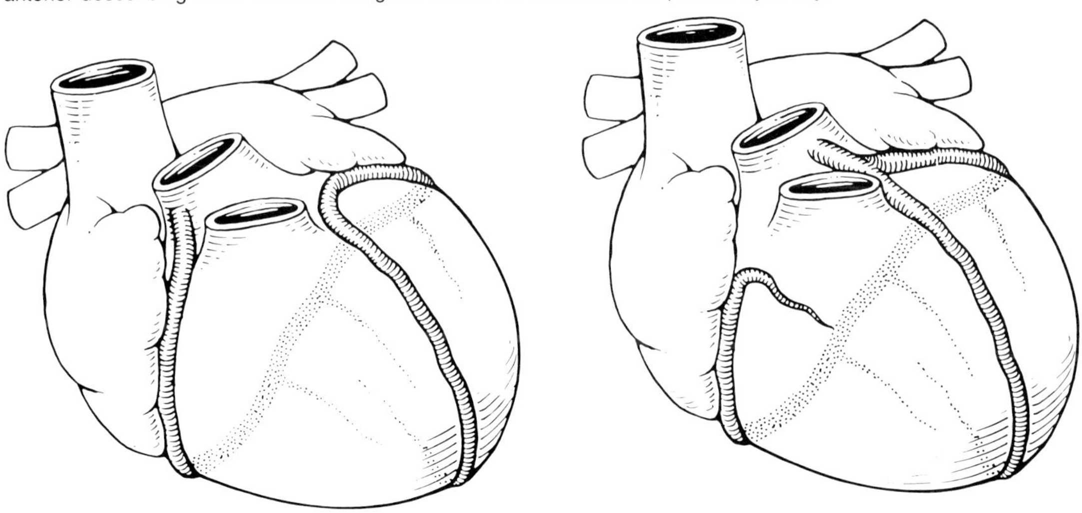

RI LI

A B

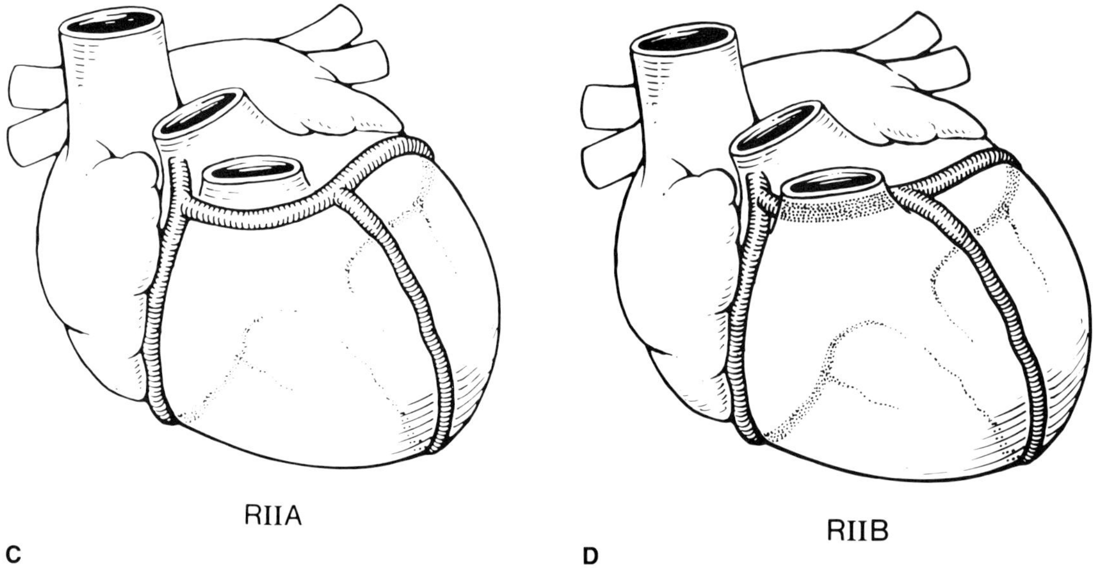

(Figure 3-13, continued)

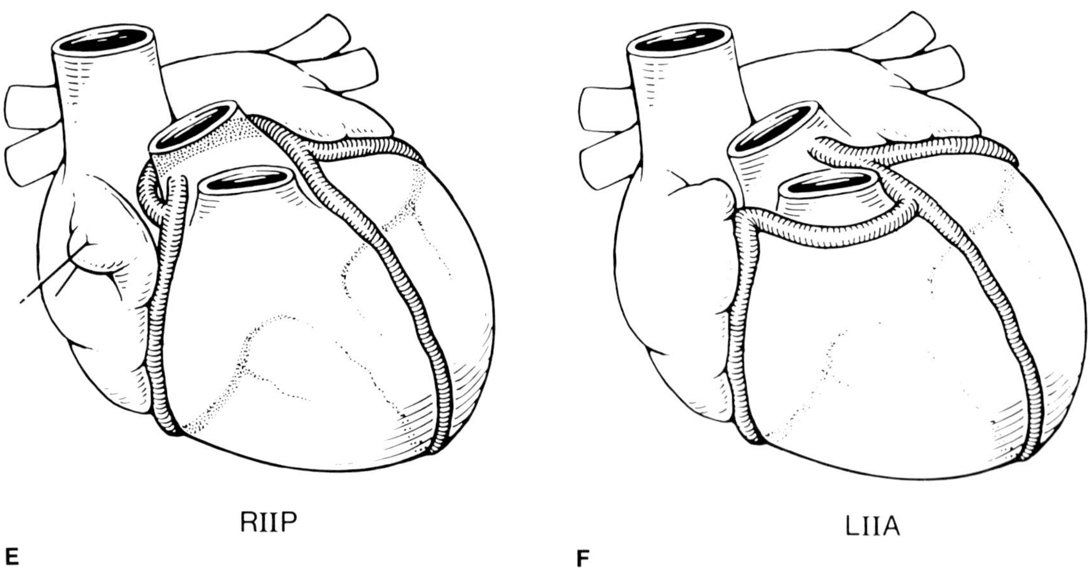

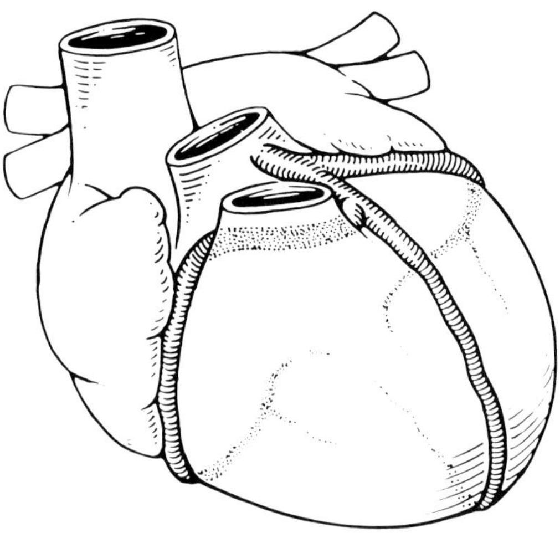

G

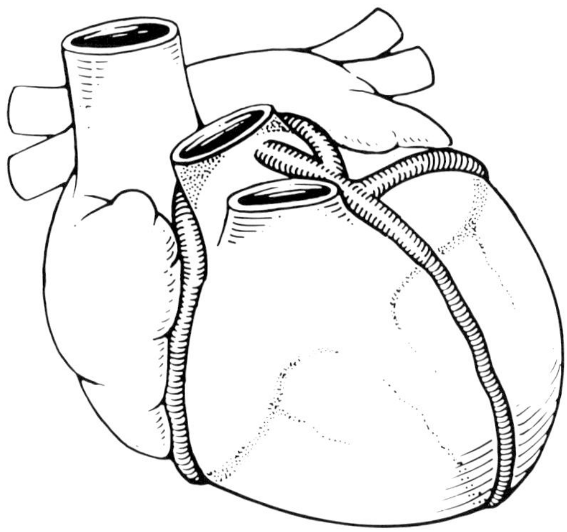

H

(Figure 3-13, continued)

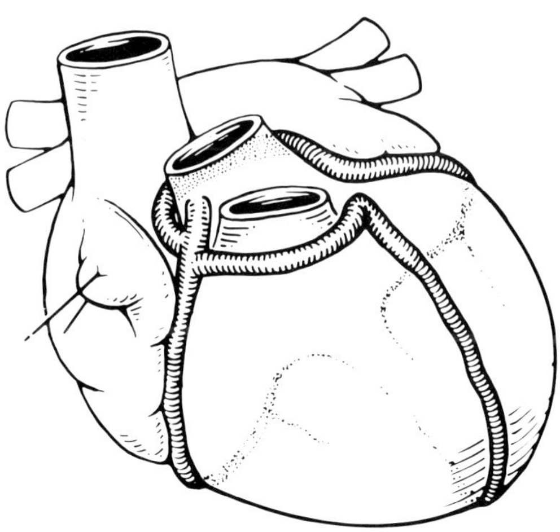

I

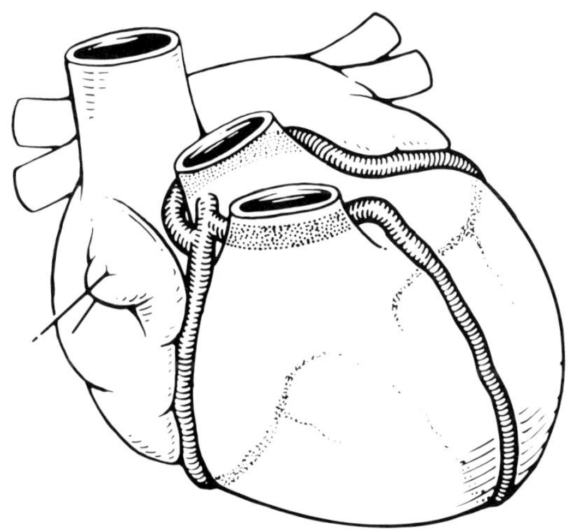

J

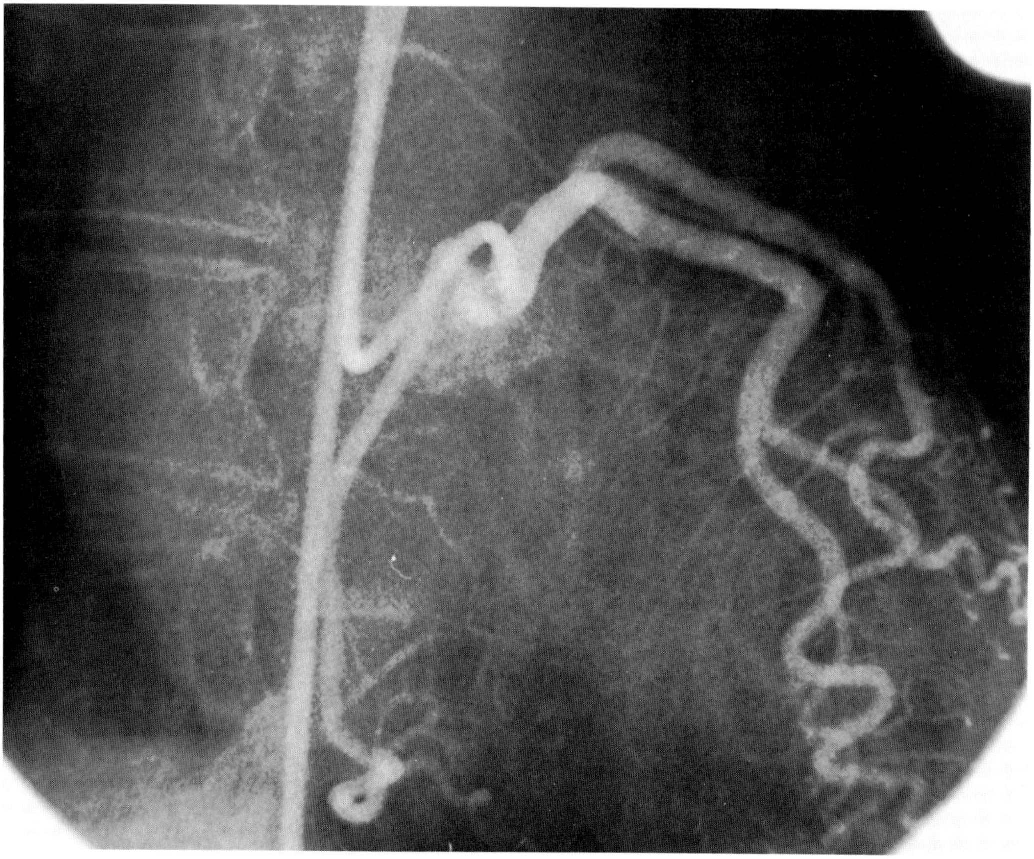

A

Figure 3-14 Coronary arteriogram in patients with single coronary arteries. In type RIIB (defined in Fig. 3-13) the left coronary artery arises from the right coronary sinus and passes between the great vessels, shown in right anterior oblique view (*a*). In (*c*) RIIA is shown in right anterior oblique view with the left coronary artery passing anterior to the pulmonary artery. In (*b*) and (*d*) LIIB is shown in right anterior and left anterior views, respectively.

into the main pulmonary artery. At surgery a continuous thrill has been noted over the dilated right coronary artery that supplies the anomalous left coronary artery. The pansystolic murmur of mitral regurgitation may be present. Signs of biventricular heart failure may occur.

On a chest x-ray the heart may extend to the left lateral chest wall indicating a left ventricular aneurysm. The left atrium may be large, and pulmonary edema may be present in the infant. In the adult and adolescent, heart size may be normal or mildly enlarged.

In 80 percent of a series of 50 cases with anomalous left coronary artery from the pulmonary artery, the electrocardiogram showed anterolateral myocardial infarction. Deep (greater than 4 mm) rather than broad Q waves occurred in leads I aV_L and V_4 to V_6. Nearly all cases had T-wave inversion, and 40 percent had ST-segment elevation in these leads. Left axis deviation is common. A deep S wave in lead V_1 and a tall R wave in leads V_5 and V_6 may be noted in the older child. The horizontal loop of the vectorcardiogram is clockwise and posteriorly oriented, reflecting posterobasal left ventricular hypertrophy. An ECG exercise test in the adult with anomalous left coronary artery may

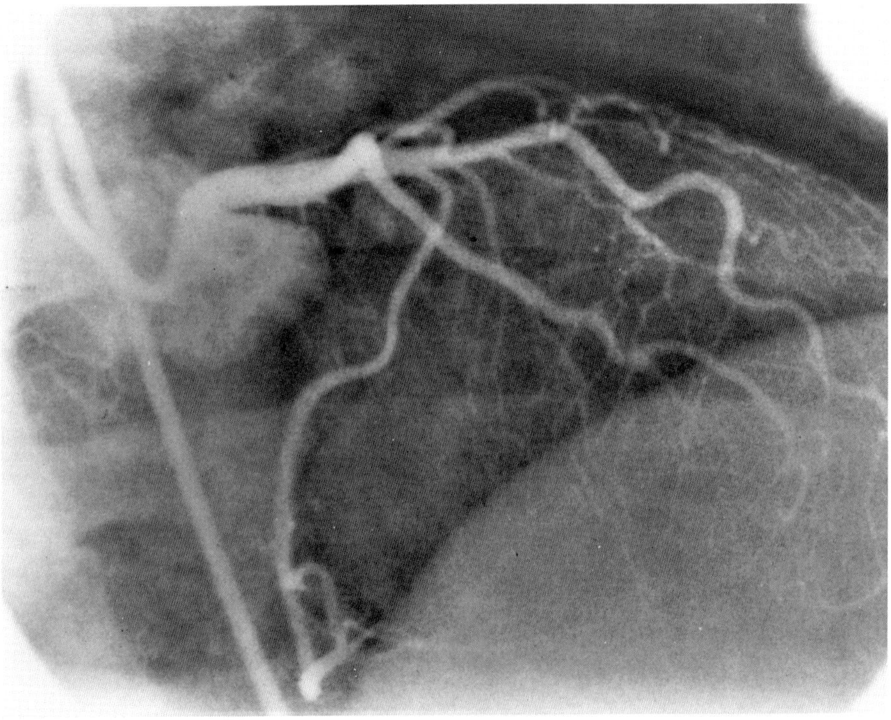

B

show ischemic ST-segment depression.[38] The echocardiogram shows an enlarged left atrium and left ventricle with poor septal and anterior left ventricular wall motion.[39,40] A right coronary artery dilated at its origin may be seen (Fig. 3-16). In a 14-year-old patient we operated on, the first pass rest and stress study showed mild diffuse hypokinesis at rest with inferior apical akinesis and severe anterior hypokinesis with exercise (Fig. 3-17). The thallium scan in this patient showed anterior wall defects in the mid-apical region with partial reperfusion at redistribution. Similar findings have been reported in the literature.[39,41] A nuclear scan is useful in separating global from regional ischemic or perfusion problems.

Cardiac Catheterization and Coronary Arteriography

The pulmonary capillary and pulmonary artery pressures are within normal limits unless significant left ventricular and mitral valve dysfunction are present. Pulmonary vascular resistance is within normal limits. The blood oxygen saturation step-up in the pulmonary artery is usually small since the volume of left-to-right shunt is usually small in comparison to clinically detectable intracardiac shunts from septal defects. The intercoronary artery pressure in the anomalous left coronary artery is the same as pulmonary artery systolic pressure, commonly 30 mmHg. Following clamping of the left coronary artery at the pulmonary artery ostium the systolic pressure in the left coronary artery rises to systemic levels (Fig. 3-18).[42] Retrograde flow to the pulmonary artery through the left coronary artery may amount to a flow of 1 L/min. Following pericardial patching of the left ostium of anomalous left coronary artery to pulmonary artery and aortic grafting to the detached left coronary artery, the flow through the vein graft measured 550 to 750 mL/min.[43] Similar high graft flows were noted in

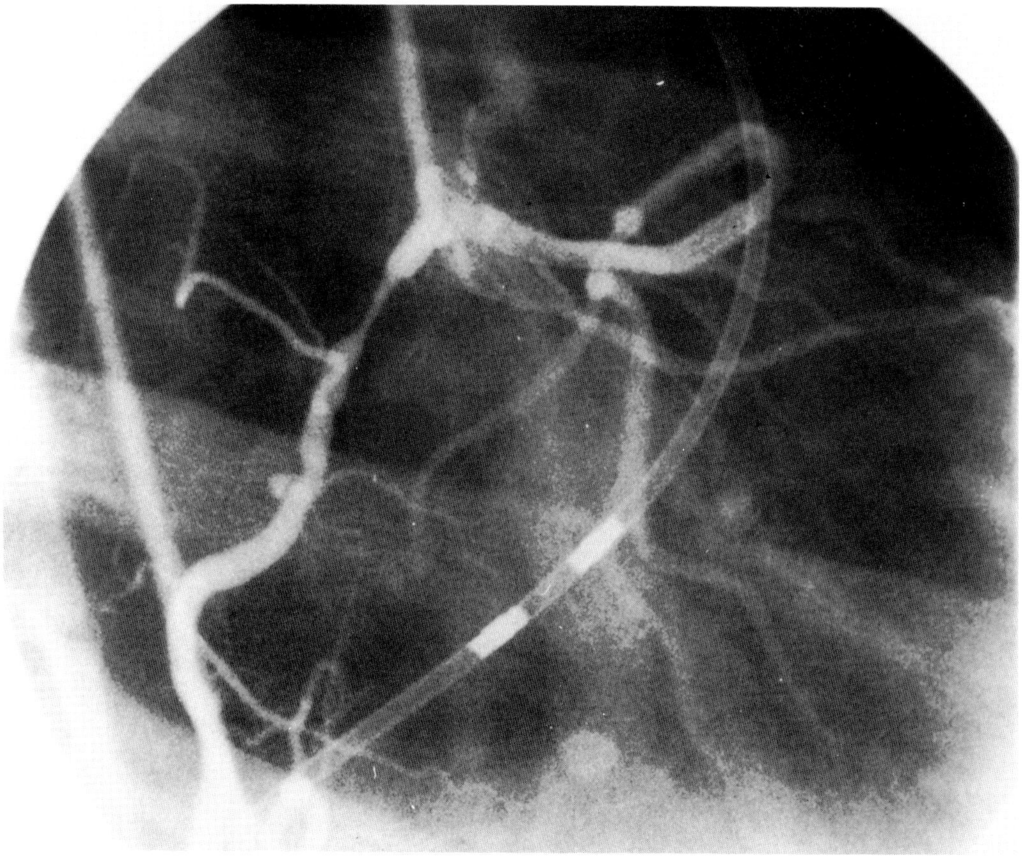

C *(Figure 3-14, continued)*

two other 40-year-old patients along with a new diastolic murmur postoperatively.[44,45]

Following an aortic root injection only the right coronary artery opacifies initially (Fig. 3-19). Its multiple collaterals then fill the entire left coronary artery retrogradely, and contrast medium appears in 0.5 s in the main pulmonary artery via the anomalously placed main left coronary artery (Fig. 3-19*b*). The sequence is even more dramatically outlined following a selective injection of contrast medium into the ostium of the dilated right coronary artery. The left ventricular angiogram shows anterolateral, septal, and apical hypokinesis. Significant mitral regurgitation may be present, reflecting papillary muscle dysfunction.

The differential diagnosis includes myocarditis, endocardial fibroelastosis, or in cases with a continuous murmur, patent ductus arteriosus or ventricular septal defect with aortic regurgitation. If poor left ventricular function or mitral regurgitation is unexplained in the catheterization of a child or adolescent, anomalous left coronary artery from the pulmonary artery should be considered. Even then if a poor-quality aortogram is performed, the fact that the left coronary artery fills via right coronary artery collaterals may be missed, or a false diagnosis of right coronary artery–to–pulmonary artery fistula may be made.

Rarely, only the left circumflex arises anomalously from the pulmonary artery.[46,47] Both the

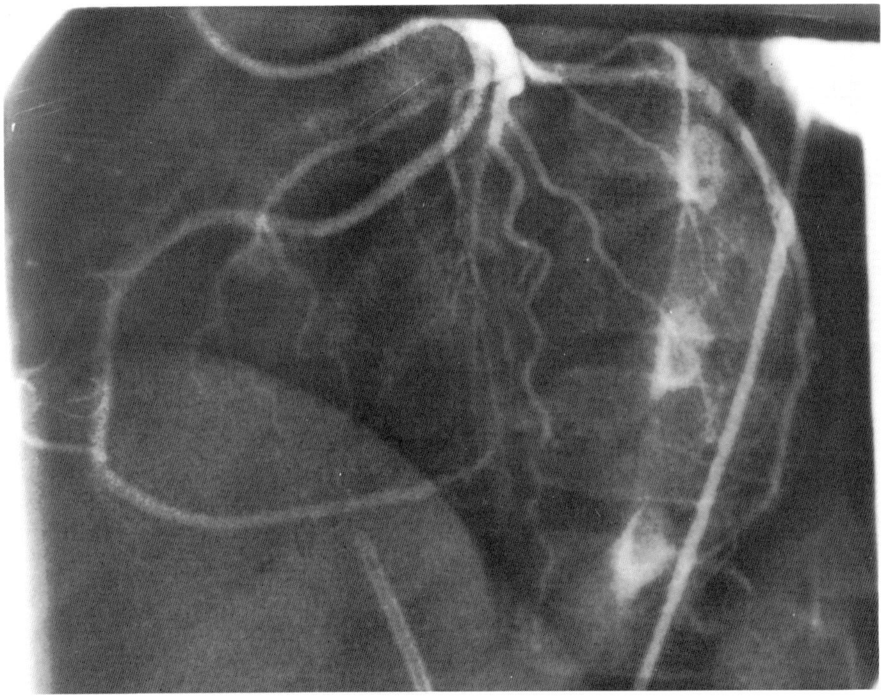

D *(Figure 3-14, continued)*

Figure 3-15 Artist's sketch in operating room showing the usual posterior origin of the anomalous left coronary artery from the main pulmonary artery (PA). *(Courtesy of Grace PR, Angelini P, Cooley DA: Aortic implantation of anomalous left coronary artery arising from pulmonary artery, Am J Cardiol, 39:608, 1977.)*

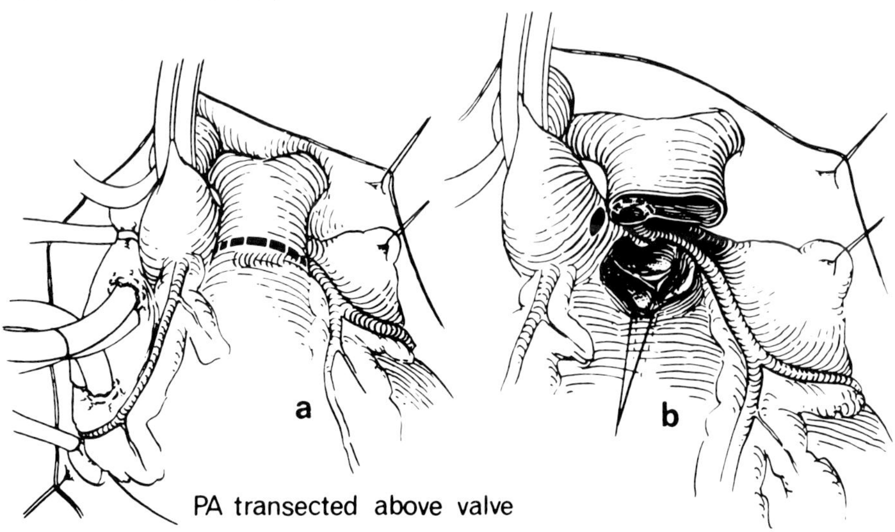

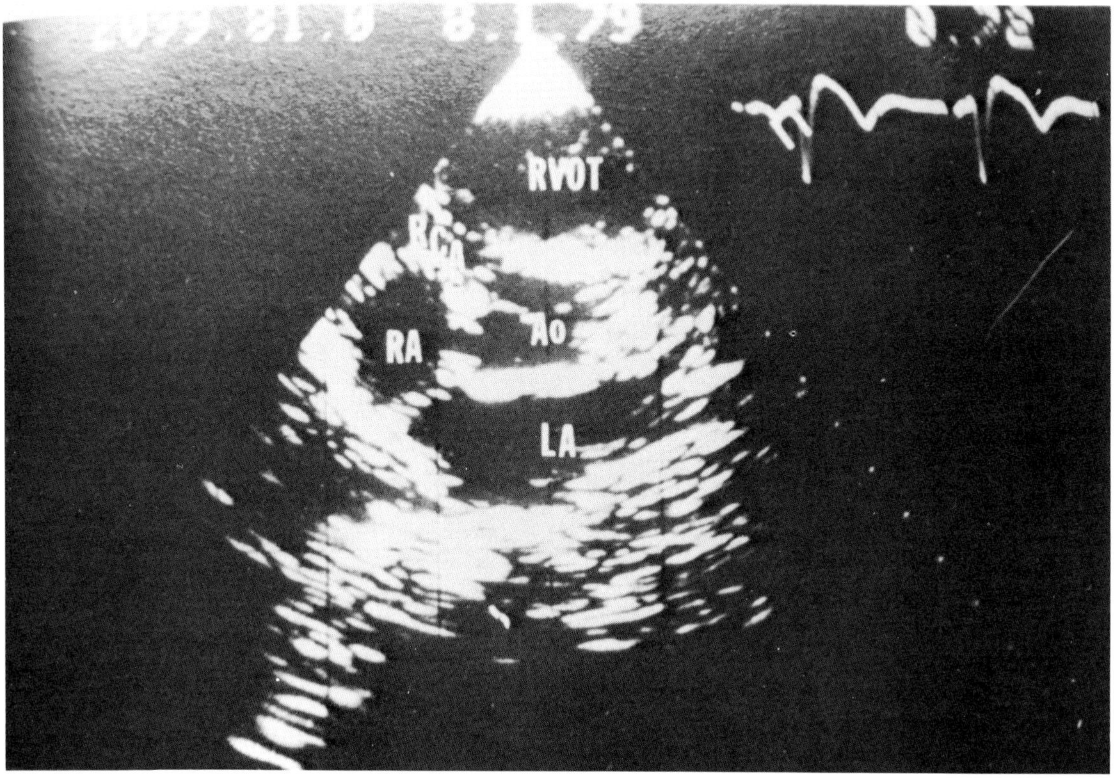

Figure 3-16 Short-axis echocardiogram image. The anomalous left coronary artery arising from the main pulmonary artery is not seen, but the right coronary artery which is dilated at its origin from the aorta is imaged. AO = aorta, LA = left atrium, RA = right atrium, RVOT = right ventricular outflow tract. *(Courtesy of Sahn DJ, Anderson F: Dimensional Anatomy of the Heart. Wiley & Sons, New York, 1982.)*

right coronary artery and the left anterior descending artery arise from the right aortic sinus and provide collateral flow to the circumflex artery. We have noted significant stenosis of the main pulmonary artery (50-mm peak systolic gradient) following surgical removal of the anomalous left coronary artery from the pulmonary artery. Surgical restoration of a normal two–coronary artery circulation is desirable in most cases. After surgery several patients have shown negative exercise tolerance tests, and one of our patients and some reported by other physicians had marked increase in LV ejection fraction[48] (e.g., a 3-year-old child showed a rise from .24 to .70 after a subclavian–to–left coronary artery graft).

CORONARY ARTERIOVENOUS FISTULA

The coronary artery or its branch that connects directly to the right atrium or ventricle, the pulmonary artery, or the coronary sinus forms a coronary-cameral or coronary arteriovenous fistula (CAVF). In Keith's study CAVF occurred in 0.07 percent of a population of 15,104 with congenital heart disease.[29] Nine cases of CAVF were operated on between 1961 and 1971 at the Mayo Clinic in contrast to 450 cases of patent ductus.[50] Sones reported 13 cases of CAVF in 6000 consecutive coronary angiograms at the Cleveland Clinic.[51] CAVF results from the failure of embryonal intramyocardial sinusoids to obliterate or, in the case of the

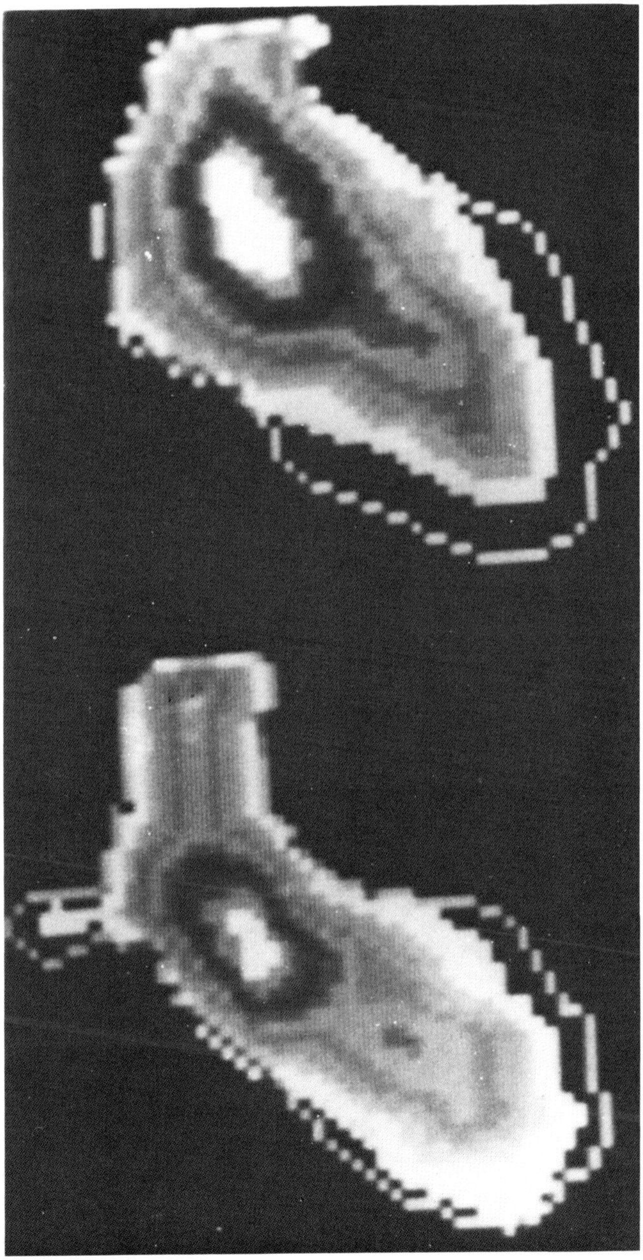

Figure 3-17 Frontal projection first pass nuclear left ventricular angiogram in a 15-year-old girl with ALCAPA. At rest (*top*) we see mild diffuse hypokinesis and during upright bicycle exercise (*bottom*) anteroapical akinesis with significant diffuse hypokinesis. Referral was made at 4 years of age when cardiomegaly was noted on chest x-ray prior to tonsillectomy. She has a small left-to-right shunt and a normal right coronary artery. Ligation and coronary artery bypass graft surgery were successfully performed.

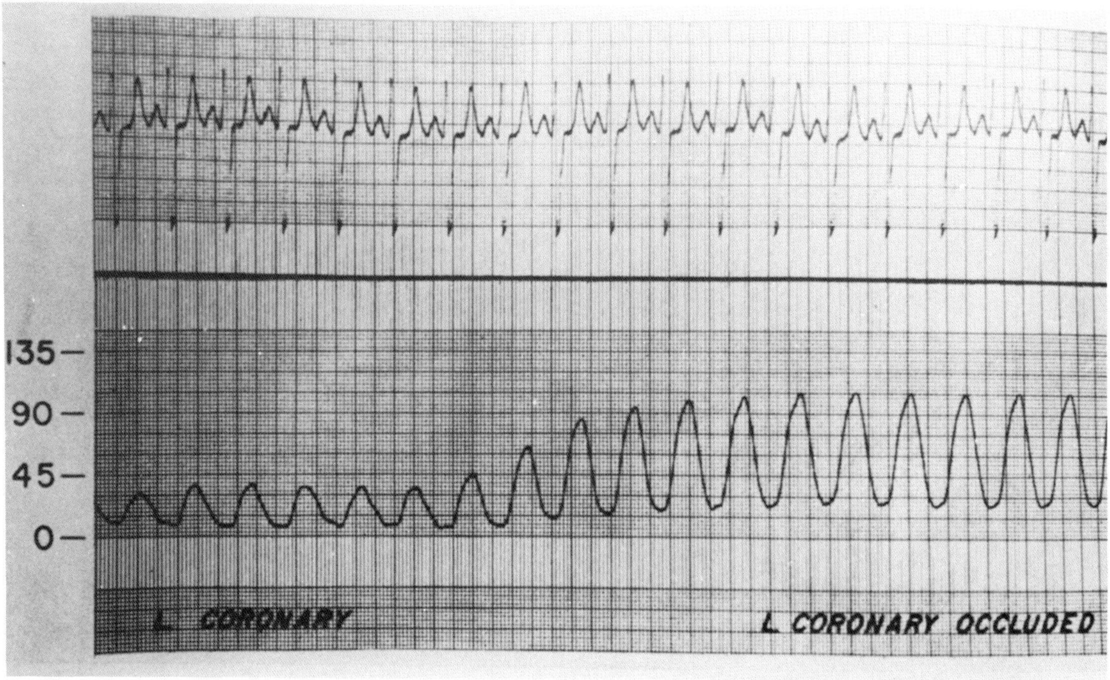

Figure 3-18 Left coronary artery (LCA) pressure tracing and ECG lead III before (35/10 mmHg) and after (105/30 mmHg) occlusion of the left coronary artery at its origin from the main pulmonary artery in a 45-year-old person with angina. No change was noted in the electrocardiogram following ligation of the proximal left coronary artery. *(Courtesy of Baue AE, Baum S, Blakemore WS, et al: A later stage of anomalous coronary circulation with origin of the left coronary artery from the pulmonary artery, Circulation, 36:878, 1967.)*

pulmonary artery, small accessory or supernumerary conal arteries from the main pulmonary artery connect with branches of the proximal right and/or left coronary arteries (Figs. 3-20 and 3-21). Of all CAVF, 5 percent are bilateral.[52] Of all bilateral CAVF, one-half enter the main pulmonary artery.[53] The preponderance of bilateral CAVF to the main pulmonary artery suggests a high persistence of bilateral conal arteries or a Vieussens' annulus opening into the anterior main pulmonary artery.

Over one-half of the CAVF are supplied by branches of the right coronary artery.[54] The site of insertion is usually the right ventricle or the right atrium followed in frequency by the coronary sinus, main pulmonary artery, and superior vena cava.[55] Other types of CAVF include a circumflex artery entering a persistent left superior vena cava,[56,57] a large left atrial circumflex artery connecting with the apical pulmonary artery branch of the right upper lobe via a bronchial collateral,[58] a double fistula to both the right atrium and the right ventricle, and a fistula from the sinus node artery from the right or left coronary artery to the right atrium–superior vena cava junction.

The feeding coronary artery is grossly dilated (up to 5 cm in diameter) (Fig. 3-22). It is elongated, serpentine, and in the adult, especially, segmental saccular bulging occurs in the arterial wall as well as sporadic calcification. Mural thrombi, occlusion, or distal embolization is rare. The fistulous artery usually ends by tapering into a single opening (these have the largest flow) (Fig. 3-23). There may also be multiple opening sites via multiple looping vessels. The ostium is less affected by systole in an atrial or venous channel than in the ventricle.

In a series of 75 cases of CAVF terminating in the right atrium three types were noted[59]: (1) In 19

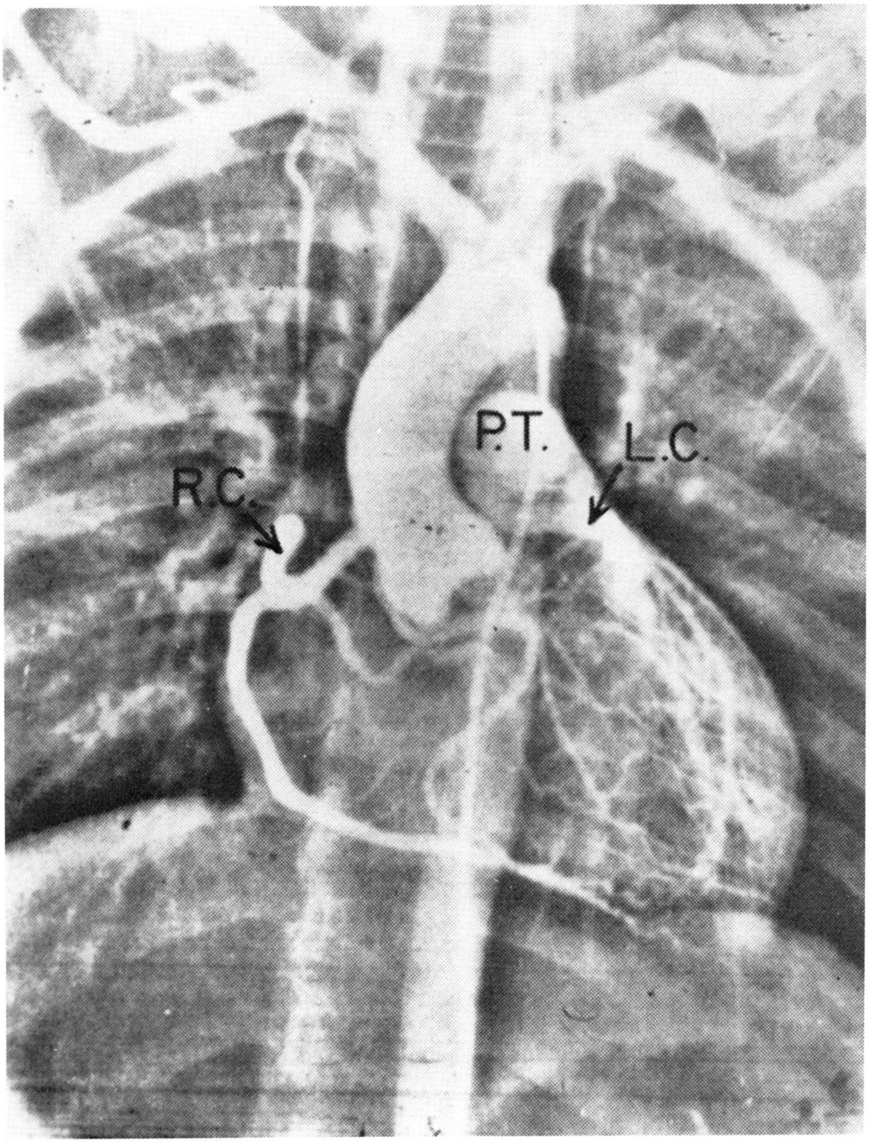

A

Figure 3-19 (*a*) Aortogram in frontal view showing the (arrow) origin of left coronary artery (LC) from the pulmonary trunk (PT); the right coronary artery (RC) arises normally. *(Courtesy of Edwards JE: Congenital Heart Disease: Correlation of Pathologic Anatomy and Angiocardiography, Saunders, Philadelphia, 1965.)* (*b*) Composite diagram in a 29-year-old woman showing opacification of the dilated right coronary artery and collaterals by aortography in the left anterior oblique view and retrograde flow through the anomalous left coronary artery with filling of the main pulmonary artery. Ant. desc. = anterior descending, AO = aorta, LCA = left coronary artery, PA = pulmonary artery, Post. descending = posterior descending, RCA = right coronary artery, Ventric. = ventricular. *(Courtesy of Likar I, Criley JM, et al: Anomalous left coronary artery arising from the pulmonary artery in an adult, Circulation, 33:727, 1966.)*

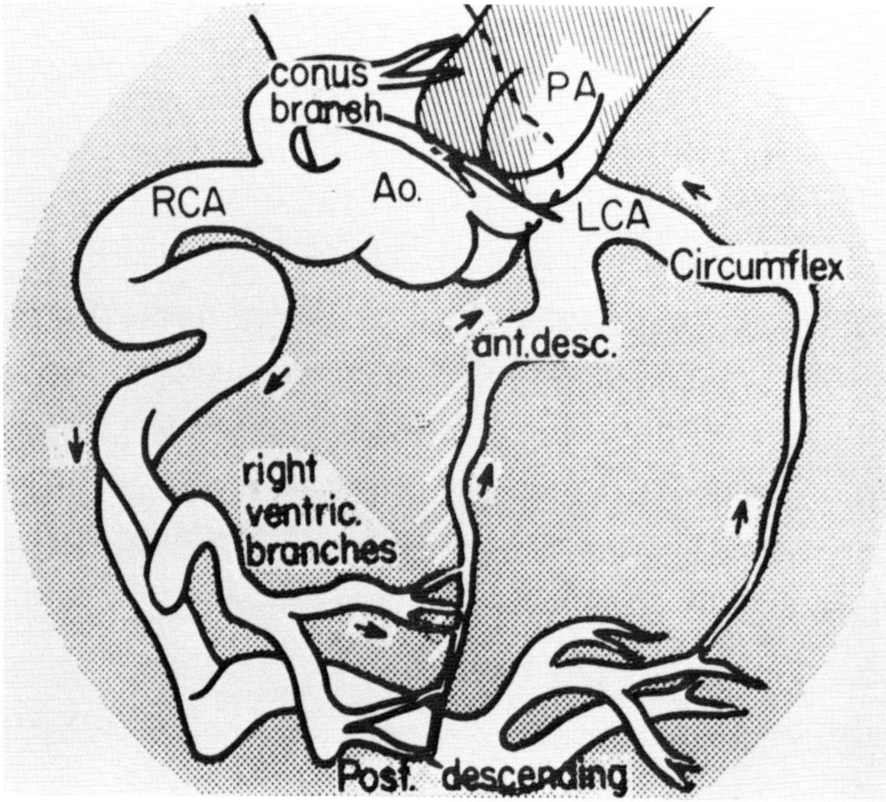

B *(Figure 3-19, continued)*

Figure 3-20 Diagrams (*a,b*) of the development of the coronary arteries. Small aberrations can result in communications between the main pulmonary artery and branches from either the right or left coronary artery or both. Dev. = developing. *(Courtesy of Becker AF, Anderson RH: Pathology of Congenital Heart Disease, Butterworths, London, 1981, p 371.)*

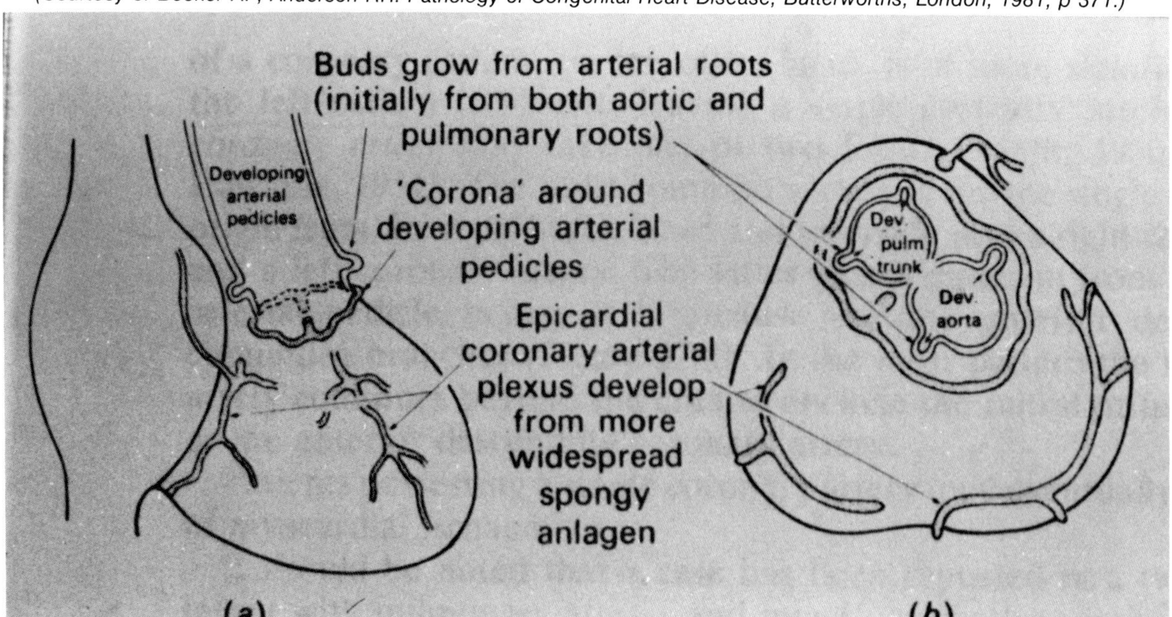

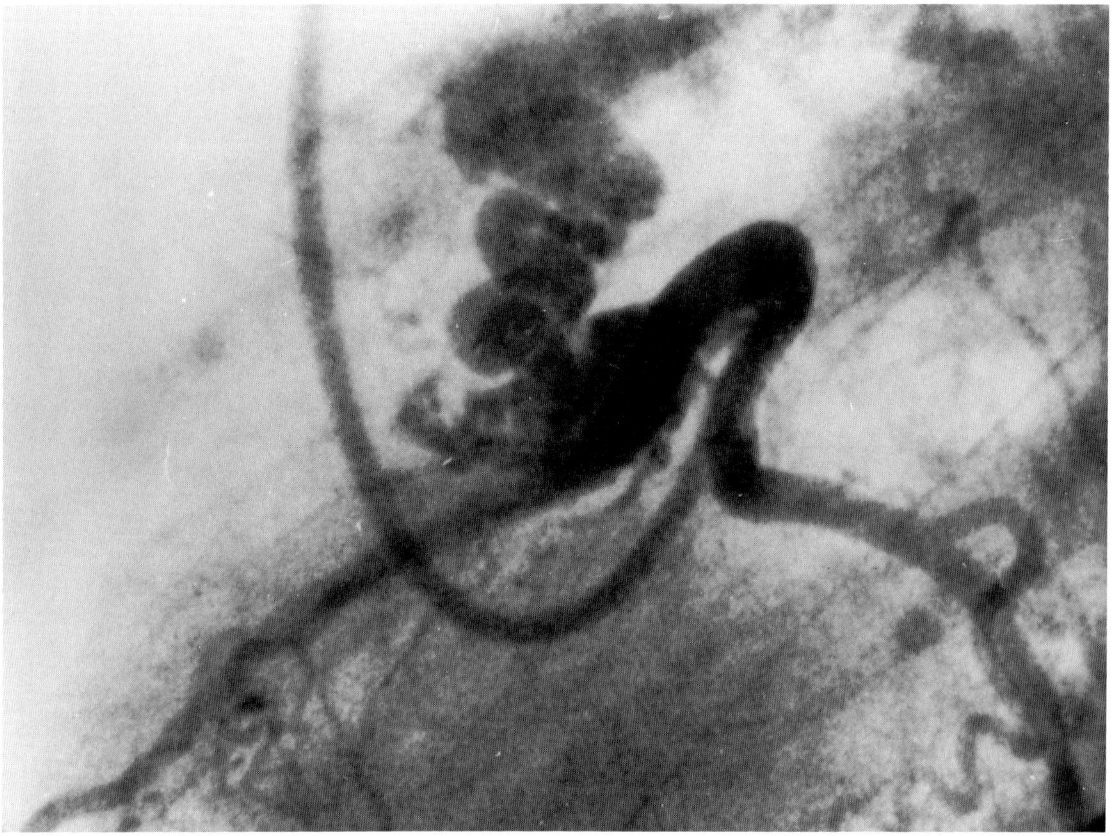

Figure 3-21 Selective left coronary artery angiogram in the lateral projection. A tortuous conuslike branch of the left anterior descending enters the superiorly positioned main pulmonary artery.

cases, a short right coronary artery branch from the main right coronary artery extends to the right atrial appendage or anterior right atrial wall near the tricuspid valve (Fig. 3-24): (2) in 39 cases the sinus node branch of the right (19 cases) or left (20 cases) coronary artery passes to the superior vena cava or to the posterior atrial surface; (3) in 10 cases the right or left coronary artery ends in the posterior surface of the right atrium along the atrioventricular (AV) groove. In seven cases of CAVF to the coronary sinus the feeding artery was the left circumflex in four and the right coronary artery in three.[60] CAVF to the right ventricle may be supplied by both the right and the left coronary artery.

Most patients with CAVF are asymptomatic. Some observers have noted that one-half of the patients develop symptoms of ventricular dysfunction or angina with increasing age.[61] In our experience angina and heart failure, however, are rare even in old age unless there is associated coronary artery or valve disease or hypertrophic cardiomyopathy. It is known, however, that AV fistulas in the limbs can cause ischemic symptoms distal to the fistula. Indeed, in a 23-year-old with right coronary artery–to–coronary sinus fistula a nontransmural myocardial infarction has been described presumably secondary to diversion of flow from the high-resistance myocardial capillaries to the low-resistance fistula.[62]

A continuous murmur, soft and superficial, is heard at the site of the fistula. Thus, a fistula entering the coronary sinus is best heard in the back, and a fistula to the main pulmonary artery or to the

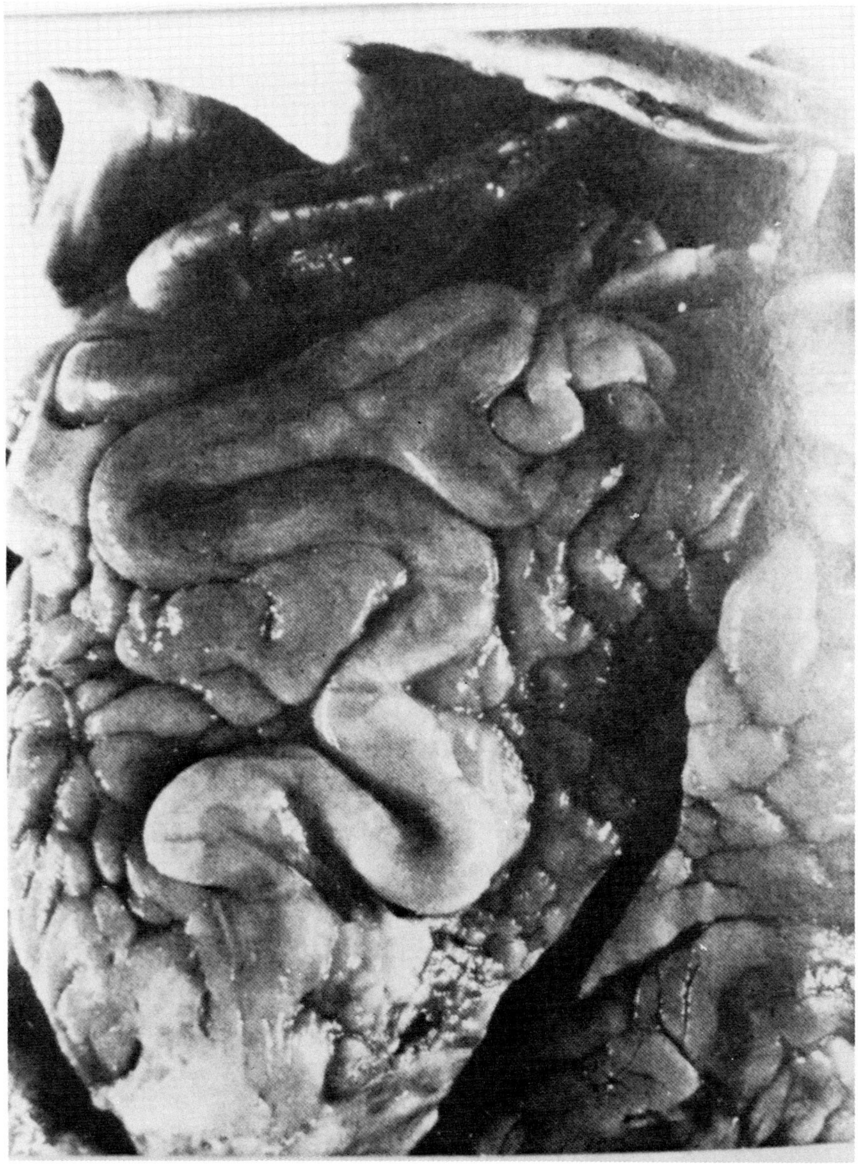

Figure 3-22 The heart of a 62-year-old man at postmortem. The anterior surface has elongated, serpentine, dilated coronary arteries, related to multiple coronary arterioventricular fistulas to both ventricles from both coronary arteries. *(Courtesy of Rose AG: Multiple coronary arterioventricular fistulae, Circulation, 58:178, 1978.)*

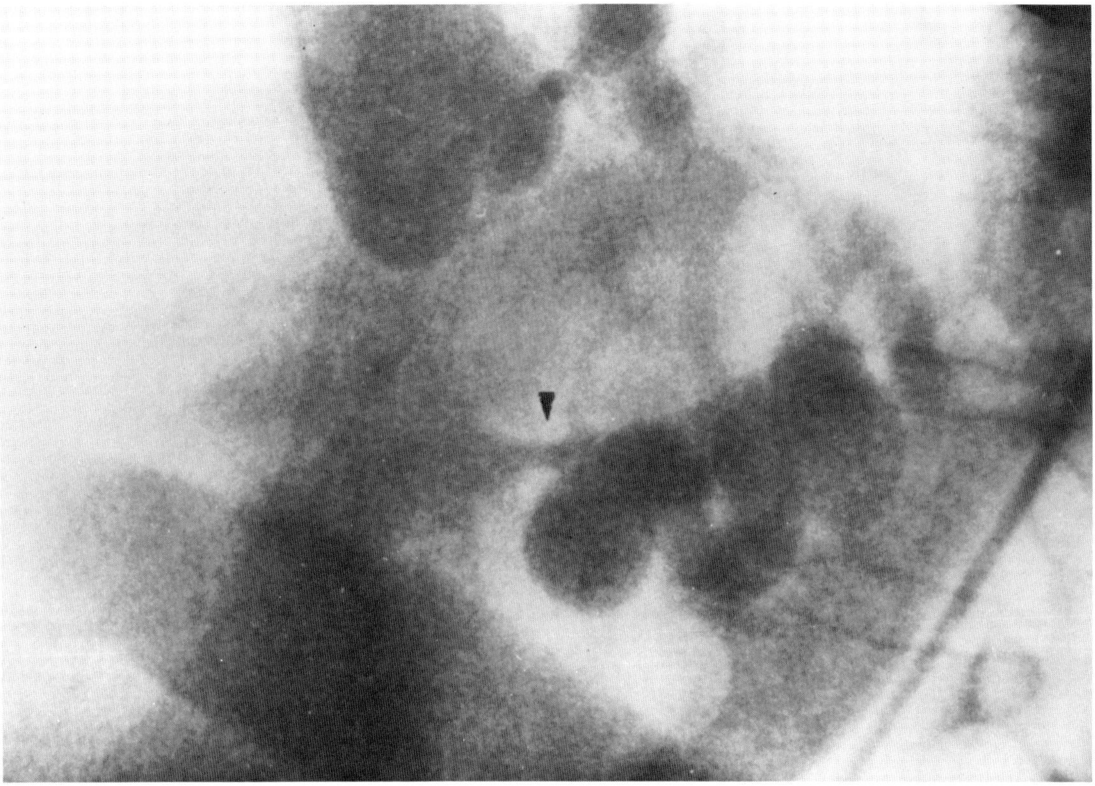

Figure 3-23 Selective left coronary artery angiogram in the left anterior oblique projection. The circumflex artery is dilated and tortuous. The fistula is a tubular channel as it enters the lower right atrium near the coronary sinus *(arrow)*. Asymptomatic 57-year-old mother of 10 children whose internist detected a faint high-pitched continuous murmur in the interscapular area during a routine visit for mild hypertension.

high right ventricular outflow tract is best heard in the second left interspace, simulating the murmur of patent ductus arteriosus. Right atrial and right ventricular CAVF are heard away from the ductus area. Described variations in the intensity of the continuous murmurs in systole and diastole have not been personally useful in defining the site of the fistula.

The x-ray is within normal limits in most cases. Occasionally, increased pulmonary blood flow is noted, or right coronary artery dilation may present as a double bulge on the border of the right side of the heart, or calcification of the wall of the aneurysmal coronary artery is present. The electrocardiogram is usually within normal limits. Left ventricular hypertrophy is uncommon.

Two-dimensional echocardiography defined a 2.5 × 1.5 cm thin-walled channel within the right ventricular muscle supplied by a large left anterior descending coronary artery.[63] The fistula opening into the lateral right ventricular free wall was 3 mm in diameter, yielding a small 10 percent shunt. The dilated coronary sinus may be identified by echocardiography as has been described in children in whom all or part of the pulmonary venous return enters the coronary sinus.[64] Dilated coronary arteries near the aortic root have been visualized.[65]

Pressures on the right side of the heart are normal; occasionally mild pulmonary artery hypertension is noted. If the coronary sinus is the site of the CAVF, the catheter tip may enter it readily,

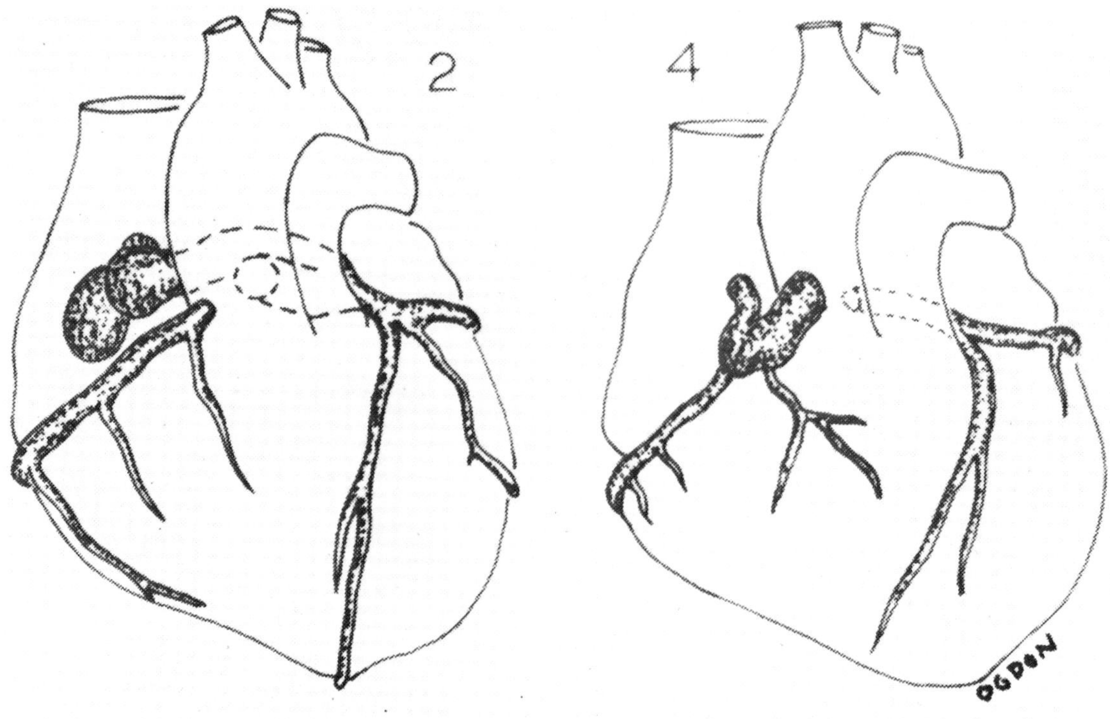

Figure 3-24 Diagram of sinus node artery to right atrium coronary arterioventricular fistula. The origin of the sinus node artery may be from either the left or right coronary artery. *(Courtesy of Ogden JA, Stance JC Jr: The anatomic variability of coronary arterial fistulae termination in the right and left atria, Chest, 65:78, 1974.)*

and selective blood sampling from it and the great and middle cardiac veins can be obtained. Oximetry is used to confirm the site of the emptying of the fistula and to quantitate its flow. The pulmonary flow–systemic flow ratio is usually 1.5:1 or less, exceeding 2:1 in rare cases.[61] Normally 10 percent of the cardiac output supplies the coronary artery tree; in a CAVF there is a 1.5:1 ratio: 50 percent of the cardiac output passes through the fistula. In the operating room shunts of 700 to 1800 mL/min have been measured. An acute model using a left circumflex–to–pulmonary artery fistula in a dog yielded a 1.1:1 pulmonary flow–systemic flow ratio. Proximal left circumflex coronary blood flow increased from 31 to 97 mL/min, and distal coronary blood flow decreased from 28 to 21 mL/min. These shunts were well-tolerated with no detectable change in stroke volume, cardiac output blood pressure, or LVDPDT (the first derivative of the left ventricular pressure curve).

Selective coronary or single or biplane aortic root injection shows in a dramatic display the origin and course of the dilated artery supplying the fistula. The tortuous sigmoid channel may obscure its exact site of termination by lying over the entry site (Fig. 3-25). The artery may so dwarf its normal coronary artery companions that its identity is not clear. For example, a large sinus node artery arising from the left circumflex to empty into the right atrium may not be recognized as the sinus node artery (Fig. 3-26). If the flow through the fistula is large, a conventional selective coronary arteriogram hand injection of 10 mL of contrast medium may be inadequate due to marked dilution. A pres-

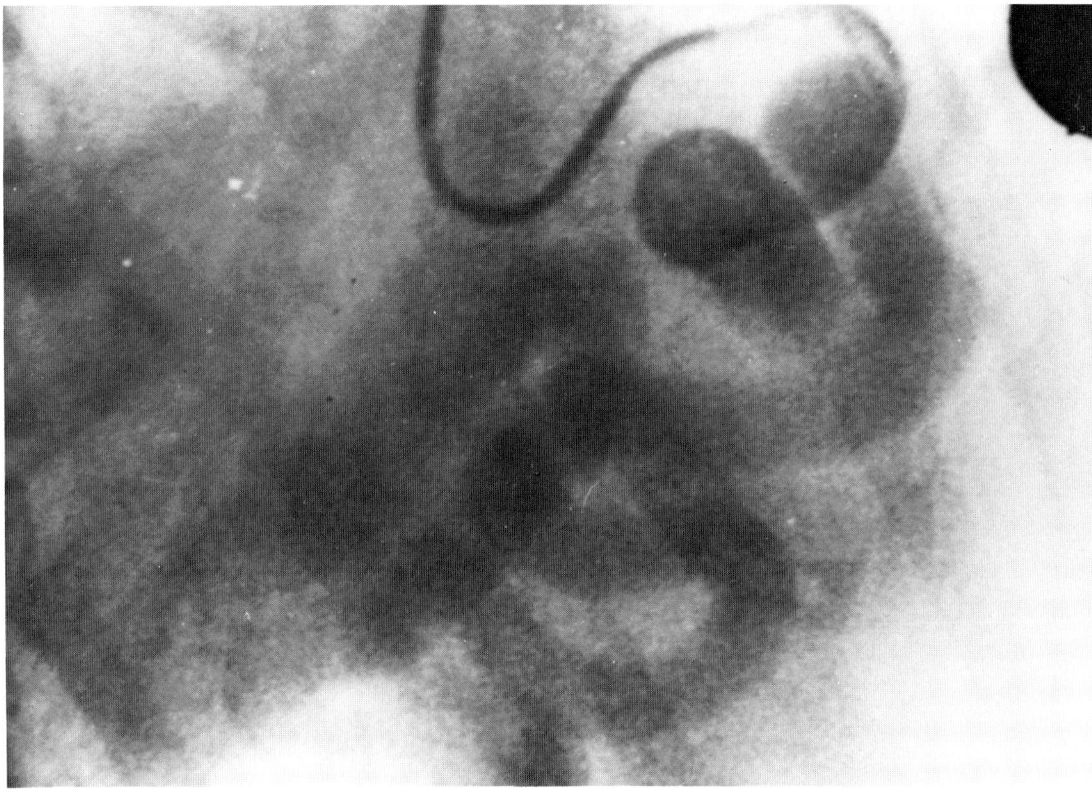

Figure 3-25 Selective left coronary artery arteriogram in a 67-year-old female who was undergoing catheterization prior to mitral valve replacement for severe mitral regurgitation secondary to myxomatous degeneration with chordal rupture. There is extreme dilation, elongation, and tortuosity of the left circumflex branch of the left coronary artery. The fistual orifice enters the distal third of the coronary sinus.

sure injector may be used, delivering 15 to 25 mL selectively into the involved coronary artery or 50 mL into the aortic root.

The natural history of CAVF is reasonably well known. Survival with CAVF to seventh and eighth decades has been reported. In an autopsy group, 9 of 13 were greater than 53 years of age. A 50-year-old man with CAVF to the main pulmonary artery and a 2:1 shunt and normal pulmonary artery pressure showed no change in his catheterization 13 years later. Subacute bacterial endocarditis is of low incidence, approximately 4 percent. Thrombosis or rupture of the CAVF is rare. Spontaneous closure of a right coronary artery–to–right ventricular fistula was documented by catheterization in a 5-year-old, as was the regression of dilation of the right coronary artery and circumflex coronary arteries.[66] Occlusion by atherosclerosis may occur in the adult. In the years after successful closure of CAVF, the coronary artery may still remain large and dilated.

The differential diagnosis of CAVF most commonly includes small patent ductus arteriosus or ruptured sinus of Valsalva aneurysm. Acquired causes of CAVF include coronary artery bypass grafting to a coronary vein[67]; rarely, after myocardial infarction; and blunt or perforating trauma, including gunshot wound, ice pick stab, and steering wheel injury.[69–70a] It has been suggested that CAVF may occur secondary to coronary athero-

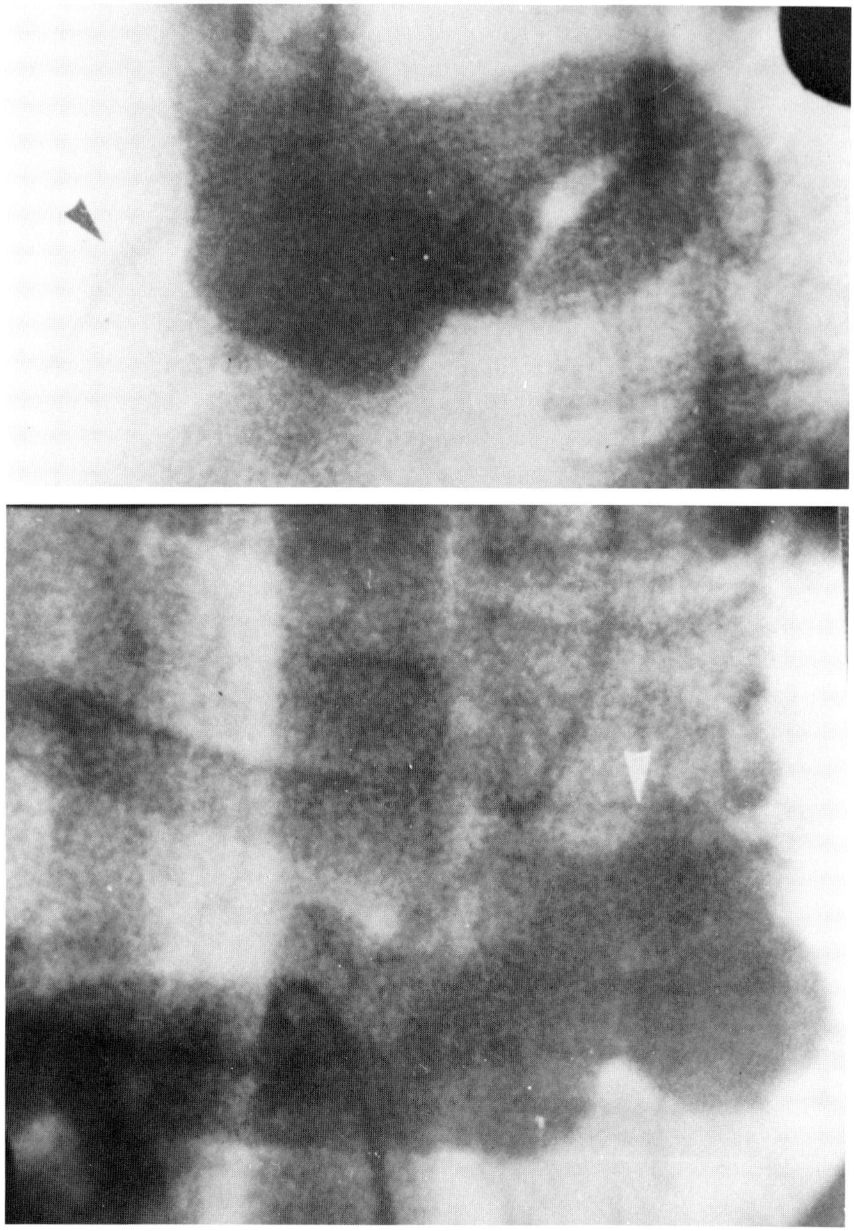

Figure 3-26 Aortic root injection in a young woman in left anterior oblique view (*top*) and right anterior oblique view (*bottom*). A dilated main left coronary artery and proximal left coronary artery gives off a large sinus node artery that courses rightward and posteriorly to enter the right atrium near the superior vena cava orifice. Black arrow points to the right coronary artery; white arrow points to the upper right atrium.

sclerosis.[70b] A right atrial cavernous hemangioma fed by both coronary arteries showed puddling of contrast medium in the right atrial wall and a very small shunt and was confused with a CAVF.[71]

Fistula of Coronary Artery to Left Atrium or Left Ventricle

Coronary artery fistulas to the left side of the heart are uncommon. Of 172 patients with CAVF 8 percent emptied into the left side of the heart; in 10 patients to the left atrium, and in 3 patients to the left ventricle. In another series of 88 cases of atrial CAVF, 72 entered the right atrium or the right atrial superior vena cava junction, and 16 entered the left atrium.[59]

In a group of seventeen patients with coronary artery fistula to the left ventricle (LV), the left coronary artery was involved in seven, the right coronary artery in four, and both coronary arteries in six. Three patients had chest pain postulated to be secondary to left ventricular steal from the right coronary artery tree.[72] These communications tend to be silent, as only three had a continuous murmur.[72,73] Eight patients had an enlarged heart on chest x-ray. A 1.5-mm depression in the ST segment was noted 3 minutes after exercise without pain in a 59-year-old woman with left coronary artery–to–LV fistula; the thallium scan after exercise was normal in this patient and in another 53-year-old woman.[72] The coronary artery involved in the fistula was dilated, tortuous, and elongated. In 17 cases of coronary artery fistula to the LV the termination in the LV had multiple fistulas in 9 and a single fistulous opening in 8.[72] In a 49-year-old man both coronary arteries gave branches via the distal right coronary artery and distal LAD, joining to a single "venous" channel that emptied into the LV near the mitral valve.[74] Shunt flow is generally not well quantitated but is likely to be small. Following coronary arteriography the left ventricular cavity may show a feathered striate pattern suggesting multiple intramural fistulas (Fig. 3-27). Successful closure of left coronary artery to LV fistula has been performed for recurrent chest pain and left ventricular hypertrophy.[75,76]

ANOMALOUS RIGHT CORONARY ARTERY FROM THE PULMONARY ARTERY

Rarely the right coronary artery arises from the main pulmonary artery (ARCAPA) and follows a normal distribution. This anomaly is much less common and serious than anomalous left coronary artery from the pulmonary artery (ALCAPA). The majority of cases have no clinical evidence of ischemia or infarction in the distribution of the right coronary artery. Potentially a right coronary artery steal could result in compromising left coronary artery flow distally. A 17-year-old girl was found at autopsy to have occlusion by thrombus of the left coronary artery.[77] Of a group of 19 cases of ARCAPA reported in the literature 12 of 19 were diagnosed at autopsy.[78] Of 19, 7 were diagnosed by coronary angiography or aortography; 3 had associated congenital heart disease: the first, an atrial septal defect, the second, ventricular septal defect and aortopulmonary window, and the third, tetralogy of Fallot with patent ductus. The right coronary artery is large, serpentine, and thin-walled. In the adult, atherosclerosis has been noted only in the left coronary. In three cases the pulmonary flow–systemic flow ratio was 1.7, 1.8, and 2.7. The last value may result in volume overload of the left ventricle. In one case 84 percent of microspheres injected into the left coronary artery reached the lung, suggesting a large shunt with estimated blood flow through the right coronary artery at 1300 mL/min. Normal blood flow is 85 mL/min per 100 myocardium.[79]

At angiography this lesion might be mistaken for coronary AV fistula to the main pulmonary artery because of the generalized dilatation of the coronary arteries. One can avoid this confusion by attention to the anatomic sequence of filling following a technically satisfactory selective left coronary arteriogram.

CORONARY ARTERY ATRESIA OR HYPOPLASIA

Atresia or hypoplasia of the main left or right coronary artery is a rare cause of ischemic heart disease

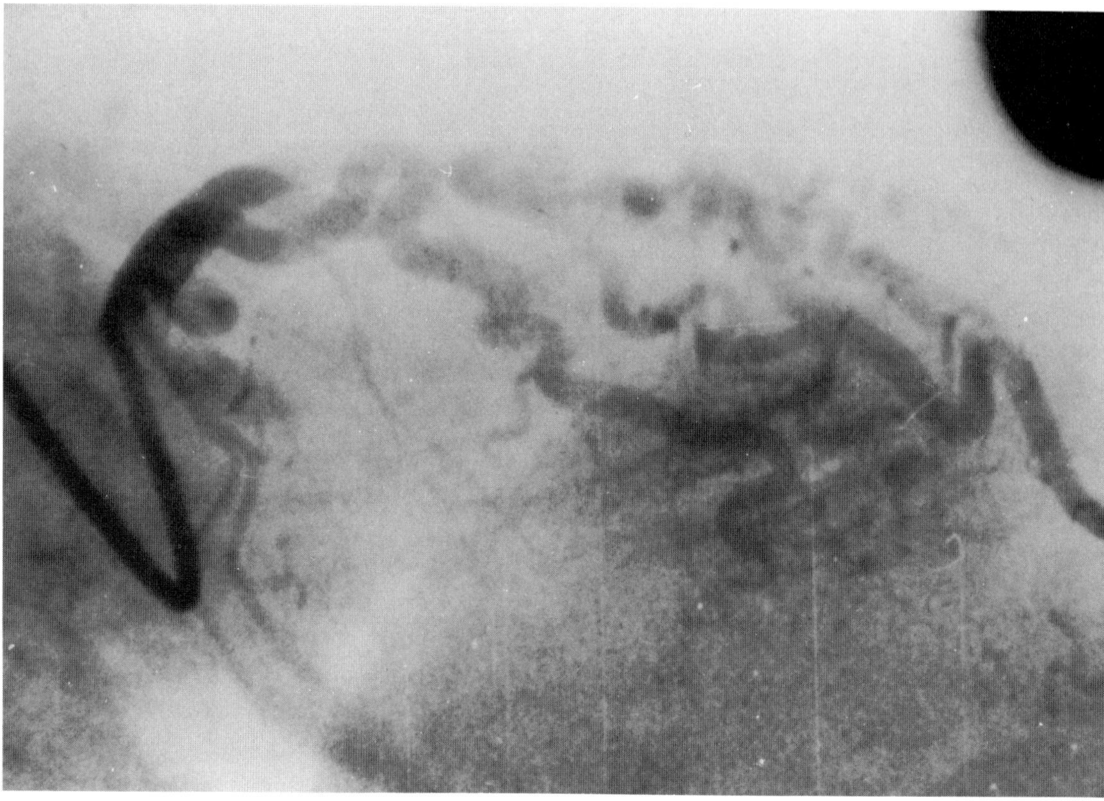

Figure 3-27 Selective left coronary artery injection in a 62-year-old female in the right anterior oblique view with cranial angulation shows a left coronary artery–to–left ventricular fistula. A striate pattern of left ventricular filling is noted, suggesting predominantly direct coronary-cameral communications.

in infancy and childhood.[2,80,81] Survival to adulthood depends on the development of adequate collateral flow from the other main coronary artery. Survival to old age has been reported in one patient with atresia of the left main coronary artery who developed atherosclerotic stenosis of the coronary arteries which provided collateral flow with resultant increase in ischemic symptoms and eventually death.[82] Atresia of the proximal portion of either main coronary artery may produce findings resembling those of single coronary artery or anomalous origin of the coronary artery from the pulmonary artery, and misdiagnosis has been reported.[80] Successful bypass surgery has been reported in patients with atresia of the left main coronary artery.[83] Congenital membrane–like structures extending across the left sinus of Valsalva, isolating the left main coronary artery, have been reported with successful surgical correction.[84] Atresia of the left main coronary artery has been reported in association with pulmonary atresia[81] (see "Pulmonary Atresia" below).

CONGENITAL CORONARY ARTERY ANEURYSMS

Isolated congenital coronary aneurysms are rarely diagnosed ante mortem. Dysplasia of the arterial media is the presumed etiology; however, it is difficult in most cases to exclude arteritis due to drug, toxin, infection, or autoimmune process. Coronary artery aneurysms in childhood have been associated with sudden death,[85] myocardial infarction,[86] angina pectoris,[86,87] rupture,[88] thrombosis,[86,89] and embolism. Coronary artery aneurysms may produce a shadow which protrudes from the heart border on chest roentgenograms,[85] and "eggshell" calcification may be present. Treatment of these congenital coronary aneurysms with coronary bypass surgery with and without proximal ligation has been attempted.[86,90]

VARIATIONS OF THE CORONARY ARTERIAL PATTERN IN PATIENTS WITH CONGENITAL HEART DEFECTS

The principal purpose of defining coronary artery distribution is to forewarn the surgeon of important epi- or intramyocardial aberrant coronary arteries passing through a potential ventriculotomy site. It is the responsibility of the cardiologist to provide this data routinely at the time the diagnostic catheterization study is obtained and reviewed. Biplane aortography in the oblique projection is the traditional technique employed by the pediatric cardiologist to outline the coronary arteries, while the adult cardiologist employs selective coronary arteriography.[91]

In a complex congenital heart defect, coronary arteriography may be useful in identifying whether a ventricle is the anatomic right or left ventricle. In this effort the epicardial course of the coronary

Figure 3-28 Artist's sketch of the heart of a patient with tetralogy of Fallot; the anomalous left anterior descending (3) originates from the right coronary artery (1) and crosses the right ventricular outflow track passing proximal to a dilated right ventricular infundibula chamber (4). The left coronary artery (2) is small. *(Courtesy of Blake HA, Manion WC, et al: Coronary artery anomalies, Circulation, 30:937, 1964.)*

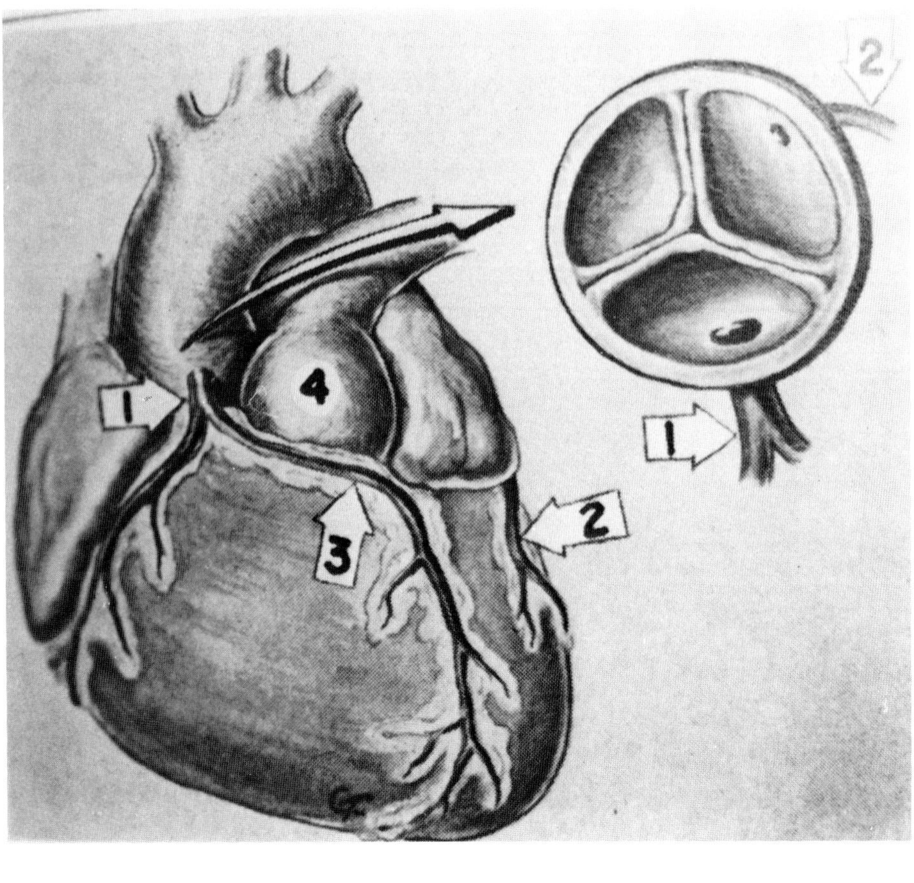

arteries is more useful than the site of takeoff from the aorta.[92]

The origin of the coronary arteries from the aortic sinuses may differ from the normal in congenital heart disease. Orientation of the aortic sinuses in transposition of the great arteries (TGA) varies depending on whether the aorta is in an oblique, side-by-side, or anteroposterior relation to the pulmonary artery. Thus, in TGA with an oblique position, the origin of the right coronary artery is from the posterior aortic sinus; the right aortic sinus is the noncoronary sinus.

Tetralogy of Fallot

The coronary artery distribution should be defined (by selective coronary arteriography or an excellent aortic root injection) during diagnostic catheterization in the patient with tetralogy of Fallot who will require a right ventriculotomy for repair. The study is especially important in those patients under 2 years of age. The purpose of the study is to detect a large left coronary artery or left anterior descending or conus branch that may be crossing the right ventricular outflow tract after its origin from the right coronary artery or the right aortic sinus and thus may be subject to interruption, especially if its course is intramyocardial or is obscured by a pad of fat tissue[93] (Figs. 3-28 and 3-29). The prevalence of this anomaly (most commonly the left anterior descending from the right coronary) is approximately 4 to 7 percent.[94,95] In 40 of 109 cases of tetralogy of Fallot the conus artery was large

Figure 3-29 Selective right coronary artery injection in an 18-year-old male with tetralogy of Fallot. The anomalous left anterior descending (arrow) arises from the right coronary artery crossing the right ventricular conus, thence entering the anterior interventricular groove.

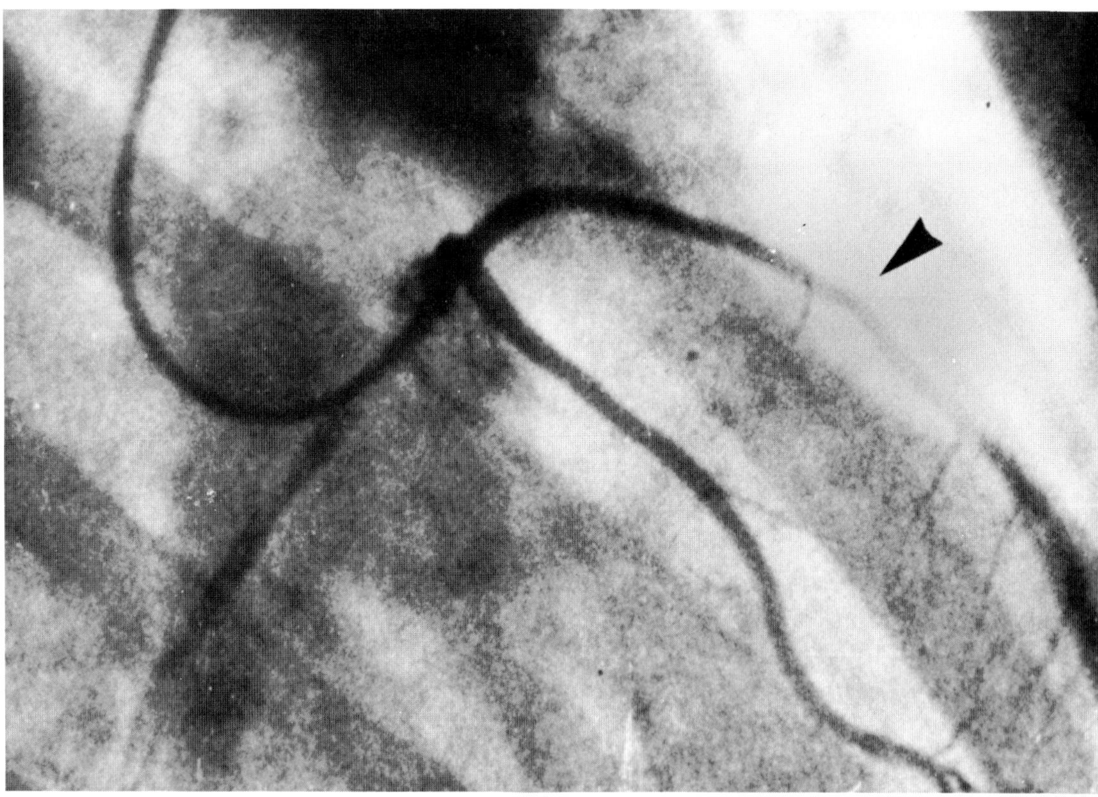

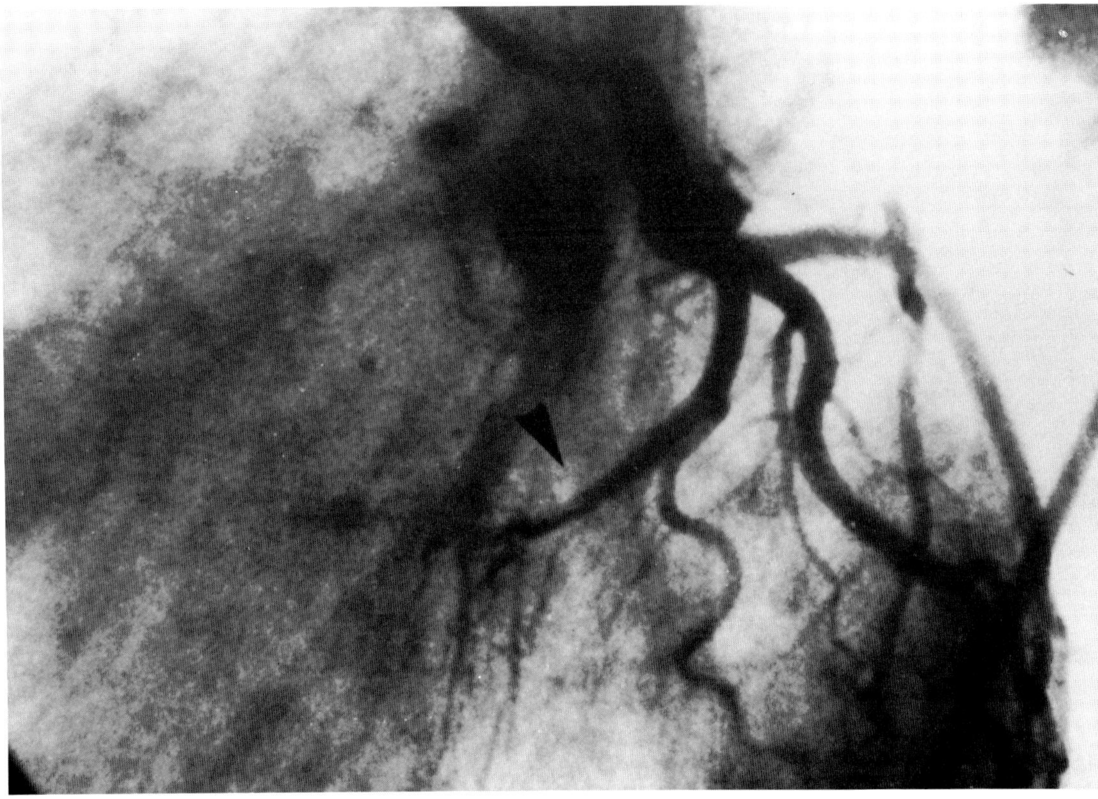

A

Figure 3-30 Selective coronary angiograms in 57-year-old man with tetralogy of Fallot. (*a,b*) Left coronary artery injections in left anterior oblique and right anterior oblique projections. The abbreviated left anterior descending terminates in a large first septal perforator (arrow). (*c*) Right coronary artery injection in the right anterior oblique view. The right coronary artery is prominent; a large right ventricular branch is noted. The arrow points to an anomalous coronary artery arising from the proximal right coronary artery and traversing the right ventricular outflow tract to supply the mild and distal left anterior descending artery distribution.

and elongated. One of our 58-year-old patients with tetralogy of Fallot had a split supply to the left anterior descending (LAD) distribution. The LAD to the mid and distal anterior interventricular groove arose from the proximal right coronary artery, while the proximal LAD rose normally from the left coronary artery (Fig. 3-30).

Another major coronary anomaly in tetralogy of Fallot occurs when a single coronary artery arises from either the left or the right aortic sinus.[94,96,97] In this event the left coronary or the right coronary artery, respectively, may cross the right ventricular infundibulum. In 109 cases of tetralogy of Fallot studied at autopsy two patients had a single coronary artery arising from the right aortic sinus and seven had the LAD arising from the right aortic sinus or the right coronary artery; in five cases the right ventricular outflow tract was crossed high at the base of the main pulmonary artery, and in two cases the artery crossed the mid or proximal portion of the right ventricular outflow tract.[94]

Aortic root injection was not satisfactory in outlining the coronary arteries in 10 of 94 studies of children with tetralogy of Fallot; the percentage

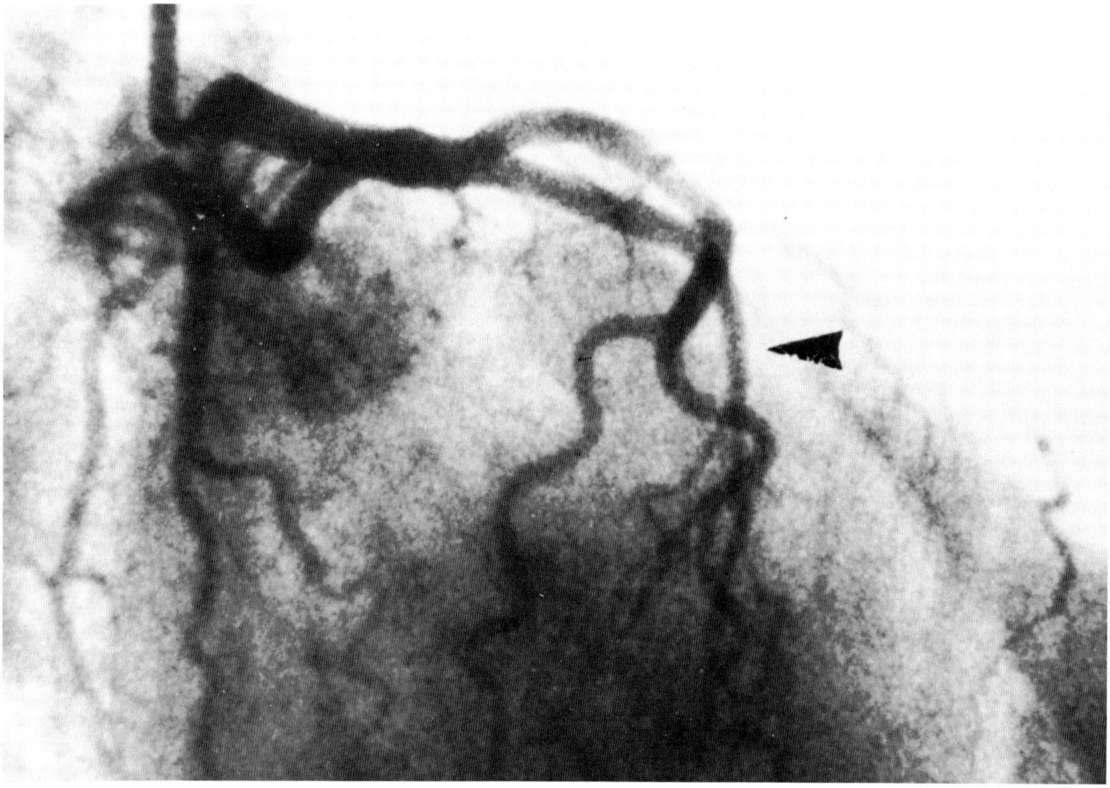

B *(Figure 3-30, continued)*

may even be higher in the adolescent or adult patient if this technique is used.[98] In children an injection of 0.5 to 1 mL of contrast medium per kilogram of body weight is used for ascending aortography and nonselective opacification of the coronary arteries. Selective aortic root angiography can be made at catheterization of the right side of the heart if the overriding aorta is entered via a ventricular septal defect. In several cases we have selectively hand-injected the left coronary artery ostia via the venous catheter that is passed antegrade into the aortic root across the ventricular septal defect.

Outlining the coronary arteries seems mandatory in a patient who has had a previous cardiotomy since pericardial thickening may hide the epicardial coronary artery. It is of interest that in a group of 27 surgical cases with anomalous coronary artery 21, or 80 percent were male.[99] In performing selective coronary arteriography in the patient with tetralogy of Fallot the following anatomic point should be kept in mind: Looking up through the aortic valve the aortic root may be rotated clockwise, so that the right aortic sinus and right coronary artery may arise anteriorly and leftward in comparison to the normal patient.

Transposition of the Great Arteries

In patients with transposition of the great arteries (TGA) the right aortic sinus gives off no coronary artery[100] (Fig. 3-31). In two-thirds of cases the posterior sinus gives off the right coronary artery and the left sinus, the left coronary artery.[101] One-fourth of patients with transposition of the great arteries have an anomalous left circumflex arising from the proximal right coronary artery or the posterior sinus.[102] In these cases the left anterior descending rises from the left aortic sinus. In a small

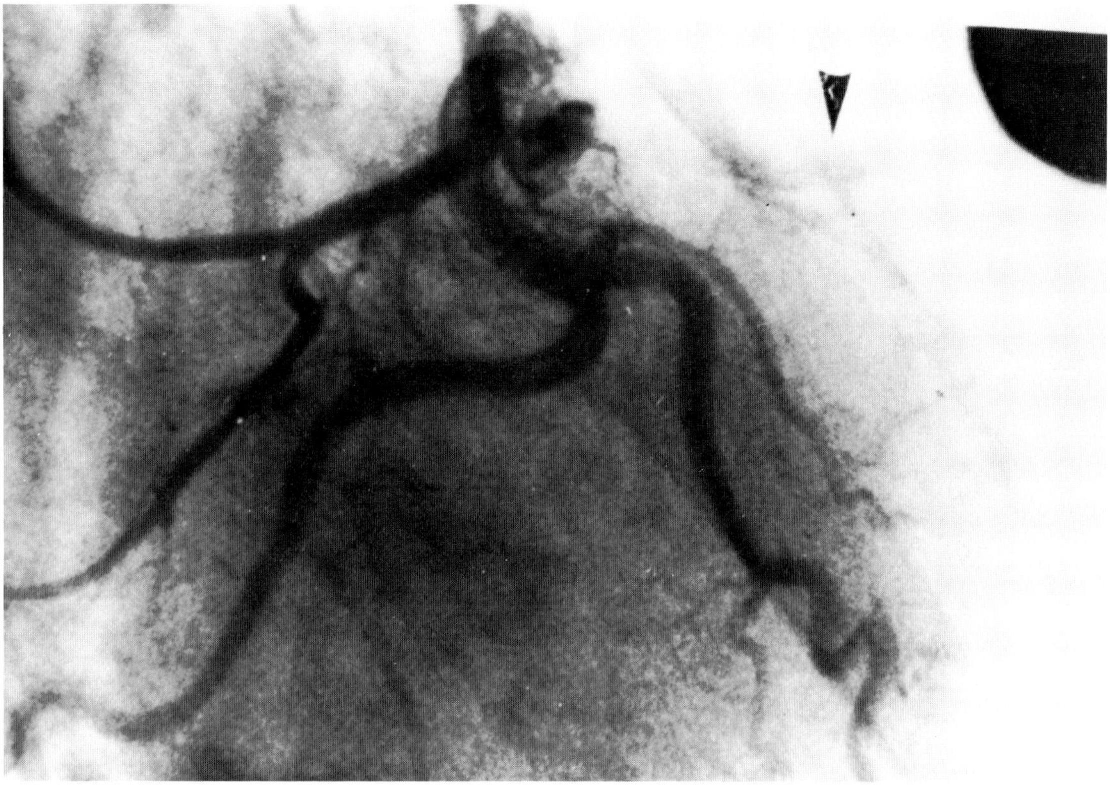

C *(Figure 3-30, continued)*

number of patients with transposition of the great arteries a single coronary artery arises from the posterior sinus or less commonly from the left aortic sinus. Coronary anatomy must be known if a Rastelli conduit is to be placed from the ventricle to the pulmonary artery. Of 23 patients with TGA and left ventricular outflow obstruction, sixteen had an anomalous coronary artery that could have been injured by ventriculotomy.[101]

Pulmonary Atresia with Intact Ventricular Septum

In patients with pulmonary atresia and intact ventricular septum the right ventricle is a small, thick-walled cavity with, in over one-half cases, a competent tricuspid valve. Systemic or suprasystemic right ventricular systolic pressure enables blood to leave the right ventricle via the myocardial sinusoidal and intertrabecular spaces that communicate with the left coronary artery tree (Fig. 3-32). Following selective right ventricular angiography the contrast medium is forced through the sinusoids into the left coronary artery tree, and retrograde flow into the aorta is identified (Fig. 3-33). In one of our infants asystole occurred secondary to the large dose of contrast medium entering the coronary artery tree following right ventricular injection. In one case the right ventricular infundibular cavity connected with the epicardium via a large, single, tapering channel (from 11 to 5 mm in circumference), thence joining the distal left main coronary artery.[103] The walls of the left coronary artery were cordlike and thickened; there was intimal fibrous narrowing not seen in the right coronary artery. In some of these cases the left main coronary artery may be three times greater in di-

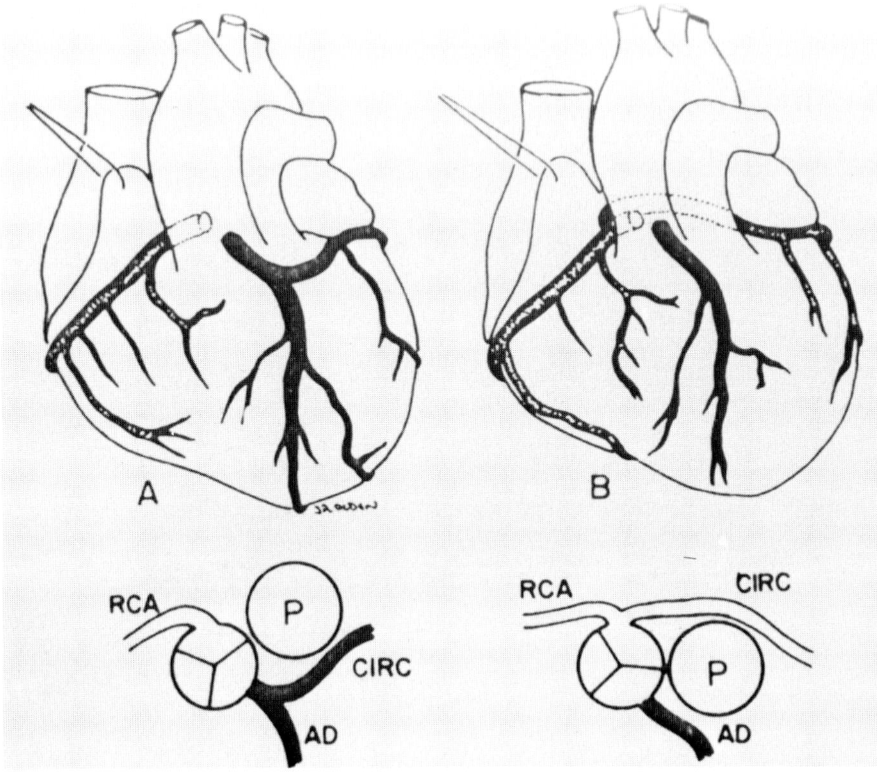

Figure 3-31 Sketches of two common coronary artery patterns in transposition of the great arteries with oblique (*a*) and side-by-side (*b*) great vessel relationship. Note that the right coronary artery arises from the posterior aortic sinus with or without the circumflex coronary artery. The right aortic sinus contains no coronary ostium. The left anterior descending arises from the left aortic sinus. AD = anterior descending artery, Circ = circumflex artery, P = pulmonary artery, RCA = right coronary artery. *(Courtesy of Ogden JA, Stansel HC Jr: Roentgenographic manifestations of congenital coronary artery disease, Am J Roentg, 113:538, 1977.)*

ameter than the right coronary artery. Rarely the proximal left main coronary artery may be absent in pulmonary atresia.[104] In these patients the retrograde flow may impede normal coronary artery diastolic filling. A patent ductus arteriosus can lead to a coronary steal in this group. Recent myocardial infarction affecting the left ventricular papillary muscle has been described.

In patients with pulmonary atresia and ventricular septal defect the coronary arteries may supply the pulmonary artery bed with collateral circulation. In one of our teenage patients with pulmonary atresia and ventricular septal defect the left main coronary artery provided a large branch to the main pulmonary artery that served as the sole source of systemic collateral blood flow to the lung maintaining an arterial oxygen saturation of 89 percent in a pulmonary flow–systemic flow ratio of 2:1.

Univentricular Heart Including Tricuspid Atresia

In 20 of 21 autopsied cases of univentricular heart (main chamber of the left ventricular type with an anterior outlet chamber) large parallel branches of the right coronary artery crossed the right ventricular outflow tract[105] (Fig. 3-33). In 13 cases these vessel branches had been injured in the septation and/or cardiac conduit procedure. The longitudinal

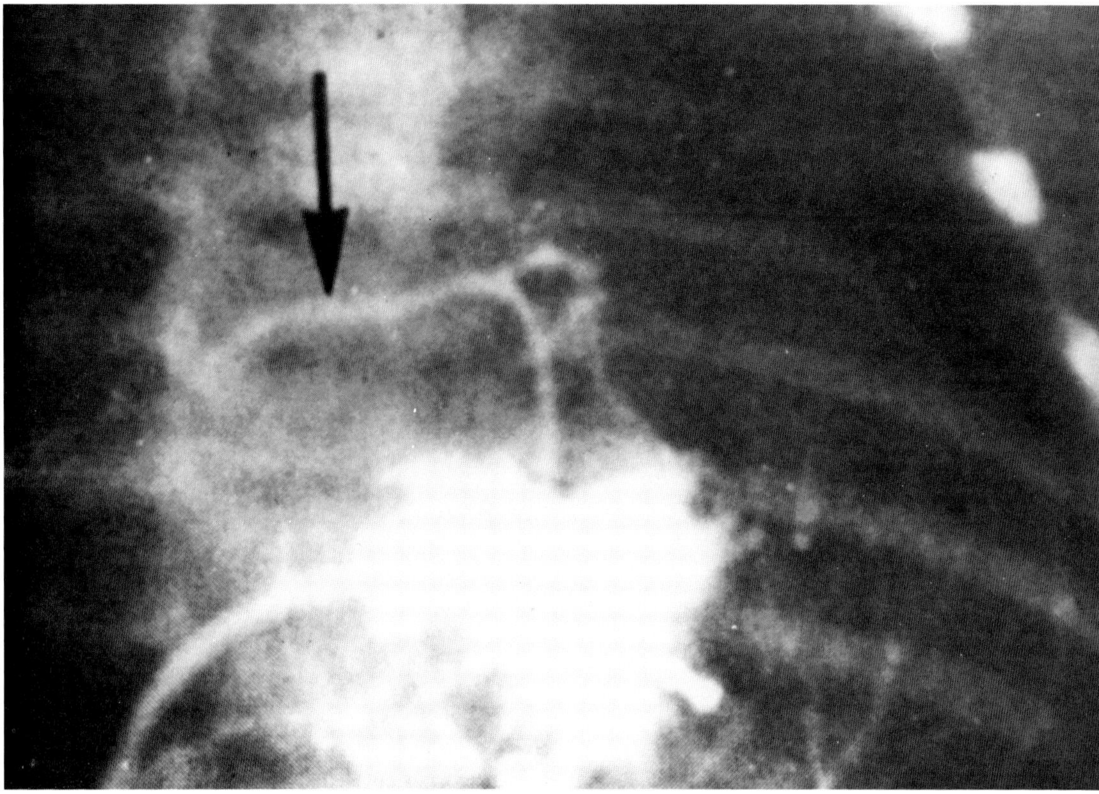

Figure 3-32 Selective right ventricular injection opacifies the left coronary artery retrograde via intramyocardial sinusoids in a patient with pulmonary atresia and intact ventricular septum. Arrow points to left coronary artery which later filled the ascending aorta. *(Courtesy of Cornell SH: Myocardial sinusoids in pulmonary valvular atresia, Radiology, 86:421, 1966.)*

margins of the outlet chamber were defined delimiting branches from the right and left coronary arteries, the right being more prominent. The anterior aortic sinus of the transposed aorta is the noncoronary sinus. The left coronary and right coronary arteries arise from their respective posterior right and left sinuses. A typical coronary artery pattern occurred in five hearts. The coronary artery distribution in tricuspid atresia is similar to that of double-inlet left ventricle.[106]

Congenitally Corrected Transposition of the Great Arteries

In congenitally corrected transposition of the great arteries (CCTGA) the atria are in normal position. The great arteries are transposed so that the ascending aorta is to the left and anterior to the main pulmonary artery and the ventricles with their respective atrioventricular valves are inverted.[107] Thus, the distribution of the coronary arteries is reversed in keeping with the ventricular inversion (Fig. 3-34). The anterior aortic sinus is the noncoronary sinus. The morphologically left coronary artery arises from the right posterior–oriented aortic sinus and supplies the pulmonary ventricle, which is the anatomic left ventricle.[108] The morphologically right coronary artery arises from the left posterior aortic sinus and supplies the systemic ventricle, which is the anatomic right ventricle (Fig. 3-34).

Truncus Arteriosus

The most common truncal origins regardless of the number of cusps for the coronary ostia were as follows: in 19 of 31 cases of truncus arteriosus (61

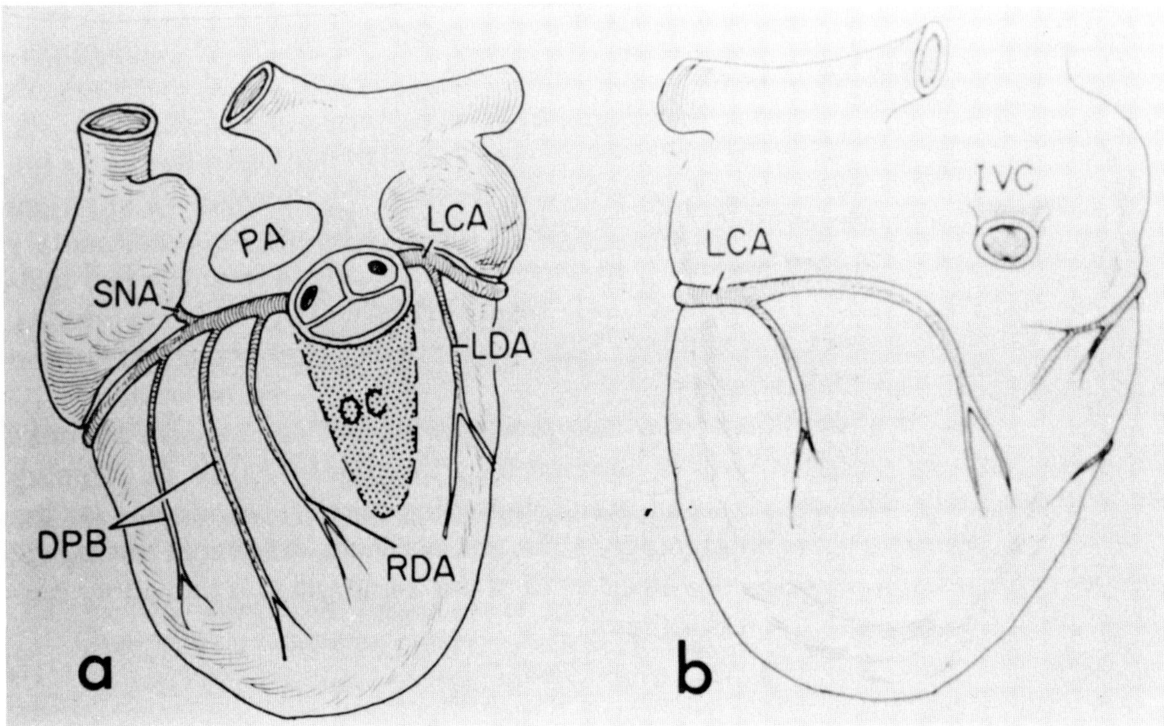

Figure 3-33 Sketch of the front (*a*) and back (*b*) of a common epicardial coronary artery pattern in univentricular heart with *L*-transposition of the great arteries and a left-sided outlet chamber (OC) bracketed by the right delimiting and left descending arteries (R and LDA). Note the multiple epicardial delimiting parallel branches over the ventriculotomy site for a septation procedure. SNA = sinus node artery, IVC = inferior vena cava, DPB = delimiting parallel branches. *(Courtesy of Keeton BR, Lie JT, et al: Anatomy of coronary arteries in univentricular hearts and its surgical implications, Am J Cardiol, 43:569, 1979.)*

percent) the left coronary artery arose from the left posterior aspect of the truncus.[109] Only very rarely may the left coronary artery ostium be high near the origin of the pulmonary artery from the truncus. In 15 of 31 cases with a tricuspid valve (48 percent) the right coronary artery arose from the right truncal sinus (Fig. 3-35). Other variations are described.[110] The right coronary artery may give off several large anterior diagonal branches inferior and parallel to the conus artery[111] (Fig. 3-36). Since the right ventriculotomy incision for repairing the ventricular septal defect and also for suturing a conduit between the right ventricle and the pulmonary artery may cross this area, the surgeon should be alerted of this angiographic finding. In 78 percent of all cases the truncal valve in this group consisted of three cusps.

Double-Outlet Right Ventricle

In double-outlet right ventricle the origin of both great arteries is entirely or predominantly from the right ventricle. In 14 cases of double-outlet right ventricle, two patients with aberrant coronary artery were noted. One patient had two left anterior descending arteries, one from the left and one from the right aortic sinus. In the second patient the right coronary artery arose as a branch of the left coronary artery; an accessory left anterior descending coronary artery came from the right coronary sinus. The coronary artery pattern should be studied for

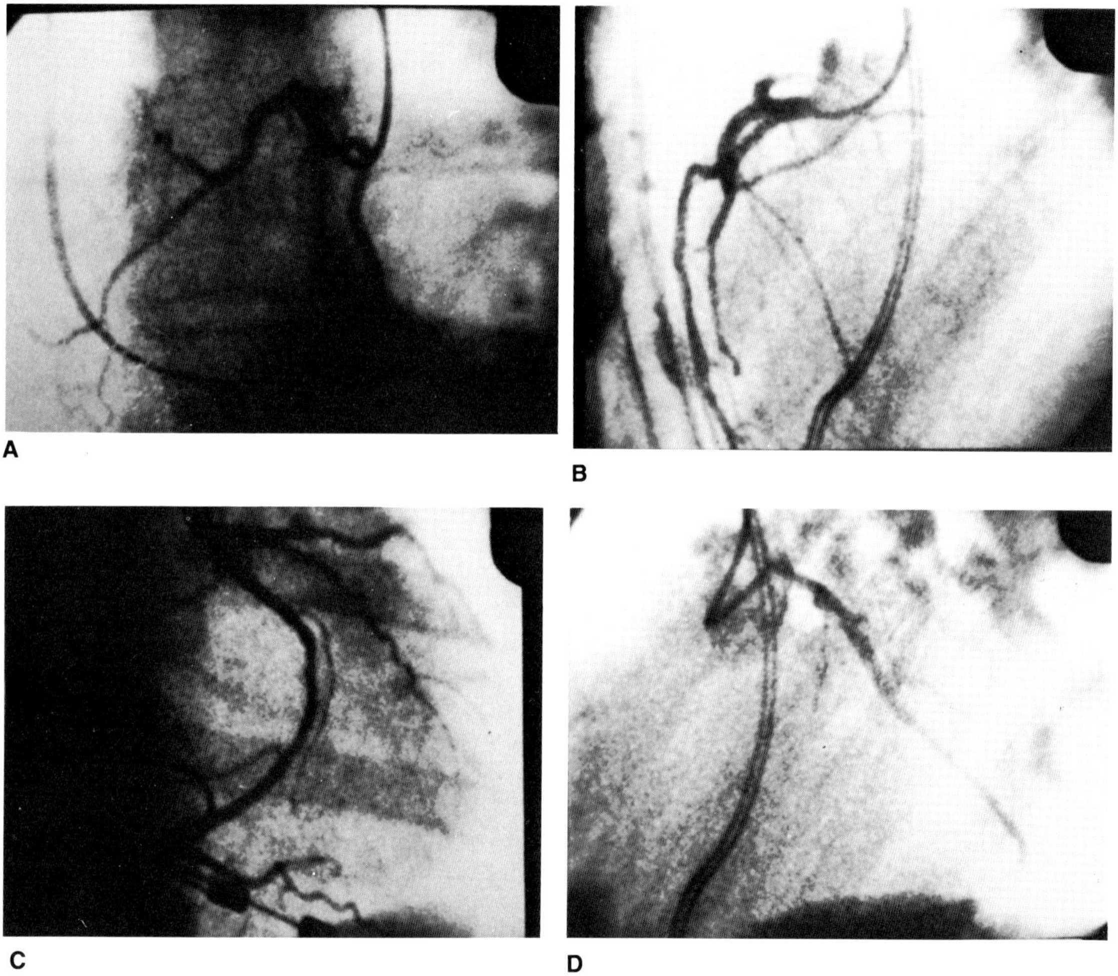

Figure 3-34 Prints of selective anterior (*a,c*) and lateral (*b,d*) views of the (*a*) and (*b*) left, (*c*) and (*d*) right coronary arteries in a 36-year-old housewife with isolated congenitally corrected transposition of the great arteries. The left coronary artery arises from the right posterior aortic sinus and supplies the pulmonary (anatomic left) ventricle. The right coronary artery arises from the left posterior aortic sinus and supplies the systemic (anatomic right) ventricle. The anterior aortic sinus is the noncoronary sinus. A bipolar endocardial catheter is noted in the pulmonary ventricle. *(Courtesy of Masden RR, Franch RH: Isolated congenitally corrected transposition of the great arteries, in Hurst JW (ed): Update III: The Heart, McGraw-Hill, New York, 1980, pp 59–84.)*

any large artery which crosses the right ventricular outflow tract at the site of ventriculotomy.[111–113]

Bicuspid Aortic Valve

In an autopsy group of 50 cases with congenital bicuspid aortic valve the left coronary artery rose from a high takeoff at or above the sinotubular ridge in 44 percent compared to 20 percent in a control group. The incidence of aortic origin of the conus artery was 33 percent in both groups. This is in the range reported in normal individuals, i.e., 23 to 50 percent.[114]

Left coronary artery dominance is known to be increased in isolated aortic stenosis and in bicuspid

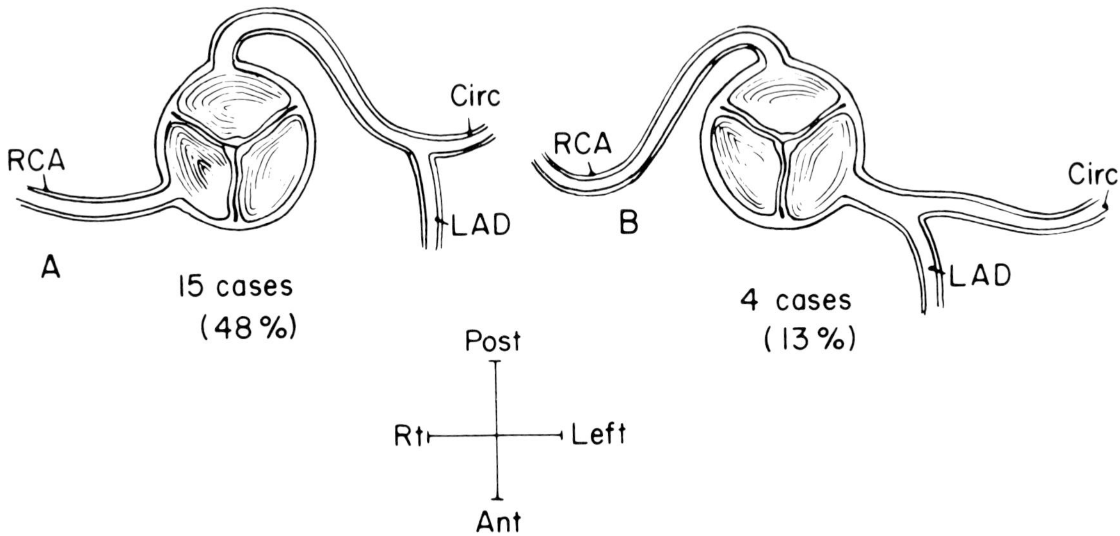

Figure 3-35 Two patterns of coronary artery anatomy in thirty-one patients with truncus arteriosus with a tricuspid truncal valve. Circ = circumflex artery, LCA = left coronary artery, RCA = right coronary artery. *(Courtesy of Anderson KR, McGoon DD, Lie JT: Surgical significance of coronary arterial anatomy in truncus arteriosus communis, Am J Cardiol, 41:76, 1978.)*

Figure 3-36 Sketch of the anterior surface of the heart in a patient with truncus arteriosus. Prominent branches of the right coronary artery (RC) cross diagonally over the potential site of a ventriculotomy for a conduit implantation in the right ventricle. Circ = circumflex artery, LAD = left anterior descending artery, LC = left coronary artery. *(Courtesy of Anderson KR, McGoon DD, et al: Surgical significance of coronary arterial anatomy in truncus arteriosus communis, Am J Cardiol, 41:76, 1978.)*

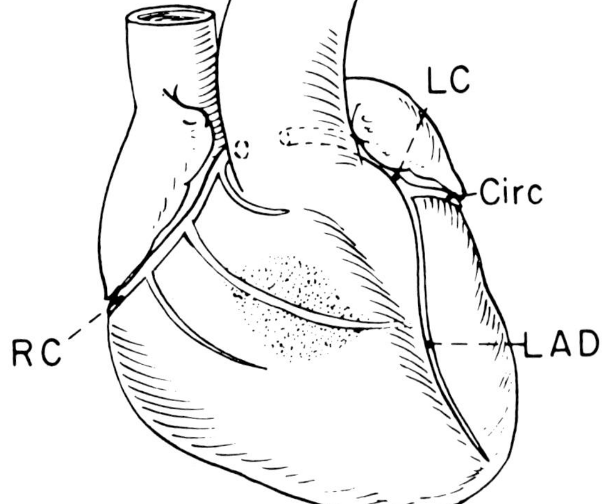

aortic valve.[115] It occurred in 26 percent of the 50 cases with bicuspid aortic valve, well above the prevalence in the normal population (10 percent). The left main coronary artery was shorter in hearts with left coronary artery dominance than in those with right or codominance.

Supravalvular Aortic Stenosis and Coarctation of the Aorta

In supravalvular aortic stenosis the coronary ostia are subject to high systolic pressure and potential encroachment by the intimal aortic disease associated with the stenotic lesion. In one of our 16-year-old patients who died at the dinner table extensive intimal irregularity and atherosclerosis was noted in both coronary arteries.

In patients with coarctation of the aorta under 30 years of age the coronary arteries may show intimal changes, medial hypertrophy, and atheromas of varying degree.[116]

Supravalvular Mitral Stenosis

Supravalvular mitral stenosis is an unusual cause of obstruction between the left atrium and left ven-

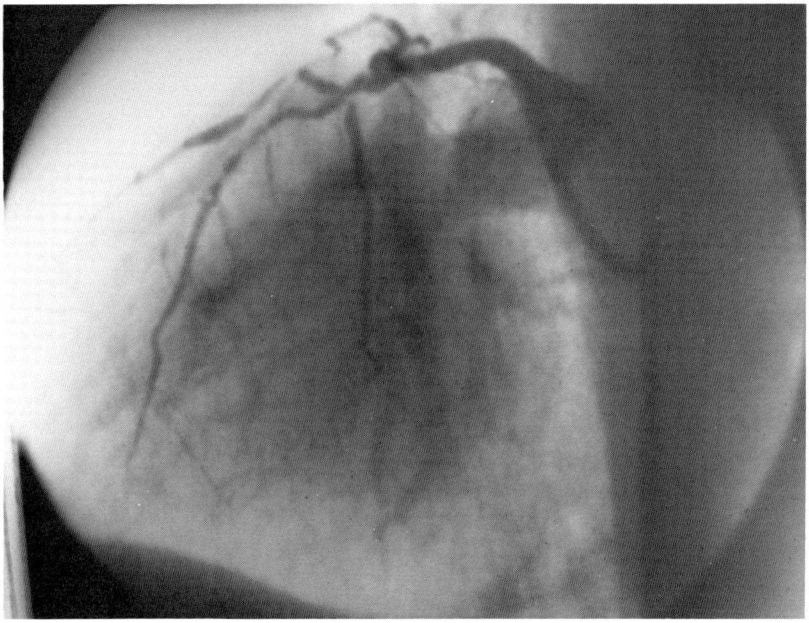

A

Figure 3-37 Situs inversus. Left anterior oblique view of left coronary arteriogram (*a*), right coronary arteriogram (*b*), and left ventriculogram (*c*).

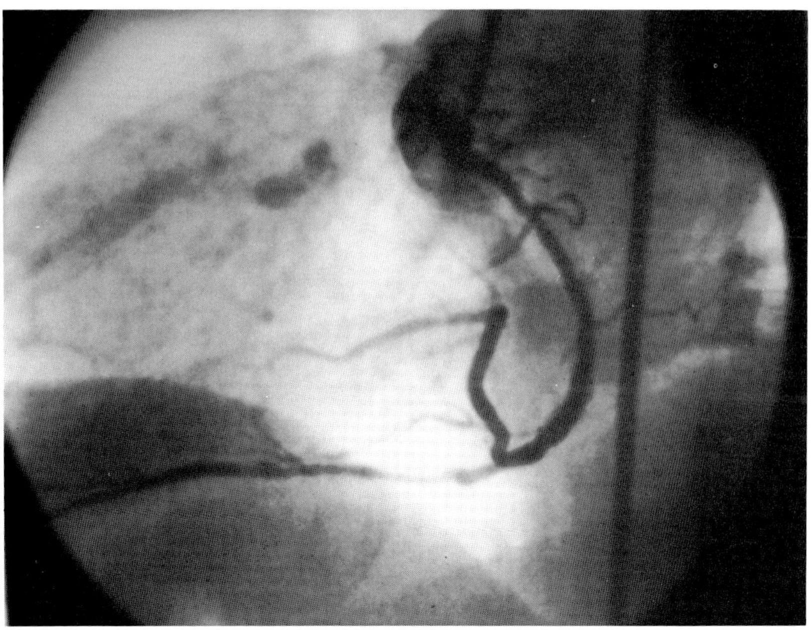

B

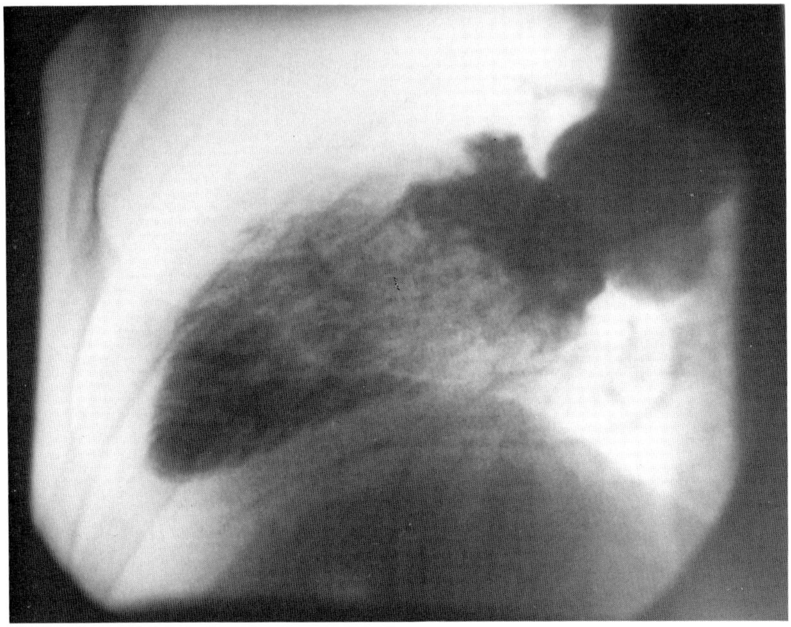

C (Figure 3-37, continued)

tricle. The supravalvular ridge is a fibrous encircling diaphragm or shelf that may be formed by the sulcus at the site of attenuation of left atrial myocardium. In a 2-month-old the circumflex artery of a left dominant system was enfolded in the ridge; excision of the latter would have transected this major artery.[117]

Superoinferior Ventricular Heart (Crisscross Pattern)

In superoinferior ventricular heart the interventricular septum is horizontal; the anatomic left ventricle is inferior and the anatomic right ventricle is superior. The atria are in relative normal position and thus bear a crisscross relation to their respective ventricles. Complete or congenitally corrected transposition of the great arteries or double-outlet right ventricle are three associated congenital malformations that are commonly noted. The coronary artery pattern is as described for these entities. This anatomic arrangement is surgically correctable, and therefore the coronary pattern needs to be carefully defined.[118]

Situs Inversus

Patients with situs inversus have a mirror image coronary circulation which is otherwise not different from normal situs. Catheterization of adult patients with this condition has presented no special problem other than reversing one's orientation. Sones, Judkins, or multipurpose catheters have been used successfully (Fig. 3-37).

REFERENCES

1 Donaldson RM, Raphael M, Radley-Smith R, Yacoub MH, Ross DN: Angiographic identification of primary coronary anomalies causing impaired myocardial perfusion. Cathet Cardiovasc Diagn, 9:237, 1983.
2 Vlodaver Z, Neufeld HN, Edwards JE: Pathology of coronary disease. Semin Roentgenol, 7:376, 1972.
3 Ogden JA: Congenital anomalies of the coronary arteries. J Cardiol, 25:474, 1970.
4 Engel HJ, Torres C, Page HL Jr: Major variations in anatomical origin of the coronary arteries: Angiographic observation in 4,250 patients without

associated congenital heart disease. Cathet Cardiovasc Diagn, 1:157, 1975.

5 Benge W, Martins JB, Funk DC: Morbidity associated with anomalous origin of the right coronary artery from the left sinus of Valsalva. Am Heart J, 99:96, 1980.

6 Antopol W, Kugel MA: Anomalous origin of the left circumflex coronary artery. Am Heart J, 8:802, 1933.

7 Donaldson RM, Raphael MJ: Missing coronary artery: Review of technical problems in coronary arteriography resulting from anatomical variants. Br Heart J, 47:62, 1982.

8 Kimbiris D, Iskandrian AS, Segal BL, Bemis CE: Anomalous aortic origin of the coronary arteries. Circulation, 58:606, 1978.

9 Chaitman BR, Lesperance J, Saltiel J, Bourassa MG: Clinical, angiographic, and hemodynamic findings in patients with anomalous origin of the coronary arteries. Circulation, 53:122, 1976.

10 Page HL Jr, Engel HJ, Campbell WB, Thomas CS Jr: Anomalous origin of the left circumflex coronary artery: Recognition, angiographic demonstration, and clinical significance. Circulation, 50:768, 1974.

11 Patterson FK: Sudden death in a young adult with anomalous origin of the posterior circumflex artery. South Med J, 75:748, 1982.

12 Roberts WC, Morrow AG: Compression of anomalous left circumflex coronary arteries by prosthetic valve fixation rings. J Thorac Cardiovasc Surg, 57:834, 1969.

13 Levin DC, Fellows KE, Abrams HL: Hemodynamically significant primary anomalies of the coronary arteries: Angiographic aspects. Circulation, 58:25, 1978.

14 McManus BM, Waller BF, Jones M, Epstein SE, Roberts WC: The case for preoperative coronary angiography in patients with tetralogy of Fallot and other complex congenital heart disease. Am Heart J, 103:451, 1982.

15 Heuser RR, Achuff SC, Brinker JA: Inadvertent division of an anomalous left anterior descending coronary artery during complete repair of Tetralogy of Fallot: 22-Year follow-up. Am Heart J, 103:430, 1982.

15a Sacks JH, Londe SP, Rosenbluth A, Zalis EG: Left main coronary bypass for aberrant (aortic intramural) left coronary artery. J Thorac Cardiovasc Surg, 73:733, 1977.

16 Moodie DS, Gill C, Loop FD, Sheldon WC: Anomalous left main coronary artery originating from the right sinus of Valsalva: Pathophysiology, angiographic definition, and surgical approaches. J Thorac Cardiovasc Surg, 80:198, 1980.

16a Mustafa I, Gula G, Radley-Smith R, Durrer S, Yacoub M: Anomalous origin of the left coronary artery from the anterior aortic sinus: A potential cause of sudden death. Anatomic characterization and surgical treatment. J Thorac Cardiovasc Surg, 82:297, 1981.

17 Cohen LS, Shaw LD: Fatal myocardial infarction in an 11-year-old boy associated with a unique coronary artery anomaly. Am J Cardiol, 19:420, 1967.

18 Benson PA: Anomalous aortic origin of coronary artery with sudden death: Case Report and Review. Am Heart J, 79:254, 1970.

19 Cheitlin MD, DeCastro CM, McAllister HA: Sudden death as a complication of anomalous left coronary origin from the anterior sinus of Valsalva. Circulation, 50:780, 1974.

19a Chaitman BR, Lesperance J, Saltiel J, Bourassa MG: Clinical, Angiographic and hemodynamic findings in patients with anomalous origin of the coronary arteries. Circulation, 53:122, 1976.

20 Liberthson RR, Dinsmore RE, Fallon JT: Aberrant coronary artery origin from the aorta: Report of 18 patients. Review of literature and delineation of natural history and management. Circulation, 59:748, 1979.

21 Thompson SI, Vieweg WV, Alport JS, Hagan AD: Anomalous origin of the right coronary artery from the left sinus of Valsalva with associated chest pain: Report of two cases. Cathet Cardiovasc Diagn, 2:397, 1976.

22 Roberts WC, Siegel RJ, Zipes DP: Origin of the right coronary artery from the left sinus of Valsalva and its functional consequences: Analysis of 10 necropsy patients. Am J Cardiol, 49:863, 1982.

22a Brandt B III, Martins JB, Marcus ML: Anomalous origin of the right coronary artery from the left sinus of Valsalva. N Engl J Med, 309:596, 1983.

23 Ogden JA, Goodyer AVN: Patterns of distribution of the single coronary artery. Yale J Biol Med, 43:11, 1970.

24 Sharbaugh AH, White RS: Single coronary artery: Analysis of the anatomic variation, clinical importance, and report of five cases. JAMA, 230:243, 1974.

25 Lipton MJ, Barry, Williah H, Obrez, Ivo, Silverman JF, Wexler L: Isolated single coronary artery: Diagnosis, angiographic classification, and clinical significance. Radiology, 130:39, 1979.
26 Smith JC: Review of single coronary artery with report of 2 cases. Circulation, 1:1168, 1950.
27 Joswig BC, Warren SE, Vieweg WV, Hagan AD: Transmural myocardial infarction in the absence of coronary arterial luminal narrowing in a young man with single coronary arterial anomaly. Cathet Cardiovasc Diagn, 4:297, 1978.
28 Spring DA, Thomsen JH: Severe atherosclerosis in the "Single Coronary Artery": Reports of a previously undepicted pattern. Am J Cardiol, 31:663, 1973.
29 Keith JD, Rowe RD, Vlad P: *Heart Disease in Infancy and Childhood* (3d ed). Macmillan, New York, 1978, p 1014.
30 Wilcox WD, Hagler DJ, Lie JT, Danielson GK, Smith HC, Fulton RE: Anomalous origin of left coronary artery from pulmonary artery in association with intracardiac lesions: Report of two cases. J Thorac Cardiovasc Surg, 78(1):12–20, 1979.
31 Driscoll DJ, Garson A Jr, McNamara DG: Anomalous origin of the left coronary artery from the right pulmonary artery associated with complex congenital heart disease. Cathet Cardiovasc Diagn, 8:55, 1982.
32 Pinsky WW, Gillette PC, Duff DF, et al: Anomalous origin of left coronary artery from the pulmonary artery with ventricular septal defect. Circulation, 57:1026, 1978.
33 Wesselhoeft H, Fawcett JS, Johnson AL: Anomalous origin of the LCA from the pulmonary trunk: A review of 140 cases with seven further cases. Circulation, 38:403, 1968.
34 Nora JJ, McNamara DG, Hallman GL, Sommerville RS, Cooley DA: Medical and surgical management of anomalous origin of the left coronary artery from the pulmonary artery. Pediatrics, 42:405, 1968.
35 Akhtar N, et al: Anomalous origin of left coronary artery from pulmonary artery in adults. J Thorac Cardiovasc Surg, 66:112, 1973.
36 Sabiston DC Jr, Floyd WL, McIntosh HD: Anomalous origin of the left coronary artery from the pulmonary artery in adults. Arch Surg, 97:963, December 1968.
37 Arcinegos E, Farooki ZQ, Hakimi M, Green EW: Management of anomalous left coronary artery from the pulmonary artery. Circulation, 62:I-180, 1980.
38 Flamm MD, Stinson EB, Hultgren HW, Shumway NE, Hancock EW: Anomalous origin of the left coronary artery from the pulmonary artery. Circulation, 38:113, 1968.
39 Wasserman LS, Eshaghpour E, Takahashi O, Iskandrian A, Kotler MN: The noninvasive assessment of anomalous origin of the left coronary artery from the pulmonary artery. Cathet Cardiovasc Diagn, 5:85, 1979.
40 Shapiro J: Echocardiogram in infants with anomalous origin of the left coronary artery from the pulmonary artery. Pediatr Cardiol, 1:23, 1979.
41 Finley JP, Howan-Giles R, Gilday AL, et al: Thallium-201 myocardial imaging on anomalous left coronary artery arising from the pulmonary artery. Circulation, 41:1043, 1970.
42 Baue AE, Baum S, Blakemore WS, Zinsser NF: A later stage of anomalous coronary circulation with origin of the left coronary artery from the pulmonary artery. Circulation, 36:878, 1967.
43 Wilson CL, Diabal PW, Holeyfield RW, et al: Anomalous origin of the left coronary artery from the pulmonary artery. J Thorac Cardiovasc Surg, 73:887, 1977.
44 Chaitman BR, Bourassa MG, Lesperance J: Anomalous left coronary artery from pulmonary artery: 8-Year follow up after SVG bypass graft. Circulation, 51:552, 1975.
45 Thomas CSJr, Campbell WB, Alford WCJr, Burrus GR, Stoney WS: Complete repair of anomalous origin of the left coronary artery in the adult. J Thorac Cardiovasc Surg, 66:439, 1973.
46 Honey M, Lincoln JCR, Osborne MP, deBono DP: Coarctation of aorta with right aortic arch. Report of surgical correction in two cases: One with associated anomalous origin of left circumflex coronary artery from the right pulmonary artery. Br Heart J, 37:937, 1975.
47 Chaitman BR, Bourassa MG, Lesperance S, et al: Aberrant course of LAD coronary artery associated with anomalous left circumflex origin from the pulmonary artery. Circulation, 52:955, 1973.
48 Levitsky S: Anomalous LCA in the infant: Recovery of LV function following early direct aortic implantation. J Thorac Cardiovasc Surg, 79:598, 1980.
49 Yoshida Y, Emmanouilides GC, Nelson RJ, Bay-

len BG, Criley JM: Anomalous origin of the left coronary artery from the pulmonary artery. Cathet Cardiovasc Diagn, 6:293, 1980.
50 Edis AJ, Schattenberg TT, Feldt RH, Danielson GK: Congenital coronary artery fistula. Mayo Clin Proc, 47:567, 1972.
51 Effler DB, Sheldon WC, Turner JJ, Groves LK: Coronary arteriovenous fistulas: Diagnosis and surgical management. Report of fifteen cases. Surgery, 61:41, 1967.
52 Levin DC, Fellows KE, Abrams HL: Hemodynamically significant primary anomalies of the coronary arteries. Circulation, 58:25, 1978.
53 Baim DS, Kline H, Silverman JF: Bilateral coronary artery–pulmonary artery fistulas. Circulation, 65(4):810, 1982.
54 Lowe JE, Oldham HNJr, Sabiston DCJr: Surgical management of congenital coronary artery fistulas. Ann Surg, 194:373, 1981.
55 Upshaw CBJr: Congenital coronary arteriovenous fistula: Report of a case with an analysis of seventy-three reported cases. Am Heart J, 63:399, 1962.
56 Gailbraith AJ, Werner D, Cutforth RH: Fistula between left coronary artery and superior vena cava. Br Heart J, 46:99, 1981.
57 Gensini GG, Palacio A, Buonanno C: Fistula from circumflex coronary artery to superior vena cava. Circulation, 33:297, 1966.
58 Spindola-Franco H, Weisel A, Delman AJ: Anastomoses between the coronary and bronchial arteries. Radiology, 126:25, 1978.
59 Ogden JA, Stansel HC Jr: The anatomic variability of coronary arterial fistulae termination in the right and left atria. Chest, 65:76, 1964.
60 Ogden JA, Stansel JC Jr: Coronary arterial fistulas terminating in the coronary venous system. J Thorac Cardiovasc Surg, 63:172, 1972.
61 Liberthson RR, Sagar K, Berkoben JP, Weintraub RM, Levine FH: Congenital coronary arteriovenous fistula: Report of 13 patients, review of the literature and delineation of management. Circulation, 59:849, 1979.
62 Bishop JO, Mathur VS, Gwinn GA: Congenital coronary artery fistula and myocardial infarction. Chest, 65:233, 1974.
63 Reeder GS, Tajik AJ, Smith HC: Visualization of coronary artery fistula by two-dimensional echocardiography. Mayo Clin Proc, 55:185, 1980.
64 Rodgers DM, Wolf NM, Barrett MJ, et al: 2-D echocardiographic features of coronary arteriovenous fistula. Am Heart J, 104:872, 1982.
65 Yoshibawn J, Katao H, Yonagehara K, et al: Noninvasive visualization of the dilated main coronary arteries in coronary artery fistulas by cross-sectional echocardiography. Circulation, 65:600, 1982.
66 Mahoney LT, Schieken RM, Lauer RM: Spontaneous closure of a coronary artery fistula in childhood. Pediatr Cardiol, 2:311, 1982.
67 Klinke WP, Pepine CJ, Conti CR: Demonstration of an inadvertently created aorto-coronary venous anastomosis: Evidence against the clinical effectiveness of retrograde coronary venous perfusion. Cathet Cardiovasc Diagn, 5:367–370, 1979.
68 Phillips PA, Libanoff AJ: Arteriovenous communication associated with obstructive arteriosclerotic coronary artery disease and myocardial infarction. Chest, 65:106, 1974.
69 Siepser SL, Kaltman AJ, Mills N, Pughkem T, Fox AC: Coronary collateral flow after traumatic fistula between right coronary artery and right atrium. N Engl J Med, 287:754, 1972.
70 Austin SM, Applefeld MM, Turney SZ, Mech KF: Traumatic left anterior descending coronary artery to right ventricle fistula: Report of two cases. South Med J, 70:581, 1977.
70a McLarin CW, Douglas JS Jr, King SB III: Asymptomatic continuous murmur due to acquired coronary artery to right ventricular fistula. Natl Med Ass J, 73:447, 1981.
70b King SB III, Schoonmaker FW: Coronary artery to left atrial fistula in association with severe atherosclerosis and mitral stenosis: Report of surgical repair. Chest, 67:361, 1975.
71 Raabe DS Jr, Fischer JC, Brandt RL: Cavernous hemangioma of the right atrium: Presumptive diagnosis by coronary angiography. Cathet Cardiovasc Diagn, 2:389, 1976.
72 Vogelbach KH, Edmiston WA, Stenson RE: Coronary artery–left ventricular communications: A report of two cases and review of the literature. Cathet Cardiovasc Diagn, 5:159, 1979.
73 Ahmed SS, Haider B, Regan TJ: Silent left coronary artery–cameral fistula: Probable cause of myocardial ischemia. Am Heart J, 104:869, 1982.
74 MacMillan RM, Meister SG, Frankl WS: Congenital coronary arteriovenous fistula: A diagnostic challenge. Cathet Cardiovasc Diagn, 4:183, 1978.

75 Housman LB, Morse J, Litchford B, Stein R, et al: Left ventricular fistula as a cause of intractable angina pectoris. JAMA, 240:372, 1978.

76 Midell AI, Bermudez GA, Replogle R: Surgical closure of LCA-LV fistula. J Thorac Cardiovasc Surg, 74:199, 1977.

77 Wald S, Stonecypher K, Baldwin BB, Nutter DO: Anomalous origin of the right coronary artery from pulmonary artery. Am J Cardiol, 27:677, 1981.

78 Bermudez MD, Abdelnur R, Midell AI, Replogle R: Anomalous origin of the right coronary artery from the pulmonary artery with large left-to-right shunt. Cathet Cardiovasc Diagn, 5:371, 1979.

79 Mintz GS, Iskandrian AS, Benis CE et al: Myocardial ischemia in anomalous origin of the right coronary artery from the pulmonary trunk. Am J Cardiol, 51:610, 1983.

80 Byrum CJ, Blackman MS, Schneider B, Sondheimer HM, Kavey RW: Congenital atresia of the left coronary ostium and hypoplasia of the left main coronary artery. Am Heart J, 99:354, 1980.

81 Blackman MS, Schneider B, Sondheimer Henry M: Absent proximal left main coronary artery in association with pulmonary atresia. Br Heart J, 46:449, 1981.

82 Fortuin NJ, Roberts WC: Congenital atresia of the left main coronary artery. Am J Med, 50:385, 1971.

83 Mullins CE, El-Siad G, McNamara DG, Cooley DA, Treistman B, Garcia E: Atresia of the left coronary artery ostium: Repair by saphenous vein graft. Circulation, 64:989, 1972.

84 Gibson R, Nihill MR, Mullins CE, Cooley DA, Sandiford FM, McNamara DG: Congenital coronary artery obstruction associated with aortic valve anomalies in children: Report of two cases. Circulation, 64:857, 1981.

85 Wilson CS, Weaver WF, Zeman ED, Forker AD: Bilateral nonfistulous congenital coronary arterial aneurysms. Am J Cardiol, 35:319, 1975.

86 Mattern AL, Baker WP, McHale JJ, Dixon EL: Congenital coronary aneurysms with angina pectoris and myocardial infarction treated with saphenous vein bypass graft. Am J Cardiol, 30:906, 1972.

87 McMartin DE, Stone AJ, Franch RH: Multiple coronary-artery aneurysms in a child with angina pectoris. N Engl J Med, 290:669, 1974.

88 Kalke B, Edwards JE: Localized aneurysms of the coronary arteries. Angiology, 19:460, 1968.

89 Rose DF: Congenital aneurysm of the coronary artery with thrombosis and death. South Med J, 64:607, 1971.

90 Ghahramania A, Iyengar R, Cunha D, et al: Myocardial infarction due to congenital coronary arterial aneurysm (with successful saphenous vein bypass graft). Am J Cardiol, 29:863, 1972.

91 Fellows KE, Smith J, Kean JF: Preoperative angiocardiography in infants with tetralogy of Fallot: Review of 36 cases. Am J Cardiol, 47:1279, 1981.

92 VanPraagh R, Durnin RE, Jockin H, et al: Anatomically corrected malposition of the great arteries (S,D,L). Circulation, 51:20, 1975.

93 Friedman S, Ash R, Klein D, Johnson J: Anomalous single coronary artery complicating ventriculotomy in a child with cyanotic congenital heart disease. Am Heart J, 59:140, 1960.

94 Meng CCL, Friedrich AO, Lev M: Coronary artery distribution in tetralogy of Fallot. Arch Surg, 90:363, March 1965.

95 Fellows KE, Freed MD, Keane JF, et al: Results of routine preoperative coronary angiography in tetralogy of Fallot. Circulation, 51:561, 1975.

96 White RI Jr, Frech RS, Castaneda A, Amplatz K: The nature and significance of anomalous coronary arteries in tetralogy of Fallot. Am J Roentgenol, 114(2):350, 1972.

97 Dabezzi RP, Capuoli G, Aiazzi L, et al: Distribution and anomalies of coronary arteries in tetralogy of Fallot. Circulation, 61:95, 1980.

98 Hurwitz RA, Smith W, King H, Girod DA, Caldwell RL: Tetralogy of Fallot with abnormal coronary artery: 1967 to 1977. J Thorac Cardiovasc Surg, 80:129, 1980.

99 Berry BE, McGoon DC: Total correction for tetralogy of Fallot with anomalous coronary artery. Surgery, 74:894, December 1973.

100 Elliot LP, Amplatz K, Edwards JE: Coronary arterial patterns in transposition complexes. Am J Cardiol, 17:362, 1966.

101 Shaher RM, Puddie GC: Coronary arterial anatomy in complete transposition of the great vessels. Am J Cardiol, 17:355, 1966.

102 Rowlatt UF: Coronary artery distribution in complete transposition. JAMA, 179:269, 1962.

103 O'Connor WN, Cottrill CM, Johnson GL, Noonan JA, Todd EP: Pulmonary atresia with intact ventricular septum and ventriculocoronary communi-

cations: Surgical significance. Circulation, 65:805, 1982.

104 Blackman M, Schneider B, Sondheimer HM: Absent proximal left main coronary artery in association with pulmonary atresia. Br Heart J, 46:449, 1981.

105 Keeton BR, Lie JT, McGoon DC, et al: Anatomy of coronary arteries in univentricular hearts and its surgical implications. Am J Cardiol, 43:569, 1979.

106 Deanfield JE, Tommasini G, Anderson RH, MacCartney FJ: Tricuspid atresia: Analysis of coronary artery distribution and ventricular morphology. Br Heart J, 48:485, 1982.

107 Masden RR, Franch RH: Isolated congenitally corrected transposition of the great arteries, in Hurst JW (ed): *Update III: The Heart*. McGraw-Hill, New York, 1980, pp 59–84.

108 Shea PM, Lutz JF, Vieweg WVR, Coceoran FH, et al: Selective coronary arteriography in congenitally corrected transposition of the great arteries. Am J Cardiol, 44:1201, 1979.

109 Anderson KR, McGoon DC, Lie JT: Surgical significance of the coronary arterial anatomy in truncus arteriosus communis. Am J Cardiol, 41:76, 1978.

110 Shrivastava S, Edwards JE: Coronary arterial origin in persistent truncus arteriosus. Circulation, 55:551, 1977.

111 Udoff EJ, Roland JM, White RI Jr: Coronary artery anomaly in double-outlet right ventricle. Am J Roentgenol, 131:210, 1978.

112 McManus BM, Waller BF, Jones M, Epstein SF, Roberts WC: The case for preoperative coronary angiography in patients with tetralogy of Fallot and other complex congenital heart diseases. Am Heart J, 102:451, 1982.

113 Sridaromont S, Feldt R, Ritter DG, Davis GD, Edwards JE: Double outlet RV: Hemodynamics and anatomic correlations. Am J Cardiol, 38:85, 1976.

114 Lerer PK, Edwards WD: Coronary arterial anatomy in bicuspid aortic valve: Necropsy study of 100 hearts. Br Heart J, 46:142, 1981.

115 Higgins CB, Wexter L: Reversal of dominance of the coronary arterial system in isolated aortic stenosis and bicuspid aortic valve. Circulation, 52:292, 1975.

116 Vlodaver Z, Neufeld HN: The coronary arteries in coarctation of the aorta. Circulation, 37:449, 1968.

117 Huhta JC, Edwards WD, Danielson GK: Supravalvular mitral ridge containing the dominant left circumflex coronary artery. J Thorac Cardiovasc Surg, 81:577, 1981.

118 Schneeweiss A, Shem-Tov A, Neufeld HN: Coronary arterial pattern in superoinferior ventricular heart: Implications on significance of morphogenesis of this anomaly. Br Heart J, 46:559, 1981.

Chapter 4

Pathoanatomy of the Coronary Arteries

John S. Douglas, Jr., M.D.
Spencer B. King III, M.D.

PATHOANATOMY OF CORONARY ATHEROSCLEROSIS

The Atheroma

The clinical importance of atherosclerotic plaque in the coronary arteries relates either to its space-occupying characteristics, which produce narrowing of the artery, or its thrombogenic potential. Atherosclerotic lesions have a characteristic morphology and may be classified as fatty streaks, fibrous plaques, or complicated plaques. Fatty streaks, which appear in the late teens, are ubiquitous, yellowish, nonobstructing collections of lipid-laden cells of smooth muscle origin and extracellular lipid and have no clinical sequelae other than as a possible precursor of the fibrous plaque. It has been suggested that fibrous plaques originate from fatty streaks, but the absence of fibrous plaques in certain anatomic sites where fatty streaks are common indicates that all fatty streaks do not progress to fibrous plaques, and some data suggest that none do.

Stages in the development of coronary atherosclerosis are shown in Fig. 4-1. The fibrous plaque is grossly white in appearance and extends into the lumen of the coronary artery, where progressive increase in size compromises the arterial lumen with a resultant alteration in blood flow. The fibrous plaque is composed of an accumulation of smooth muscle cells laden with lipid, extracellular lipid, and cell debris covered by a fibrous cap (Fig. 4-2). Progression to an advanced or complicated lesion occurs as a result of progressive cell degeneration, intrusion of blood elements into the lesion from the lumen and media, and ultimately, calcification. The central necrotic core is rich in cholesterol esters and may have visible cholesterol crystals. Lesions become increasingly complex as

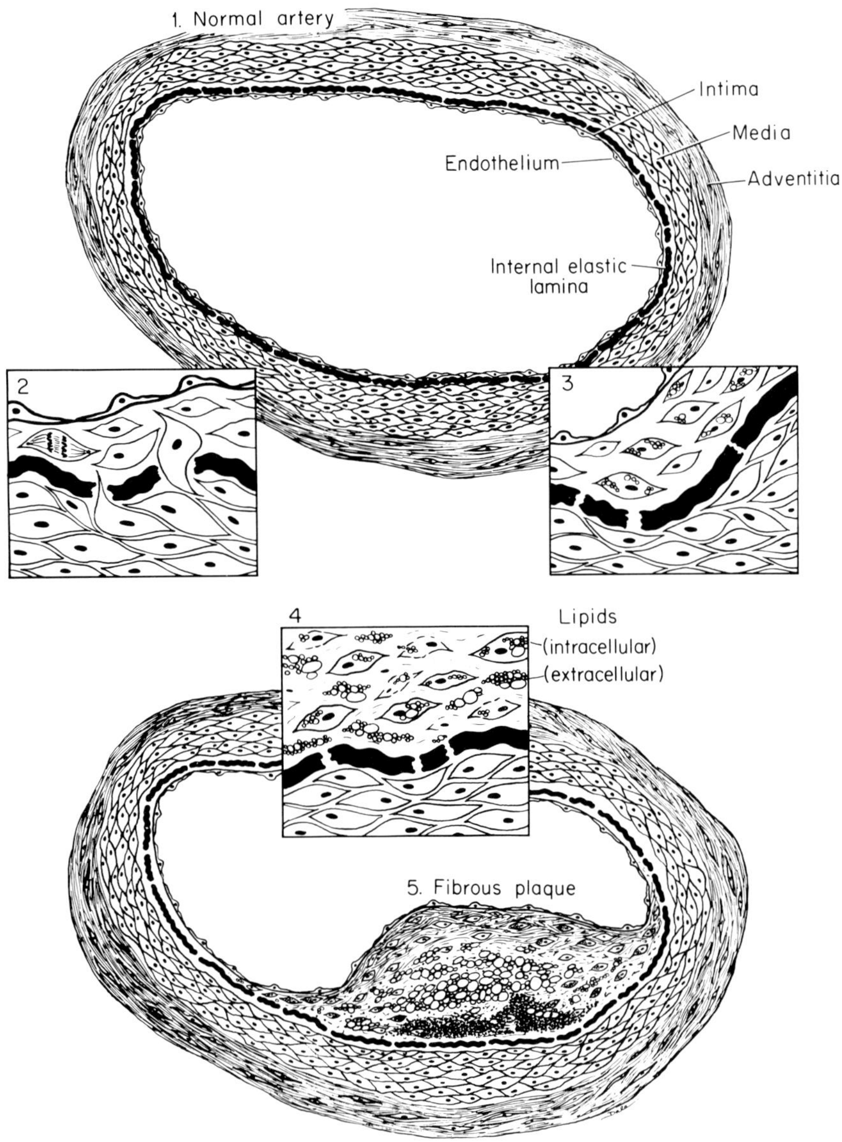

Figure 4-1 A series of possible stages in the development of the various lesions of atherosclerosis. (1) The appearance of a normal muscular artery and its component layers: The intima bounded by endothelium and internal elastic lamina, the media, and the adventitia. In children and young adults the intima is thin and contains only an occasional smooth muscle cell; with age it slowly and uniformly increases in thickness and cell content. (2) The first phase of a developing lesion in atherosclerosis; a focal thickening of the intima consists of an increase in smooth muscle cells and extracellular matrix. Smooth muscle cells are shown proliferating within the intima; two are in the process of migrating through fenestrae of the internal elastic lamina. Subsequent to or possibly concomitant with intimal smooth muscle proliferation, accumulation of intercellular lipid deposits (3) or extracellular lipid (4), or both, occurs resulting in a fatty streak. A fibrous plaque (5) may result from a continued accumulation of a connective tissue cap covering increased numbers of smooth muscle cells laden with lipids, extracellular lipid, and cell debris overlying a deeper extracellular pool of lipid. A complicated lesion may form as a result of continuing cell degeneration, ingress of blood constituents, and calcification superimposed upon the elements present in the fibrous plaque. *(From Glomset JA, Russell R: Atherosclerosis and the arterial smooth muscle cell, Science, 180:1332, 1973. Reproduced with permission of author and publisher.)*

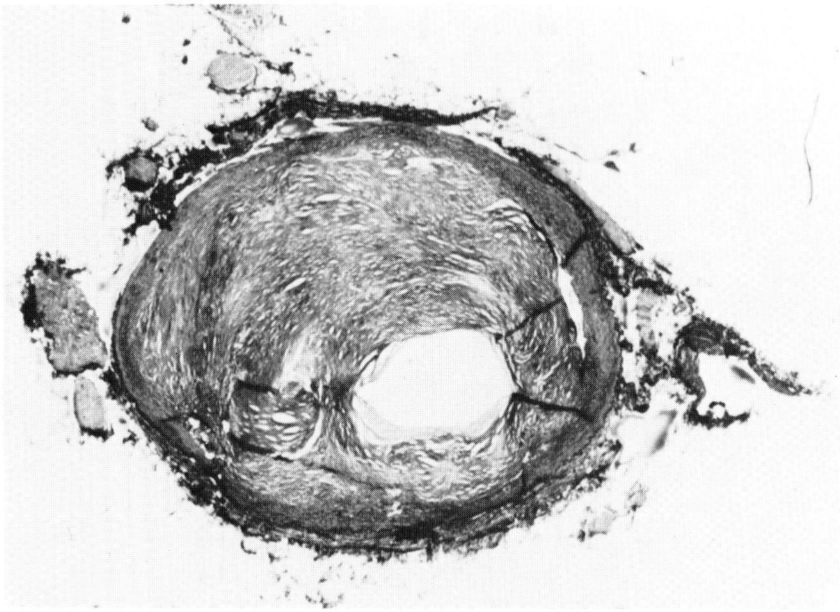

Figure 4-2 Photomicrograph of a fibrous plaque in a coronary artery causing major luminal narrowing and eccentricity. *(From Hurst JW, King SB III, Walter PF, Friesinger GC, Edwards JE: Atherosclerotic heart disease: Angina pectoris, myocardial infarction, and other manifestations of myocardial ischemia, in Hurst JW (ed-in-chief): The Heart (5th ed), McGraw-Hill, New York, 1982, p 10–11. Reproduced with permission of author and publisher.)*

further hemorrhage and calcification occur. Rupture of the fibrous cap at the intimal surface may occur, with exposure of the necrotic core of thromboplastic substances (Fig. 4-3). Thrombus formation on the surface of the ulcerated plaque may result in an acute arterial occlusion and acute myocardial infarction. Thrombi may lyse spontaneously or organize and lead to an increase in plaque size. The process of plaque rupture may liberate the necrotic core, with reduction in the volume of the plaque as the contents of the core are embolized distally. As the atherosclerotic process continues,

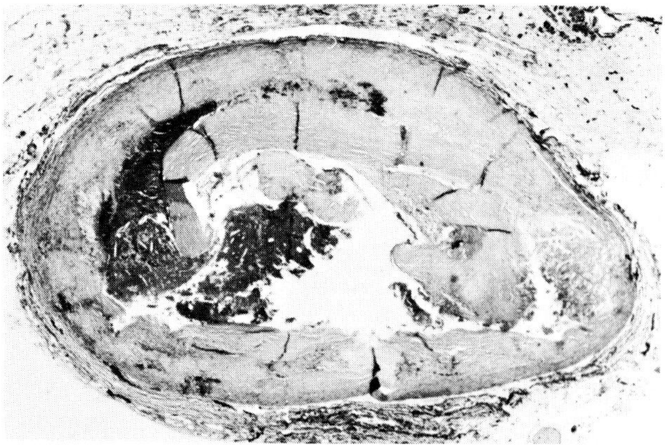

Figure 4-3 Photomicrograph of an atherosclerotic coronary artery. At the extreme left of the illustration is a focus of hemorrhage within the atherosclerotic intima. There has been rupture of the overlying connective tissue, with extrusion of atheromatous material into the lumen of the vessel. Such material may embolize. Also, the process of the intimal hemorrhage with rupture of the overlying tissue may serve as a nucleus of thrombosis. *(From Hurst JW, King SB III, Walter PF, Friesinger GC, Edward JE: Atherosclerotic heart disease: Angina pectoris, myocardial infarction, and other manifestations of myocardial ischemia, in Hurst JW (ed-in-chief): The Heart (5th ed); McGraw-Hill, New York, 1982, p 10–12. Reproduced with permission of author and publisher.)*

the smooth muscle of the media frequently atrophies, with resultant ectasia or occasionally frank aneurysm formation.

Since the atherosclerotic process is progressive, capable of inducing sudden or gradual alterations in anatomy, findings at one point in time may differ strikingly from those at another. Progression of a lesion to total vessel occlusion, recanalization of an occluded vessel, regression of a lesion, and healing of an ulceration or localized arterial dissection may occur.

Distribution of Atheroma

The distribution of atherosclerosis along the course of the coronary arteries is of critical importance clinically due to the ability to surgically bypass or perform angioplasty for proximal disease. Early pathological studies noted a tendency for more proximal involvement. Vlodaver and Edwards reported that obstructive atherosclerotic lesions were localized to the proximal portion of the left anterior descending coronary artery in 76 percent of the patients while 17 percent had equal proximal and distal disease and 7 percent had only distal disease.[1] The distribution of disease in the circumflex coronary artery paralleled that of the anterior descending artery. Disease in the mid–right coronary artery exceeded all sites in frequency in this early study, but in a later study Vlodaver reported that disease was equally frequent in the proximal and middle segments of the right coronary artery with relative sparing of the distal segment.[2] Our observation in over 20,000 coronary arteriograms supports these early pathological observations. The frequency of significant atherosclerotic lesions in proximal segments of all three coronary arteries exceeds that in the distal segments by factors exceeding a range of 3 to 5:1 (see Chap. 13). Although atherosclerosis may be a focal disease, once the disease becomes manifest clinically, it is characteristic that lesions are multiple and have a strong tendency to involve more than one coronary artery.

Angiographic Assessment

Necropsy studies indicate that rather diffuse proliferative thickening of the intima occurs in patients with clinically severe coronary artery disease.[3,4] Arnette et al. reported that 90 percent of 465 5-mm segments of coronary arteries examined in 10 patients with fatal coronary artery disease had greater than 25 percent cross-sectional narrowing and 75 percent had over 50 percent narrowing as defined by the degree of luminal obliteration within the internal elastic membrane on histological examination. These observations, although in undistended postmortem arteries, indicate that diffuse intimal thickening does occur with coronary atherosclerosis and that regions of focal luminal narrowing which appear to be only 50 percent reduced by angiography may be 75 percent reduced from the original lumen diameter defined by the internal elastic membrane on histological examination. This would result in angiographic underestimation of the degree of coronary artery narrowing. Several studies suggest, however, that aging, poststenotic turbulence, and the atherosclerotic process may result in significant dilatation of the medial layer of the artery.[5,6] If the internal elastic membrane is then used to define the normal lumen, there will be an overestimation of the appropriate diameter of the lumen by the histological method just as the angiographic method may lead to underestimation of its size. Comparing quantitative angiographic methods with pressure-injected postmortem coronary artery specimens, Brown et al. obtained an excellent correlation between computer-predicted angiographic luminal area and planimetered absolute luminal areas,[7] validating the clinical utility of angiographic methods.

Other potential sources of angiographic error derive from the fact that the distribution of the intimal lesion of atherosclerosis is usually not circumferential. Rather, one arc of the vessel is characteristically more involved.[1] The asymmetrical accumulation of the atheroma in the vessel wall accounts for the common eccentric position of the lumen. As seen on histological sections cut through the atheromatous vessel, the appearance of the lumen is commonly noted to be that of an exaggerated ellipse, and may be frankly slitlike or irregular in shape, even stellate. Vlodaver[1] reported that in unselected sections of atherosclerotic coronary arteries, these slitlike lumina occurred in 29 percent of sections, whereas the incidence of central and eccentric lumina was 30 and 40 percent, respectively. The importance of the slitlike lumen is that the degree of stenosis may be underestimated angiographically since the artery would be seen as severely narrowed only in the angiographic projection that parallels the long axis of the slit. Similarly, the crescent-shaped lumen, a variant of the slitlike lumen, may not appear significantly narrowed in any view. In both the slitlike and crescent-shaped lumen, lucency due to reduced concentration of contrast medium in the diseased segment may be the only clue. Vlodaver et al. in a study correlating postmortem histological and angiographic findings noted that slitlike lumina were present as postmortem examination in 68 percent of 22 segments taken from areas of angiographic underestimation (false-negative reading) and in 33 percent in areas of agreement.[2] Segments prone to angiographic underestimation were the midsegment of the right coronary artery, the left main coronary artery, and the proximal one-half of the circumflex coronary artery. However, the validity of these observations on postmortem coronary arteries, which were fixed and embedded in a nonpressurized state, has been questioned. Liu[8] studied arterial luminal shape in severely diseased arteries which were fixed under physiological pressure and found that 62 percent of narrowed lumina were round or oval with a major-to-minor axis ratio of less than 2.0. Only 9 percent of all diseased lumina had a major-to-minor axis ratio of over 3, and none greater than 5. They stated "in contrast to the general belief, truly slitlike lumina did not exist in our series; this is probably due to proper distension of the lumen in the arteries studied." Brown et al.,[9] in a quantitative angiographic study, reported that 95 percent of diseased lumina studied had a ratio of minimum diameters (d min RAO/d min LAO) between 0.73 and 1.33, and none below 0.55 or above 1.55. These observations were "not consistent with the natural occurrence of very many slitlike lesions" and suggested that the diseased arterial lumen in vivo adopted a configuration that minimized flow resistance, that is, a round-to-oval configuration. These studies emphasized that casual examination of the postmortem specimen is not neccessarily the gold standard for determining coronary arterial luminal narrowing.

In a study comparing angiography, pathological examination, and regional myocardial blood flow, Marcus et al. reported finding unobstructed coronary angiograms and only modest impairment of myocardial perfusion despite the presence of obstructive lesions of the coronary arteries on pathological examination. The studies lead the authors to state that the undistended vessel examined pathologically differs from the physiological state, where the atherosclerotic lesion is outwardly displaced by luminal pressure. The authors hypothezied that medial atrophy associated with atherosclerotic process contributed to this outward displacement.[10]

WHAT CONSTITUTES SIGNIFICANT STENOSIS?

In the clinical evaluation of patients with coronary artery disease, it becomes important to define that degree of luminal stenosis that constitutes a significant lesion. Two important aspects of this consideration are the *hemodynamic effects* of the luminal narrowing and the *prognostic significance* of the stenosis. The latter estimate incorporates such factors as the risk of progression of disease and untoward cardiac events. Levin attempted to define angiographic morphological features of coronary stenosis associated with increased risk of coronary artery occlusion.[11] Irregular borders of the stenosis and intraluminal lucencies correlated with the presence of a ruptured or hemorrhagic plaque, a partially occluding or recanalized thrombus, or a combination thereof and suggested a poor prognosis. Factors determining the hemodynamic effect of the coronary stenosis have been the subject of intense investigation,[12–15] but there is no general agreement on the degree of narrowing that constitutes a "significant" stenosis.

Based on fundamental equations describing fluid mechanics of coronary artery stenoses, it has been pointed out that the *minimal luminal diameter is the primary determinant of the hemodynamic impact of a lesion.*[13,14] Coronary resistance is inversely proportional to the fourth power of vessel diameter. Although percent stenosis (which incorporates the normal adjacent luminal diameter as the denominator) is theoretically a less precise estimate of hemodynamic impact than minimal diameter, percent stenosis has evolved as a useful clinical expression of disease severity. The American Heart Association committee report recommended that 80 percent reduction in luminal diameter be considered a significant lesion based on the fact that pressure gradients at surgery were present only with lesions of this magnitude.[16] Potential problems of angiographic underestimation due to diffuse intimal disease of the "normal" adjacent vessel wall and overestimation of stenosis due to vessel ectasia are apparent and have been discussed previously. Experimental studies[17] using open chest dogs have shown that resting coronary artery blood flow remains normal until coronary artery luminal diameter reduction exceeds 85 percent (Fig. 4-4). Lesser degrees of stenosis were compensated for by reduction in coronary arteriolar resistance. When the coronary peripheral vascular bed was fully dilated, hyperemic flow was reduced when luminal diameter narrowing exceeded 45 percent equivalent to 70 percent cross-sectional stenosis. That is, a 45 percent diameter narrowing became a "signifi-

Figure 4-4 The relation of resting mean blood flow (dotted line) and hyperemic flows (solid line) to percentage of arterial diameter reduction. Flows are expressed as ratios to control resting mean values at the beginning of the experiment. The shaded area represents the range of values measured in individual dogs: r = correlation coefficient; SQ DEV = mean square of deviations. *(From Gould KL, Lipscomb K, Hamilton GW: Physiologic basis for assessing critical coronary stenosis, Am J Cardiol, 33:87, 1974. Reproduced with permission of author and publisher.)*

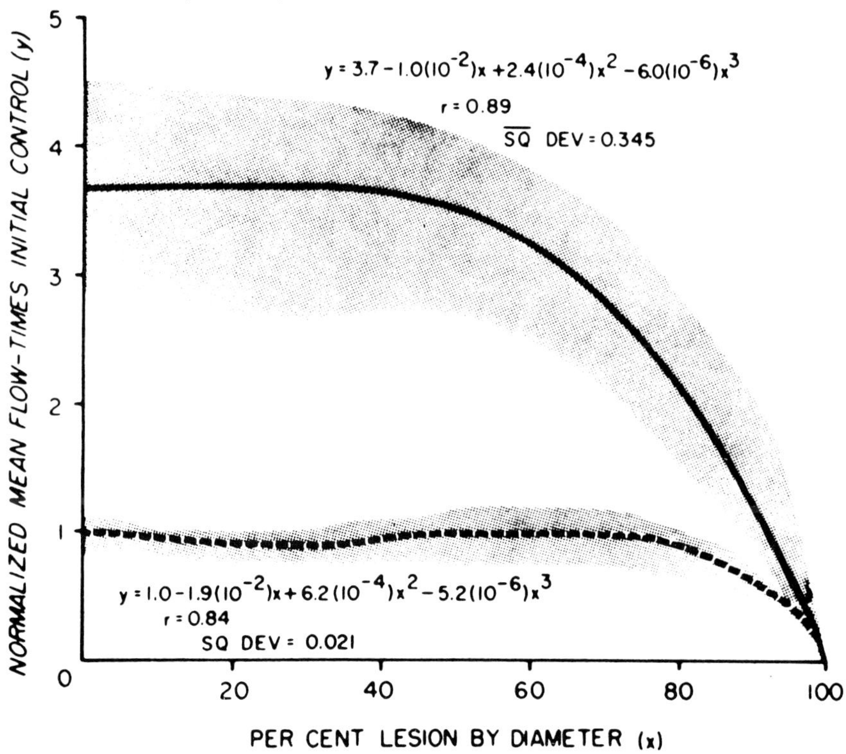

cant'' stenosis at high coronary flow rates. This report and others[12] show that small changes in luminal diameter in vessels with over 80 percent stenosis may produce large changes in pressure gradient and reduction in coronary blood flow.

Confirmatory clinical data has been reported in studies correlating exercise-induced ischemia as detected by myocardial perfusion scintigraphy and blood pool imaging techniques with coronary angiography. Massie[18] studied 25 patients and noted that in 8 of 9 patients with cross-sectional stenosis less than 70 percent, myocardial images were normal; in 14 of 16 patients with over 70 percent stenosis, scans were abnormal. Peterson et al.,[19] using pressure gradients determined at coronary angioplasty and percent coronary stenosis determined at coronary angiography, found that stenoses of 75 percent and pressure gradients of 40 best separated patients into subgroups with and without evidence of exercise ischemia by radionuclide angiography. The impact of stenosis length on coronary blood flow has been the subject of some debate. Logan[12] reported that 10-fold increases in stenosis length produced only modest changes in coronary flow. Feldman, however, showed convincingly that short 40 to 60 percent narrowings had no significant resting hemodynamic effect, but increasing the length of the narrowings to 10 to 15 mm consistently resulted in significant pressure gradients and flow reductions[20] (see Fig. 4-5).

The above experimental data are consistent with clinical observations that anginal symptoms usually do not occur with less than 50 percent cross-sectional stenosis, that they may be present with over 75 percent stenosis, and that angina at rest is usually associated with over 90 percent stenosis. The relationship between resistance and luminal cross-sectional area demonstrates that in far-advanced disease slight progression can produce significant hemodynamic changes.

EFFECTS OF CORONARY ARTERIAL VASOMOTOR TONE

It has been suggested and demonstrated in patients that ''normal'' variations in coronary arterial smooth muscle tone superimposed upon fixed atherosclerotic lesions may produce clinical ischemic events.[21–23] This phenomenon may explain the development of rest pain in patients with subcritical lesions and therefore may be a cause for angiographic underestimation of the importance of a given atherosclerotic lesion (see Fig. 4-6). The importance of this phenomenon and its frequency are unknown. Some have suggested that a dynamic interaction between the pathological features of atherosclerosis and ''normal'' amounts of coronary smooth muscle shortening account for the clinical features in a majority of patients with ischemic heart disease.[22] Preliminary studies attempting to address this problem have suggested that changes in coronary vasomotor tone superimposed on fixed lesions may not be a common cause of variable angina threshold and coronary reserve.[24]

The development of excessive coronary arterial tone, that is, frank coronary artery spasm, is exhibited in its purest form in the variant angina patient who has angiographically normal coronary arteries which spontaneously or on pharmacological or other provocation undergo marked constriction with focal luminal obliteration, angina, and ST-segment elevation.[25–29] Coronary spasm has been amply documented as a cause of spontaneous[30–32] or exertion-induced myocardial ischemia,[33–35] myocardial infarction,[36–39] arrhythmia,[40–42] syncope,[43] and sudden death.[44,45] The primary mechanism is a decrease in regional coronary blood flow due to focal vasoconstriction. Coronary spasm frequently occurs at a segment of the coronary artery that has atheromatous involvement.[46,47] Prostacyclin (PGI 2), which may regulate regional myocardial blood flow by its vasodilator effect, has been shown to be in reduced concentration in the intima in and around an atheroma, and this may sensitize this area to the development of smooth muscle contraction.[47] In contrast, an important vasoconstrictor, thromboxane A2, is synthesized by platelets and released during platelet activation and may locally stimulate coronary artery spasm. Its metabolites have been reported to be elevated in patients with coronary artery spasm.[48] The details of these and other proposed pathophysiolog-

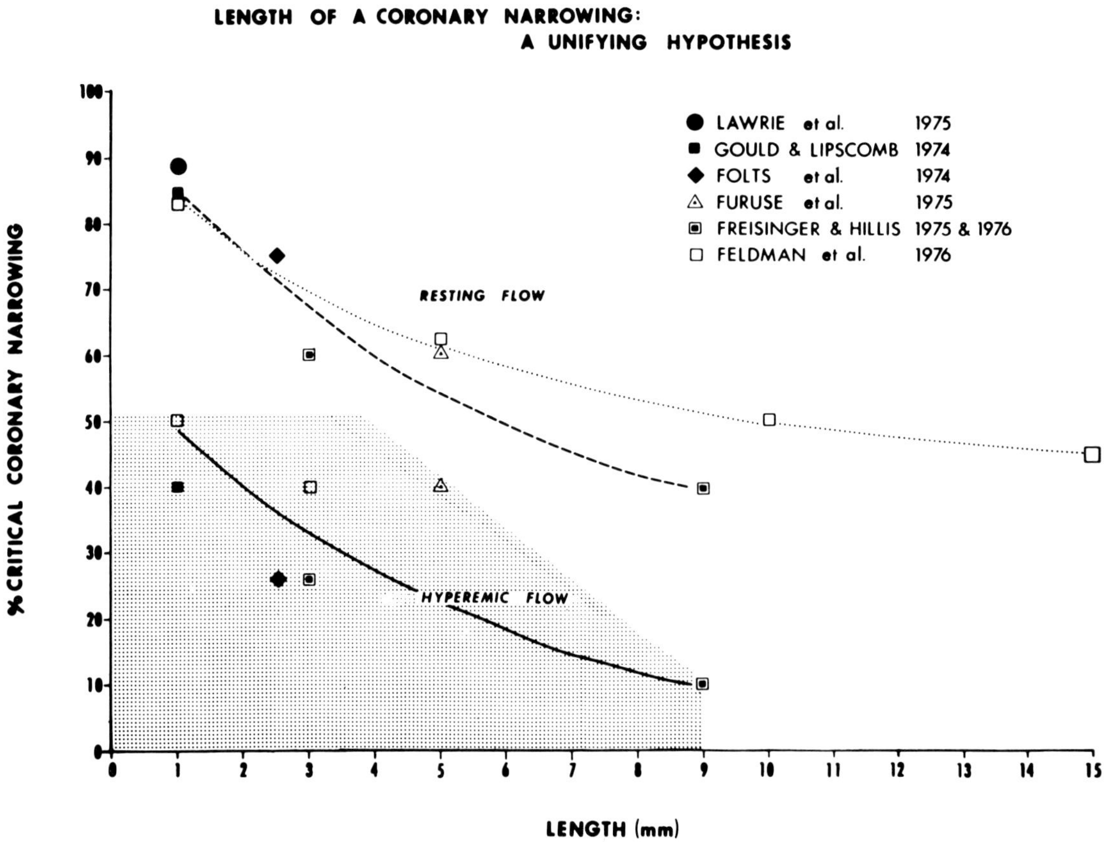

Figure 4-5 This figure illustrates the role that narrowing length plays in determination of critical coronary narrowing. Data at rest and during reactive hyperemia from a number of investigations were analyzed with regard to length of narrowing (horizontal axis) and plotted against the reduction in diameter reported to alter flow significantly (vertical axis). *From Feldman RL, Nichols WW, Pepine CJ, Conti CR: Hemodynamic significance of the length of a coronary arterial narrowing. Am J Cardiol, 41:865, 1978.)*

ical interactions in coronary spasm are amply described elsewhere.[47–53]

Recognizing coronary spasm is clinically important since specific therapy with calcium antagonists will eliminate symptoms in 70 percent and reduce the symptoms in another 20 percent of patients.[54] Usual therapy of angina pectoris with beta-blocking agents may exacerbate and rarely relieves symptoms due to coronary artery spasm.[55] In addition, percutaneous balloon angioplasty is less effective in the presence of coronary artery spasm due to a higher recurrence of stenosis,[56] and coronary bypass surgery[57] or other surgical procedures[58] are usually not indicated in the absence of significant fixed atherosclerotic stenosis. The long-term outlook for patients with coronary artery spasm on medical treatment is excellent. Bott-Silverman and Heupler[59] reported no cardiac deaths in a long-term follow-up, and Waters[60] noted almost 50 percent of patients had spontaneous remission and could be weaned from medical treatment.

The diagnosis of coronary artery spasm is an angiographic one; however, only a small proportion of patients have spontaneous coronary spasm during coronary arteriography. Waters in a consecutive series of 162 variant angina patients noted only 32 had spontaneous spasm during the study,[61] and Maseri noted only 17 of 107 patients had spon-

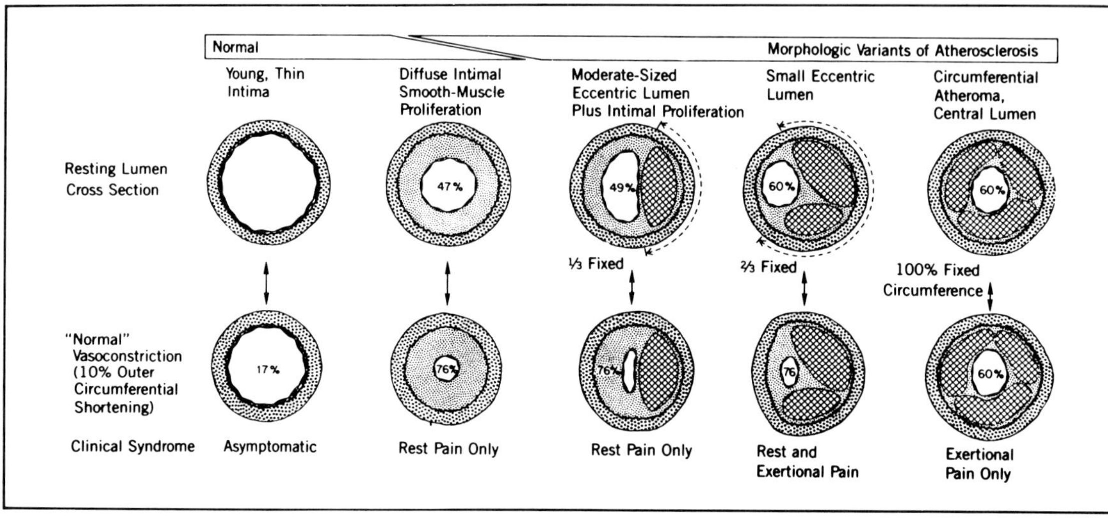

Figure 4-6 Morphologic spectrum of normal and diseased coronary artery cross sections. In regions where smooth muscle viability and flexibility are retained, 10 percent isovolumetric outer circumferential shortening caused dramatic changes in lumen caliber. Size of resting and constricted lumen in each section determines associated anginal syndrome. *(From Brown BG: Coronary vasospasm: Observations linking the clinical spectrum of ischemic heart disease to the dynamic pathology of coronary atherosclerosis, Arch Intern Med, 141:716, 1981.)*

taneous spasm at coronary arteriography.[62] Provocative testing with ergonovine maleate has evolved as the method of choice in attempting to document the presence of coronary artery spasm.[27,28,61,64] Ergonovine produces coronary artery constriction in a dose-related manner. Constriction by approximately 20 percent is observed in most patients with normal coronary arteries. A positive test consists of marked focal constriction of the coronary artery associated with chest pain. ST-segment elevation is common, although ST-segment depression may occur. In most cases, coronary artery spasm is promptly relieved by intracoronary or sublingual nitroglycerin. Death has been reported as a complication of ergonovine testing due to irreversible coronary artery spasm.[63] Other methods of provocative testing, such as exercise testing and a cold pressor test have been advocated, but Waters in comparing these three techniques found ergonovine to be a much more sensitive test.[62]

Since there is some inherent risk in administering ergonovine, considerable judgment is necessary in determining which patients may benefit since there are no generally accepted guidelines for its administration. Serious complications of ergonovine testing due to irreversible spasm have occurred most often in patients with histories compatible with coronary artery spasm, that is, rest angina and ST-segment elevation, and in patients to whom larger doses of ergonovine were administered. For these reasons, we have not felt it necessary to give ergonovine provocation in those patients with bona fide ST-segment elevation with angina whose coronary arteriogram appears normal. When coronary spasm is strongly suspected but confirmation by provocative testing is needed, small increments of ergonovine beginning with as little as 0.025 mg are administered with nitroglycerin 200 μg ready for intracoronary administration. If right coronary artery spasm is suspected, a transvenous pacemaker is inserted first. Virtually all patients with a positive ergonovine test will respond to a cumulative dose of 0.2 mg. Contraindications to ergonovine are acute myocardial infarction, high-grade stenosis of a major epicardial coronary artery, significant narrowing of the left main coronary artery, severe hypertension, or severe aortic stenosis.

WHAT EFFECTS DO COLLATERALS HAVE?

Although the coronary artery is an end artery with respect to its microcirculation, extensive arterial anastomotic communications exist from birth linking major coronary trunks and branches. These interarterial anastomoses, which exceed 100 μm in diameter in the normal heart, progressively enlarge as a long-range adaptation to coronary atherosclerosis. Normally, collaterals are not demonstrated angiographically unless there is complete or subtotal occlusion of one coronary artery resulting in a substantial blood pressure gradient between distal arteries. However, collaterals may rarely be visualized during forceful and excessive injections of contrast medium through a catheter wedged in the mouth of a coronary artery.

Following acute occlusion of a coronary artery, indexes of collateral function—peripheral coronary pressure and blood flow into the ischemic area—show a variable, but small, collateral circulation. Consequently, severe myocardial ischemia and/or infarction are the usual result of major coronary arterial occlusion in humans. It is unclear why some patients develop myocardial infarction with coronary occlusion while others with similar anatomy do not, but collateral function must be an important determinant. In patients with normal coronary arteries, mean peripheral coronary pressure is roughly 20 percent of aortic pressure,[65] whereas symptomatic patients undergoing coronary bypass surgery have been shown to have peripheral coronary pressure of 25 to 40 percent of aortic blood pressure.[65,66] During percutaneous coronary angioplasty it has been shown that the peripheral coronary artery pressure of totally occluded arteries is significantly higher than it is for arteries with less than complete occlusion.[67] Intraoperative[68] and coronary angiographic studies[69] of patients with chronic coronary artery disease have estimated collateral flow at 50 to 80 percent of normal basal levels.

Although collateral flow is difficult to study in humans, it is clear that collaterals preserve myocardial tissue, although to a variable and limited degree.[70] One has only to observe the coronary arteriogram of a patient with triple vessel occlusion and normal left ventricular function to be convinced. In clinical studies the presence of collaterals has been associated with smaller infarctions,[71–72a] a greater likelihood that nitroglycerin will improve contraction abnormalities of the left ventricle,[73] the presence of exercise defects on thallium-201 myocardial perfusion imaging,[74] and with better myocardial salvage following streptokinase thrombolysis for acute myocardial infarction[75] even when the procedure is delayed.[76] Patients with good collateral function as evidenced by a high peripheral coronary artery pressure at percutaneous coronary angioplasty are less likely to suffer severe left ventricular damage when emergency surgery is done for acute coronary occlusion complicating the angioplasty procedure. It has been suggested and seems plausible that collateral function may protect against a lethal outcome of myocardial infarction.[77]

Well-developed collaterals have been considered to function in a manner comparable to a 90 percent stenosis, that is, allowing relatively normal resting myocardial blood flow, but with a severely limited capacity to augment flow during conditions of increased demand, as with exercise.[78] Therefore patients with substantial myocardium served by collateral flow commonly have signs and symptoms of ischemia. However, in contrast to the situation that exists with a 90 percent stenosis, collateral flow from a patent neighboring artery is not subject to acute occlusion and is therefore associated with a more stable condition.

For the coronary angiographer, the presence or absence of collaterals has several implications: (1) Collaterals indicate severe disease. Collateral filling of a coronary artery without apparent high-grade proximal obstruction implies that the stenosis was simply overlooked and further evaluation is indicated. (2) Absence of any collateral filling of an apparently occluded artery is unusual and dictates a need to look further. Several possibilities exist: (a) The occlusion may have been quite recent. (b) The coronary artery supplying collateral flow may not have been selectively injected. A knowledge of routes of collateral flow is required to ensure that this does not occur (see below). (c) Nitroglycerin administration may be needed to enhance collateral filling to allow visualization. (d) Absence of an artery on angiography and no evidence of collateralization raises the possibility that the artery may not be occluded, but simply arising anomalously. Similarly, failure to demonstrate collateral filling of an occluded artery receiving an apparently occluded bypass graft suggests that the graft was not injected and should be searched for further. (3) The presence of a rich collateral network to a poorly contracting left ventricular wall segment suggests the presence of viable muscle. Left ventriculography following nitroglycerin may show improved wall motion, and thallium-201 myocardial perfusion imaging commonly indicates ischemic muscle in this setting.

Development of coronary artery collaterals may occur throughout the coronary arterial tree, connecting all three major coronary arteries. However, coronary collaterals are most common within the interventricular septum and interatrial septum, at the apex of the heart, over the right ventricle, and between the atrial branches. Collaterals that bridge branches of the same major coronary artery are *intracoronary collaterals* and those that bridge major coronary arteries are *intercoronary collaterals*. While there is no established classification of collaterals, it is helpful to consider collateral routes to the major coronary arteries roughly in their order of frequency of occurrence.

Collateral Flow to Occluded Left Anterior Descending Coronary Artery

Intracoronary communications to the distal left anterior descending coronary artery (LAD) occur via (1) small threadlike periobstruction communications which may be enlarged vaso vasorum, (2) collaterals diagonal to LAD (Fig. 4-7*e*), or (3) septal collaterals (Fig. 4-7*b*). *Intercoronary* collateral circulation to the distal anterior descending artery includes (1) anastomosis between the right ventricular branches of the right coronary artery and the anterior descending (Fig. 4-7*a*); (2) anastomosis from the conus artery or Vieussens' annulus (Fig. 4-7*d*) (It is important to note that the conus artery arises as a separate orifice in 50 percent of instances, and selective injection of the small conus artery may be required.); and (3) anastomosis from the posterior descending artery via the septum (Fig. 4-7*g*) or around the apex of the heart to the anterior descending artery (Fig. 4-7*f*); also (4) obtuse marginal arteries may communicate with the diagonal arteries with retrograde flow to the anterior descending, or obtuse marginals may communicate with the anterior descending artery directly (Fig. 4-7*c*) and (5) the AV-node artery may communicate via septal branches with the anterior descending artery.

Collateral Flow to Occluded Right Coronary Artery

Intracoronary collateral flow may include the following: (1) There may be small bridging arteries around the occlusion. (2) Communications between right ventricular branches are common (Fig. 4-8*d*). (3) Kugel's artery, the arteria anastomotica auricularis magna to the atrioventricular (AV) node, may pass from the proximal right or circumflex coronary artery via the interatrial septum to the distal right coronary artery (Fig. 4-8*e*). (4) Less frequently, the posterior descending artery is supplied by right ventricular branches (Fig. 4-8*h*). (5) Rarely the sinus node branch of the right coronary artery communicates with the distal right coronary by circuitous atrial branches (Fig. 4-8*i*).

Intercoronary collaterals include the following: (1) The distal right coronary artery may receive collaterals via the septum from the anterior descending artery (Fig. 4-8*a*) or around the apex from the LAD (Fig. 4-8*f*) or from the LAD via right ventricular branches (Fig. 4-8*j*). (2) Collaterals may course from the circumflex coronary artery in the AV groove to the distal right coronary artery (Fig. 4-8*b*) or from obtuse marginal branches on the posterolateral surface of the left ventricle to the posterior descending artery (Fig. 4-8*c*). The left atrial

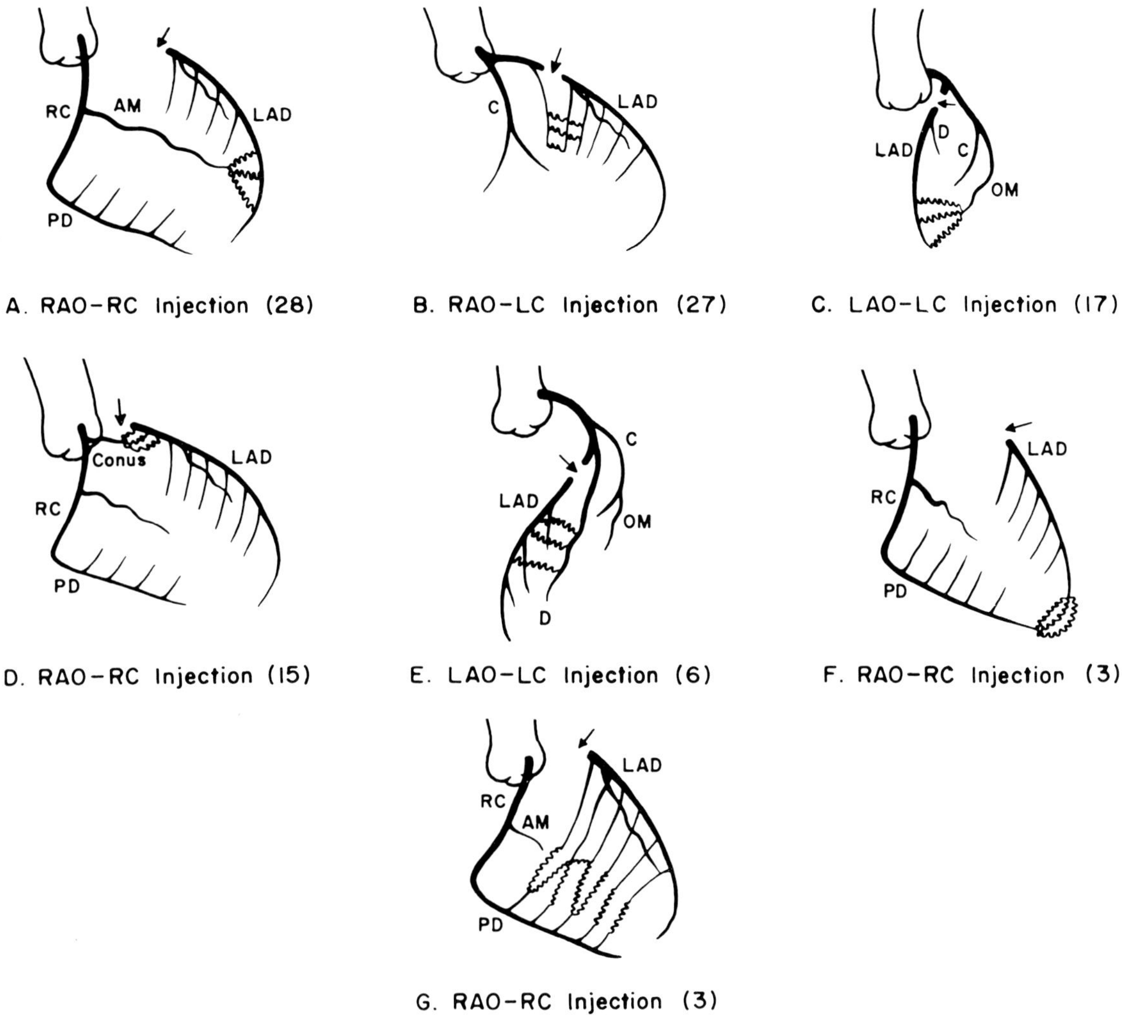

Figure 4-7 Routes of collateral supply in left anterior descending coronary artery (LAD) occlusion (a–g). RAO = right anterior oblique projection, LAO = left anterior oblique projection, LC = left coronary artery, RC = right coronary artery, D = diagonal branch of the left anterior descending coronary artery, AM = anterior marginal branch of the right coronary artery, OM = obtuse marginal branch of the circumflex coronary artery, LAD = left anterior descending artery, PD = posterior descending artery, C = circumflex, Numbers in parenthesis signify frequency with which the given collateral root occurred in this series. *(From Levin DC: Pathways and functional significance of the coronary collateral circulation, Circulation, 50:831, 1974. Reproduced with permission of the author and the American Heart Association.)*

circumflex is a common communicator between the circumflex and right coronary artery (Fig. 4-8*g*).

Collateral Flow to an Occluded Distal Circumflex Coronary Artery

Collateral routes of flow to an occluded distal circumflex coronary artery include the following: *Intracoronary* collaterals are (1) bridging arteries around the occlusion, (2) left atrial circumflex artery (Fig. 4-9*a*) and (3) obtuse marginal to obtuse marginal communications (Fig. 4-9*b*). *Intercoronary* collaterals can involve (1) communication from diagonal to obtuse marginal bridging the LAD and circumflex systems (Fig. 4-9*c*), or (2) the posterior

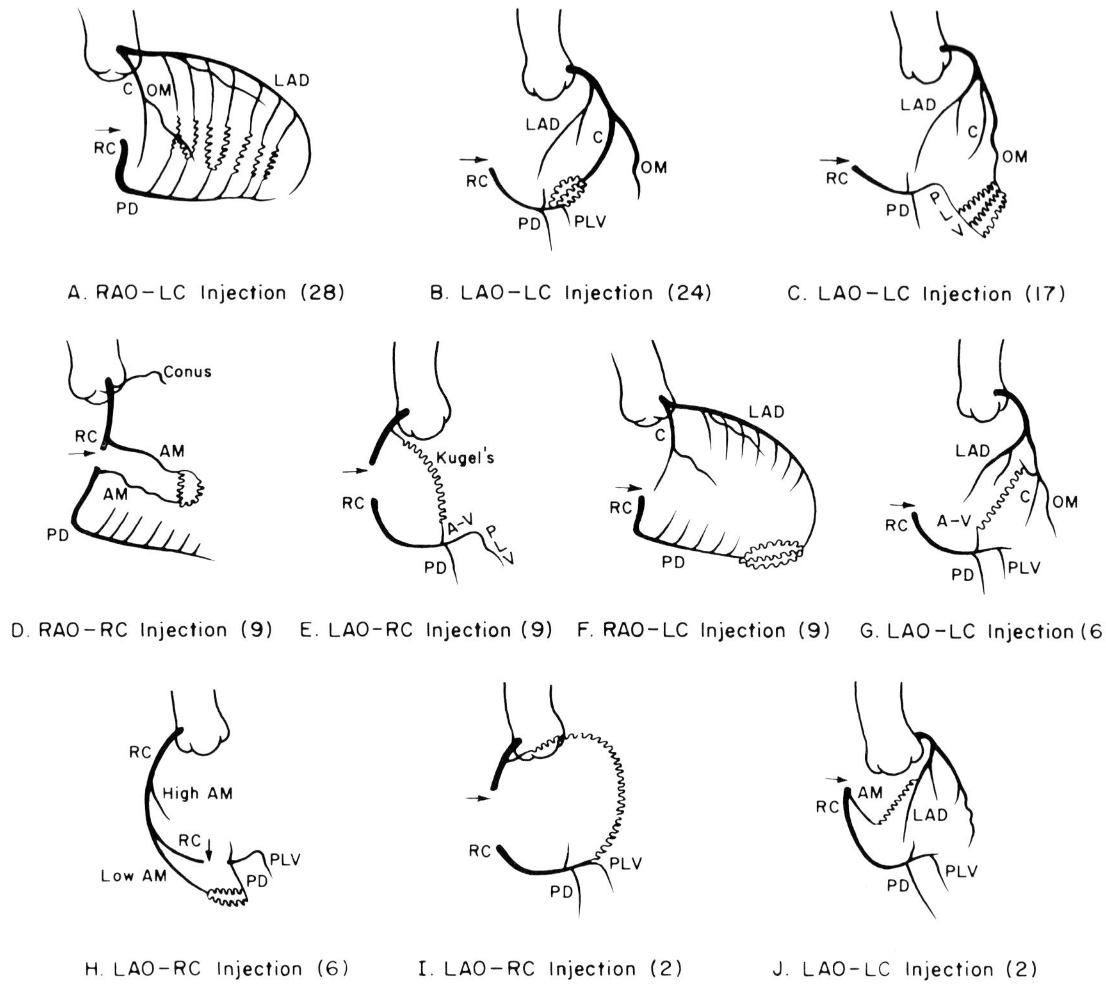

Figure 4-8 Routes of collateral supply in right coronary artery occlusion (a–j). Abbreviations as in Fig. 4-7. A-V = artery to the atrioventricular node; PLV = posterior left branch of the right coronary artery. *(From Levin DC: Pathways and functional significance of the coronary collateral circulation, Circulation, 50:831, 1974. Reproduced with permission of the author and the American Heart Association.)*

descending (Fig. 4-9*d*) or left ventricular branch of the right coronary artery (Fig. 4-9*e*) collateralizing the circumflex or obtuse marginal branches.

MYOCARDIAL BRIDGING

Bridging of epicardial coronary arteries by left ventricular myocardium is a relatively common finding at autopsy and is recognized at angiography by systolic compression of the intramyocardial segment of the artery (see Fig. 4-10). Bridging is found almost exclusively in the left anterior descending coronary artery, and the junction of the proximal and middle thirds is the most common site. Morales et al.[79] reported that 27 percent of consecutive autopsies had an intramyocardial left anterior descending coronary segment, and Kramer in a careful analysis of 658 otherwise normal coronary arteriograms at the Cleveland Clinic reported that 12 percent had myocardial bridges; 1.7 percent of

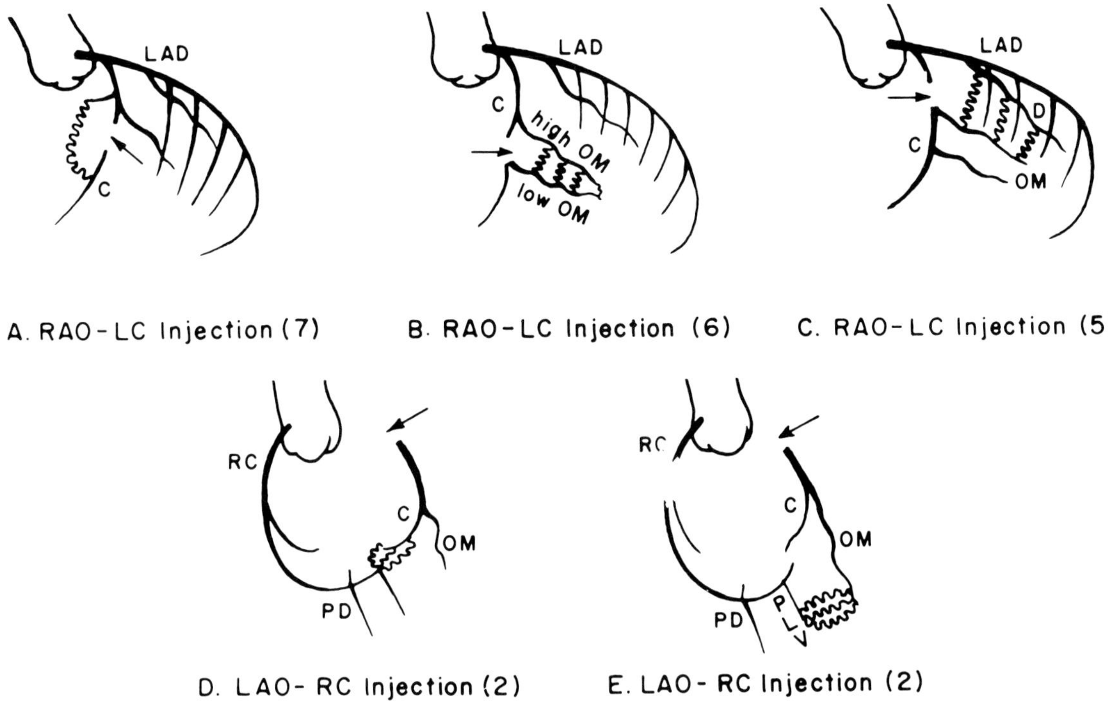

Figure 4-9 Routes of collateral supply in circumflex coronary artery occlusion (a–e). Abbreviations as in Figs. 4-7 and 4-8. *(From Levin DC: Pathways and functional significance of the coronary collateral circulation, Circulation, 50:831, 1974. Reproduced with permission of the author and the American Heart Association.)*

the total had systolic compression of over 50 percent.[80] This incidence of systolic compression is virtually identical to the 1.6 percent rate reported in 313 consecutive angiograms reviewed by Ishimori et al.[81] Myocardial bridges are known to occur more frequently in hypertrophic cardiomyopathy. Kitazume et al. reported that in a consecutive series of patients with hypertrophic cardiomyopathy given angiograms 30 percent had myocardial bridges, and in 15 percent systolic compression of over 50 percent occurred.[82] The angiographic morphology of the systolic narrowing was analyzed by Brugada et al.[83] Patients without hypertrophic cardiomyopathy showed a smooth and progressive constriction of the coronary artery up to the point of maximal stenosis, giving a "rat-tail" appearance. The systolic narrowing of the coronary artery in patients with hypertrophic cardiomyopathy had a scalloped or "sawfish" appearance which the authors postulated was due to the disorganized arrangements of hypertrophied muscle fibers characteristically seen in hypertrophic cardiomyopathy.

Myocardial bridging may be an important source of angiographic error if the compressed segment is misinterpreted as a fixed stenosis. Intramyocardial segments also present a technical problem for the cardiac surgeon. Deeply intramyocardial anterior descending coronary arteries may be inaccessible, and complications such as perforation into the right ventricle may occur during attempts to locate these vessels.

Fortunately, the outlook for most patients with myocardial bridging is excellent. Long-term follow-up of a total of 101 patients at the Cleveland Clinic revealed no myocardial infarctions or cardiac deaths,[80,82] and this correlates with our clinical experience suggesting that myocardial bridging is a benign variant of normal. However, in recent

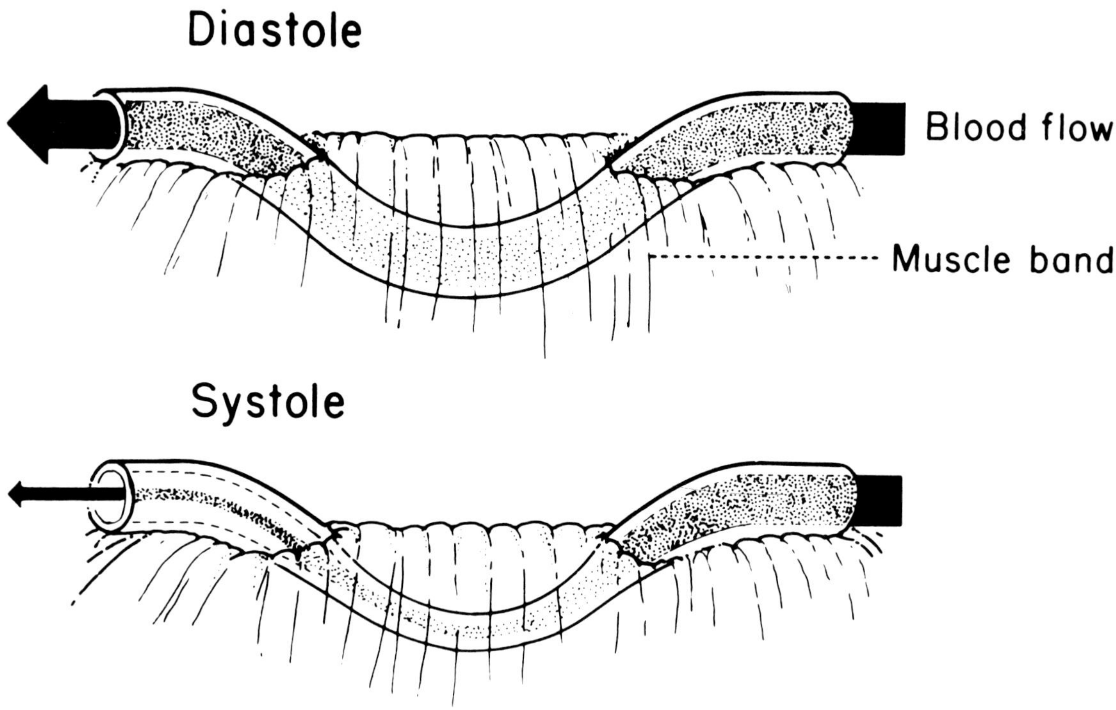

Figure 4-10 Artist's sketch of myocardial bridge. When the epicardial coronary artery is embedded in the myocardium, systolic contraction occludes the vessel to varying degrees. *(From Gorlin R: Dynamic vascular factors in the genesis of myocardial ischemia, J Am Coll Cardiol, 1:897, 1983, with permission of the author and publisher.)*

years myocardial bridging has been implicated in case reports as a primary or contributing factor in the genesis of myocardial ischemia, myocardial infarction, ventricular fibrillation, complete heart block, and sudden death. Noble observed 11 patients with angina pectoris and bridging of the left anterior descending coronary artery; four of five patients with over 75 percent systolic narrowing developed ischemic ECG changes and abnormal lactate production or extraction with pacing tachycardia,[84] and surgical removal of these bridges significantly relieved angina pectoris.[84,85,87]

Development of a reversible thallium defect[86] in patients with only myocardial bridging further implicates bridging as a source of myocardial ischemia, although coronary artery spasm is difficult to exclude conclusively. Faruqui et al. reported one patient with ventricular fibrillation and myocardial infarction,[85] and Morales[79] described three patients who died suddenly during exercise in whom myocardial bridging of the left anterior descending artery and evidence of septal ischemia was obtained. The evidence strongly suggests that in certain rare patients myocardial bridging may alter flow sufficiently to produce myocardial ischemia and its consequences. In three patients with sudden death, all had a dominant left coronary artery system and diminutive right coronary artery supply to the diaphragmatic surface of the heart. Factors contributing to the development of ischemia in this setting are the presence of a large volume of myocardium supplied by the compressed artery, marked compression of the artery by the overlying bridge, and sympathetic stimulation with an increased inotropic state and tachycardia and a resultant marked decreased time for diastolic filling. With an increased myocardial oxygen demand caused by exercise, a critical imbalance between demand and supply of myocardial blood flow may result in myocardial ischemia, arrhythmia, and even sudden death.[88] In Fig. 4-11 the coronary arteriogram, left ventriculogram, and electrocardiogram of a young male with myocardial infarction, systolic bridging of the left anterior descending coronary artery, and otherwise normal coronary arteries are shown.

COMPLICATIONS OF CORONARY ATHEROSCLEROSIS

Acute Myocardial Infarction

Myocardial infarction is the most common serious complication of coronary atherosclerosis. Necropsy and angiographic studies show multivessel obstruction in a majority of patients,[89–93] although rare individuals experience myocardial infarction with coronary arteries which are normal by radiographic and necropsy examination.[94–97] Angiographic studies performed during the early hours of acute myocardial infarction have shed new light on the pathoanatomy of this disorder by pointing out the high frequency of occluding coronary thrombi, supporting a causal role of thrombosis in the genesis of acute myocardial infarction.[98] DeWood has reported a total of 517 patients studied within 24 hours of transmural infarction; 80 percent seen within 6 hours had angiographic evidence of thrombus compared to 59 percent seen within 6 to 12 hours and 54 percent within 12 to 24 hours.[99]

Figure 4-11 A 31-year-old male was referred for coronary arteriography because of persisting chest pain at rest and with effort which occurred 3 months following anterior septal myocardial infarction. The electrocardiogram (*a*) and left ventriculogram (*b,c*) showed evidence of a large anterior-apical myocardial infarction. However, the left coronary artery in diastole (*d*) and the right coronary artery were normal. Mild to moderate compression of the mid–left anterior descending coronary artery (LAD) occurred during systole (*e*). Following infusion of isoproterenol, the end-diastolic appearance of the LAD remained normal (*f*); however, marked compression of the mid–LAD occurred during systole resulting in virtual obliteration of the lumen (*g*), chest discomfort, and transient bundle branch block.

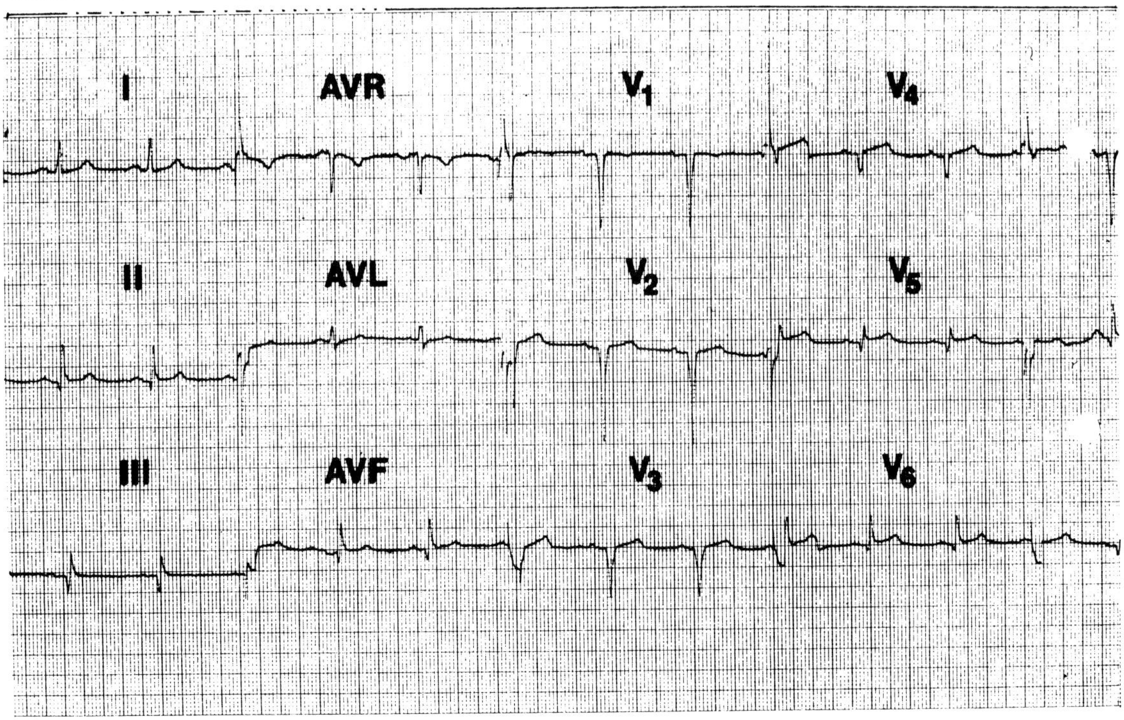

A

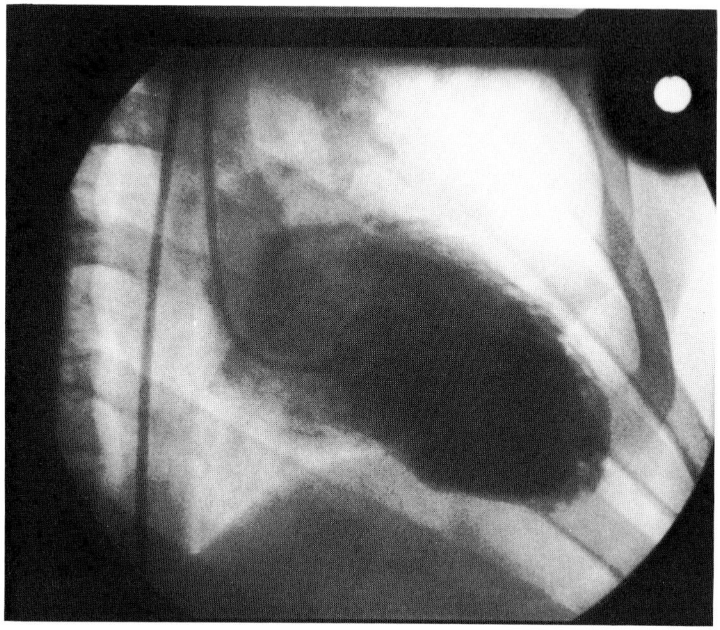

B

(Figure 4-11, continued)

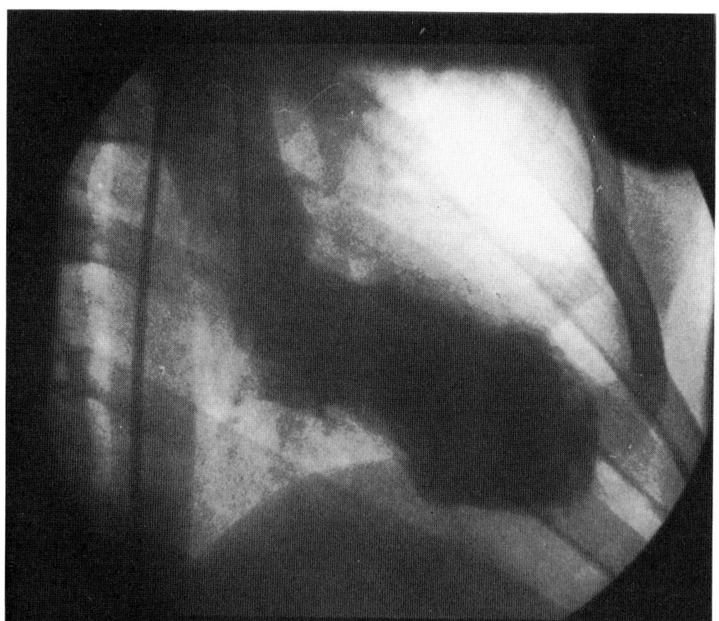

C

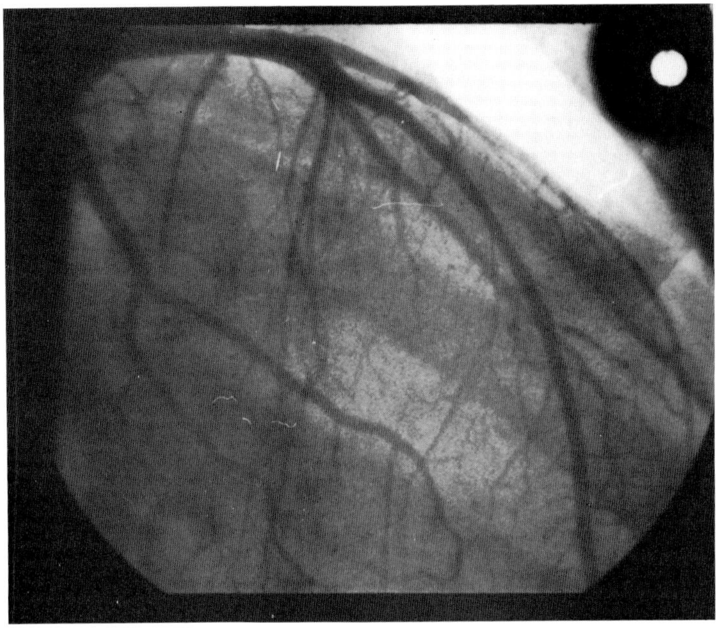

D (Figure 4-11, continued)

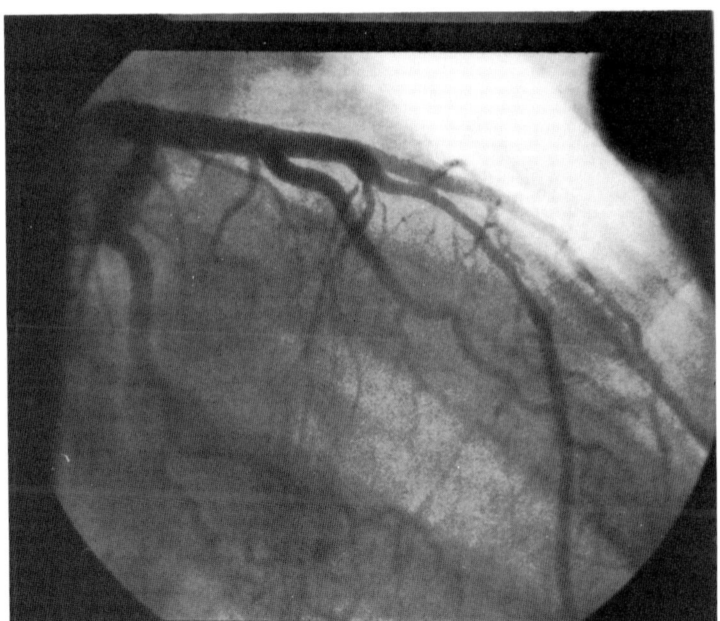

E

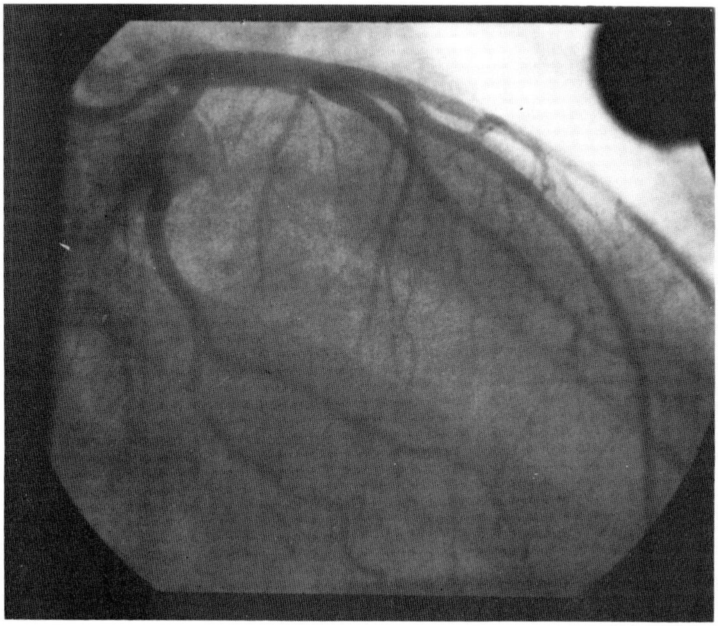

F

(Figure 4-11, continued)

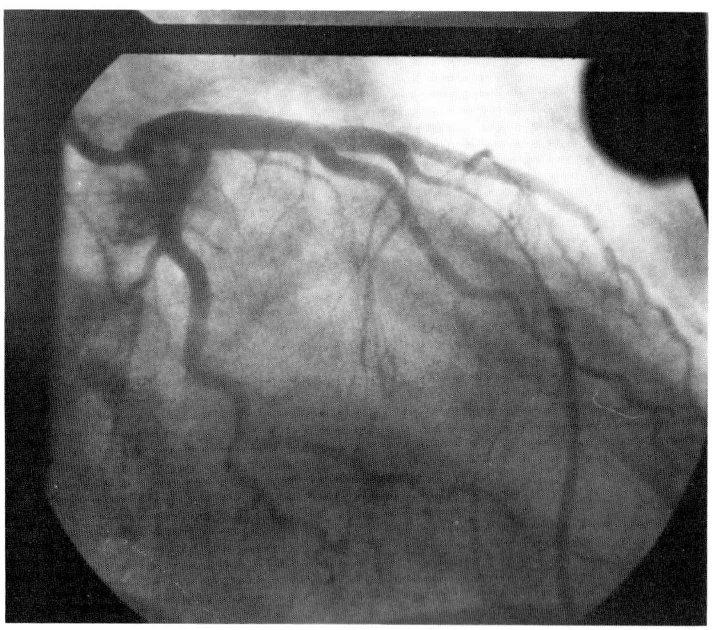

G

Pathological studies of acute myocardial infarction report that in 80 to 90 percent of acute occlusions, ulcerated plaques, or intimal erosions can be identified underlying the thrombus[100,101] Dynamic interactions of platelets, atherosclerotic plaque, and coronary spasm have been suggested as contributing factors to thrombotic coronary artery occlusion in acute myocardial infarction.[102–104] Transmural infarctions are commonly associated with complete coronary occlusion and nontransmural infarctions with high-grade coronary artery stenosis. In the latter condition, transient interruption of coronary flow by thrombus with rapid lysis, coronary spasm, or hypoperfusion due to arrhythmia or systemic hypotension are possible mechanisms. Myocardial pathology of nontransmural infarction is that of reperfusion necrosis with patchy accordianlike condensation of sarcomeres as contrasted with the coagulation necrosis most apt to occur with permanent coronary occlusion.[105,106] Unrestrained calcium entry into the cell is the apparent basis for reperfusion myocardial necrosis, and calcium antagonists have been advocated for use in the early phase of myocardial infarction and in cardiopulmonary bypass to minimize reperfusion injury.[107–109] Because of the common presence of high-grade proximal coronary stenosis in nontransmural infarction, the risk of coronary occlusion and reinfarction is substantial.[110–112] In a recent prospective study of 350 patients from Barnes Hospital, 42 percent of patients with nontransmural infarction experienced reinfarction, and the mortality rate in patients with reinfarction was 34 percent.[110] Distribution of the occluded coronary artery determines site of infarction in most instances. That is, occlusion of the left anterior descending coronary artery causes infarction in the anteroseptal, apical, and variable amounts of inferoapical left ventricle. Occlusion of the right coronary artery produces inferior, inferoseptal, and right ventricular infarction, and occlusion of the circumflex leads to lateral wall and variable inferior infarction, depending on the distribution of the artery. If the occluded artery is a source of collateral flow, infarction frequently occurs at a site remote from the occlusion; that is, occlusion of the left anterior descending artery, which collateralizes the distal right coronary artery, may produce inferior wall infarction.

Myocardial infarction most often involves the left ventricle and the interventricular septum. Occlusion of a major coronary artery results in a transmural gradient of ischemia, with the more ischemic subendocardium portion of the left ventricle experiencing cell death first. Infarction of the right ventricle and atria occurs in a minority of patients with left ventricular infarction and rarely as an isolated event.[113–116] The low oxygen demand, thin wall (which allows diffusion of oxygen from intracavitary blood), and rich coronary collateral network of these structures protect from ischemic damage even though obstructive disease in the perfusing coronary arteries is quite frequent. Manifestations of atrial infarction, more common in the right atrium, include atrial arrhythmias and mural thrombus formation with pulmonary and systemic embolization. Features of right ventricular infarction, which occur in 25 percent of inferobasal infarctions, include elevated systemic venous pressure in the absence of pulmonary congestion, systemic arterial hypotension, decreased right ventricular (RV) ejection fraction on radionuclide ventriculography, ventricular fibrillation complicating temporary RV pacing, and frequent hemodynamic improvement after volume expansion carried out in spite of elevated venous pressure.[117–119]

Coronary artery and left ventricular pathoanatomy are primary determinants of prognosis after infarction. Clinical strategies are directed at identifying those patients with significant residual "jeopardized" myocardium in order that revascularization may be carried out where appropriate in order to avoid reinfarction and its consequences. Clinical clues to the presence of jeopardized myocardium and a poor prognosis are postinfarction angina,[120] nontransmural infarction,[110–112] evidence of ischemia on stress electrocardiography or radionuclide testing,[121,122,124] and complex ventricular arrhythmias, although the latter is more often an indicator of severe left ventricular damage than of ischemia.

Postinfarction patients with these clues need coronary arteriography and evaluation for possible revascularization procedures. Whether all patients with uncomplicated transmural infarction should have further testing to stratify risk is a matter of some controversy because of the added cost and small risk of the additional procedures.[123–127] However, the group of postinfarction patients is extremely heterogeneous, so much so that only with further testing can those patients with unfavorable pathoanatomy be identified.

Left Ventricular Aneurysm

This complication of myocardial infarction is reported to occur in 15 percent of patients who survive.[128] However, the ability to recognize aneurysm varies widely, depending on whether one is at the autopsy table,[129–131] in the operating room,[132–136] using angiography,[137–140] or using bedside clinical methods.[130,131] In addition, uniformly accepted criteria for diagnosing left ventricular aneurysm are lacking. Cabin and Roberts[141] define left ventricular aneurysm as "a localized cavitary (other than when filled with thrombus) protrusion of left ventricular free wall." They further define *anatomic* aneurysm as a "localized protrusion of left ventricular free wall in both ventricular systole and diastole" and a *functional* aneurysm as a "protrusion only during ventricular systole" (see Fig. 4-12).

An anatomic aneurysm may be "true" or "false." A true aneurysm has a wide mouth, and its wall, which was the former left ventricular wall, is made up of necrotic muscle and/or fibrous tissue. A false aneurysm has a narrow neck and is the result of cardiac rupture and confinement of the hematoma by pericardial tissue. Its wall is composed of parietal pericardium and organized hematoma and does not contain myocardial fibers. False aneurysms may rupture; true aneurysms do not have this tendency. At autopsy, only anatomic aneurysms are recognized to be aneurysmal. Anatomic aneurysms are irreversible consequences of a remote infarction. Functional aneurysms are recognized at operation, during angiography, or by noninvasive techniques such as echocardiography (but not at autopsy) and may be irreversible, when composed of fibrous tissue, or reversible, if viable myocardium remains.

True left ventricular aneurysms occur at the anterior apical segment of the left ventricle 80 percent of the time and average 4 cm in diameter.[128] Inferior left ventricular aneurysms are rare in clinical practice because of frequent posterior medial papillary muscle involvement in large inferior infarctions with consequent cardiogenic shock and early death.[136,142] When left ventricular aneurysms do not interfere significantly with mitral valve function, the primary hemodynamic effects are on systolic function of the left ventricle, although diastolic function is usually abnormal. Systolic function is reduced due to loss of contractile elements and "stealing" of stroke volume by the bulging aneurysm in systole.[143] The noninvolved myocardium compensates by increased fiber shortening and hypertrophy, but when approximately 20 percent of the surface area of the ventricle becomes nonfunctional, ventricular dilatation occurs with resultant increase in wall stress and oxygen requirements in the residual myocardium.[18,137] Congestive heart failure ensues when the aneurysm is large and/or the residual myocardium is damaged or functions poorly due to ischemia. In patients without overt congestive heart failure, the long-term outlook is primarily determined by the quality of the coronary arteries perfusing the remaining myocardium. The primary cause of death is reinfarction.[128,145] Recent data on the natural history of left ventricular aneurysms from the CASS study suggest that the prognosis of patients is not as bleak as suggested from early autopsy studies. The survival of patients in this study at 4 years was 71 percent.[138]

Although 50 percent of aneurysms contain thrombus, the incidence of distal embolization is less than 5 percent, and routine anticoagulation is not required.[141,146] This low incidence of embolization contrasts with the higher incidence observed

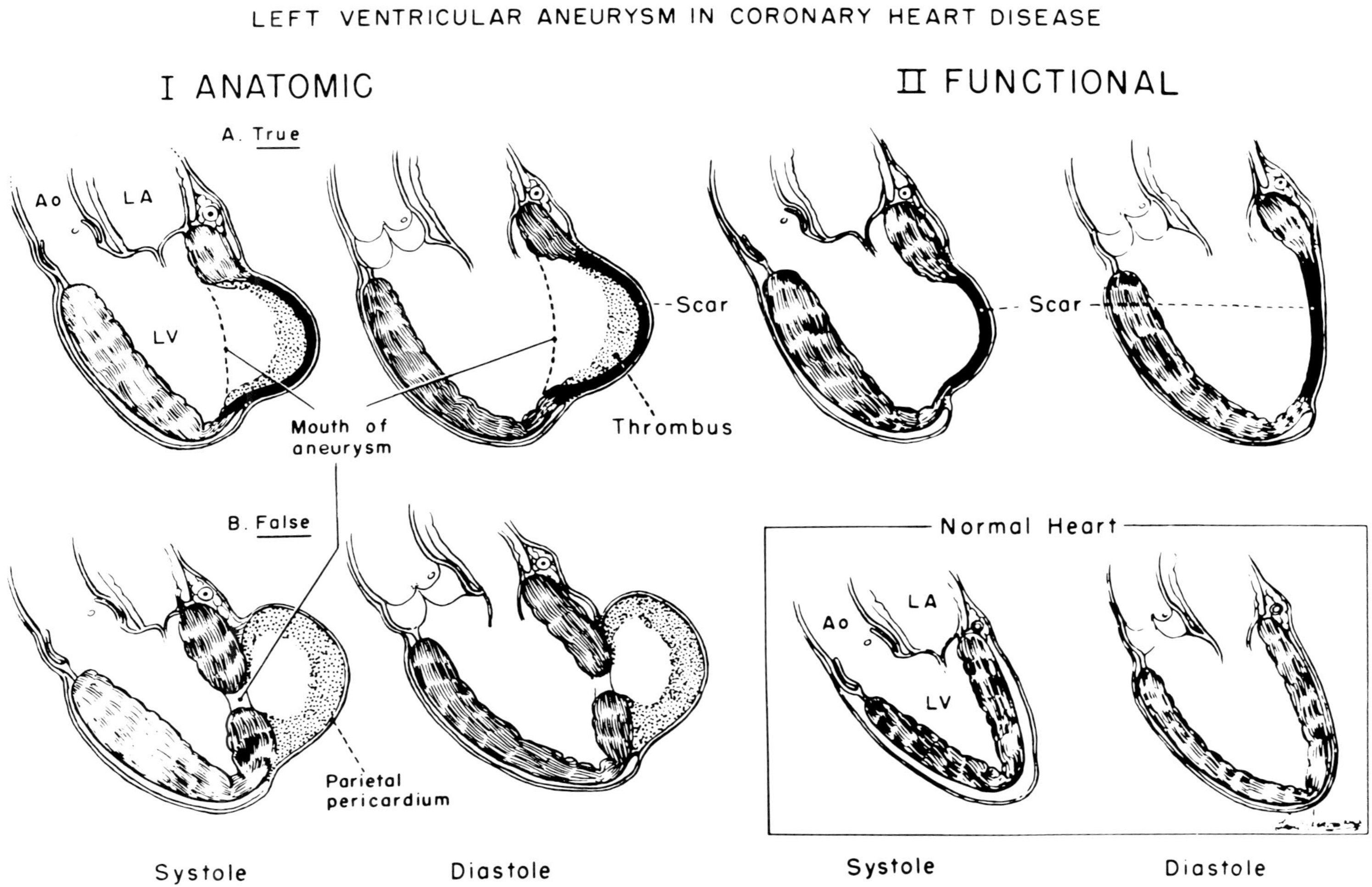

Figure 4-12 Diagrams of hearts in systole and diastole with true (*a*) and false (*b*) anatomic and functional left ventricular aneurysms and healed myocardial infarction. A diagram of the normal heart in systole and diastole is shown for comparison. The true anatomic left ventricular aneurysm protrudes outside the expected left ventricular silhouette during both systole and diastole and has a mouth that is as wide or wider than the maximal diameter of the aneurysm. A true aneurysm may or may not contain thrombus and virtually never ruptures once healing has occurred. The false anatomic left ventricular aneurysm protrudes during both systole and diastole, but has a mouth that is considerably smaller than the maximal diameter of the aneurysm. The false anatomic aneurysm represents a penetration of the wall of the ventricle, has a wall that is made up of parietal pericardium, frequently contains thrombus, and often ruptures. The functional left ventricular aneurysm protrudes only during ventricular systole and is made up of fibrous tissue with or without myocardial tissue. Ao = aorta; LA = left atrium, LA = left ventricle. *(From Cabin HS, Roberts WC: Left ventricular aneurysm, intraaneurysmal thrombus and systemic embolus in coronary heart disease, Chest, 77:586, 1980, with permission of the authors and publisher.)*

in idiopathic and ischemic cardiomyopathy, where there is global hypokinesia. Malignant arrythmia due to a reentry mechanism which is usually located at the border of the aneurysm has been effectively treated by aneurysmectomy[147–149] and more recently by endocardial mapping procedures and endocardial resection.[150–153]

Current indications for isolated left ventricular aneurysmectomy are refractory congestive heart failure, recurrent thromboembolism in spite of anticoagulation, and left ventricular false aneurysm.[154] The goal in aneurysmectomy for congestive heart failure is reduction in left ventricular end-diastolic volume with lowering of wall stress, reduction of the stealing effect on stroke volume, and reduction in mitral regurgitation. Most published studies show excellent improvement in symptoms following left ventricular aneurysmectomy.[133,136,155,156] The greatest improvement understandably occurs in patients with large, thin-walled aneurysms.[143,155] For patients with isolated left anterior descending coronary disease and discrete anterior apical aneurysm operative mortality rate is reported to be 3 to 5 percent,[156] whereas patients with multivessel disease and impaired residual contractile function have an operative mortality rate of about 12 percent with a 7-year survival rate of about 55 percent.[133]

Cardiogenic Shock

Patients with acute myocardial infarction and shock or left ventricular power failure have a survival rate of less than 10 percent on pharmacological therapy alone[157] and at autopsy exhibit necrosis of at least 40 percent of the left ventricle.[158,159] The majority of patients have triple vessel coronary artery disease[160] and show evidence of stepwise loss of functional myocardium by marginal extension of the infarction.[161] Occasionally, left ventricular paralysis due to global ischemia can be reversed by surgical revascularization, balloon angioplasty, or thrombolytic therapy.[162–164] Some patients with pump failure, shock, and congestive heart failure are found to have surgically correctable lesions such as severe mitral insufficiency, subacute left ventricular rupture with tamponade, ruptured ventricular septum, or rarely an acutely aneurysmal infarction, which may be resected with benefit. In the largest series of patients operated upon for shock and acute myocardial infarction using the intraaortic balloon pump, 47 percent survived.[165] The outlook of patients treated nonsurgically but with intraaortic balloon pump remains poor; in six reports a total of 36 of 164 patients (22 percent) survived.[157,166–172]

Interventricular Septum Perforation

Rupture of the interventricular septum is a devastating event complicating anteroseptal and inferior infarctions with roughly equal frequency.[173–176] The coronary arterial pathoanatomy is occlusion of the septal blood supply, that is, the anterior descending and/or the dominant posterior coronary artery, usually the right coronary artery (see Fig. 2-3). In 25 to 40 percent of septal ruptures, single vessel coronary disease is present.[174–176] Extensive transmural necrosis (usually involving over 25 percent of the left ventricle) and poor or absent collaterals are important factors in the pathogenesis of septal rupture.[173] Although septal rupture is rare, complicating 1 to 2 percent of myocardial infarctions,[173] it is the most common severe mechanical complication of acute myocardial infarction seen clinically in which there is time for surgical intervention.

Perforation of the septum occurs within the first week following a first myocardial infarction (usually 2 to 4 days after infarction) and is signalled by sudden change in clinical course with development of heart failure, hypotension or frank cardiogenic shock, and appearance of a new pansystolic murmur and thrill.[173–176] The degree of hemodynamic deterioration is determined by the extent of infarction, particularly the amount of right ventricular involvement, and the size of the septal defect, which determines the magnitude of the left-to-right shunt.[173,174] Bedside Swan-Ganz balloon catheterization has become standard for shunt measurement (pulmonary blood flow is usually three to four times systemic flow) and for hemodynamic monitoring. Although two-dimensional echocardiography has proved useful in documenting the presence of a ventricular septal defect,[177–179] catheterization of the left side of the heart and coronary arteriography are carried out in most centers in those patients who are sufficiently stable.

Initial attempts at surgical correction were carried out in patients surviving for several weeks after infarction,[180–182] but a majority of patients die in the few days after infarction due to progressive hemodynamic deterioration and cardiogenic shock even when aggressive medical therapy is utilized. With improvement in surgical techniques, early surgical repair became a possibility, although the risk of surgery remains high.[183–194]

Cardiogenic shock, resulting in a 70 percent operative mortality rate in our center and others,[174,176] and right ventricular infarction are primary determinants of survival following surgical repair of postinfarction septal ruptures.[174] Patients in cardiogenic shock treated medically virtually all die, and there is a tendency for rapid deterioration in patients who are apparently stable following septal rupture. This has led some to advocate immediate surgery for ruptured ventricular septum.[174a,174b] Others have attempted stabilization of patients and postponement of surgery if stability can be achieved.[195,196] In those patients who survive 3 weeks after infarction, the operative risk is 10 to 20 percent.[174,176]

If the intraaortic balloon pump is needed to achieve stability, abrupt clinical deterioration is common, and this period of brief stability should be used in our opinion to perform cardiac catheterization and plan surgery. We attempt early surgical repair of septal rupture (combined with coronary bypass when indicated) in patients with cardiogenic shock and severe pulmonary edema requiring intraaortic balloon pumping for support. In the rare patient who stabilizes relatively easily on aggressive medical therapy with vasodilators, optimal timing of surgery is controversial, and we do not have a standardized approach. The much reduced operative mortality rate at 3 weeks after infarction must be weighed against the tendency for abrupt hemodynamic deterioration and for sudden death, both well-recognized complications of septal rupture. When a decision is made to delay surgery to allow healing to occur, intensive monitoring and the capability for abrupt surgical intervention are maintained. Treatment of patients with postinfarction septal rupture has remained an extremely vexing problem.

Acute Mitral Regurgitation

Acute mitral regurgitation with congestive heart failure and/or cardiogenic shock in the setting of acute myocardial infarction can be due to papillary muscle rupture or dysfunction or distortion of the spatial relationships of intrinsically normal components of the mitral apparatus by ventricular wall motion abnormalities.[175,197–202] Prompt diagnosis, vasodilator therapy, intraaortic balloon pumping, and mitral valve replacement with or without coronary revascularization may improve an otherwise poor outlook, although the risk of surgery remains high.

Papillary muscle rupture, which involves the posterior medial papillary muscle five times more frequently than the anterior lateral papillary muscle,[175] occurs with equal frequency in subendocardial and transmural infarctions and in the presence of single vessel disease about 50 percent of the time.[201] Acute right coronary occlusion is reported to be twice as common as circumflex occlusion in rupture of the posteromedial papillary muscle,[200] but circumflex occlusion predominates in our experience. Rupture commonly occurs 2 to 7 days after infarction, and the infarction involves less than 25 percent of left ventricular myocardium in most patients.[200] Rupture may involve all of a papillary muscle (total rupture) or only one or several heads of a papillary muscle (partial rupture) (Fig. 4-13). Vlodaver and Edwards reported equal frequency of total and partial papillary muscle rupture[175] but noted that the anterior lateral papillary muscle, represented by a solitary mass, usually ruptured completely whereas the posteromedial papillary muscle, composed of several independent heads, commonly had partial rupture. Rupture of an entire papillary muscle is generally viewed as incompatible with life; rupture of a single

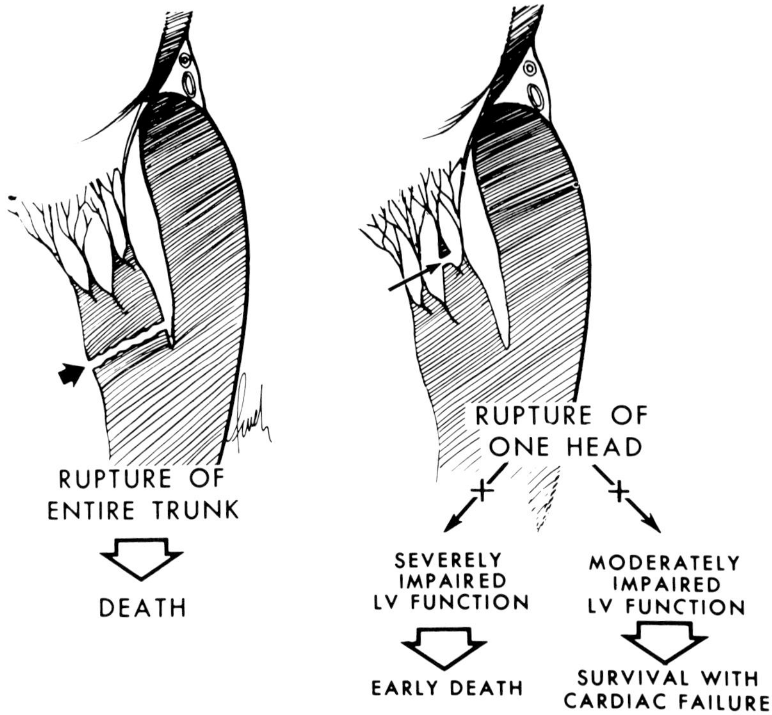

Figure 4-13 Diagrammatic representation of the types and possible consequences of papillary muscle rupture during acute myocardial infarction. Rupture of the entire trunk (*left*) is probably incompatible with survival in any patient because the support of both valve leaflets is destroyed. With rupture of one of the heads of the papillary muscle (*right*), survival may depend on the extent to which the function of the left ventricle has been impaired by the myocardial infarction. With severely impaired left ventricular function, the additional burden of mitral regurgitation may be intolerable. If left ventricular (LV) function is good, survival is possible for weeks and months, but congestive heart failure develops. *(Reproduced from Roberts WC, Perloff JK: Mitral valvular disease: A clinicopathologic survey of the conditions causing the mitral valve to function abnormally, Ann Intern Med, 77:939, 1972, with permission of the authors and publishers.)*

head of a papillary muscle may produce moderate mitral regurgitation and chronic congestive heart failure (Fig. 4-13).

Clinical findings are variable; a loud decrescendo systolic murmur is usually heard, but the murmur may be unimpressive in severe acute mitral regurgitation due to early equalization of left atrial and left ventricular systolic pressures. Electrocardiograms, in our experience, commonly do not show definite evidence of infarction; 9 of 14 patients had ST-T–interval or T-wave abnormalities only.[202a] Two-dimensional echocardiography has been reported to be useful in distinguishing papillary muscle dysfunction (hypokinetic, echo-dense papillary muscle) from rupture (flail mitral leaflet: visualization of the tip of the papillary muscle attached to chordae).[203,204] In the presence of severe mitral regurgitation, left ventriculography frequently shows relatively complete left ventricular emptying due to low-pressure runoff into the left atrium.

Surgical treatment with mitral replacement and coronary bypass within 30 days of infarction has a reported mortality rate exceeding 30 percent,[202a,205,206] but few if any patients with severe hemodynamic impairment survive on medical treatment alone, and acute deterioration from an apparently stable condition is common.[201] We recommend early surgery in patients with acute severe mitral regurgitation with uncontrolled congestive heart failure or cardiogenic shock.

Left Ventricular Rupture

Perforation of the free wall of the left ventricle, reported in 10 to 20 percent of fatal myocardial infarctions,[207] is roughly 10 times as common as papillary muscle or ventricular septal rupture.[208] Abrupt tamponade, electromechanical dissociation and death usually occur, but small left ventricular tears producing less acute tamponade occur rarely and are amenable to therapy.[209–215] Ventricular rupture—a result of loss of myocardial tensile strength, the pulling and sheer forces of adjacent normal myocardium, and intracavitary pressure—usually occurs at 3 to 5 days, but rarely up to 3 weeks after infarction.[207] The mechanism of rupture is dissection of an intramural hematoma in a sometimes serpentine fashion to the anterior septal, lateral, and inferior epicardial surfaces with equal frequency.[175] Thinning and regional dilatation of the infarcted segment, documented at autopsy[216,217] and in two-dimensional echocardiographic studies in living patients,[218] predisposes to rupture, as does advanced age, female sex, steroid therapy, hypertension, transmural infarction, and the absence of collaterals, myocardial fibrosis, and hypertrophy.[207,208]

Ventricular rupture is most common with large infarctions, but may occur with small infarctions when absence of collaterals permits rapid transmural necrosis with early regional thinning and dilatation.[217] Most patients have multivessel coronary occlusion or occlusion of the left anterior descending coronary artery.[207] Cobbs et al., recognizing electromechanical dissociation as a relatively specific and quickly recognizable sign of cardiac rupture, attempted repair of three ventricular perforations secondary to myocardial infarction with two long-term survivors.[209] In both survivors, pericardiocentesis confirmed the diagnosis and improved hemodynamics substantially, affording time for emergency surgical repair. Intravascular volume expansion[215,219] and intraaortic balloon pumping[210] may offer temporary circulatory support.

In incomplete left ventricular rupture, subacute tamponade with hypotension and distended neck veins may simulate biventricular infarction, and both conditions can cause pulsus paradoxus and equalization of diastolic pressures of the right side of the heart and pulmonary capillary wedge pressure. Determination of the presence of a hemopericardium by needle aspiration, echocardiography, carbon dioxide, or contrast angiography is imperative. Greenburg suggests that the loss of diastolic "Y" descent of the right atrial pressure tracing is evidence of tamponade even if biventricular infarction is present.[214] Outlook of survivors of surgical repair may be excellent since many patients with left ventricular rupture are experiencing their first infarction and have only moderate-sized infarctions.

PATHOANATOMY OF AORTOCORONARY SAPHENOUS VEIN GRAFTS

The pathoanatomy of aortocoronary saphenous vein grafts is dissimilar to that of native coronary arteries and is dependent on the time interval since implantation.[220–225] Ultrastructural studies of veins removed from the legs show the endothelium to be promptly denuded in a majority of cases. Within 24 hours of surgery, vein grafts show fibrin and platelet deposition on their surface. Mural thrombi form in vein grafts and lead to occlusion of 10 to 20 percent of vein grafts within 1 month. Early studies suggest that platelet inhibitory drugs may have a significant effect on the incidence of early graft occlusion.[226] Virtually all grafts develop intimal fibrous thickening or hyperplasia within 1 month of surgery, and subsequent progression of this intimal change is highly variable between cases and in a given patient with more than one vein graft. It has been suggested that the fibrous plaque which develops within weeks of surgery is a normal reparative phenomenon resulting from endothelial injury at the time of surgery, but that the propagation of the fibrous plaque as time goes on represents continued trauma related to increased pressure within the graft. The magnitude of the intimal thickening has been shown to be proportional to the caliber of the coronary artery distal to the anastomosis, and it has also been suggested that the intimal thickening is a remodeling process by which the vein graft approximates the size necessary to accommodate the distal runoff.[225] As time passes, the presence of moderate to marked intimal proliferation in vein grafts is a usual finding, but this process is compatible with good conduit function if the residual lumen is of sufficient size. In spite of the universal finding of intimal hyperplasia, complete vein graft occlusion by this process is rarely reported.

In our experience and in that of others,[227,228]

early vein graft *stenosis* usually occurs at the anastomosis of the saphenous vein to the coronary artery. This problem presents most often as a recurrence of angina 3 to 4 months postoperatively and appears to be the result of failure to perform a precise surgical anastomosis. The pathology of this lesion is uncertain, but it is probably a result of accumulation of products of thrombosis. This lesion is of particular interest because of the potential impact of platelet active agents in its prevention. In addition, percutaneous balloon angioplasty has proved to be an excellent treatment effecting a lasting correction in most cases.[229]

Atherosclerosis of vein grafts, identified as intimal foam cell accumulation or frank plaque, is rarely found for the first few years postoperatively[225]; however, Smith and Geer reported that veins examined over 3 years postoperatively had atherosclerotic changes in 70 percent of cases and that vein graft atheromas were noted to be extremely friable. Plaque rupture was the cause of late thrombotic graft occlusion. A study of 152 saphenous vein grafts examined 1.5 to 6 years postoperatively by Stolte et al. led to the conclusion that "long segment" stenoses commonly had a component of intimal hyperplasia, whereas, "short segment" stenoses were usually caused by atheroma.[230] Although these "short segment" stenoses may in many cases be amenable to percutaneous balloon angioplasty, the friability of vein graft atheromas make distal embolization a potential threat.

REFERENCES

1 Vlodaver Z, Edwards JE: Pathology of coronary atheroclerosis. Prog Cardiovasc Dis, 14:256, 1971.

2 Vlodaver Z, Frech R, Van Tassel RA, Edwards JE: Correlation of the antemortem coronary arteriogram and the postmortem specimen. Circulation, 47:162, 1973.

3 Roberts WC: The coronary arteries and left ventricle in clinically isolated angina pectoris: A necropsy analysis. Circulation, 54:388, 1976.

4 Arnett EN, Isner JM, Redwood DR, Kent KM, Baker WP, Ackerstein H, Roberts WC: Coronary artery narrowing in coronary heart disease: Comparison of cine angiographic and necropsy findings. Ann Intern Med, 91:350, 1979.

5 Learoyd BM, Taylor MG: Alterations with age in the viscoelastic properties of human arterial walls. Circ Res, 18:278, 1966.

6 Roberts CS, Roberts WC: Cross-sectional area of the proximal portions of the three major epicardial coronary arteries in 98 patients with different coronary events: Relationship to heart weight, age, and sex. Circulation, 62:953, 1980.

7 Brown BG, Bolson E, Frimer M, Dodge HT: Quantitative coronary arteriography: Estimation of dimensions, hemodynamic resistance, and atheroma mass of coronary artery lesions using the arteriogram and digital computation. Circulation, 55:329, 1977.

8 Liu LB, Richardson T, Holt JH, Taylor CB: Luminal eccentricity and deformity in atherosclerotic coronary arteries. Paroi Arterielle, 3:167, 1976.

9 Brown BG, Peterson RB: Computer-assisted measurements of coronary artery stenosis. Circulation, 60:1196, 1979 (reply to Letter to the Editor).

10 Marcus ML, Armstong ML, Heistad DD, Eastham CL, Mark AL: Comparison of three methods of evaluating coronary obstructive lesions: Postmortem arteriography, pathologic examination and measurement of regional myocardial perfusion during maximal vasodilation. Am Cardiol, 49:1699, 1982.

11 Levin DC, Fallon JT: Significance of the angiographic morphology of localized coronary stenosis: Histopathologic correlations. Circulation, 66:316, 1982.

12 Logan SE: On the fluid mechanics of coronary artery stenosis. IEEE Trans Biomed Eng, 22:321, 1975.

13 Mates RE, Gupta RL, Bell AC, Klocke FJ: Fluid dynamics in coronary artery stenosis. Circ Res, 42:152, 1978.

14 McMahon MM, Brown BG, Cukingnan R, et al: Quantitative coronary angiography: Measurement of the critical stenosis in patients with unstable angina and single vessel disease without collaterals. Circulation, 60:106, 1979.

15 Harrison DG, White CW, Hiratzka LF, et al: Can

the significance of a coronary stenosis be predicted by quantitative coronary angiography? Circulation, 64 (suppl IV):IV-160, 1981.

16 American Heart Association Committee Report: A reporting system on patients evaluated for coronary artery disease. Circulation, 51:7, 1975.

17 Gould KL, Lipscomb K, Hamilton GW: Physiologic basis for assessing critical coronary stenosis. Am J Cardiol., 33:87, 1974.

18 Massie B, Morady F, Botvinick E, Ratskin R, Tyberg J, Parmeley W: Quantitative assessment of coronary artery stenosis: Correlation with coronary flow. Circulation, 52(suppl II):II-26, 1975.

19 Peterson RJ, King SB III, Fajman WA, Douglas JS Jr, Jones RH: Relationship of coronary artery stenosis and gradient to exercise-induced ischemia. J Am Coll Cardiol, I:673, 1983.

20 Feldman RL, Nichols WW, Pepine CJ, Conti CR: Hemodynamic significance of the length of a coronary arterial narrowing. Am J Cardiol, 41:865, 1978.

21 McAlpin RN: Contribution of dynamic vascular wall thickening to luminal narrowing during coronary artery constriction. Circulation, 60:296, 1980.

22 Brown BG: Coronary vasospasm: Observations linking the clinical spectrum of ischemic heart disease to the dynamic pathology of coronary atherosclerosis. Arch Intern Med, 141:716, 1981.

23 Epstein SE, Talbot TL: Dynamic coronary tone in precipitation, exacerbation and relief of angina pectoris. Am J Cardiol, 48:797, 1981.

24 Rouleau JL, Chatterjee K, Ports T, Parmley W: Coronary reserve and angina threshold in patients with fixed obstructive coronary artery disease: Alterations in coronary vascular tone do not play a significant role. J Am Coll Cardiol, I:672, 1983.

25 Heupler FA: Syndrome of symptomatic coronary arterial spasm with nearly normal coronary arteriograms. Am J Cardiol, 45:873, 1980.

26 Selzer A, Langston M, Ruggeroli C, et al: Clinical syndrome of variant angina with normal coronary arteriogram. N Engl J Med, 295:1343, 1976.

27 Curry RC, Pepine CJ, Sabom MB, et al: Effects of ergonovine in patients with and without coronary artery disease. Circulation, 56:803, 1977.

28 Heupler FA, Proudfit SL, Razavi M, et al: Ergonovine maleate provocative test for coronary arterial spasm. Am J Cardiol, 41:631, 1978.

29 Conti CR, Curry RC, Christie LG, et al: Clinical use of provocative pharmacoangiography in patients with chest pain. Adv Cardiol, 26:44, 1979.

30 MacAlpine R, Cattus A, Alvaro A: Angina pectoris at rest with preservation of exercise capacity: Prinzmetal's variant angina. Circulation, 47:946, 1973.

31 Oliva P, Potts D, Pluss R: Coronary arterial spasm in Prinzmetal angina: Documentation by coronary arteriography. N Engl J Med, 288:746, 1973.

32 Whiting R, Klein M, Van der Veer J, Lown B: Variant angina pectoris. N Engl J Med, 282:709, 1970.

33 Wasue H, Omote S, Takizawa A, et al: Circadian variation of exercise capacity in patients with Prinzmetal's variant angina: Role of exercise-induced coronary arterial spasm. Circulation, 59:938, 1979.

34 Weiner D, Schick E, Hood W, Ryan T: ST segment elevation during recovery from exercise: A new manifestation of Prinzmetal's variant angina. Chest, 74:133, 1978.

35 Speccha G, deServi S, Falcone C: Coronary arterial spasm as a cause of exercise-induced ST segment elevation in patients with variant angina. Circulation, 59:948, 1979.

36 Oliva PB, Breckinridge JC: Arteriographic evidence of coronary arterial spasm in acute myocardial infarction. Circulation, 56:366, 1977.

37 Johnson AD, Detwiler JH: Coronary spasm, variant angina and recurrent myocardial infarction. Circulation, 55:947, 1977.

38 Maseri A, L'Abbate A, Baroldi G, et al: Coronary vasospasm as a possible cause of myocardial infarction: A conclusion derived from a study of "preinfarction" angina. N Engl J Med, 299:1271, 1978.

39 Madias JE: The syndrome of variant angina culminating in acute myocardial infarction. Circulation 59:297, 1979.

40 Prchkov VK, Mookhergee S, Scheiss WM, et al: Variant anginal syndrome, coronary arterial spasm and ventricular fibrillation in the absence of chest pain. Ann Intern Med, 81:858, 1974.

41 Previtali M, Klersy C, Salernoja: Ventricular tachyarrhythmias in Prinzmetal's variant angina: Clinical significance and relevance to the degree and time course of ST segment elevation. Am J Cardiol, 52:19, 1983.

42 Gorfinkel H, Inglesby T, Lansing A, et al: ST

segment elevation, transient left posterior hemiblock and recurrent ventricular arrhythmias unassociated with pain; a variant of Prinzmetal's angina syndrome. Ann Intern Med, 79:795, 1973.

43 Lasser RT, DeLapaz NS: Repetitive transient myocardial ischemia, Prinzmetal's type, without angina pectoris presenting with Stokes-Adams attacks. Chest, 64:350, 1973.

44 El-Maraghi NRH, Sealey BJ: Recurrent myocardial infarction in a young man due to coronary arterial spasm demonstrated at autopsy. Circulation, 61:199, 1980.

45 Roberts WC, Curry RC Jr, Isner JM, et al: Sudden death in Prinzmetal's angina with coronary spasm documented by angiography: Analysis of three necropsy patients. Am J Cardiol, 50:203, 1982.

46 MacAlpin RN: Relation of coronary arterial spasm to sites of organic stenosis. Am J Cardiol, 46:143, 1980.

47 Moncada S, Vane JR: Arachidonic acid metabolites and the interactions between platelets and blood vessel walls. N Engl J Med, 300:1142, 1979.

48 Levy RI, Smith JB, Silver MS, et al: Detection of thromboxane B2 in the peripheral blood with Prinzmetal's angina. Prostaglandins Med, 2:243, 1979.

49 Ricci DR, Orlick AE, Cipriano PR et al: Altered adrenergic activity in coronary arterial spasm: Insight into mechanism based on study of coronary hemodynamics and the electrocardiogram. Am J Cardiol, 43:1073, 1979.

50 Berger HS, Zaret BL, Speroff L, et al: Cardiac prostaglandin release during myocardial ischemia induced by atrial pacing in patients with coronary artery disease. Am J Cardiol, 39:481, 1977.

51 Mudge GH, Grossman W, Miles RM: Reflex increase in coronary vascular resistence in patients with ischemic heart disease. N Engl J Med, 295:1333, 1976.

52 Yasue H, Touyama M, Shimamoto M, et al: Role of autonomic nervous system in the pathogenesis of Prinzmetal's variant form of angina. Circulation, 50:534, 1974.

53 Bashour TT, Ajkim O, Cheng TO: Coronary spastic angina in middle-aged women: A psychosomatic disorder? Am Heart J, 106:609, 1983.

54 Kimura E, Kishida H: Treatment of variant angina with drugs: A survey of 11 cardiology institutes in Japan. Circulation, 63:844, 1981.

55 Robertson RM: Exacerbation of vasotonic angina pectoris by propranolol. Circulation, 65:281, 1982.

56 Dangoisse V, Guiteras Val P, David PR, et al: Recurrence of stenosis after successful percutaneous transluminal coronary angioplasty. Circulation, 66(suppl II):II-331, 1982.

57 Raizner AE, Chahine RA: The treatment of Prinzmetal's variant angina with coronary bypass surgery, in Hurst JW (ed): *Update II: The Heart*. McGraw-Hill, New York, 1980, p 85.

58 Weber J, Georges-Patrick D, Chauvaud S, et al: Assessment of plexectomy in the treatment of severe coronary spasm in patients with normal coronary arteries. Am J Cardiol, 51:1072, 1983.

59 Bott-Silverman C, Heupler FA Jr: Natural history of pure coronary artery spasm in patients treated medically. J Am Coll Cardiol, 2:201, 1983.

60 Waters DD, Bouchard A, Theroux P: Spontaneous remission is a frequent outcome of variant angina. J Am Coll Cardiol, 2:195, 1983.

61 Waters DD, Miller DD, Theroux P: Determining coronary artery spasm noninvasively. J Cardiovasc Med, 7:998, 1982.

62 Maseri A, Severi S, DeNes M, et al: "Variant" angina: One aspect of a continuous spectrum of vasospastic myocardial ischemia. Pathogenic mechanisms, estimated incidence and cinical and arteriographic findings in 138 patients. Am J Cardiol, 42:1019, 1978.

63 Buston A, Goldberg S, Hirshfeld JW, et al: Refractory ergonovine induced coronary vasospasm: Importance of intracoronary nitroglycerin. Am J Cardiol, 46:329, 1980.

64 Waters DD, Szlachcic J, Bonan R: Comparative sensitivity of exercise, coldpressor and ergonovine testing in provoking attacks of variant angina in patients with active disease. Circulation, 67:310, 1983.

65 Oldham HN Jr, Rembert JC, Greenfield JC Jr, Wechsler AD, Sabiston DC Jr: Intraoperative relationships between aorto-coronary bypass graft blood flow, peripheral coronary-artery pressure and reactive hyperemia, in Maseri A, Klassen GA, Lesch M (eds): *Primary and Secondary Angina Pectoris*. Grune & Stratton, New York, 1978, pp 363–373.

66 Goldstein, RE, Michaelis LL, Morrow AG, Epstein SE: Coronary collateral function in patients without occlusive coronary artery disease. Circulation, 51:118, 1975.

67 Dervan JP, Baim DS, Cherviles J, Grossman W: Transluminal angioplasty of occluded coronary arteries: Use of a movable guide wire system. Circulation, 68:776, 1983.

68 Gorlin R: Coronary collaterals. Major Prob Intern Med, 11:59, 1976.

69 Cannon PJ, Weiss MB, Casarella WJ: Studies of regional myocardial blood flow: Results in patients with left anterior descending coronary artery disease. Semin Nucl Med, 6:279, 1976.

70 Verani MS: The functional significance of coronary collateral vessels: Anecdote confronts science. Cathet Cardiovasc Diagn 9:333, 1983.

71 Schwarz F, Schuler G, Hoffmann M, Kubler W: Recruitment of collaterals following acute coronary occlusion reduces infarct size in man. J Am Coll Cardiol, 1:591, 1983.

72 Hamby RI, Aintablian A, Schwartz A: Reappraisal of the functional significance of the coronary collateral circulation. Am J Cardiol, 38:305, 1976.

72a Nohara R, Kambara H, Murakami T, et al: Collateral function in early acute myocardial infarction. Am J Cardiol, 52:955, 1983.

73 Banka VS, Bodenheimer MM, Halfant RH: Determinants of reversible asynergy: Effect of pathologic Q waves, coronary collaterals and anatomic location. Circulation, 50:714, 1974.

74 Rigo P, Becker LC, Griffith LSC, et al: Influence of coronary collateral vessels on the results of thallium-201 myocardial stress imaging. Am J Cardiol, 44:452, 1979.

75 Mehmel HC, Schwarz F, Schuler G, Maurer W, Tillmanns H, Senges J, Kubler W: The functional result of intracoronary streptokinase therapy after myocardial infarction may be determined by collaterals. Circulation, 64(suppl IV):IV-194, 1981.

76 Rentrop P, Merx W, Mathey D, Blanke H, Rutsch W, Karsch KR: Functional results of streptokinase—Reperfusion in relation to collaterals and duration of symptoms. Circulation, 64(suppl IV):IV-194, 1981.

77 Helfant RH, Vokonas PS, Gorlin R: Functional importance of the human coronary collateral circulation. N Engl J Med, 284:1277, 1971.

78 Flameng W, Schwarz F, Hehrlein FN: Intraoperative evaluation of the functional significance of coronary collateral vessels in patients with coronary artery disease. Am J Cardiol, 42:187, 1978.

79 Morales AR, Romanelli R, Boucek RJ: The mural left anterior descending coronary artery, strenuous exercise and sudden death. Circulation, 62:230, 1980.

80 Kramer JR, Kitazume H, Proudfitt WL, Sones FM Jr: Clinical significance of isolated coronary bridges: Benign and frequent condition involving the left anterior descending artery. Am Heart J, 103:283, 1982.

81 Ishimori T, Raizner AE, Chahine RA, et al: Myocardial bridges in man: Clinical correlations and angiographic accentuations with nitroglycerin. Cathet Cardiovasc Diag, 3:59, 1977.

82 Kitazume H, Kramer JR, Krauthamer D: Myocardial bridges in obstructive hypertrophic cardiomyopathy. Am Heart J, 106:131, 1983.

83 Brugada P, Bar FWHM, De Zwaan C, et al: "Sawfish" systolic narrowing of the left anterior descending coronary artery: An angiographic sign of hypertrophic cardiomyopathy. Circulation, 66:80, 1982.

84 Noble J, Bourassa MG, Petitclerc R, Dyrda I: Myocardial bridging and milking effect of the left anterior descending coronary artery: Normal variant or obstruction? Am J Cardiol, 37:993, 1976.

85 Faruqui AMA, Maloy WC, Felner JM et al: Symptomatic myocardial bridging of coronary artery. Am J Cardiol, 41:1305, 1978.

86 Dulk KD, Brugada P, Braat S, et al: Myocardial bridging as a cause of paroxysmal atrioventricular block. J Am Coll Cardiol, 1:965, 1983.

87 Grondin P, Bourassa MG, Noble J, et al: Successful course after supra-arterial myotomy for myocardial bridging and the milking effect of the left anterior descending artery. Ann Thorac Surg, 24:422, 1977.

88 Cheitlin MD: The intramural coronary artery: Another cause of sudden death with exercise? Circulation, 62:238, 1980.

89 Blumgart HL, Schlesinger MJ, Davis D: Studies in the relationship of the clinical manifestations of angina pectoris, coronary thrombosis and myocardial infarction to the pathologic findings with particular reference to the significance of the collateral circulation. Am Heart J, 19:1, 1940.

90 Roberts WC: Coronary arteries in fatal acute myocardial infarction. Circulation, 45:215, 1972.

91 Williams RA, Cohn PF, Vokonos PS, et al: Electrocardiographic, arteriographic and ventri-

culographic correlations in transmural myocardial infarction. Am J Cardiol, 31:595, 1973.
92 Miller RR, DeMaria AN, Vismara LA, et al: Chronic stable inferior myocardial infarction: Unsuspected harbinger of high risk proximal left coronary arterial obstruction amenable to surgical revascularization. Am J Cardiol, 39:954, 1977.
93 Turner JD, Rogers WJ, Mantle JA, Rackley CE, Russell RO Jr: Coronary arteriography soon after myocardial infarction. Chest, 77:58, 1980.
94 Rosenblatt A, Seltzer A: The nature and clinical features of myocardial infarction with normal coronary arteriograms. Circulation, 55:578, 1977.
95 Khan AH, Haywood LJ: Myocardial infarction in 9 patients with radiographically patent coronary arteries. N Engl J Med, 291:425, 1974.
96 Eliot RS, Baroldi G, Leone A: Necropsy studies in myocardial infarction with minimal or no coronary luminal reduction due to atherosclerosis. Circulation, 50:1127, 1974.
97 Bulkley BH, Klacsmann PG, Hutchins GM: Angina pectoris, myocardial infarction and sudden cardiac death with normal coronary arteries: A clinicopathologic study of 9 patients with progressive systemic sclerosis. Am Heart J, 95:563, 1978.
98 DeWood MA, Spores J, Notske R, Mouser LT, Borroughs R, Golden MS, Lang HT: Prevalence of total coronary occlusion during the early hours of transmural myocardial infarction. N Engl J Med, 303:897, 1980.
99 DeWood MA, Spores J, Hensley GR, Simpson CS, Eugster GS, Sutherland KI, Grunwald RP, Shields JP: Coronary arteriographic findings in acute transmural myocardial infarction. Circulation, 68(suppl I):I-39, 1983.
100 Constantinides P: Plaque fissures in human coronary thrombosis. J Athero Res, 6:1, 1966.
101 Friedman M, Vanden B: The pathogenesis of coronary thrombosis. Am J Pathol, 48:19, 1966.
102 Oliva PB, Breckenridge JC: Arteriographic evidence of coronary arterial spasm in acute myocardial infarction. Circulation, 56:366, 1977.
103 Rentrop KP, Blanke H, Karsch KR, et al: Acute myocardial infarction: Intracoronary application of nitroglycerin and streptokinase. Clin Cardiol, 2:354, 1979.
104 Gold HK, Leinbach RC: Coronary obstruction in anterior myocardial infarction: Thrombus or spasm? Am J Cardiol, 45:483, 1980.
105 Herdson PB, Sommers HM, Jennings RB: A comparative study of the fine structure of normal and ischemic dog myocardium with specific reference to early changes following temporary occlusion of a coronary artery. Am J Pathol, 46:367, 1965.
106 Bulkley BH, Hutchins GM: Myocardial consequences of coronary artery bypass graft surgery: The paradox of necrosis in areas of revascularization. Circulation, 56:906, 1977.
107 Nayler WG, Fassold E, Yepez C: Pharmacological protection of mitochondrial function in hypoxic heart muscle: Effect of verapamil, propranolol, and methylprednisolone. Cardiovasc Res, 12:152, 1978.
108 Reimer KA, Lowe JE, Jennings RB: Effect of calcium antagonist verapamil on necrosis following temporary coronary occlusion in dogs. Circulation, 55:581, 1977.
109 Voehe PR, Helias J, Robt P, Grondin MB: Myocardial protection through cold cardioplegia with potassium or Diltiazem: Experimental evidence that Diltiazem provides better protection even when coronary flow is impaired by a critical stenosis. Circulation, 65:1078, 1982.
110 Marmor A, Geltman EM, Schechtman K, Sobel BE, Roberts R: Recurrent myocardial infarction: Clinical predictors and prognostic implications. Circulation, 66:415, 1982.
111 Cannon DS, Levy W, Cohen LS: The short- and long-term prognosis of patients with transmural and nontransmural infarction. Am J Med, 61:452, 1976.
112 Madigan NP, Rutherford BD, Frye RL: The clinical course, early prognosis and coronary anatomy of subendocardial infarction. Am J Med, 60:634, 1976.
113 Isner JM, Roberts WC: Right ventricular infarction complicating left ventricular infarction secondary to coronary heart disease: Frequency, location, associated findings and significance from analysis of 236 necropsy patients with acute and healed myocardial infarction. Am J Cardiol, 42:885, 1978.
114 Wackers FGT, Lie KI, Sokole EB, et al: Prevalence of right ventricular involvement in inferior wall infarction assessed with myocardial imaging with thallium-201 and technetium-99m pyrophosphate. Am J Med, 42:358, 1978.
115 Cushing EH, Feil HS, Stanton EJ, Wartman WB: Infarction of the cardiac auricles (atria); clinical,

pathological and experimental studies. Br Heart J, 4:17, 1942.

116 Hellerstein KH, Van Dyke AE: Atrial myocardial infarction: A contemporary view, in Hurst JW (ed): *Update IV: The Heart*. McGraw-Hill, New York, 1981, p 43.

117 Rackley CE, Russell RO, Mantle JA, et al: Right ventricular infarction and function. Am Heart J, 101:215, 1981.

118 Cintron GB, Hernandez E, Linares E, Aranda JM: Bedside recognition, incidence and clinical course of right ventricular infarction. Am J Cardiol, 47:224, 1981.

119 Sclarovsky S, Zafrir N, Strasberg B, Kracodd O, et al: Ventricular fibrillation complicating temporary ventricular pacing in acute myocardial infarction: Significance of right ventricular infarction. Am J Cardiol, 48:1160, 1981.

120 Schuster EH, Bukley BH: Early post-infarction angina: Ischemia at a distance and ischemia in the infarct zone. N Engl J Med, 305:1101, 1981.

121 Gibson RS, Watson DD, Craddock GB, et al: Predicting cardiac events after uncomplicated acute myocardial infarction: A prospective study comparing predischarge exercise thallium-201 scintigraphy and coronary angiography. Circulation, 68:321, 1983.

122 Corbett JR, Dehmer GJ, Lewis SE, et al: The prognostic value of submaximal exercise testing with radionuclide ventriculography before hospital discharge in patients with recent myocardial infarction. Circulation, 64:535, 1981.

123 Epstein SE, Palmeri ST, Patterson RE: Evaluation of patients after acute myocardial infarction: Indications for cardiac catheterization and surgical intervention. N Engl J Med, 307:1487, 1982.

124 Smith JW, Dennis CA, Gassmann A, et al: Exercise testing three weeks after myocardial infarction. Chest, 75:12, 1979.

125 Biggers JT: New directions and new uses for risk stratification in post hospital phase of acute myocardial infarction. Am J Med, 67:1, 1979.

126 Rahimtoola SH: Coronary arteriography in asymptomatic patients after myocardial infarction: The need to distinguish between clinical investigation and clinical care. Chest, 77:53, 1980.

127 Douglas JS Jr, Hurst JW: Which patients should have arteriography after acute myocardial infarction? J Cardiovasc Med, 9:219, 1984.

128 Abrams DL, Edelist A, Lurai MH, Miller AJ: Ventricular aneurysm: A reappraisal based on a study of 65 consecutive autopsied cases. Circulation, 27:164, 1963.

129 Schlichter J, Hellerstein JK, Katz LN: Aneurysm of the heart: A correlative study of one hundred and two proved cases. Medicine, 33:43, 1954.

130 Dubnow MH, Burchell HB, Titus JL: Postinfarction ventricular aneurysm: A clinicomorphologic and electrocardiographic study of 80 cases. Am Heart J, 70:753, 1965.

131 Davis RW, Ebert PA: Ventricular aneurysm: A clinical-pathologic correlation. Am J Cardiol, 29:1, 1976.

132 Cooley DA, Hallman GL, Henly WS: Left ventricular aneurysm due to myocardial infarction. Arch Surg, 88:114, 1964.

133 Loop FD, Effler DB, Navia JA, Sheldon WC, Groves LK: Aneurysms of the left ventricle: Survival and results of a ten-year surgical experience. Ann Surg, 178:399, 1973.

134 Rao G, Zikria EA, Miller WH, Samadani SR, Ford WB: Experience with sixty consecutive ventricular aneurysm resections. Circulation, 50(suppl 2):149, 1974.

135 Marco JD, Kaiser GC, Barner HE, Codd JE, William VL: Left ventricular aneurysmectomy. Arch Surg, 111:419, 1976.

136 Reddy SB, Cooley DA, Duncan JM, Norman JC: Left ventricular aneurysm: 20-Year surgical experience with 1572 patients at the Texas Heart Institute. Cardiovasc Dis Bull, 8:165, 1981.

137 Klein MD, Herman MV, Gorlin R: A hemodynamic study of left ventricular aneurysm. Circulation, 35:614, 1967.

138 Faxon DP, Ryan TJ, Davis KB, et al: Prognostic significance of angiographically documented left ventricular aneurysm from the coronary artery surgery study (CASS). Am J Cardiol, 50:157, 1982.

139 Cheng TO: Incidence of ventricular aneurysm in coronary artery disease: An angiographic appraisal. Ann Intern Med, 50:340, 1971.

140 Proudfit WL, Bruschke AVG, Sones FM Jr: Natural history of obstructive coronary artery disease: 10-Year Study of 601 nonsurgical cases. Prog Cardiovasc Dis, 21:53, 1978.

141 Cabin HS, Roberts WC: Left ventricular aneurysm, intraaneurysmal thrombus and systemic embolus in coronary heart disease. Chest, 77:586, 1980.

142 Loop FD, Effler DB, Webster JS, Groves LK:

Posterior ventricular aneurysms: Etiologic factors and results of surgical treatment. N Engl J Med, 288:237, 1973.

143 Swan HJC, Forrester JS, Diamond G, et al: Hemodynamic spectrum of myocardial infarction and cardiogenic shock. Circulation, 45:1097, 1972.

144 Feild BJ, Russell RO, Dowling JT, Rackley CE: Regional left ventricular performance in the year following myocardial infarction. Circulation, 46:679, 1972.

145 Gorlin R, Klein MD, Sullivan JM: Prospective correlative study of ventricular aneurysm: Mechanistic concept and clinical recognition. Am J Med, 42:512, 1967.

146 Simpson MT, Oberman A, Kouchoukos NT, Rogers WJ: Prevalence of mural thrombi and systemic embolization with left ventricular aneurysm: Effect of anticoagulation therapy. Chest, 77: 1980.

147 Couch OA Jr: Cardia aneurysm with ventricular tachycardia and subsequent excision of aneurysm: Case report. Circulation, 20:251, 1959.

148 Hunt D, Sloman G, Westlake G: Ventricular aneurysmectomy for recurrent tachycardia. Br Heart J, 31:264, 1969.

149 Welch TG, Fontana ME, Vasko JS: Aneurysmectomy for recurrent ventricular tachyarrhythmias. Am Heart J, 85:685, 1973.

150 Josephson NE, Harken AH, Horowitz LN: Endocardial excision: A new surgical technique for the treatment of recurrent ventricular tachycardia. Circulation, 60:1430, 1979.

151 Horowitz LN, Harken AH, Kastor JA, Josephson ME: Ventricular resection guided by epicardial and endocardial mapping for treatment of recurrent ventricular tachycardia. Circulation, 60:1430, 1979.

152 Harken AH, Horowitz LN, Josephson NE: Comparison of standard aneurysmectomy and aneurysmectomy with directed endocardial resection for the treatment of recurrent sustained ventricular tachycardia. J Thorac Cardiovasc Surg, 80:527, 1980.

153 Wiener I, Mindich B, Pitchon R: Determinants of ventricular tachycardia in patients with ventricular aneurysms: Results of intraoperative epicardial and endocardial mapping. Circulation, 65:856, 1982.

154 Cohen M, Packer M, Gorlin R: Indications for left ventricular aneurysmectomy. Circulation, 67:717, 1983.

155 Ott DA, Parravacini R, Cooley DA, et al: Improved cardiac function following left ventricular aneurysm resection: Pre and post operative performance in 150 patients. Tex Heart I J, 9:267, 1982.

156 Loop FD, Cosgrove DM: Results of ventricular aneurysmectomy. Ann J Surg, 141:684, 1981.

157 Johnson SA, Scanlon PJ, Loeb HS, Moran JM, et al: Treatment of cardiogenic shock in myocardial infarction by intra-aortic balloon counterpulsation and surgery. Am J Med, 62:687, 1977.

158 Alonso DR, Scheidt S, Post M, Killip T: Pathophysiology of cardiogenic shock; quantitation of myocardial necrosis, clinical pathologic and electrocardiographic correlation. Circulation, 48:588, 1973.

159 Page DL, Caulfield JB, Kastor JA, et al: Myocardial changes associated with cardiogenic shock. N Engl J Med, 285:133, 1971.

160 Wackers FJ, Lie KI, Becker AE, Durrer D, Wellens HJ: Coronary artery disease in patients dying from cardiogenic shock or congestive heart failure in the setting of acute myocardial infarction. Br Heart J, 38:906, 1976.

161 Gutovitz AL, Sobel BE, Roberts R: Progressive nature of myocardial injury in selected patients with cardiogenic shock. Am J Cardiol, 41:469, 1978.

162 Mundth ED, Yurckak PM, Buckley MY, et al: Circulatory assistance and emergency direct coronary artery surgery for shock complicating acute myocardial infarction. N Engl J Med, 283:1382, 1970.

163 Meyer J, Merx W, Door R, Lambertz H, et al: Successful treatment of acute myocardial infarction shock by combined percutaneous transluminal coronary recanalization (PTCR) and percutaneous transluminal coronary angioplasty (PTCA). Am Heart, J, 103:132, 1982.

164 Kennedy JW, et al: Intracoronary streptokinase in acute MI: Report from the Society for Cardiac Angiography Registry. Circulation, 68(Suppl III):III-121, 1983.

165 Mundth ED: Surgical treatment of cardiogenic shock and acute mechanical complications following myocardial infarction. Cardiovasc Clin, 2:241, 1977.

166 Mueller H, Ayres SM, Giannelli S Jr, Conklin ER, Mazzara JT, Grace WJ: Effect of isoproterenol, l-norepinephrine and intraaortic counterpulsation on hemodynamics and myocardial metabolism in shock following acute myocardial infarction. Circulation, 45:335, 1972.

167 Scheidt S, Wilner G, Mueller H, Summers D, et al: Intra-aortic balloon counterpulsation in cardiogenic shock: Report of a co-operative clinical trial. N Engl J Med, 228:979, 1973.

168 O'Rourke MF, Chang VP, Windsor HM, et al: Acute severe cardiac failure complicating myocardial infarction: Experience with 100 patients referred for consideration of mechanical left ventricular assistance. Br Heart J, 37:169, 1975.

169 Lefemine AA, Kosowsky B, Dadoff I, Black H, Lewis M: Results and complications of intraaortic balloon pumping in surgical and medical patients. Am J Cardiol, 40:416, 1977.

170 Hagemeiger F, Laird JD, Haalebos MMP, Hugenholtz PG: Effectiveness of intraaortic balloon pumping without cardiac surgery for patients with severe heart failure secondary to a recent myocardial infarction. Am J Cardiol, 40:951, 1977.

171 Willerson JT, Curry GC, Watson JT, Leshin SJ: Intraaortic balloon counterpulsation in patients with cardiogenic shock, medically refractory left ventricular failure and/or recurrent ventricular tachycardia. Am J Med, 58:183, 1975.

172 Maroko PR, Bernstein EF, Libby P, et al: Effects of intraaortic balloon counterpulsation on the severity of myocardial ischemic injury following acute coronary occlusion: Counterpulsation and myocardial injury. Circulation, 45:1150, 1972.

173 Hutchins GM: Rupture of the interventricular septum complicating myocardial infarction: Pathologic analysis of 10 patients with clinically diagnosed perforations. Am Heart J, 97:165, 1979.

174 Radford MJ, Johnson RA, Daggett WM, et al: Ventricular septal rupture: A review of clinical and physiologic features and an analysis of survival. Circulation, 64:545, 1981.

174a Gray RJ, Sethna D, Matloff JM: The role of cardiac surgery in acute myocardial infarction: I. With mechanical complications. Am Heart J, 106:723, 1983.

174b Forfar JC, Irving JB, Miller HC, et al: The management of ventricular septal rupture following myocardial infarction. J Q Med 49:205, 1980.

175 Vlodaver Z, Edwards JE: Rupture of ventricular septum or papillary muscle complicating myocardial infarction. Circulation, 55:815, 1977.

176 Cooke DB, Clements SD Jr, Hurst JW, et al: Ruptured ventricular septum due to myocardial infarction (submitted for publication).

177 Drobac M, Bilvert B, Howard R, et al: Ventricular septal defect after myocardial infarction: Diagnosis by two-dimensional contrast echocardiography. Circulation, 67:335, 1983.

178 Farcot JC, Boisanle L, Rigand M, Varde J, Bourdarias JP: Two-dimensional echocardiographic visualization of ventricular septal rupture after acute anterior myocardial infarction. Am J Cardiol, 45:370, 1980.

179 Mintz GS, Victor MF, Kotler MN, Parry WR, Segal BL: Two correctable complications of acute myocardial infarction. Circulation, 64:91, 1981.

180 Cooley DA, Belmohte BA, Zeis LB, et al: Surgical repair of ruptured interventricular septum following acute myocardial infarction. Surgery, 41:930, 1957.

181 Varnard PM, Kennedy JH: Post infarction ventricular septal defect. Circulation, 32:76, 1965.

182 Boicourt OW, Tirzmann LW, Chase JD, Starr A, McCord CW: Rupture of the infarcted interventricular septum. Circulation, 26:1321, 1962.

183 Iben AB, Pupello DF, Stinson EB, Shumway NE: Surgical treatment of postinfarction ventricular septal defects. Ann Thorac Surg, 8:253, 1969.

184 Crosby IK, Craver JM, Cramptom RS, Schrank JP, Wellons HA: Resection of acute posterior ventricular aneurysm with repair of ventricular septal defect after acute myocardial infarction. J Thorac Cardiovasc Surg, 70:57, 1975.

185 Kaplan MA, Harris CN, Kay JH, Parker DP, Magidson O: Post infarction ventricular septal rupture. Chest, 69:734, 1976.

186 Graham AF, Stinson EB, Daily PO, Harrison DC: Ventricular septal defects after myocardial infarction. JAMA, 225:708, 1973.

187 Daggett SM, Guyton RA, Mundth ED, Buckley MJH, McEnany MT, Gold KH, Leinback RC, Austen SG: Surgery for post-myocardial infarct ventricular septal defect. Ann Surg, 186:260, 1977.

188 Montoya A, KcKeever L, Scanlon P, Sullivan JH, Gunnar RM, Pifarre R: Early repair of ventricular septal rupture after infarction. Am J Cardiol, 45:345, 1980.

189 Buckley MJ, Mundth ED, Daggett WM, DeSanctis RW, Sanders CA, Austen SG: Surgical therapy for early complications of myocardial infarction. Surgery, 70:814, 1971.

190 Oldham JM, Scott SM, Dart CH, Fish RG, Claxton CP, Dillon ML, Sabiston DC: Surgical correction of ventricular septal defect following acute myocardial infarction. Ann Thorac Surg, 7:193, 1969.

191 Brandt B, Weight CB, Ehrenhaft JL: Ventricular septal defect following myocardial infarction. Ann Thorac Surg, 27:580, 1979.

192 Selzer A, Gerbode F, Kerth WJ: Clinical, hemodynamic, and surgical considerations of rupture of the ventricular septum after myocardial infarction. Am Heart J, 78:598, 1969.

193 Radford MJ, Johnson RA, Daggett WM, Fallon JT, Buckley MJ, Gold HK, Leinback RC: Ventricular septal rupture: A review of survival. Circulation, 64:545, 1981.

194 Jones EL, Tyras DH, King SB, Logue RB, Hatcher CR: Myocardial revascularization combined with intracoronary infusion of hyperosmolar solution in the early management of post-infarction ventricular septal defect. Circulation, 52:170, 1975.

195 Giuliani ER, Danielson GK, Pluth JR, et al: Post infarction ventricular septal rupture. Circulation, 49:455, 1974.

196 Kitamura S, Mendez A, Kay JH: Ventricular septal defect following myocardial infarction. J Thorac Cardiovasc Surg, 61:186, 1971.

197 Burch GE, DePasquale NP, Phillips JH: Clinical manifestations of papillary muscle dysfunction. Arch Intern Med, 112:112, 1963.

198 Roberts WC, Perloff JK: Mitral valvular disease: A clinicopathologic survey of the conditions causing the mitral valve to function abnormally. Ann Intern Med, 77:939, 1972.

199 Cheng TO, Bashour T, Adkins PC: Acute severe mitral regurgitation from papillary muscle dysfunction in acute myocardial infarction: Successful early surgical treatment by combined mitral valve replacement and aortocoronary saphenous vein bypass graft. Circulation, 46:491, 1972.

200 Wei JY, Hutchins GM, Bulkley BH: Papillary muscle rupture in fatal acute myocardial infarction: A potentially treatable form of cardiogenic shock. Ann Intern Med, 90:149, 1979.

201 Nishimura RA, Hartzel VS, Shub C, Gersh BJ, Edwards WD, Tagik AJ: Papillary muscle rupture complicating acute myocardial infarction: Analysis of 17 patients. Am J Cardiol, 51:373, 1983.

202 Morrow AG, Cohen LS, Roberts WC, Braunwald NS, Braunwald E: Severe mitral regurgitation following acute myocardial infarction in ruptured papillary muscle: Hemodynamic findings and results of operative treatment in four patients. Circulation, 37–38(suppl II):124, 1968.

202a Clements SD Jr, et al: Ruptured papillary muscle, a complication of myocardial infarction: Clinical presentation, diagnosis and treatment (submitted for publication).

203 Mintz GS, Victor MF, Kotler MN, Parry WR, Segal BL: Two-dimensional echocardiographic identification of surgically correctable complications of acute myocardial infarction. Circulation, 64:91, 1981.

204 Erbel R, Schweizer P, Bardos P, Meyer J: Two-dimensional echocardiographic diagnosis of papillary muscle rupture. Chest, 79:595, 1981.

205 Kouchoukos NT: Surgical treatment of acute complications of myocardial infarction. Cardiovasc Clin, II:141, 1981.

206 Buckley MJ, Mundth ED, Daggett WM, Gold HK, et al: Surgical management of ventricular septal defects and mitral regurgitation complicating acute myocardial infarction. Ann Thorac Surg, 16:598, 1973.

207 Bates RJ, Beutler S, Resnekof L, Anagnostopoulos CE: Cardiac rupture—Challenge of diagnosis and management. Am J Cardiol, 40:439, 1977.

208 Lee WY, Cardon L, Slodki SJ: Perforation of infarcted intraventricular septum: Report of a case with prolonged survival diagnosed antemortem by cardiac catheterization and review of the literature. Arch Intern Med, 109:731, 1962.

209 Cobbs BW Jr, Hatcher CR Jr, Robinson PH: Cardiac rupture: 3 Operations with 2 long-term survivals. JAMA, 223:532, 1973.

210 Hochreiter C, Goldstein J, Borer JS, et al: Myocardial free-wall rupture in acute infarction: Survival aided by percutaneous intraaortic balloon pump counterpulsation. Circulation, 65:1279, 1982.

211 O'Rourke MF: Subacute heart rupture following myocardial infarction—clinical features of a correctable condition. Lancet, 2:124, 1973.

212 Montegut FJ Jr: Left ventricular rupture secondary to myocardial infarction: Report of survival with surgical repair. Ann Thorac Surg, 14:75, 1972.

213 Chandraratna PAN, Imaizumi T, Pitha JV, Nanna M, Aronow WS: Prolonged survival after cardiac rupture following myocardial infarction. Chest, 81:643, 1982.

214 Greenburg MA, Gitler B: Left ventricular rupture

in a patient with coexisting right ventricular infarction. N Engl J Med, 309:539, 1983.

215 Coma-Canella I, Lopex-Sendon J, Gonzalez LN, Ferrufino O: Subacute left ventricular free wall rupture following acute myocardial infarction: Bedside hemodynamics, differential diagnosis, and treatment. Am Heart J, 106:278, 1983.

216 Hutchins GM, Bulkley BH: Expansion vs. extension: Two different types of acute myocardial infarction. Am J Cardiol, 41:1127, 1978.

217 Schuster EH, Bulkley BH: Expansion of transmural myocardial infarction: A pathophysiologic factor in cardiac rupture. Circulation, 60:1532, 1979.

218 Eaton LW, Weiss JL, Bulkley BH, Garrison JB, Weisfeldt ML: Regional cardiac dilatation after acute myocardial infarction: Recognition by two-dimensional echocardiography. N Engl J Med 300:57, 1979.

219 Kerber RE, Gascho JA, Litchfield R, Wolfson P, Ott D, Pandien NG: Hemodynamic effects of volume expansion and nitroprusside compared with pericardiocentesis in patients with acute cardiac tamponade. N Engl J Med, 307:929, 1982.

220 Spray TL, Roberts WC: Changes in saphenous veins used as aortocoronary bypass grafts. Am Heart J, 94:500, 1977.

221 Bulkley BH, Hutchins GM: Accelerated "atherosclerosis": A morphologic study of 97 saphenous vein coronary artery bypass grafts. Circulation, 55:153, 1977.

222 Unni KK, Kottke BA, Titus JL, et al: Pathologic changes in aortocoronary saphenous vein grafts. Am J Cardiol, 34:526, 1974.

223 Spray TL, Roberts WC: Status of the grafts and the native coronary arteries proximal and distal to coronary anastomotic sites of aortocoronary bypass grafts. Circulation, 55:741, 1977.

224 Lie JT, Lawrie GM, Morris GC Jr: Aortocoronary bypass saphenous vein graft atherosclerosis: An anatomic study of 99 vein grafts from normal and hyperlipoproteinemic patients up to 75 months postoperatively. Am J Cardiol, 40:906, 1977.

225 Smith SH, Geer JC: Morphology of saphenous vein–coronary artery bypass grafts: 7–116 months after surgery. Arch Pathol Lab Med, 107:13, 1983.

226 Chesebro JH, Clements IP, Fuster V, et al: A platelet inhibitor drug trial in coronary-artery bypass operations: Benefit of perioperative dipyridamole and aspirin therapy in early postoperative vein graft patency. N Engl J Med, 307:73, 1982.

227 Griffith LSC, Bulkley BH, Hutchins GM, et al: Occlusive changes at the coronary artery-bypass graft anastomosis. J Thorac Cardiovasc Surg, 73:668, 1977.

228 Moore GW, Hutchins GM: Coronary artery bypass grafts in 109 autopsied patients: Statistical analysis of graft and anastomosis patency and regional myocardial injury. JAMA, 246:1785, 1981.

229 Douglas JS Jr, Gruentzig AR, King SB III, et al: Percutaneous transluminal coronary angioplasty in patients with prior coronary bypass surgery. J Am Coll Cardiol, 2:745, 1983.

230 Stolte M, Heidbrink A, Schmuziger M: Morphology and pathogenesis of the aortocoronary bypass stenosis, in Kaltenbach M, Gruentzig A, Rentrop K, Bussmann W (eds): *Transluminal Coronary Angioplasty and Intracoronary Thrombolysis: Coronary Heart Disease IV*. Springer-Verlag, Berlin, 1982, p 167.

Chapter 5

Indications, Limitations, and Risks of Coronary Arteriography and Left Ventriculography

Spencer B. King III, M.D.
John S. Douglas, Jr., M.D.

Twenty-five years after the development of selective coronary arteriography, there remain differences of opinion as to the indications for the procedure. Some would reserve the technique for the most desperate cases with the idea that medical management is equal to any other therapy and therefore knowledge of coronary pathoanatomy is irrelevant. The prevalent current opinion among cardiologists, however, is that this knowledge can profoundly affect their decision making regarding patient management. Our view is that coronary arteriography is as essential a part of the evaluation of patients with suspected coronary artery disease as an upper gastrointestinal series is for the evaluation of patients with suspected peptic ulcer disease. If that belief is correct, the procedure should be made widely available. This would obviously affect future planning for catheterization facilities, as we believe it should.

The development of selective coronary arteriography by Mason Sones in 1958 heralded an era of unparalleled growth in the knowledge of the heart and circulation, and it spawned the development of coronary surgery and transluminal coronary angioplasty.[1] Since Sones' description, modifications and alternative methods have been developed.[2–7] With these techniques, costly errors in diagnosis could be almost eliminated. Prognosis could be put on a firm scientific footing, and therapeutic methods could be developed to correct the anatomic and physiological derangements of coronary artery disease.

Since the development of coronary arteriography, many new technologies have expanded our knowledge of coronary heart disease. Echocardiography and nuclear scintigraphy are established methods, and digital subtraction and nuclear magnetic resonance hold promise for the future, yet coronary arteriography remains the gold standard for the accurate diagnosis of and therapeutic guide to the management of coronary artery disease. In this chapter, we will discuss the indications for coronary arteriography as they developed at Emory University Hospital over the past 12 years as well as the limitations and risks of the procedure.

RELIABILITY OF CORONARY ARTERIOGRAPHY

The usefulness of coronary arteriography is related to how reliable it is in detecting coronary artery disease. Improvements in imaging systems have made possible the accurate delineation of lesions even in obese patients. Improved television systems allow for real time visualization and review by videotape that rivals the developed cine film. This capability enables the operator to make informed decisions about the need for more views prior to completion of the procedure. The most important new development has been the use of the cranially and caudally angled x-ray beam.[8–12] This has allowed direct on side visualization of all coronary arterial segments without overlap or foreshortening and has markedly improved the ability to accurately define the lesions. All manufacturers now have catheterization laboratory x-ray equipment that can achieve these views. No new laboratory should be constructed without this capability.

LIMITATIONS OF CORONARY ARTERIOGRAPHY

Despite these improvements in technical aspects of coronary arteriography, limitations remain. These are (1) lack of complete anatomic-pathological correlation; (2) interobserver variability; (3) imperfect correlation with flow; and (4) progression of disease.

Many investigators have attempted to correlate angiographic narrowings of coronary arteries with postmortem findings. A number of studies have been flawed by the use of angiograms done in the very beginning of coronary arteriography, when visualization was very poor.[13–16] However, more recent studies also find discrepancies. Some pathological studies fail to take into account postmortem changes; however, others have correlated postmortem findings following pressure injection and fixation of the coronary vessels.[17] When errors have been made in angiographic assessment of pathological findings, it is more common to underestimate the lesion than overestimate it.[18–21] A recent study found good correlation in arteries narrowed histologically by 50 percent or less and in those narrowed greater than 75 percent but found a significant underestimation in those lesions which produce 51 to 75 percent narrowing. These authors concluded that failure to obtain a normal segment of artery to compare to the stenosed segment was the most prominent cause of underestimation. One study comparing postmortem examination to coronary arteriograms done only a few months earlier found a high accuracy rate.[22] Another recent study[23] demonstrated 70 percent underestimation in vessels with 60 to 90 percent cross-sectional stenosis by histological study.

The angiographic morphology of the atherosclerotic plaque was correlated with postmortem histopathology.[24] Postmortem angiograms with findings of smooth, hourglass lesions correlated with simple plaque of fatty or fibrous composition and intact intima, while complicated stenoses with irregular borders and filling defects correlated with plaque rupture, plaque hemorrhage, superimposed thrombus, or recanalized thrombus. In vivo angiograms, of course, do not have the fine detail of postmortem studies, but with improved visualization it is sometimes possible to classify lesions by morphology as well as simply by percent stenosis.

It is not clear how much underestimation of coronary obstruction occurs because of the tendency of angiographers to utilize diameter reduction in measuring lesions rather than converting that to a cross-sectional area, which, of course, is the method used by the pathologists. The method of grading stenoses is discussed further in Chap. 3.

Interobserver and intraobserver variability in the evaluation of coronary stenoses is another important limitation of the technique.[25–27] Careful measuring of lesions and interpretation by several observers can help minimize these differences. Improved imaging techniques as described can display lesions in a clear fashion, making the differences of opinion less marked.

The degree of apparent obstruction may not correlate completely with the flow reserve. A lesion which narrows the artery by approximately 50 percent of the diameter may or may not influence one's ability to increase flow with exercise. Nuclear medicine and digital subtraction studies can help clarify the hemodynamic alterations in these borderline lesions.

Finally, the progression of coronary artery disease cannot be predicted. Coronary arteriography demonstrates a disease process that is present at one point in time. It is impossible to predict the rate of progression of these lesions.

RISKS AND BENEFITS

Risks

Before indications for coronary arteriography can be discussed, one must weigh the risk of the procedure against the benefits to be gained. There are certain inherent dangers in placing catheters in the heart chambers and coronary arteries. The most serious relate to the thromboembolic phenomenon, which may cause stroke or myocardial infarction. Fortunately the recognition of this potential danger has led to techniques of anticoagulation and vigorous flushing of the catheters in the abdominal aorta, prior to advancing them around the aortic arch, so as to dislodge any thrombotic material that has been picked up into an area where it will do no harm.[28] The high incidence of acute myocardial infarction, stroke, and arrhythmia as reported by Adams, Fraser, and Abrams in 1973 has been dramatically reduced.[29] The second study by these authors demonstrated the decrease in the mortality rate of the procedure.[30] The registry of the Society for Cardiac Angiography participating centers shows that in coronary arteriograms performed between 1978 and 1981 the risk to life was 0.125 percent.[31]

It is important in considering risks to take into account the condition of the patient. Patients who have been in cardiogenic shock or have unstable angina or recent infarction are at greater risk than those undergoing a purely diagnostic exam. At Emory University Hospital, the mortality rate in the past 5 years has been 0.05 percent, and mortality has been confined largely to those patients with severe left main coronary artery disease. Similar results were found in the survey of those patients catheterized in the combined series from the Society for Cardiac Angiography.[31] Special precautions may reduce the risk to those patients with left main disease who are the very ones with the greatest need for the procedure. In the past 5 years, morbidity at Emory University Hospital has included myocardial infarction 0.06 percent, stroke 0.07 percent, arrhythmias requiring cardioversion 0.37 percent, femoral artery occlusion 0.05 percent, and pseudoaneurysm 0.02 percent.[32] This data includes only patients who had coronary arteriograms.

The Society for Cardiac Angiography has recently registered 200,000 patients undergoing cardiac catheterization from 66 centers over a 4-year time period.[33] Of these patients 79 percent had coronary arteriograms, and 93 percent had left ventricular angiograms. Complications were death 0.15 percent, myocardial infarction 0.09 percent, stroke 0.07 percent, and vascular complications 0.5 percent. Abrams[34] has recently compiled the complication rates from a number of reports from the literature on patients reported since 1975. The mortality rate was 0.17 percent in 35,500 patients. Reports in the literature prior to 1975 showed a mortality rate of 0.44 percent on 55,640 cases. All studies from the literature seem to show improving mortality and improving complication rates as more experience is gained with coronary arteriography.

Complications are related to a number of factors. Adams and Abrams' analyses of complications made the strong point that the complications were diminished with increasing operator experience. Laboratories doing less than 100 cases per year had a much higher complication rate compared to those doing over 400 per year.[29,35] Other studies have not found a close relationship.[36] An operator with extensive experience is obviously best equipped to avoid complications or manage them effectively if they arise.

Risk for patients varies with the condition of the patient being studied. An extremely high percentage of patients dying from coronary arteriography have left main or triple vessel disease. Davis et al.[37] found severe triple vessel disease in all 12 patients who died in that series, while 5 of those patients had severe left main disease. In Bourassa and Noble's series, severe left main disease was present in all 12 patients who died.[38] Forty-six percent of the deaths in the survey by Adams and Abrams had severe left main disease,[29] and although the risk of death was 0.15 percent for all patients catheterized in the Society for Cardiac Angiographic registry, it was 0.86 percent in patients with left main disease.[33] Obviously these severely ill patients can be identified prior to catheterization in many cases, and their risk can be recognized and protective measures taken. Other complications which have been mentioned, such as cerebrovascular accident, arrhythmias, arterial occlusion, and pseudoaneurysm formation, and methods of avoiding these complications will be discussed in the chapters dealing with each specific coronary arteriographic technique.

Benefits

The benefits of coronary arteriography and left ventriculography in the management of the individual patient relates to the clinical problem that the patient presents. The true value of any test should not be determined by its ability to accurately measure some parameter but by the ability of the physician to use this knowledge to alter the course of the patient in a favorable manner. Patients who can benefit most from arteriography therefore are those who can be symptomatically improved with surgery or angioplasty, those whose life expectancy can be prolonged by surgery, and those in whom a definitive diagnosis of coronary disease or the absence of coronary disease will dramatically change their management. In the final analysis, the benefits to the patient who needs coronary arteriography can be extensive, while the cost of the procedure is now primarily financial since its safety has been well established.[30,31,39,40]

INDICATIONS FOR CORONARY ARTERIOGRAPHY FOR DIAGNOSTIC PURPOSES

Although not all patients who need coronary arteriography present with chest discomfort, this is the most common presentation. Patients who have chest discomfort fall into three categories: (1) those who have convincing angina pectoris; (2) patients who clearly do not have a myocardial ischemic pain and need no further cardiac workup to prove it; and (3) those in whom the diagnosis of coronary artery disease has been entertained but significant questions as to the presence of this condition can be raised. Many times the diagnostic dilemma posed by this third group can be solved by means other than coronary arteriography. Several examples of subsets which may require coronary arteriography for diagnostic accuracy are (1) patients with chest pain without good effort relationship and without good relief from rest or nitroglycerin; (2) persons with hyperventilation syndrome mimicking myocardial ischemia; (3) patients with gastroesophageal symptoms which cannot be distinguished from coronary disease; (4) patients with ischemic-sounding chest pain and a negative treadmill exercise test; (5) patients diagnosed as having positive exercise test because of the ST-segment changes but with no angina; (6) premenopausal females even if the history sounds convincing; (7) patients inadvisably given the diagnosis of coronary artery disease because of bundle branch block, labile T-wave changes, or high cardiac risk factor profile; and (8) patients with anxiety and depression and somatic symptoms compatible with angina; (9) diagnostic catheterization is also sometimes needed in certain persons with high-risk occupations, such as airline pilots, and in clarifying a diagnosis for employment or insurance purposes.

Coronary arteriography can be recommended in

such relatively low prevalence subsets because of the very low risk of the procedure and significant benefits to the patient if the findings are negative. The benefit of a normal coronary arteriogram to the patient formerly worried about having coronary artery disease in both emotional and economic terms cannot be overestimated. This is not to say that all patients with any type of chest discomfort should have catheterization; however, for any patients who cannot be reasonably reassured that they do not have coronary artery disease, coronary arteriography should be recommended.

Diagnostic catheterization and coronary arteriography to exclude coronary artery disease are required in some subsets of patients with rather classic-sounding angina pectoris. These are patients who fall in low-prevalence subgroups for the disease. Women of all ages, but especially younger women, have a low incidence of coronary artery disease. A group of women thought to have effort-related angina at Emory University Hospital have prevalence of disease of only 57 percent,[41] while a similar group studied at the Cleveland Clinic had a prevalence of coronary disease of 48 percent.[42] The diagnosis of coronary disease based on the history in these women would have resulted in unnecessary and potentially hazardous treatment of virtually half of the patients. Use of prevalence data in subgroups of patients based on age, sex, symptomatic status, exercise electrocardiographic tests, and radionuclear scintigraphy will be discussed later in this chapter.

The symptoms of coronary artery disease are far from classic in a high percentage of patients with severe coronary artery obstruction. These patients, of course, need to be identified so that proper treatment can be applied. The discomfort described is seldom called "pain" by the patient. The physician must search for words such as "burning," "warm feeling," "swelling," "expanding," "emptiness," "strange or funny feeling," "indigestion, need to burp," and a "feeling I can't describe." The discomfort may be limited to the jaw, the wrist, the abdomen, the back, or the shoulder rather than the chest. Myocardial ischemia may produce left ventricular dysfunction so that the primary symptom is dyspnea or weakness.

The duration is often atypical, with some discomfort lasting many minutes to hours. The personality of the patient strongly influences the expression of discomfort. Some people are like "the princess and the pea" and note every visceral feeling they have. Others train themselves to be very stoic and ignore all but the most severe discomfort. Reproduction of the feeling the patient has by exercise testing or simply by having the patient describe how he or she feels during various stressful activities is extremely valuable in sorting out symptoms. Discomfort at rest may mean very severe disease, or the opposite, that the symptoms are unrelated to coronary artery disease. Some patients have only rest discomfort. If it is sufficiently suggestive of myocardial ischemia, then diagnostic coronary arteriograms should be ordered.

INDICATIONS FOR CORONARY ARTERIOGRAMS IN PLANNING REVASCULARIZATION PROCEDURES

At this point there is little argument that angina pectoris can be improved or eliminated by saphenous vein bypass graft surgery or coronary angioplasty in anatomically suitable candidates. It is also generally accepted that bypass surgery has been successful in prolonging the life expectancy of certain subsets of patients with severe coronary artery disease.[43–45] For these reasons, it is imperative that those patients who can benefit from this therapy be identified. The patients fall into categories of those who have stable angina pectoris, those who have a variety of unstable angina syndromes, patients who are recovering following acute myocardial infarction, and asymptomatic patients identified because of other noninvasive tests.

Stable Angina Pectoris

Patients with stable angina pectoris are not a homogeneous group. At Emory University Hospital, we have found that 34 percent of the males with mild stable angina pectoris have one vessel coronary artery disease, 16 percent two vessel disease, 25 percent three vessel disease, 6 percent left main coronary artery disease, and 19 percent have no significant coronary obstruction. A high percentage of women in this subgroup had normal coronary arteriograms. This indicates that within this group of patients, there are some who are at extremely high risk and some at extremely low risk.

We believe that coronary arteriography is the preferred method for stratifying risks and clarifying therapeutic alternatives in most patients with stable angina pectoris. Exceptions include those patients who by reason of advanced age or other condition would not be candidates for revascularization. Patients with stable angina who are found to have high-risk anatomy at coronary arteriography are considered for revascularization. There are other patients with stable angina pectoris and moderate coronary disease who are not comfortable with their condition who would like to have improvement in their anginal threshold. Medical therapy is certainly helpful in this group; however, there are many persons who are intolerant of beta-blocking drugs or nitrates, and there are others whose activities, either vocational or recreational, produce angina pectoris even while on medical management.

The concept of disabling angina pectoris is one which can only be defined in the light of surgical results. When the surgical mortality rate was in the 5 percent range, as it was 10 years ago, a very significant degree of symptomatology was required for patients to admit that they were disabled. With improved surgical outlook and a risk around 1 percent and with the advent of angioplasty as an alternative, disabling angina pectoris has taken on an entirely new meaning. Many patients are unwilling to modify their lifestyle to the extent required to avoid their angina when an alternative exists which will enable them to be more physically active.

The overriding consideration in studying patients with stable angina pectoris, however, is the fact that within this subset there exist patients with a mortality risk which is high, based on the anatomic distribution of coronary artery disease, who need to be identified and treated. Randomized studies of patients with stable angina pectoris show improved survival for subsets with two or three vessel and left main disease treated surgically compared with those treated medically.[45–47]

Unstable Angina Pectoris

Little controversy exists that patients who have unstable angina syndrome should be catheterized. The change in anginal pattern usually indicates a change in the obstructive process or in myocardial oxygen demand. These unstable conditions are reflected by (1) recent onset angina, (2) progression of symptoms occurring with less and less effort, (3) the occurrence of rest pain, and (4) prolonged pains, and are grouped under the designation "unstable angina." Although all these patients are treated vigorously with medical therapy, early catheterization is indicated to identify the nature of the underlying disease process. It has long been recognized that these syndromes may herald an impending myocardial infarction.[48]

Within the group of "unstable" patients are some who do not require surgery. Severe symptoms can be produced by rather insignificant anatomic problems. Total occlusion of an artery, especially a more peripheral one or a branch on the lateral wall of the left ventricle, may produce an infarction which is undetected by the electrocardiogram. Symptoms from the occlusion may include one or more episodes of prolonged pain and may be interpreted as unstable angina. Only with the addition of the catheterization data can the whole picture be put together, a picture which may be very stable, with no more myocardium in jeopardy and a rather benign prognosis. The overriding consideration, however, in catheterizing these unstable patients is identifying those with severe obstructive disease who have large areas of jeopardized myocardium and who may be in a progressive phase of their disease. Many studies of unstable angina pectoris have shown an unacceptable mortality rate in those treated medically.[48–51]

Acute Myocardial Infarction

Although myocardial infarction would formerly have been a contraindication for coronary arteriography, there are four times at which the procedure should be considered: (1) in the very early phase if thrombolytic therapy or emergency revascularization is planned (see Chap. 16), (2) when planning emergency surgery in patients with mechanical derangements secondary to acute infarction, (3) when planning emergency surgery in patients with uncontrolled unstable angina following acute infarction, and (4) when evaluating prognosis to guide future therapy in asymptomatic patients following infarction.

Mechanical Derangements Secondary to Myocardial Infarction

Rupture of a papillary muscle or the interventricular septum following acute myocardial infarction usually produces a severe hemodynamic insult leading to congestive heart failure with pulmonary edema and cardiogenic shock. Septal rupture may be produced by either an anterior or posterior myocardial infarction, and papillary muscle rupture is usually caused by inferior or posterolateral infarction with occlusion of the circumflex artery or the left ventricular branch of the right coronary artery (see Chap. 3). The outlook for these hemodynamically unstable patients managed medically is so poor that immediate surgery is usually indicated. For that reason, catheterization and coronary arteriography, although at increased risk, is undertaken. The use of the intraaortic balloon counterpulsation devices is helpful in stabilizing the hemodynamic situation so that catheterization and coronary arteriography can be performed. Some centers have recommended emergency surgery without catheterization; however, we feel that ventriculography can better define the defects the surgeon needs to repair, and arteriography can identify areas of coronary obstruction that need to be bypassed at the time the mechanical defect is repaired.

When patients are stabilized medically following the rupture of the interventricular septum, there is a temptation to attempt to hold them in a stabilized condition with medical therapy. This would allow for demarcation of the infarction and some healing, but rapid deterioration can strike at any time and commonly does in these severely compromised patients. The decision of when to operate is a controversial and difficult one and will be strongly influenced by the ability of the available surgical team to bring these patients through surgery successfully.

Recurrent Pain Following Acute Myocardial Infarction

A group of patients with myocardial infarction who should undergo arteriography are those who have had either nontransmural myocardial infarction or a limited transmural myocardial infarction and recurrent pain which is repetitive and difficult to control (see Chap. 3). Control of symptoms following an infarction may require intensive treatment in a coronary care unit environment. Intravenous nitroglycerin, beta blockade, and, more recently, calcium antagonists are used to control symptoms. Narcotics are used with the initial episodes of pain, but if recurrent pain occurs, we would push toward early coronary arteriography. These patients should undergo catheterization to determine if there is additional jeopardized myocardium which might be salvaged by some intervention. Cardiac catheterization and coronary arteriography has been demonstrated to be safe in this group when care has been taken to minimize the length of the procedure and the contrast medium load.

Patients are selected for catheterization not because of the infarction but because the judgment has been made that additional myocardium may be in jeopardy. When these patients undergo surgery, it is not *because of* the infarction but *despite* the infarction. Studies in our center indicate that carefully selected patients in this subset can be operated on with a low mortality risk.[52,53] This is contrary to studies of patients who have undergone noncardiac surgery following a myocardial infarction; in this group the mortality rate may be high. The discrepancy can be partially explained by the fact that patients with large, complicated infarctions are usually not catheterized or operated upon, and patients are selected because of large areas of jeopardized myocardium which may be improved by the bypass operation. In noncardiac surgery, no chance for improvement exists in myocardial perfusion during the operative procedure. The anesthetic management of patients during cardiac surgery is of course exquisitely controlled with careful hemodynamic and electrocardiographic monitoring and adjustment of the parameters as necessary. Recent work by others would indicate the possibility of operating on a broader spectrum of patients with myocardial infarction with a relatively low operative and hospital mortality rate.[54–56]

Post–Myocardial Infarction Patients Without Continuing Symptoms

Patients who have had myocardial infarction usually have multivessel disease (see Chap. 3). It is also more common for patients to experience angina pectoris following myocardial infarction than for infarction to result in cessation of angina.[57,58] The prognosis of patients following infarction relates to the amount of myocardial damage suffered and also to the degree of obstruction in the coronary arteries serving the remaining viable myocardium. The most productive area of investigation is in patients who have had relatively small infarctions based on electrocardiographic and enzymatic criteria. Since most patients with subendocardial infarction have not damaged large areas of the left ventricular myocardium, they are in at least equal jeopardy of reinfarction and subsequent mortality as those with transmural infarction. These have become ideal candidates for early investigation.[59,60] We believe it is prudent to do coronary arteriography as a screening procedure several weeks following a myocardial infarction even in the absence of recurrent angina.

This is a controversial topic only because of the increase in costs of "routine" postinfarction catheterizations. It is clear, however, that some asymptomatic postinfarction patients are at high risk for cardiac events in the first year, and one form of risk stratification is needed. Others have advocated submaximal stress electrocardiography, radionuclide ventriculography, and/or thallium-201 imaging to screen patients. We believe, however, that in most patients the increased information obtained by coronary arteriography is worth the increased cost. Patients excluded from this recommendation would be elderly patients, those with associated disease which makes surgical intervention unlikely, and those with massive left ventricular destruction with congestive heart failure who have septal or papillary muscle rupture or a large ventricular aneurysm excluded by noninvasive means.

Asymptomatic Patients

Coronary artery disease exists in many asymptomatic individuals, and sudden cardiac death may be the first presentation. For these reasons a safe and reliable screening test for coronary disease has long been sought. It is economically unfeasible to recommend coronary arteriography as a screen for all individuals; however, there are subgroups of asymptomatic individuals in whom the prevalence of disease is markedly increased. Treadmill exercise testing in asymptomatic patients is now frequently carried out as part of a routine physical examination or prior to beginning physical conditioning programs. The incidence of false-positive treadmill tests in asymptomatic individuals is high, and therefore they should not be labeled as having coronary disease without first carrying out coronary arteriography. A markedly positive test with greater than 2-mm ST-segment depression on the exercise electrocardiogram, however, may herald severe coronary obstructive disease such as left main artery obstruction and therefore identify patients at a very high risk. Some patients have severe coronary artery disease and yet are insensitive to any discomfort. Diabetics are notorious in this regard. Other screening tests such as thallium scanning with exercise and first pass or multigaited exercise ventriculography are capable of identifying patients with asymptomatic coronary artery disease. These alternative methods of screening are frequently used prior to coronary arteriography in patients who are asymptomatic. Other asymptomatic categories have been discussed under the heading "Indications for Coronary Arteriography for Diagnostic Purposes."

USE OF LESS INVASIVE METHODS FOR SCREENING FOR CORONARY ARTERY DISEASE

In screening for coronary artery disease, one starts with the history, the age, and the sex of the patient. From this simple information, some index of prevalence of the disease in that population can be predicted.

As Bayes' theorem indicates, the predictive value of a normal or abnormal test result is directly related to the prevalence of the disease in the population studied. *Sensitivity* measures the percentage of people with disease who have an abnormal test, and *specificity* measures the percentage of people with no disease who have a normal test. These two indexes really measure the worth of the test, but do not predict whether the patient will have disease or not. The *predictive value of an abnormal test* is the percent of abnormal responders who truly have disease, and the *predictive value of a normal test* is the percent of normal responders who have no disease. This is directly related to the prevalence of disease in the population tested. The predictive value is therefore the index that is clinically helpful in deciding whether to order a test or not in a specific patient.

Exercise Electrocardiographic Tests

Exercise electrocardiographic testing has an overall sensitivity of 60 to 70 percent and a specificity near 90 percent.[61] Sensitivity is greater with multivessel disease and is less with single vessel disease. False-positive tests are increased in patients with vasoregulatory abnormalities, posture-induced or hyperventilation-induced ST-segment changes, resting baseline ST-T–interval changes, and in women. Marked, greater than 2-mm, ST-segment depression occurring early in exercise is a rather specific sign for coronary artery disease. The predictive value of exercise electrocardiographic testing, however, relates to the prevalence of disease in the population studied. Froelicher showed (Table 5-1) the relationship of pretest odds to posttest odds of disease in several subsets of coronary artery disease depending on the outcome of the test. Since the positive test simply moves us further in the direction of ordering coronary arteriography, it is actually the predictive value or posttest odds of a negative test that is of clinical value. If this prediction of no disease is high enough, then catheterization can be avoided.

One can see that a negative test reduces the chance of disease only mildly in patients with angina from 90 to 75 percent. Even in patients with atypical angina or others with a fifty-fifty pretest chance of disease, a negative test only reduces the chance of disease to 25 percent, still a diagnostic dilemma. In those patients with a low pretest likelihood of disease, such as those with nonanginal pain and asymptomatic patients, a negative test results in only a 2 to 4 percent risk of coronary disease being present. With this low chance of disease, one can reassure the patient and avoid coronary arteriography with confidence.

An exercise test as a screening procedure should therefore be ordered if the finding of a normal test will enable the physician to reassure the patient at that point without the need for further workup. If it is clear before the exercise test is ordered that even if a normal test is obtained it will still be necessary to go further with a workup, then the exercise test is superfluous.

Exercise Radionuclear Tests

Exercise thallium scanning and exercise radionuclear ventriculography have added to the sensitivity and specificity of the exercise electrocardiogram. The best published figures, however, would show that sensitivity and specificity are no greater than 90 percent.[62–64] If these tests are applied to patients who are in the high-prevalence population, then little advantage is obtained, since the chance of coronary disease is so high to begin with that a positive test would add little and a negative test would not eliminate the possibility of coronary dis-

	Pretest odds	Likelihood ratio	Posttest odds	Posttest probability
Anginal	9:1	Abnormal test (× 7)	63:1	$\left(\frac{63}{64}\right) = 98\%$
		Normal test (× 3)	9:3	$\left(\frac{9}{12}\right) = 75\%$
Atypical anginal	1:1	Abnormal test (× 7)	7:1	$\left(\frac{7}{8}\right) = 88\%$
		Normal test (× 3)	1:3	$\left(\frac{1}{4}\right) = 25\%$
Nonanginal	1:9	Abnormal test (× 7)	7:9	$\left(\frac{7}{16}\right) = 44\%$
		Normal test (× 3)	1:27	$\left(\frac{1}{28}\right) = 4\%$
Asymptomatic	1:19	Abnormal test (× 7)	7:19	$\left(\frac{7}{26}\right) = 27\%$
		Normal test (× 3)	1:57	$\left(\frac{1}{58}\right) = 2\%$

Table 5-1 Calculation of probability of coronary artery disease (CAD) showing how the clinical presentation affects the probability after exercise testing. The pretest odds were determined from angiographic and epidemiologic data, and the likelihood ratios are based on a sensitivity of 70 percent and a specificity of 90 percent for the ECG response to exercise test. (*Adapted from Froelicher VF: Techniques of exercise testing, in Hurst JW (ed)*: The Heart (5th ed). *McGraw-Hill, New York, 1982, p 1731*, with permission of the author.)

ease. On the other hand, in relatively low-prevalence populations, a negative test might well eliminate the need for coronary arteriography because the predictive value of a negative test would bring the chance of coronary disease to such a low level that the patient and physician would both be willing to forego any further testing (Fig. 5-1).

An example of a high-prevalence situation in which screening tests are unnecessary would be that of a 55-year-old male patient with a typical history of exertional chest discomfort relieved by rest. The prevalence of coronary disease in this subset would be approximately 90 percent. A positive radionuclear exam would increase the chance of disease up to about 99 percent, but a negative test would reduce the risk only to about 60 to 70 percent. One can see that a negative test would not eliminate the need for coronary arteriography, since the chance is still strong that coronary disease exists. At the other end of the spectrum is a female patient, age 40, who has chest discomfort which, although containing some of the features of angina pectoris, occurs without a good effort relationship and is not relieved by rest or nitroglycerin. The prevalence of disease in such a patient is difficult to establish; however, of all females with atypical chest pain catheterized at our institution, prevalence was under 20 percent. In this situation, a negative radionuclear exercise exam would bring the risk of coronary disease well under 5 percent and might eliminate the need for further testing.

Whereas exercise stress test and radionuclear stress test have a distinct place in cardiology and give additional information regarding function not available on coronary arteriograms, their usefulness as screening procedures is related to the prevalence of disease in the population from which the patient comes. They would seem to be valuable in patients who are in the mid- to lower-prevalence population and are virtually of no use as screening tests in those patients with clear-cut angina pectoris. In those situations, the most cost-effective way to evaluate the patient is to move directly to coronary arteriography.

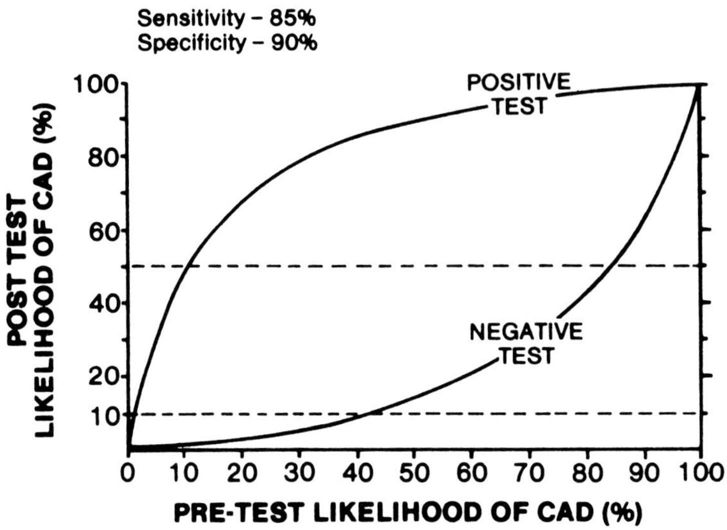

A

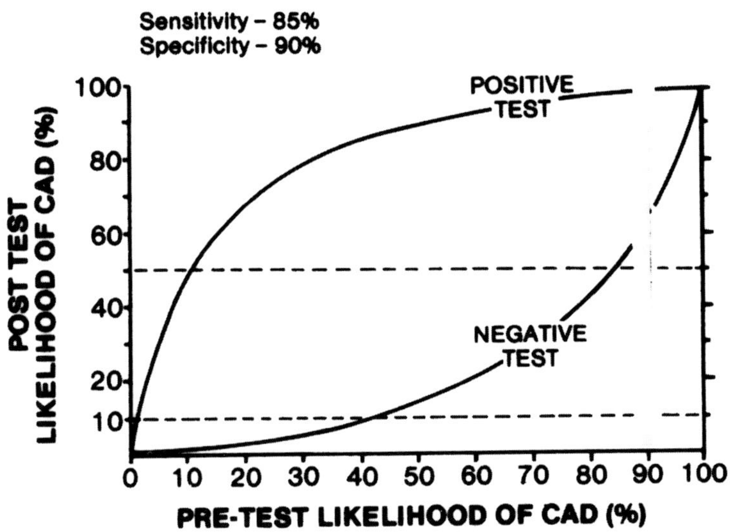

B

Figure 5-1 Chart of pretest and posttest likelihood for coronary artery disease (CAD) using radionuclear techniques. These results are based on an assumed sensitivity of 85 percent and specificity of 90 percent. (*a*) Illustrates the relationship between the pretest likelihood of coronary artery disease based on epidemiologic and angiographic data and the posttest likelihood of disease following the radionuclear exam. The effects of a positive radionuclear exercise test or a negative test are illustrated. (*b*) Patients with angina pectoris and a 90 percent pretest likelihood of coronary disease will have that likelihood reduced to only the mid–60 percent range by virtue of a negative test. (*c*) Patients with mid-range pretest likelihood of disease such as women with exercise and rest angina will have that risk reduced to 15 to 18 percent by virtue of a negative test. (*d*) Patients with a low pretest likelihood of disease such as those with atypical chest pain not thought to be of ischemic origin will have the likelihood of disease reduced to 3 to 4 percent by virtue of a negative exercise nuclear exam.

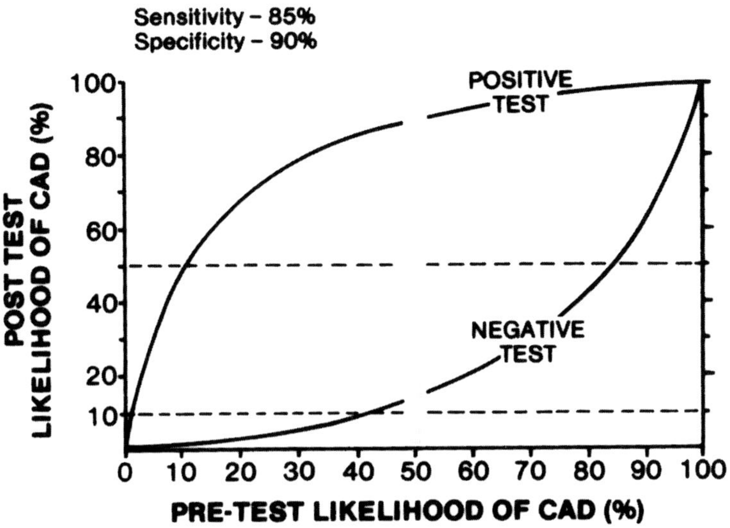
Sensitivity – 85%
Specificity – 90%
POSITIVE TEST
NEGATIVE TEST
POST TEST LIKELIHOOD OF CAD (%)
PRE-TEST LIKELIHOOD OF CAD (%)
0
10
20
30
40
50
60
70
80
90
100

C

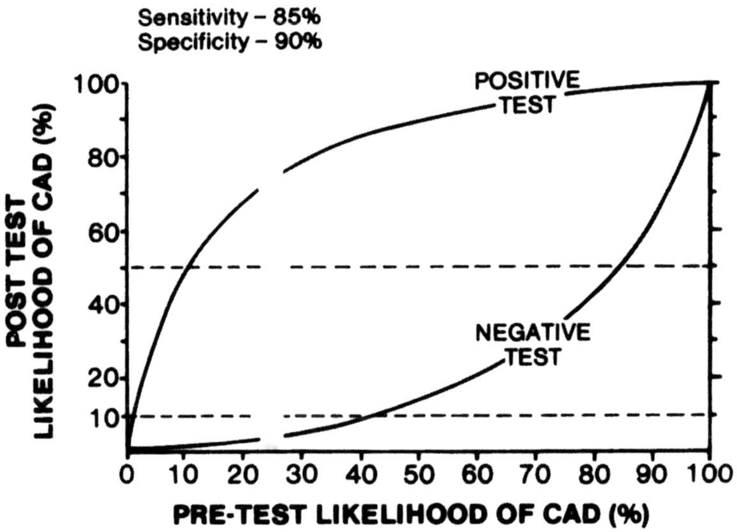
Sensitivity – 85%
Specificity – 90%
POSITIVE TEST
NEGATIVE TEST
POST TEST LIKELIHOOD OF CAD (%)
PRE-TEST LIKELIHOOD OF CAD (%)
0
10
20
30
40
50
60
70
80
90
100

D

REFERENCES

1 Sones FM Jr, Shirey EK: Cine coronary arteriography. Mod Concepts Cardiovasc Dis, 31:735, 1962.

2 Rickets HJ, Abrams JL: Percutaneous selective coronary cine arteriography. JAMA, 181:620, 1962.

3 Amplatz K: Techniques of coronary arteriography. Circulation, 27:101, 1963.

4 Gensini GG: Coronary arteriography. Prog Cardiovasc Dis, 6:155, 1963.

5 Amplatz K, Formanek G, Stranger P, et al: Mechanics of selective coronary artery catheterization via femoral approach. Radiology, 89:1040, 1967.

6 Judkins MP: Selective coronary arteriography, part 1: A percutaneous transfemoral technique. Radiology, 89:815, 1967.

7 Schoonmaker FW, King SB: Coronary arteriography by the single catheter percutaneous femoral technique: Experience in 6,800 cases. Circulation, 50:735, 1974.

8 Lesperance J, Saltiel J, Peticlerc R, et al: Angulated views in the sagittal plane for improved accuracy of cine coronary angiography. AJR, 121:565, 1974.

9 Sos TA, Lee JG, Lovin DG, et al: New lordotic projection for improved visualization of the left coronary artery and its branches. AJR, 121:575, 1974.

10 Aldridge HE: Better visualization of the asymptomatic lesion in coronary arteriography using cranial and caudal angulated projections. Chest, 71:502, 1977.

11 Frederick PR, Fry WH, Russell JG, et al: Longitudinal angulation in coronary arteriography: Apparatus and evaluation. Cathet Cardiovasc Diagn, 71:502, 1977.

12 King SB III, Douglas JS Jr, Morris DC: New angiographic views for coronary arteriography, in Hurst JW (ed): *Update IV: The Heart*. McGraw-Hill, New York, 1980.

13 Gray CR, Hoffman HA, Hammond WS, Miller KM, Oseasohn RO: Correlation of arteriographic and pathologic findings in coronary arteries in man. Circulation, 26:494, 1962.

14 Littman D, Dean D, Crowley F, Gelson I, Williams J: Clinical coronary angiography. Am J Cardiol, 7:570, 1961.

15 Sloman G, Hare WSC: Clinical application of coronary angiography. Med J Aust, 47:611, 1960.

16 Eusterman JJ, Achor RWP, Kincaid OW, Brown ALL Jr: Atherosclerotic disease of the coronary arteries: A pathologic-radiologic correlative study. Circulation, 26:1288, 1962.

17 Staiger J, Dieckmann H, Adler CP, Barmeyer J, Sandritter W: Postmortem angiographic and pathologic-anatomic findings in coronary heart disease: A comparative study using planimetry. Cardiovasc Interven Radiol, 3:1, 1980.

18 Kemp HG, Evans H, Elliott WC, Gorlin R: Diagnostic accuracy of selective coronary cinearteriography. Circulation, 36:526, 1967.

19 Vlodaver Z, Frech R, Van Tassel RA, Edwards JE: Correlation of the antemortem coronary arteriogram and the postmortem specimen. Circulation, 47:162, 1973.

20 Schwartz JN, Kong Y, Hackel DB, Bartel AG: Comparison of angiographic and postmortem findings in patients with coronary artery disease. Am J Cardiol, 36:174, 1975.

21 Arnett EN, Isner JM, Redwood DR, Kent KM, Baker WP, Ackerstein H, Roberts WC: Coronary artery narrowing in coronary heart disease: Comparison of cineangiographic and necropsy findings. Ann Intern Med, 91:198, 1979.

22 Murphy ML, Galbraith JE, de Soyza N: The reliability of coronary angiogram interpretation: An angiographic-pathologic correlation with a comparison of radiographic views. Am Heart J 97:578, 1979.

23 Staiger J, Dieckmann H, Adler CP, Barmeyer J, Sandritter W: Postmortem angiographic and pathologic-anatomic findings in coronary heart disease: A comparative study using planimetry. Cardiovasc Intervent Radiol, 3:1, 1980.

24 Levin DC, Fallon JT: Significance of the angiographic morphology of localized coronary stenoses: Histopathologic correlations. Circulation, 66:316–320, August 1982.

25 Bjork L, O'Keefe A: Estimation of coronary artery stenosis. Acta Radiol [Diagn] (Stockh), 17:777, 1976.

26 Zir LM, Miller SW, Dinsmore RE, Gilbert JP, Harthorne JW: Interobserver variability in coronary angiography. Circulation, 53:4, 1976.

27 Myers MG, Shulman HS, Saibil EA, Naqui SZ: Variation in measurement of coronary lesions on 35 and 70 mm angiograms. AJR, 130:913, 1978.

28 Takaro T, Hultgren HN, Littman D, et al: An analysis of deaths occurring in association with coronary arteriography. Am Heart J, 86:587, 1973.

29 Adams DF, Fraser DB, Abrams HL: The complications of coronary arteriography. Circulation, 48:609, 1973.

30 Abrams HL, Adams DF: The complications of coronary arteriography. Circulation, 52(suppl 2):27, 1975.

31 Kennedy JW: Complications associated with cardiac catheterization and angiography. Report of the Registry Committee of the Society for Cardiac Angiography, in Coronary Artery Disease Today. Proceedings of an international symposium, Utrecht, May 25–27, 1981.

32 Emory University Clinic Cardiac Data Bank. Report, 1983.

33 Kennedy JW: Report of the Registry Committee, Society for Cardiac Angiography. Annual meeting, Scottsdale, Arizona, May 12, 1983.

34 Abrams HL: Complications of coronary arteriography, in Abrams HL (ed): *Coronary Arteriography—A Practical Approach*. Little, Brown, Boston, 1983.

35 Davis K, Kennedy JW, Kemp HG Jr, Judkins MP, Gosselin AJ, Killip T: Complications of coronary arteriography from the collaborative study of coronary artery surgery (CASS). Circulation, 59:1105, 1979.

36 Hansing CE: The risk and cost of coronary angiography: II. The risk of coronary angiography in Washington state. JAMA, 242:735, 1979.

37 Davis K, Kennedy JW, Kemp HG Jr, Judkins MP, Gosselin AJ, Killip T: Complications of coronary arteriography from the collaborative study of coronary artery surgery (CASS). Circulation, 59:1105, 1979.

38 Bourassa MG, Noble J: Complication rate of coronary arteriography: A review of 5250 cases studied by a percutaneous femoral technique. Circulation, 53:106, 1976.

39 Adams DF, Abrams HL: Complications of coronary arteriography: A follow-up report. Cardiovasc Radiol, 2:89, 1979.

40 King SB III: Atherosclerotic coronary heart disease–coronary arteriography, in Hurst JW (ed): *The Heart* (5th ed). McGraw-Hill, New York, 1982, p 1054.

41 Douglas JS Jr, Hurst JW: Limitations of symptoms in the recognition of coronary atherosclerotic heart disease, in Hurst JW (ed): *Update III: The Heart*. McGraw-Hill, New York, 1982, p 1054.

42 Proudfit WL, Shirey EK, Sones FM Jr: Selective cine coronary arteriography: Correlation with clinical findings in 1,000 patients. Circulation, 33:901, 1966.

43 Hurst JW, King SB III, Logue RB, et al: The value of coronary bypass surgery. Controversies in cardiology: Part I. Am J Cardiol, 142:308, 1978.

44 Hurst JW, King SB III: Prolongation of life by coronary bypass surgery, in Hurst JW (ed): *Update II: The Heart*. McGraw-Hill, New York, 1980, p 141.

45 Takaro T, Hultgren HN, Lipton MJ, et al: The VA cooperative randomized study of surgery for coronary arterial occlusive disease. II: Subgroup with significant left main lesions. Circulation, 54(suppl 3):107, 1975.

46 Gunnar RM, Loeb HS, Palec R, et al: Improved survival in patients with chronic angina pectoris treated surgically: Report of a randomized prospective study of aorto-coronary bypass from Heinz, Illinois, in JW Hurst (ed): *Update II: The Heart*. McGraw-Hill, New York, 1980, p 205.

47 National Institutes of Health Consensus-Development Conference Statement, Special Report. Coronary artery bypass surgery: Scientific and clinical aspects. N Engl J Med, 304:680, 1981.

48 Gazes PC, Mobley EM, Farris MH Jr, et al: Preinfarction (unstable) angina: A prospective study. Ten year follow-up. Circulation, 48:331, 1973.

49 Bertolasi CA, Tronge JE, Mon GA, Turri D, Lugones MI: Clinical spectrum of "unstable angina." Clin Cardiol, 2:113, 1979.

50 Unstable Angina Pectoris: National Cooperative Study Group to Compare Medical and Surgical Therapy: (I) Report of protocol-patient population, Am J Cardiol, 37:896, 1976; (II) In-hospital experience and initial follow-up, Am J Cardiol, 42:839, 1978.

51 Alison HW, Russell RO Jr, Mantle JA, Kouchoukos NT, Moraski RE, Rackley CE: Coronary anatomy and arteriography in patients with unstable angina pectoris. Am J Cardiol, 41:204, 1978.

52 Jones EL, Waits TF, Craver JM, et al: Coronary bypass with relief of persistent pain following acute myocardial infarction. Ann Thorac Surg, 32:33, 1981.

53 King SB III: The role of coronary arteriography in the management of the patient with acute myocardial infarction. Primary Care, 8:415, 1981.

54 Maddigan MP, Rutherford BD, Barnhorst DA, et al: Early saphenous vein grafting after subendocardial infarction: Immediate surgical results and late prognosis. Circulation, 56(suppl 2):1, 1977.

55 Aintablian A, Hamby RI, Weisz D, et al: Results of aorto-coronary bypass grafting in patients with subendocardial infarction: Late follow-up. Am J Cardiol, 42:183–186, 1978.

56 Wiener L: Selection of patients treated surgically with evolving myocardial infarction, in Rahimtoola

SH (ed): *Cardiovascular Clinics: Coronary Bypass Surgery*. Davis, Philadelphia, 1977, p 23.

57 Kannel WB, Feinleib M: Natural history of angina pectoris in the Framingham study. Am J Cardiol, 29:154–162, 1972.

58 Amsterdam EA, Lee G: Relationship of myocardial infarction to presence of angina pectoris in patients with coronary heart disease: Lack of abolition of angina by infarction. Clin Cardiol, 1:31–34, 1978.

59 Dussia EE, Cromartie D, McCraney J, et al: Myocardial infarction with and without laboratory documentation: One year prognosis. Am Heart J, 92:148–151, 1976.

60 Schroeder JS, Lamb IH, Hu M: Do patients in whom myocardial infarction has been ruled out have a better prognosis after hospitalization than those surviving infarction? N Engl J Med, 301:1–5, 1980.

61 Froelicher VF: Techniques of exercise testing, in Hurst JW (ed): *The Heart* (5th ed). McGraw-Hill, New York, 1982, p 1726.

62 Ritchie J, Zaret B, Strauss H, et al: Myocardial imaging with thallium-201: A multicenter study in patients with angina pectoris or acute myocardial infarction. Am J Cardiol, 42:345, 1978.

63 Rerych S, Scholtz P, Newmann G, et al: Cardiac function at rest and during exercise in normals and in patients with coronary heart disease: Evaluation by radionuclide angiography. Ann Surg, 187:449, 1978.

64 Strauss HW, McKusick KA, Prohost GM: Cardiovascular nuclear medicine, in Hurst JW (ed): *Update I: The Heart*. McGraw-Hill, New York, 1979, p 329.

Chapter 6

Coronary Arteriography and Left Ventriculography: Sones Technique

Frederick Heupler, Jr., M.D.

Dr. F. Mason Sones, Jr., introduced selective coronary arteriography by the brachial artery approach at The Cleveland Clinic in 1958.[1] In the 1960s the percutaneous femoral technique of coronary arteriography was introduced and rapidly gained popularity. The advantages of the Sones technique over the percutaneous femoral method are as follows: (1) Only one catheter is necessary to visualize both coronary arteries, the left ventricle, and aortocoronary bypass grafts; (2) this method can be used in patients with severe obstructive disease of the iliofemoral system; (3) the procedure can be done on an outpatient basis, since the patient can be ambulatory immediately; (4) the depth of insertion of the catheter tip into the left coronary artery can be better controlled; and (5) the catheter tip can be rapidly shifted from one coronary artery to the other (important in the patient with coronary artery spasm).

Today, the mortality risk of coronary arteriography by the Sones technique is no more than 0.1 percent in many laboratories and 0.07 percent in our laboratory. This low mortality rate can be achieved by well-trained angiographers who are familiar with the procedure. It is the purpose of this chapter to help familiarize the student of angiography with the methods, equipment, and complications associated with the Sones technique of selective coronary arteriography. The information contained in this chapter is a compilation of ideas generated by Dr. F. Mason Sones and his colleagues at The Cleveland Clinic.

EVALUATION OF THE PATIENT FOR CATHETERIZATION

The angiographer should approach the arteriographic procedure as a clinical consultant, not a technician. After the angiographer has reviewed the patient's history, physical examination, electrocardiogram, chest x-ray, and routine laboratory studies, it should be possible to assess the indications for catheterization and the type of procedure appropriate for that particular patient. Before an elective catheterization, the angiographer should evaluate the patient for uncontrolled congestive heart failure, arrhythmias, endocarditis, hypokalemia, digitalis toxicity, and other medical conditions which increase the risk of the procedure. The patient should be adequately hydrated before and after the catheterization.

The angiographer should evaluate the patient's brachial and radial pulses before catheterization. If the brachial pulses are unequal in the arms, or if a loud subclavian bruit is present, the blood pressure should be checked in both arms. A blood pressure differential of more than 20 mmHg should alert the angiographer to use the arm with the higher pressure because of the possibility of a subclavian artery stenosis.

The angiographer should attempt to gain the confidence of the patient and be reassuring regarding the procedure. The patient should be informed of the risks involved and the reasons for performing the catheterization.

CATHETERIZATION LABORATORY PERSONNEL AND EQUIPMENT

During the coronary arteriographic procedure, we commonly use at least two assistants. The first assistant helps during catheter insertion, administration of medicines, high-pressure injections, and closure of the wound. The second assistant obtains equipment, changes film, observes the monitor screen for arrhythmias and pressure changes, and activates the electrocardiographic and pressure recording devices.

A 2 × 3 foot table contains the sterile supplies needed for the procedure (Fig. 6-1). A manifold is connected to the injection system as described in Fig. 6-2. A single electrocardiographic lead (usually lead II) is monitored by continuous display on a screen located adjacent to the fluoroscopy screen. Pressures at the catheter tip are displayed continuously on the same screen as the electrocardiogram. An external defibrillation unit is located in immediate proximity to the catheterization table (Fig. 6-3).

The choice of cinefluoroscopy equipment is determined by the uses for which it is intended. A 6-inch amplifier is optimal for coronary arteriography. If a large (9-inch) amplifier is utilized, some compromise must be made in the image quality. However, this amplifier permits better visualization of larger structures, as needed in pulmonary arteriograms, aortograms, and angiograms of dilated cardiac chambers.

We prefer a single plane rotating C-arm assembly, with the x-ray tube mounted below the table and a 6-inch image intensifier and camera mounted above (Fig. 6-3). The entire C-arm assembly can be controlled easily by a handle held in the operator's left hand. The patient lies on a portable table which may be pivoted to the right or left to obtain angulated views. Biplane cinefluoroscopy equipment has the advantage of permitting simultaneous visualization of a coronary artery in two different views with only one coronary injection. This feature is desirable for coronary angioplasty procedures. For routine coronary arteriography, the advantages of a biplane system are outweighed by the disadvantages: (1) poorer picture quality; (2) increased radiation exposure; (3) difficulty in positioning both amplifiers simultaneously; (4) higher initial installation costs; and (5) increased bulk.

Fluoroscopic and cine images are viewed on a closed-circuit television system designed especially for medical image intensifiers. The video signal may be stored on videotape or disks for subsequent playback. For routine coronary arteriography, video playback is usually unnecessary, but it is important for coronary angioplasty and intracoronary streptokinase procedures.

In a large-volume laboratory, the patient may receive initial preparation and cutdown as well as closure and dressing of the wound in an inexpensive anteroom. This patient can then be transported on the portable table into the catheterization lab-

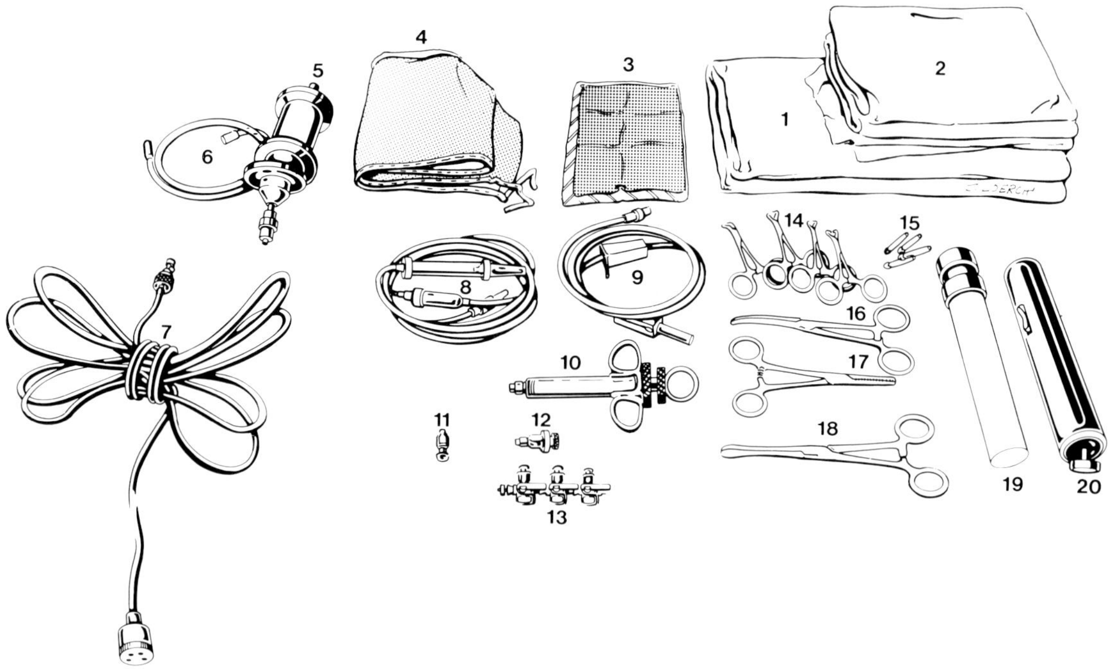

A

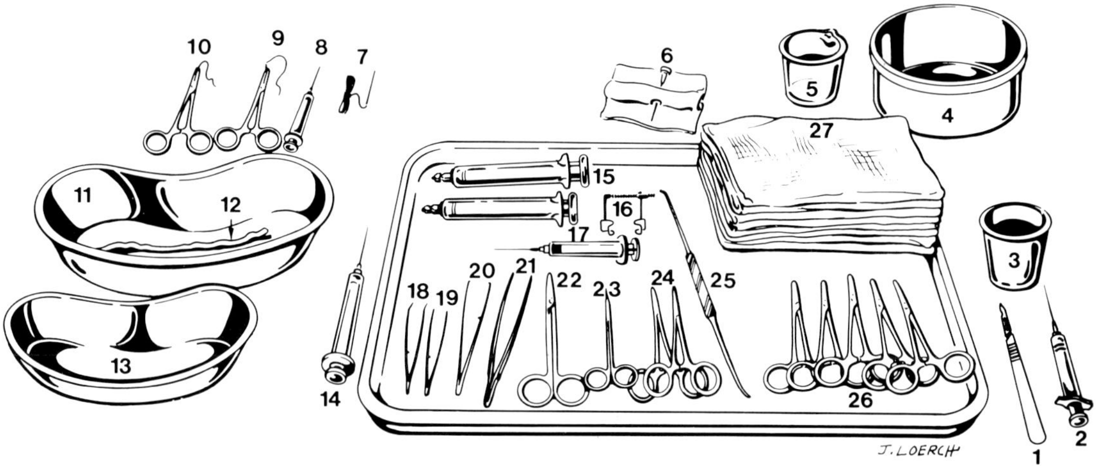

B

Figure 6-1 *(a)* Back table supplies prior to catheterization: (1) large sheet for draping patient, (2) four large towels to drape cutdown site, (3) plastic cover for shield over table-control handle, (4) surgical cap to cover amplifier, (5) power injector syringe, (6) extension tubing, (7) pressure transducer, (8) and (9) plastic tubing for dextrose and for contrast solution, (10) syringe for coronary injections, (11) metal cap for pressure transducer, (12) rotating adapter for catheter, (13) three-way manifold, (14) towel clips, (15) safety pins, (16) large curved hemostat, (17) Kocher clamp, (18) sponge forceps, (19) light bar, (20) table-control handle.

(b) Back table supplies during catheterization: (1) scalpel, (2) lidocaine syringe, (3) container with 2% lidocaine, (4) large basin for boiling water for catheters, (5) beaker for norepinephrine or other solutions, (6) no. 21 1½-inch needle, (7) needle and suture to close skin wound, (8) syringe with 1 mg atropine, (9) hemostat with rubber band, (10) needle holder with no. 5-0 polyester suture for artery, (11) large empty kidney basin, (12) umbilical tape for retracting artery, (13) small kidney basin containing heparinized dextrose solution, (14) syringe with 10 mL (5000 units) heparin solution, (15) empty 20-mL syringes, (16) Weiner eye speculum, (17) syringe with 5 mL (2.0 mg) nitroglycerin solution, (18) Nugent curved utility forceps, (19) fine delicate dressing forceps, (20) skin forceps, (21) tissue forceps, (22) suture scissors, (23) curved eye scissors, (24) curved mosquito hemostats, (25) probe, (26) straight hemostats, (27) sponges, 4 × 8 inches.

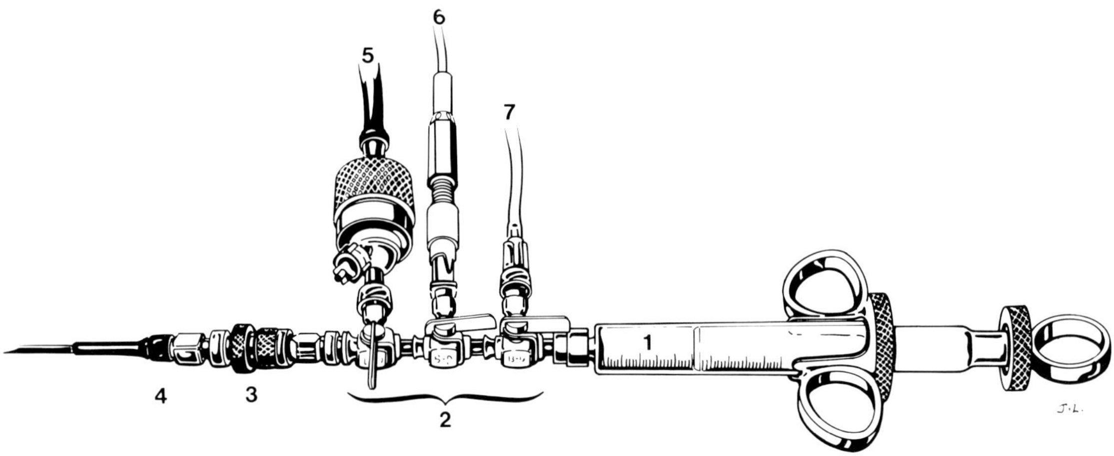

Figure 6-2 Catheter-manifold-syringe assembly: (1) syringe, (2) three-way manifold, (3) rotating adapter, (4) catheter, (5) pressure transducer, (6) tubing to dextrose solution, (7) tubing to contrast solution.

Figure 6-3 Catheterization laboratory equipment: (1) portable radiolucent bed, (2) control handle for C-arm, (3) rotating C-arm, (4) x-ray tube, (5) image intensifier, (6) movie camera, (7) sterile light bar, (8) defibrillator, (9) pressure and ECG monitor, (10) fluoroscopy screen.

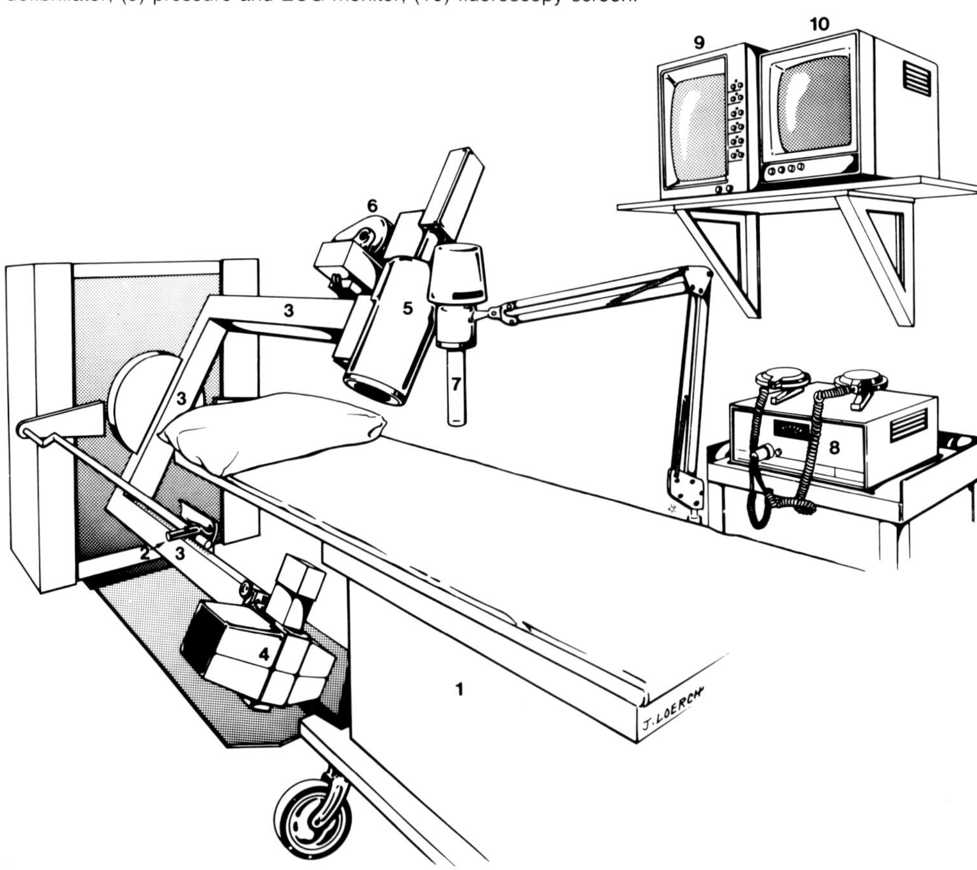

oratory for arteriography while another patient is being prepared in the anteroom. This "carousel" system of patient rotation permits optimal time utilization of the expensive cineangiographic equipment.

RADIATION EXPOSURE WITH THE SONES TECHNIQUE

Radiation exposure to the angiographer and assistants arises primarily from radiation which is scattered in the patient during fluoroscopy and cineangiography. With C-arm equipment, the operator is exposed to minimum scatter radiation in the direct path of the primary x-ray beam (during right anterior oblique projection for the right arm approach). Studies in the left anterior oblique projection produce significantly higher scatter radiation exposure to the operator.[2]

During an average coronary arteriogram by the Sones technique with a C-arm system, 80 percent of the total radiation exposure to the angiographer is due to the cine study and 20 percent to the fluoroscopy. If cineradiography is performed at a film speed of 60 frames per second, the total radiation dose is 1.8 times higher compared to the use of 30 frames per second. Since the higher film speed provides only minimal extra useful information, the film speed should be limited to 30 frames per second in most coronary arteriograms.[2]

Radiation exposure does not affect all organ systems equally. For the angiographer, radiation dosages to the corneas and thyroid gland are the most important considerations. A table-mounted lead shield (Fig. 6-4) decreases radiation dosage to the eyes by 70 percent, the thyroid by 80 percent, and the legs by 90 percent when used in conjunction with a Philips Cardiodiagnost C-arm unit (Table 6-1). With this system, an angiographer may perform at least 50 catheterizations per week (using average exposure figures) without exceeding the maximum dosage to the eyes or thyroid gland as recommended by the National Council on Radiation Protection and Measurements (NCRP).[2]

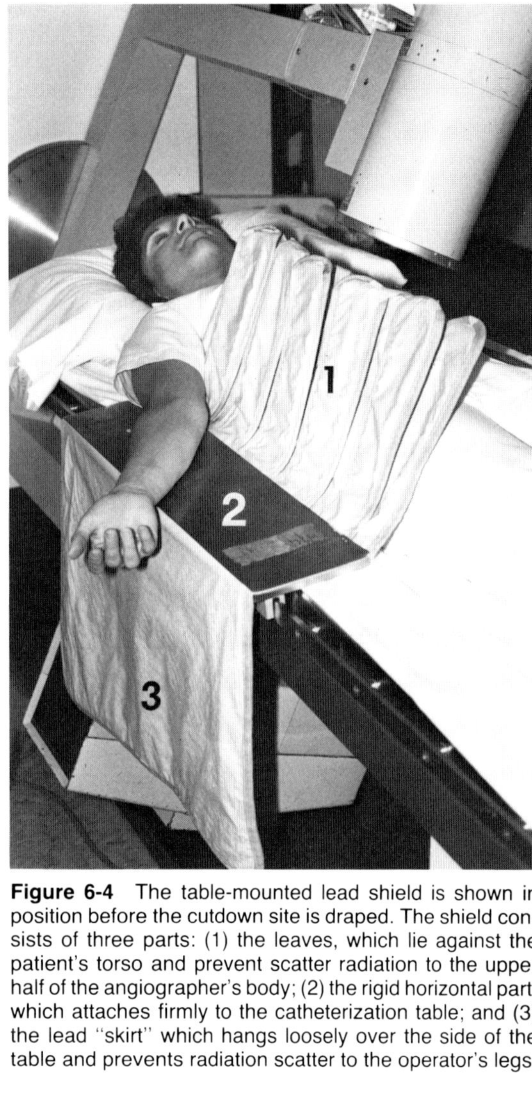

Figure 6-4 The table-mounted lead shield is shown in position before the cutdown site is draped. The shield consists of three parts: (1) the leaves, which lie against the patient's torso and prevent scatter radiation to the upper half of the angiographer's body; (2) the rigid horizontal part, which attaches firmly to the catheterization table; and (3) the lead "skirt" which hangs loosely over the side of the table and prevents radiation scatter to the operator's legs.

SELECTION OF CATHETER

Numerous catheters are available for the brachial approach for coronary arteriography and for associated procedures such as left ventriculography, aortography, and internal mammary arteriography. Those most commonly used are listed in Fig. 6-5 and Table 6-2. Structurally, all cardiac catheters can be divided into (1) the extruded type, which is a homogeneous hollow plastic tube usually made

Table 6-1 Radiation Exposure During Cardiac Catheterization*

Organ	NCRP maximum (mR†/week)	Average exposure (mR/examination)	
		No shield	Shield
Eyes	100	6	1.9
Thyroid	300	8.3	1.4
Lower legs	300	13.1	1.0

*Average time per examination = 12.7 minutes of fluoroscopy and 110 s of ciné at 30 frames per second.
†mR = milliroentgens; NCRP = National Council on Radiation Protection and Measurement.
SOURCE: Adapted from Balter et al., Circulation, 58:925–932, 1978.

of polyethylene or polyurethane (e.g., the Judkins coronary catheter) and (2) the woven type, composed of a woven tube of Dacron or nylon which is coated with a radiopaque plastic (e.g., the Sones catheter) (Fig. 6-6).

The Sones catheter (Figs. 6-5 and 6-6, and Table 6-2) is available in a variety of lengths, diameters, and compositions, but the one most commonly used in our laboratory is the no. 8 French 80-cm Sones type I catheter with a style B curve.* The no. 8 French shaft permits adequate torque control and rapid delivery of contrast material, and the more flexible no. 5 French tapered tip permits gentle placement of the catheter tip into the ostium of the coronary artery. Several modifications of the basic Sones catheter have been introduced to improve torque control (Fig. 6-6). When pressed against the aortic valve, the Sones type I catheter forms a loop approximately 1½ inches long, which is ideal for catheterization of the coronary arteries in the average adult. The Sones catheter permits adequate left ventriculography and aortography in most cases; however, the end hole causes it to "whip" during high-pressure injections, and the tapered tip limits the rate of injection.

The Shirey left atrial catheter (Fig. 6-5 and Table 6-2) was designed for retrograde transmitral catheterization of the left atrium in patients with mitral stenosis, but it is also suitable for ventriculography and aortography.[3] The shorter taper (7.5 cm long)

*United States Catheter and Instrument Corporation, Billerica, Mass.

Figure 6-5 Major catheters used for the brachial technique. The catheter tips are magnified to demonstrate the configuration of the end holes and side holes.

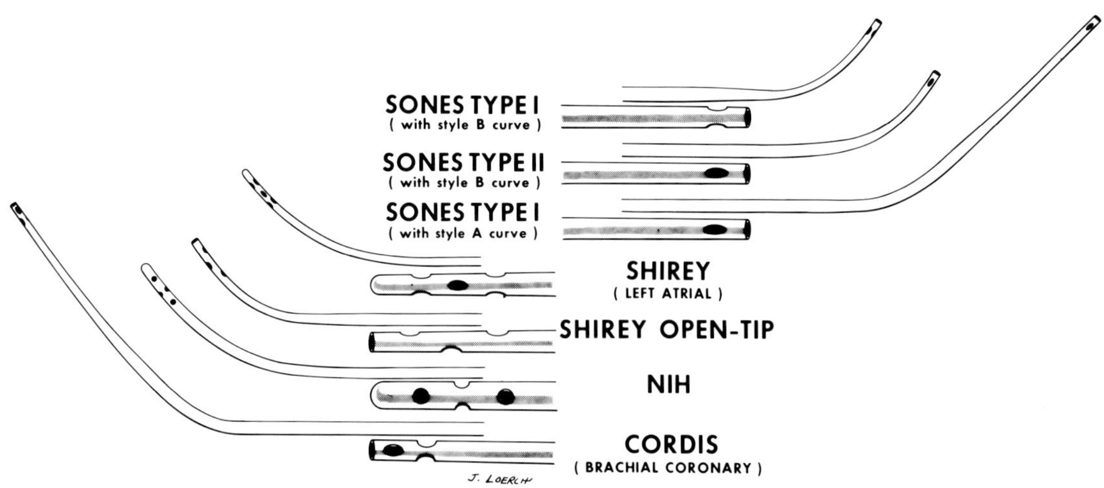

Table 6-2 Basic Catheters for the Sones Technique

Name	Length, cm	Diameter, French	Tapered tip Length, cm	Tapered tip Diameter, French	Holes End	Holes Side	Uses*
Sones type I†	80; 100	7; 8	3.8	5	Yes	2	SCA; LV; Ao
Sones type II	80; 100	7; 8	2.5	5	Yes	2	SCA with narrow aortic root; LV; Ao
Shirey	80	8	7.5; 10	5; 6	No	6	LA; LV; Ao
Shirey open tip	80	8	7.5	6	Yes	6	Cerebral angiography; SCA with dilated aortic root
NIH	80; 100	7; 8	–	–	No	6	LV; Ao

*SCA = selective coronary arteriography; LV = left ventriculography; Ao = aortography; IMA = internal mammary arteriography; LA = left atrium.
†Available with a preformed style A curve (7.5 cm from the tip) and style B curve (3.8 cm from the tip).

is used for normal or mildly dilated left ventricles, and the longer taper (10 cm long) for markedly dilated left ventricles. Since the standard Shirey left atrial catheter has no end hole, it is unlikely to recoil out of the left atrium during atriography. There is a Shirey left atrial catheter with an end hole, which is used for carotid arteriography and occasionally for coronary arteriography when the aortic root is extremely dilated.

The NIH catheter (Fig. 6-5 and Table 6-2) per-

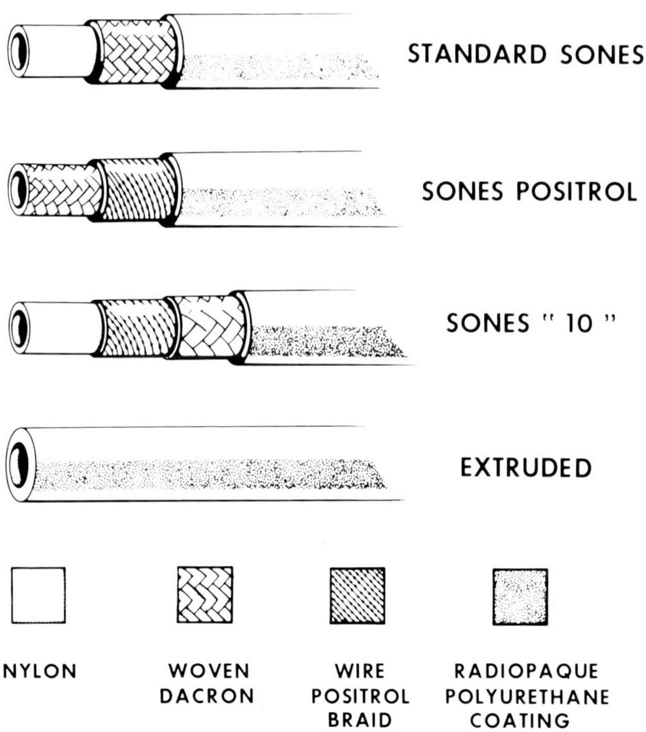

Figure 6-6 The structures of commonly used brachial catheters. The Sones Positrol and Sones "10" catheters each incorporate a wire braid which permits better torque control. The extruded catheter is a homogeneous hollow plastic tube, which may also contain a wire braid.

mits injection of large volumes under high pressure, since it has large side holes, no end hole, and no taper. This catheter is ideal for ventriculography in patients with a dilated left ventricle or severe mitral regurgitation and for aortography.

The Cordis brachial coronary catheter (Fig. 6-5) is similar to the Sones catheter, except that it has four side holes. This catheter has the advantage of extreme flexibility and memory, which permit the angiographer to preshape the catheter. It is used primarily for selective internal mammary artery visualization in our laboratory.

ARTERIAL CUTDOWN AND CLOSURE

The patient should be positioned on the catheterization table with a board taped behind the elbow to keep the arm straight. Every attempt should be made to keep the patient comfortable and calm. A sedative is administered routinely before the procedure. Electrocardiographic limb leads are attached, and a single lead is monitored continuously. The laboratory personnel prepare the skin over the cutdown site with an antiseptic solution and drape the area. The arterial cutdown is then performed (Fig. 6-7). The major risk of the arterial cutdown is injury to the median nerve, which lies medial and slightly posterior to the brachial artery (Fig. 6-8). The patient should be instructed to notify the physician immediately on sensation of "electric shock" or pain radiating down into the fingers. These symptoms usually mean that the median nerve has been contacted.

After completion of the catheterization and re-

Figure 6-7 Isolation and cannulation of the brachial artery. *(a)* The cutdown site is over the brachial artery at the level of the median epicondyle. *(b)* The artery is isolated by blunt dissection with curved mosquito hemostats. *(c)* Umbilical tapes are placed around the artery for traction. *(d)* Heparin solution is injected distally. *(e)* An arteriotomy is performed with curved eye scissors. *(f)* The catheter is then passed into the artery. *(g)* A rubber band encircles the catheter and artery proximally to prevent backflow of blood around the catheter (optional).

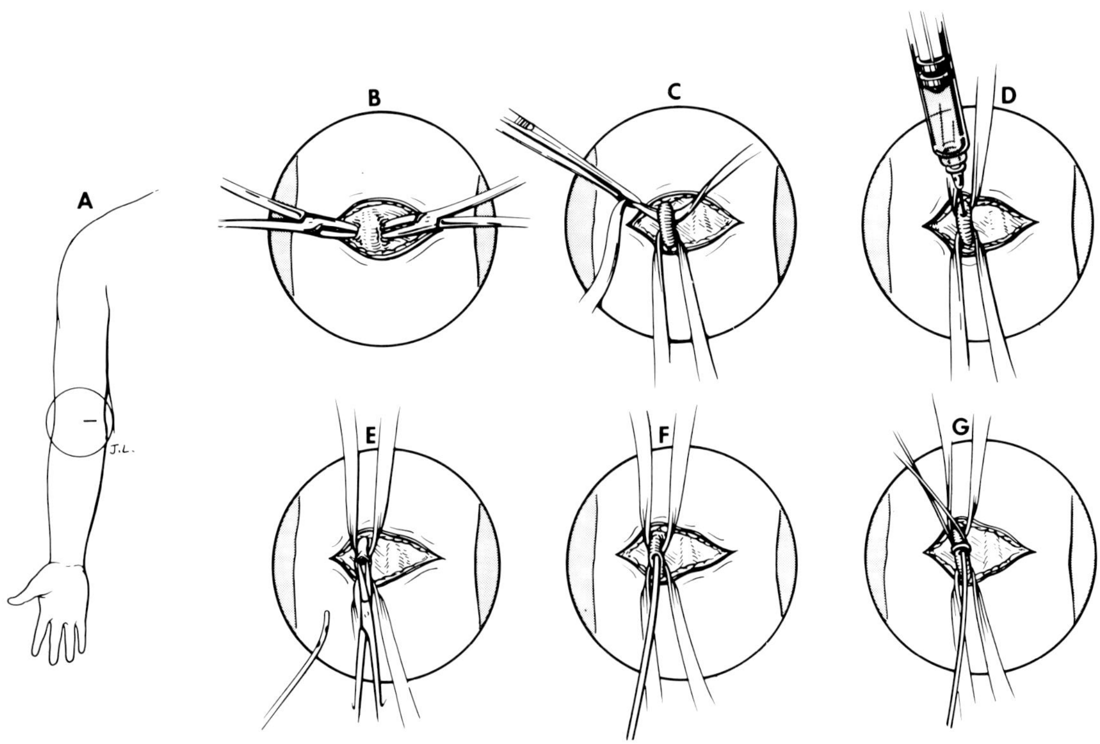

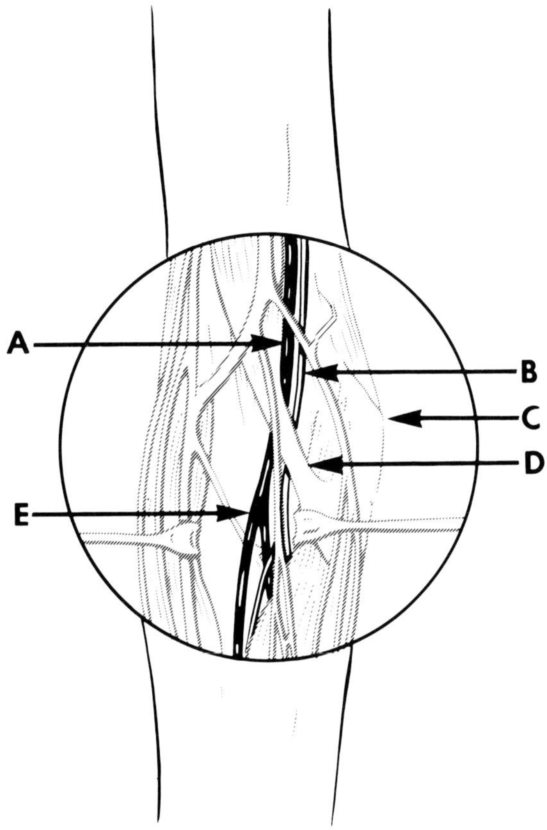

Figure 6-8 Anatomy of the right antecubital fossa. The brachial artery (*a*) lies lateral and anterior to the median nerve (*b*). The brachial artery at the level of the medial epicondyle (*c*) passes beneath the biceps aponeurosis (*d*) before it bifurcates (*e*) into radial and ulnar branches.

moval of the catheter from the artery, the angiographer should ensure vigorous flow from the proximal and distal ends of the artery. When flow from the distal end is sluggish or absent, gentle passage of a small probe into the distal artery usually permits vigorous return of blood. An operator unable to obtain retrograde blood flow from the distal artery may either close the artery and evaluate for patency or pass a Fogarty thrombectomy catheter into the distal artery. Because of the potential for producing intimal damage with this catheter, the angiographer should receive instruction from a vascular surgeon in its proper use. After thrombectomy, heparin should again be flushed into the distal artery.

We usually use the "purse-string" method to close the brachial arteriotomy (Fig. 6-9). This technique produces mild transverse narrowing of the artery at the closure site, but it permits an adequate pulse to remain in more than 95 percent of patients. In patients with small arteries, a transverse closure is preferred (Fig. 6-10). After the skin incision is closed and covered with a compression dressing, the patient should keep the arm straight for 1 hour, after which the elbow should be flexed regularly to prevent stiffness.

INTRODUCTION OF THE CATHETER INTO THE HEART

The angiographer should stand with the fluoroscopy foot switch immediately available, the table-

Figure 6-9 Purse-string closure of the brachial arteriotomy. The no. 5-0 Tevdek suture encircles the arteriotomy and is then closed in a purse-string fashion. The lateral sutures must be placed close to the edge of the arteriotomy in order to minimize the lateral narrowing which occurs with this type of closure.

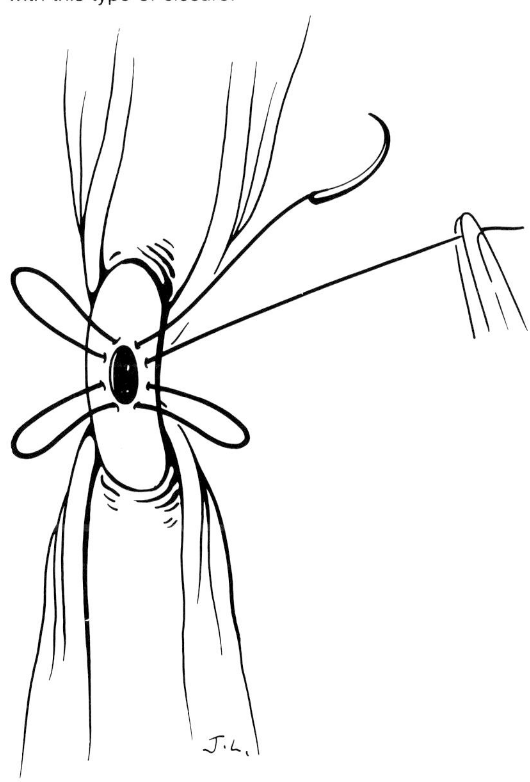

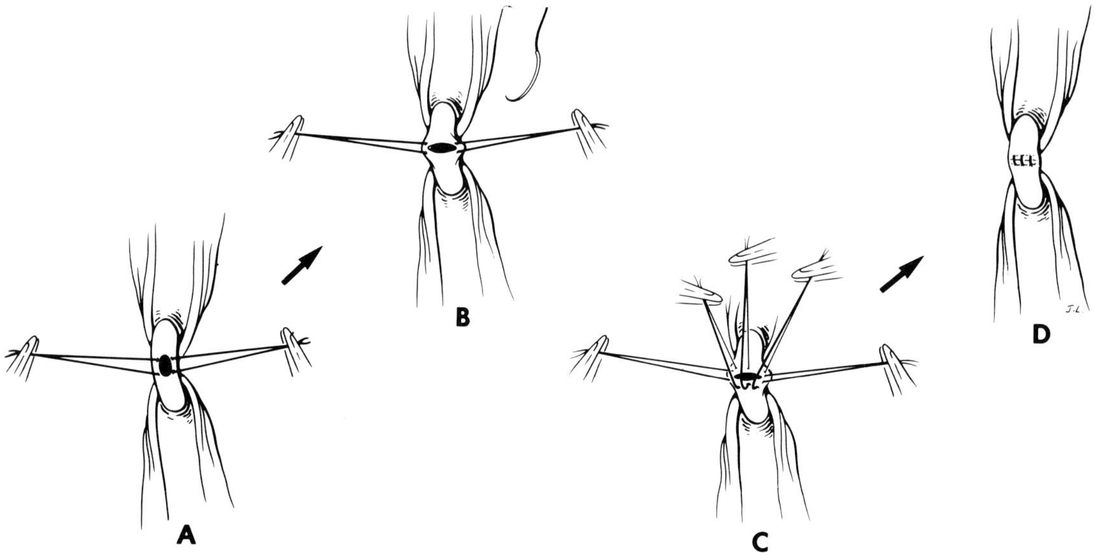

Figure 6-10 Transverse closure of arteriotomy. *(a)* "Stay sutures" are placed at 3:00 and 9:00 after arterial clamps (not shown) are positioned above and below the arteriotomy; *(b)* when these sutures are pulled, the arteriotomy becomes a transverse slit; *(c)* three interrupted sutures result in approximation of the edges; and *(d)* after closure, no transverse narrowing of the artery is present.

control handle within easy reach, and the catheter-manifold assembly to the front. The fluoroscopy screen and the screen with the electrocardiogram and pressure tracings should be in direct view of the angiographer, so that changes in rhythm and pressure during catheter manipulation will be detected. The nurse assistant should constantly observe the two video screens and notify the operator immediately of any major changes in rhythm or pressure.

The operator rotates the catheter with the left hand and the swivel with the right hand. When a catheter lies in the left coronary sinus, clockwise rotation of the shaft displaces the tip of the catheter anteriorly into the right sinus, and counterclockwise rotation displaces it posteriorly and to the left into the noncoronary sinus (Fig. 6-11). When the catheter tip lies in the aortic root, a 90° rotation applied externally commonly results in less than 90° rotation internally at the tip of the catheter. This is due to delay in transmission of torque, which is related to the physical properties of the catheter and the degree to which the brachial artery restricts rotation of the catheter. Rapid in-and-out motion of the catheter over a few millimeters will assist in transmitting the torque. Once the catheter tip has been rotated to the desired location, it often continues rotating in the same direction, even though no more torque is applied. This is because of delayed transmission of torque which is "stored" in the catheter from previous rotations. To prevent this "overshoot," the operator should partially reverse the torque once the catheter tip has been rotated to the desired spot. After the catheter has been in the arterial circuit for 5 to 10 minutes, it becomes noticably "softer." This produces slower transmission of torque and makes the catheter less likely to maintain a loop when the catheter is withdrawn. A certain amount of stiffness may be temporarily restored to the catheter by slowly flushing through 10 mL of cool saline solution.

During passage of the catheter from the brachial arteriotomy to the left ventricle, the catheter tip commonly enters branches of the brachial or subclavian artery. The angiographer should advance the catheter forward gently, and upon meeting re-

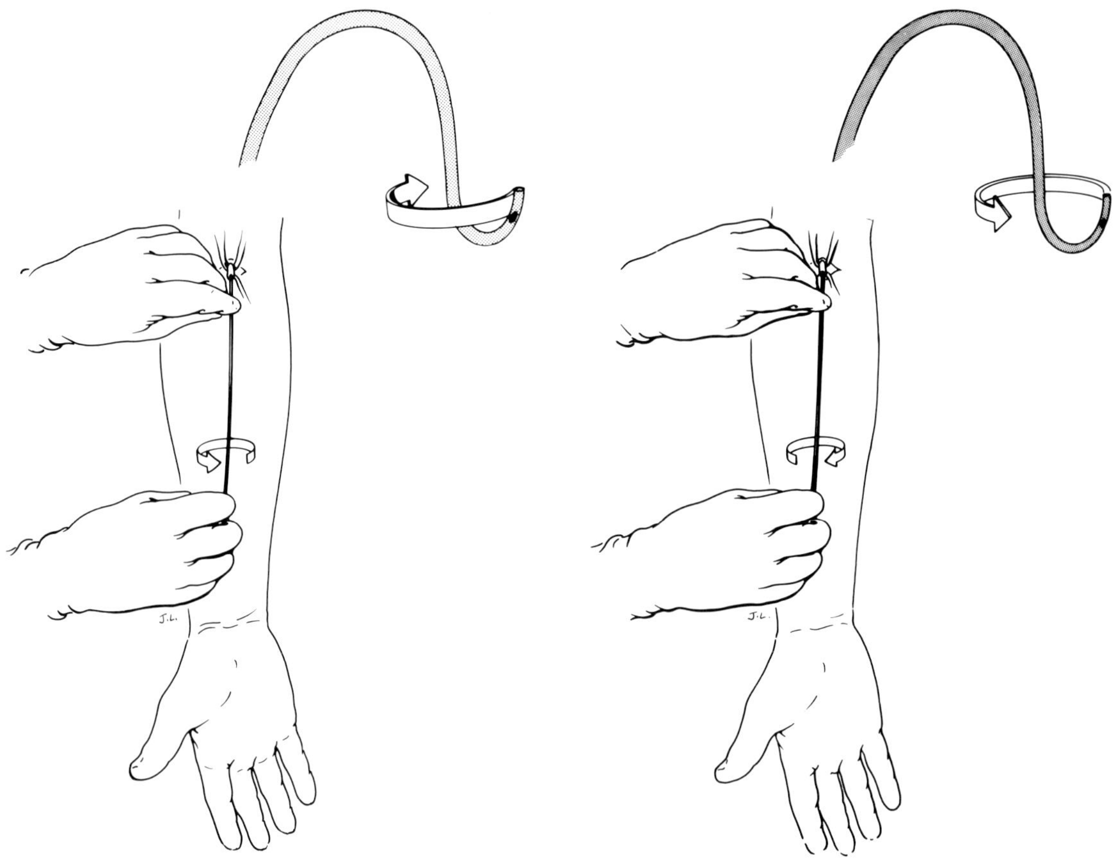

A B

Figure 6-11 The relation between the external manipulation of the catheter and the internal displacement of the catheter tip at the level of the aortic sinuses of Valsalva when the catheter is rotated *(a)* clockwise, and *(b)* counterclockwise.

sistance, pull back, rotate the catheter, and advance gently again. Once the catheter has reached the subclavian artery, it should be advanced only under fluoroscopic observation. Often, the catheter tip passes superiorly into the vertebral artery rather than into the innominate. This can usually be overcome by (1) rotating the catheter to face inferiorly; (2) having the patient turn the head to the left and inspire; and (3) removing the pillow from under the head. The angiographer should never attempt to force the catheter into the ascending aorta. A 0.035-cm safety J-spring guidewire, passed through the tip of the Sones catheter, facilitates passage from the subclavian artery into the ascending aorta. This is particularly helpful in patients with a tortuous subclavian artery, which is common in hypertensive and elderly people. When the innominate artery arises high in the aortic arch or when a retroesophageal subclavian artery is present, the catheter tip tends to enter the descending aorta. In both situations, entry into the ascending aorta can be facilitated by a J-spring guidewire and by advancing the catheter during deep inspiration.

Severe arterial spasm, which is more likely to occur in a small brachial artery, may (1) cause arm pain; (2) delay transmission of torque along the catheter; and (3) interfere with in-and-out motion of the catheter tip. When the spasm is severe enough

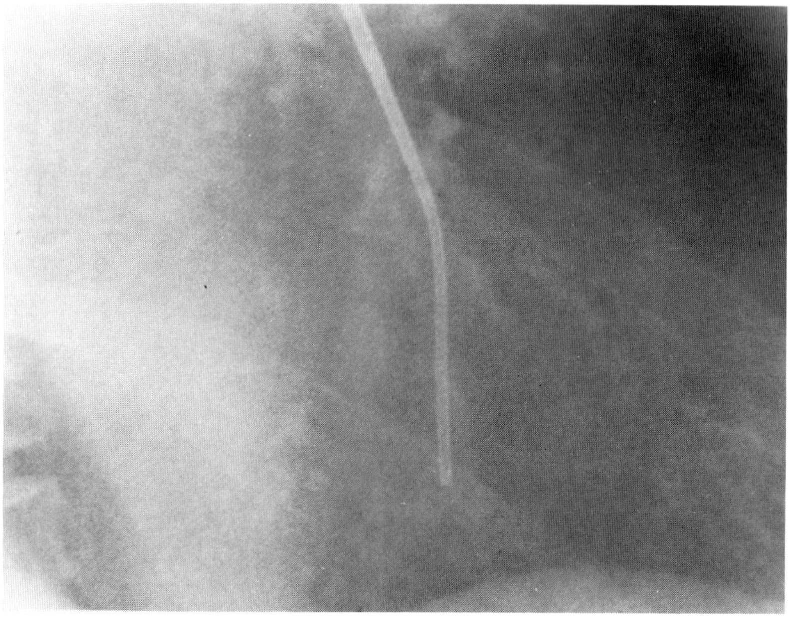

A

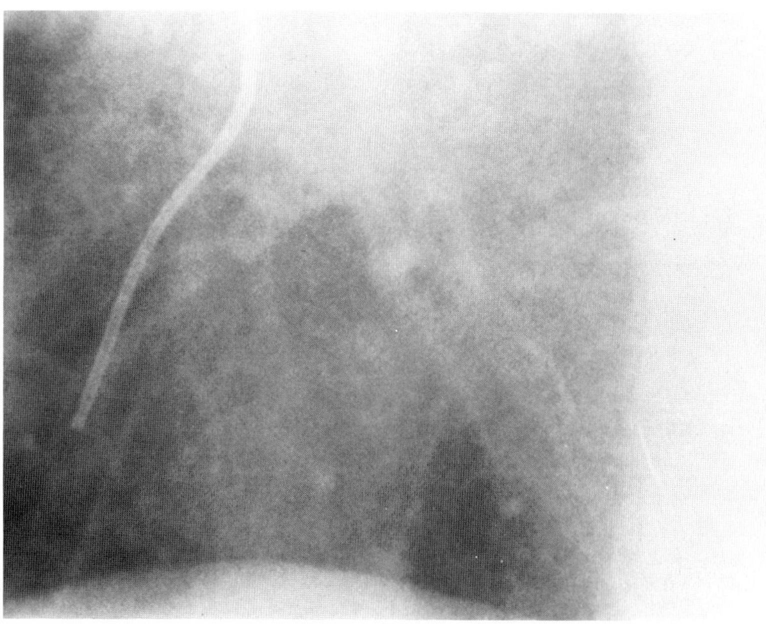

B

Figure 6-12 Inadvertent entry of the Sones catheter into the right coronary artery instead of the left ventricle. In the 35° right anterior oblique (RAO) projection *(a)*, the tip of the Sones catheter has passed several centimeters below the level of the aortic sinuses of Valsalva, and it appears to lie in the left ventricle. In the 45° left anterior oblique (LAO) projection *(b)*, the catheter tip is aimed in the wrong direction to enter the left ventricle, and it is therefore probably in the right coronary artery. Injection of contrast material in the 45° LAO projection *(c)* demonstrates that the catheter is deep inside the right coronary artery. Note that the initial part of the right coronary artery is directed almost vertically downward (arrows), and this permits the catheter tip to inadvertently enter the right coronary artery. In the 45° LAO projection *(d)*, the tip of the catheter faces away from the right coronary artery and toward the spine when it is within the left ventricle.

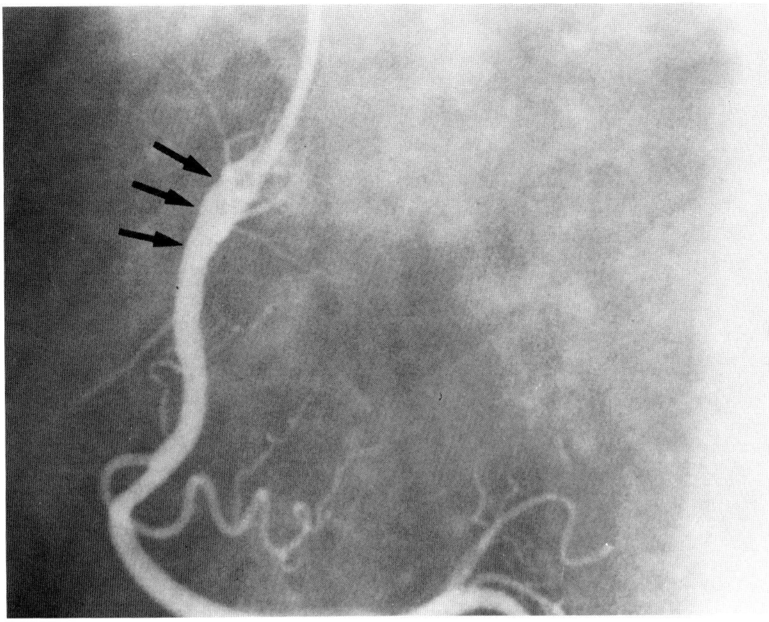

C

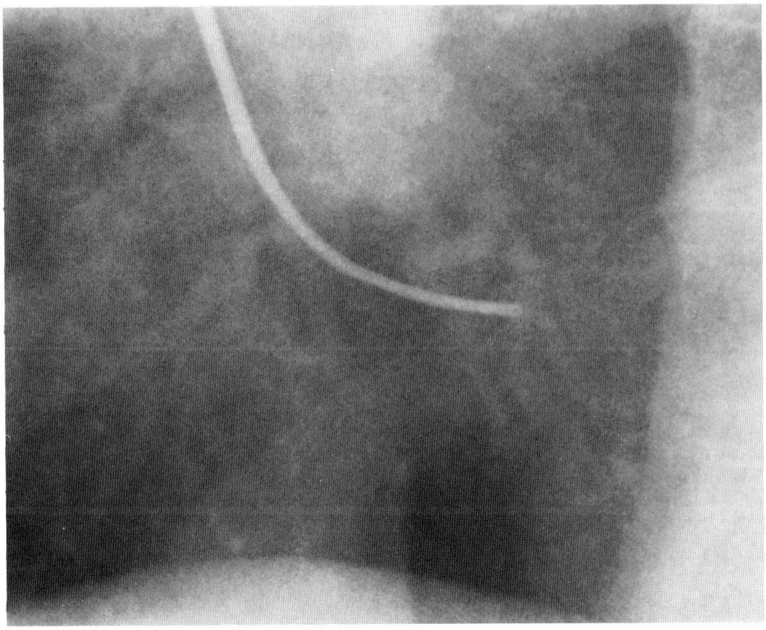

D

to interfere with the catheterization procedure, relaxation of the artery may be achieved by removing the catheter from the artery and administering small intravenous doses of a tranquilizer. After several minutes, when the patient has become more relaxed, the catheter should be reintroduced. Rarely, it may be necessary to use a narrower catheter.

Once the catheter is in the ascending aorta, it should be advanced into the left ventricle during fluoroscopy in a 45° left anterior oblique (LAO) projection. This view separates the origins of the coronary arteries and permits the angiographer to avoid inadvertent insertion of the catheter into either the right or the left coronary artery (Fig. 6-12).

In order to pass the Sones catheter retrograde across the aortic valve, the angiographer should form a long loop by pushing the catheter tip against the aortic valve. The next step is to gently and rapidly move the catheter up and down against the aortic valve in the LAO projection, while rotating the catheter clockwise. The catheter tip should be kept away from the ostium of the left coronary artery. If the patient has a severe ostial left main trunk obstruction, repeated trauma with the catheter tip could induce coronary spasm or dissection. Once the tip of the Sones catheter enters the left ventricle, it should be directed away from the ventricular septum or lateral wall in order to avoid premature beats.

The Sones catheter will not pass across a severely stenotic aortic valve with a loop. In order to cross such a valve, the angiographer should direct the tip of the catheter toward the aortic valve and advance it gently but rapidly forward during systole, synchronizing the forward movement of the catheter with the QRS complex, the upstroke of the aortic pressure curve, or the downward movement of the calcified aortic valve. A forceful jet through a stenotic aortic valve may displace the soft, flexible tip of the Sones type I catheter away from the valve. In this situation, the stiffer no. 7 French NIH catheter or the Sones Positrol catheter may be required.

CATHETERIZATION OF THE LEFT CORONARY ARTERY

In the horizontal plane the right coronary sinus faces directly anteriorly, the left sinus 120° posteriorly to the left, and the noncoronary sinus 120° posteriorly to the right (Fig. 6-13). The left coronary artery arises from the left and posteriorly,

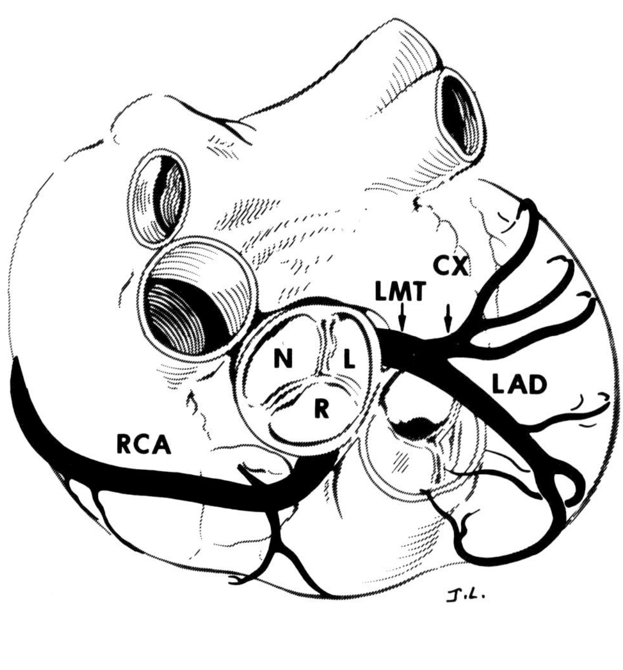

Figure 6-13 The aortic root and coronary arteries from above. R, L, and N = right, left, and noncoronary sinuses, respectively, RCA = right coronary artery, LMT = left main trunk, LAD = left anterior descending artery, CX = circumflex artery.

approximately 25° posterior to the frontal plane, and then passes anteriorly, so that its long axis is nearly parallel to the frontal plane. The right coronary artery arises almost directly anteriorly and then passes sharply to the right until it reaches the atrioventricular groove, where it curves inferiorly toward the crux. The three coronary sinuses do not lie in the same horizontal plane, but are tilted to the right and posteriorly. As a result, the left coronary sinus is the highest (most cranial), the right coronary sinus slightly lower, and the noncoronary sinus lowest.[4]

In order to catheterize the left coronary artery, the angiographer must usually perform two separate maneuvers: one to enter the left sinus, and a second to enter the left coronary ostium. When the Sones catheter is passed into the aortic root, it usually enters the noncoronary sinus. In order to enter the left coronary sinus, the angiographer usually performs one of the seven basic maneuvers illustrated in Fig. 6-14.

Once the catheter tip has entered the left sinus, it usually lies *anterior* and *inferior* to the ostium of the left coronary artery. This is because the long

Figure 6-14 Seven maneuvers to enter the left coronary sinus, 45° left anterior oblique projection. *(a)* Aim the tip of the catheter toward the left coronary sinus (1); abruptly advance the catheter tip while the patient is in inspiration until it impinges on the left coronary cusp (2); then advance the catheter to form a loop with the tip in the left coronary sinus (3).

(b) Form a long loop in the ascending aorta, aiming the catheter tip toward the left sinus (1); advance the catheter until the tip enters the left sinus (2); then withdraw the catheter slightly until the tip falls into the sinus (3). *(Continued on p. 152)*

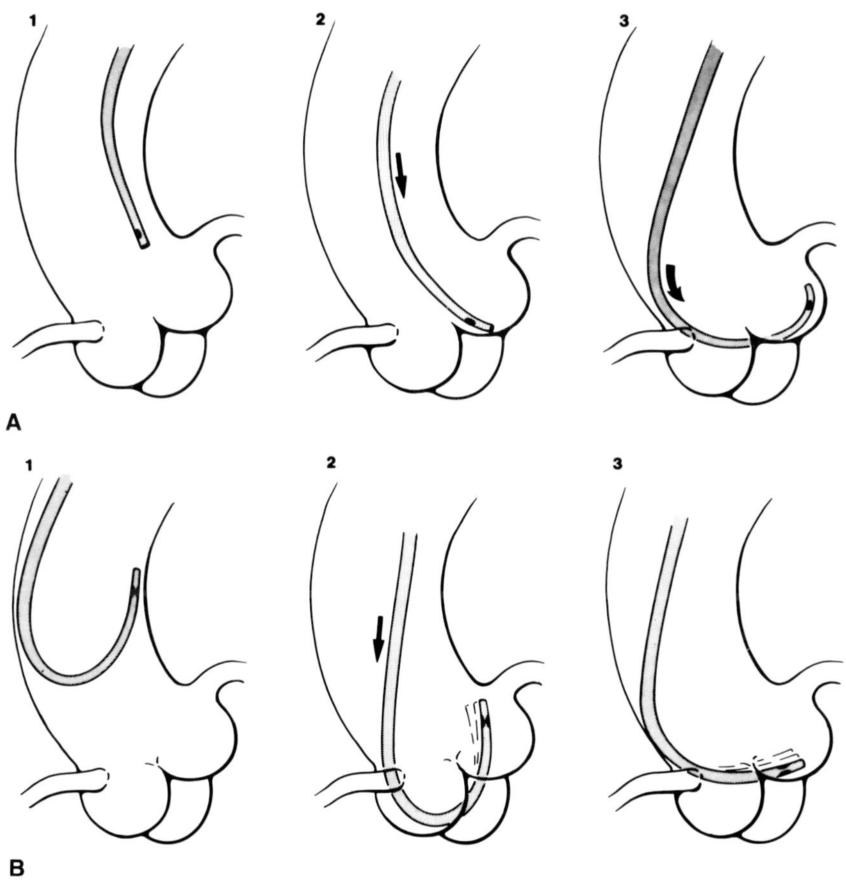

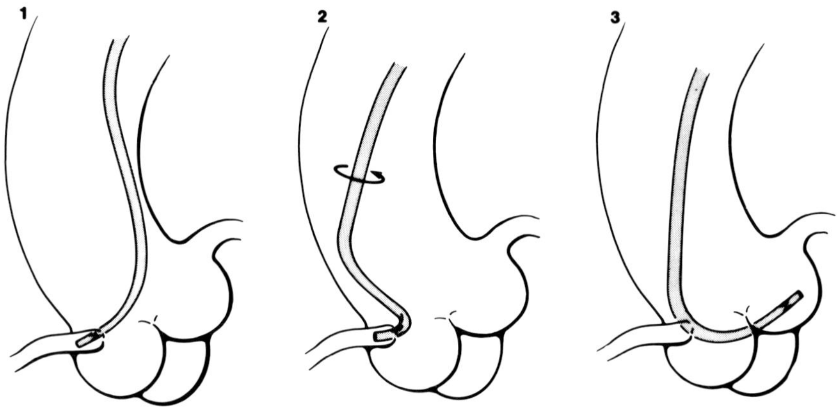

C

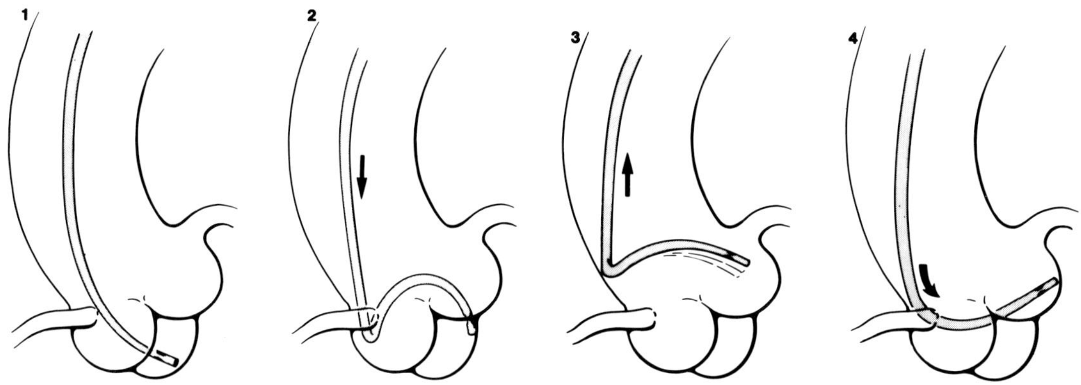

D

(Figure 6-14, continued)

(c) When the catheter tip lies in the right coronary artery or sinus (1) or when it is immediately above the sinus, rotate counterclockwise (2) until it twists into the left sinus (3).

(d) When the catheter tip lies in the noncoronary sinus (1), advance the catheter forming a "double loop" (2); rapidly withdraw the catheter 2 or 3 cm, permitting the distal loop to "uncoil" (3), and quickly advance the catheter, pushing the tip into the left sinus (4).

(e) When the catheter tip lies in the left ventricle, aim the tip toward the left coronary sinus (1); rapidly withdraw the catheter tip into the aortic root (2), and immediately advance the catheter, pushing the tip into the left sinus (3).

(f) When the catheter tip lies in the noncoronary sinus (1), aim it toward the left sinus; advance the catheter until it reaches the left sinus (2); then withdraw the catheter slightly, rotating clockwise (3).

(g) Form a long loop in the noncoronary sinus (1); rotate clockwise (2) until the tip falls into the left sinus (3).

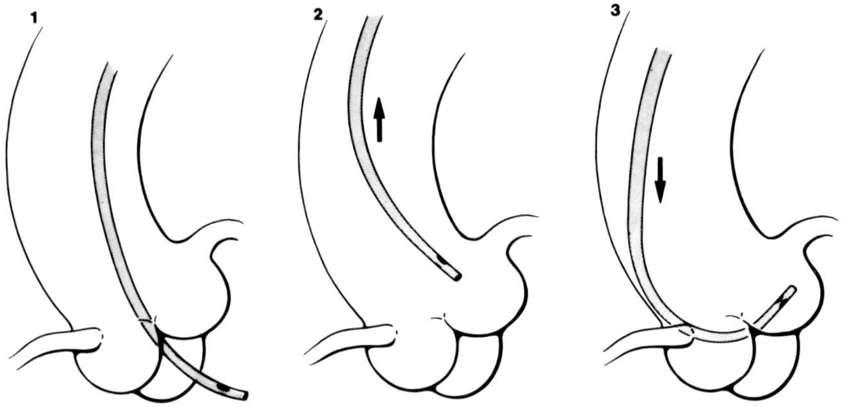

E

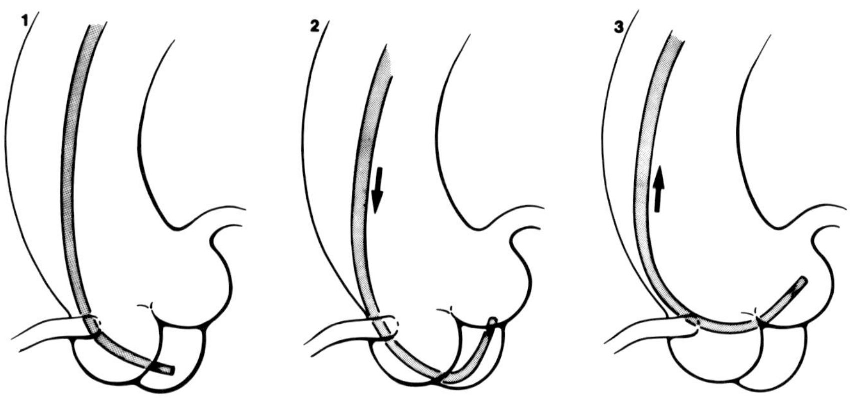

F

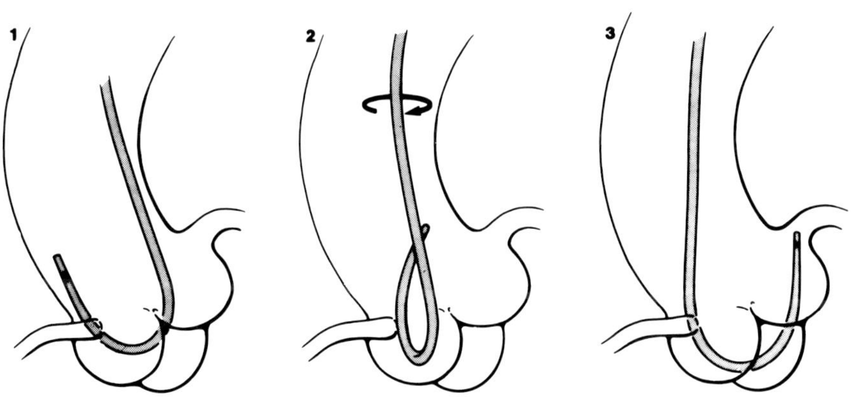

G

axis of the aortic root is tilted posteriorly and superiorly, and therefore the ostium of the left coronary artery lies in the most posterior and superior portion of the sinus. The angiographer should look for calcium in the left main trunk or anterior descending artery to help in finding the ostium of the left coronary artery.

The techniques for manipulating the Sones catheter into the left coronary ostium in either the long-loop or short-loop position are illustrated in Fig. 6-15. In the long-loop position, the tip of the catheter lies in the left main trunk, and the loop is "seated" in the noncoronary sinus. This position has the advantage of stability, but is more difficult to obtain, especially in a dilated aortic root. In the short-loop position, the tip of the catheter lies inside the left main trunk, and the loop lies free in the aortic root, with the terminal 1½ cm of the catheter directed horizontally or slightly upward. The short-loop position is easier to obtain and permits the angiographer to maneuver the catheter deeper into the left main trunk and to selectively enter either the anterior descending or circumflex artery. However, the short-loop position permits the catheter tip to fall more deeply into the artery than desired, and the catheter also tends to fall out of the left main trunk during powerful injections.

Since the left main trunk is angulated anteriorly, the catheter tip faces the posterior wall of the left main trunk as it enters the ostium. Clockwise rotation of the catheter causes the tip to rotate anteriorly and to enter more deeply into the left main trunk. This position increases the stability of the catheter tip and permits optimal visualization of the left coronary artery. If the catheter is not well positioned in the left main trunk, injections of contrast material may simulate an ostial left main trunk obstruction (Fig. 6-16).

Figure 6-15 Long-loop technique for catheterization (CATH) of the left coronary artery (LCA) in left anterior oblique *(a)* and right anterior oblique *(b)* projections. When the catheter tip lies in the left sinus, the catheter is advanced to lengthen the loop (1). The catheter is then advanced farther and rotated counterclockwise until the tip reaches the ostium of the left coronary artery (2). The catheter is then advanced farther and rotated clockwise (3) into the left main trunk. Short-loop technique for catheterization of left coronary artery in left anterior oblique *(c)* and right anterior oblique *(d)* projections. When the catheter tip lies in the left sinus, the catheter is advanced to lengthen the loop (1). The catheter is then advanced farther and rotated counterclockwise until the tip points toward the ostium of the left coronary artery (2). The catheter is then abruptly withdrawn about 2 cm and rotated clockwise (3), which causes the tip to impinge on the coronary ostium. Clockwise rotation (4) then advances the catheter tip into the left main trunk.

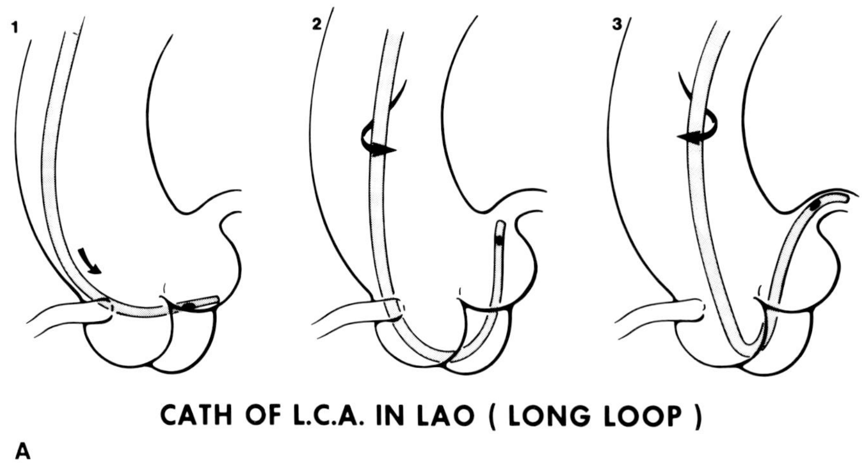

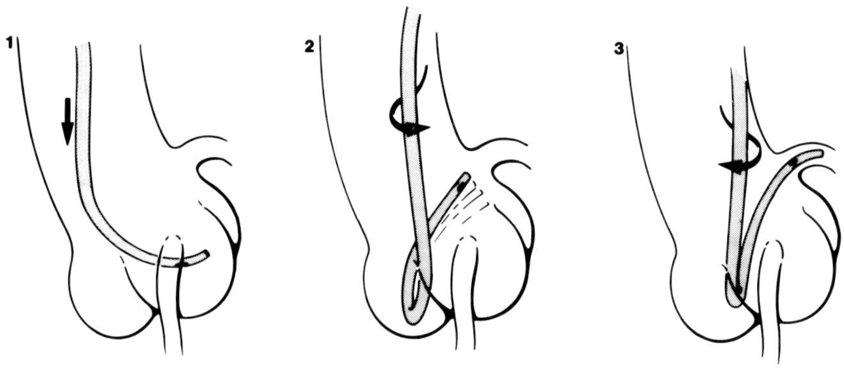

CATH OF L.C.A. IN RAO (LONG LOOP)

B

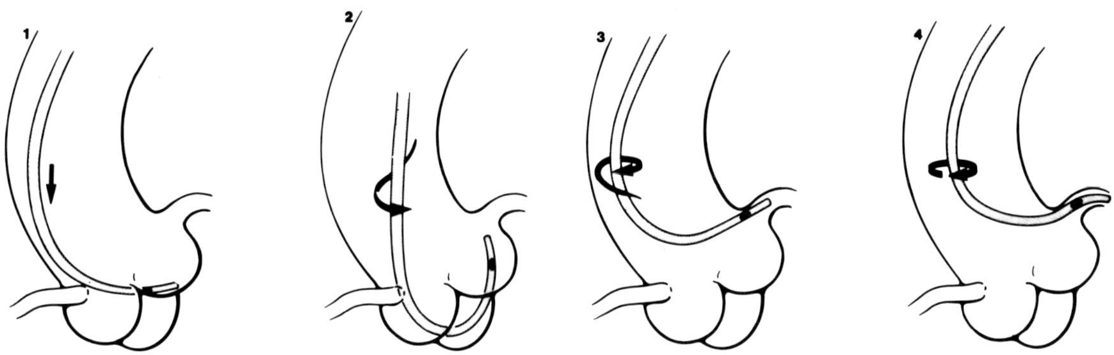

CATH OF L.C.A. IN LAO (SHORT LOOP)

C

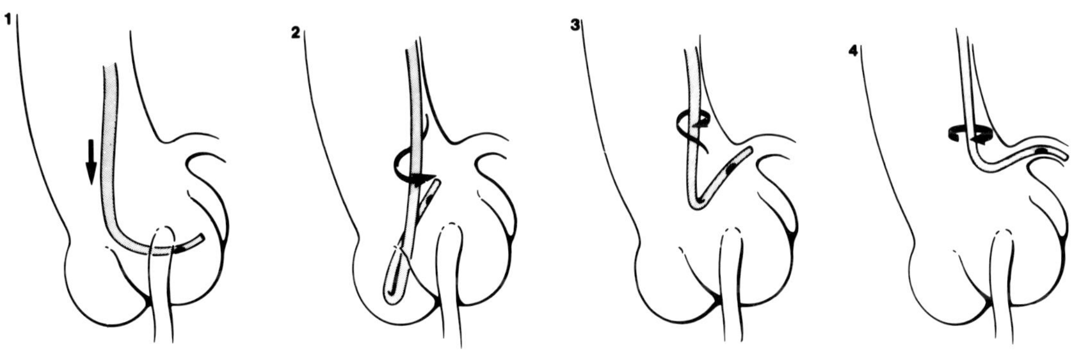

CATH OF L.C.A. IN RAO (SHORT LOOP)

D

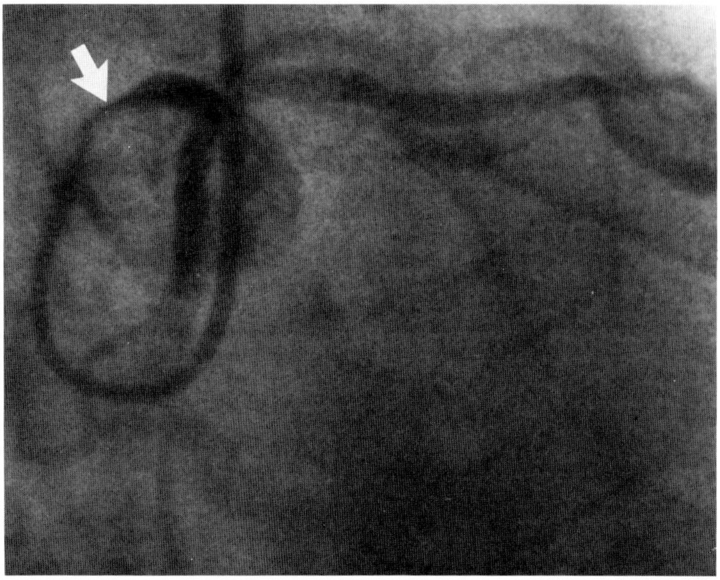

A

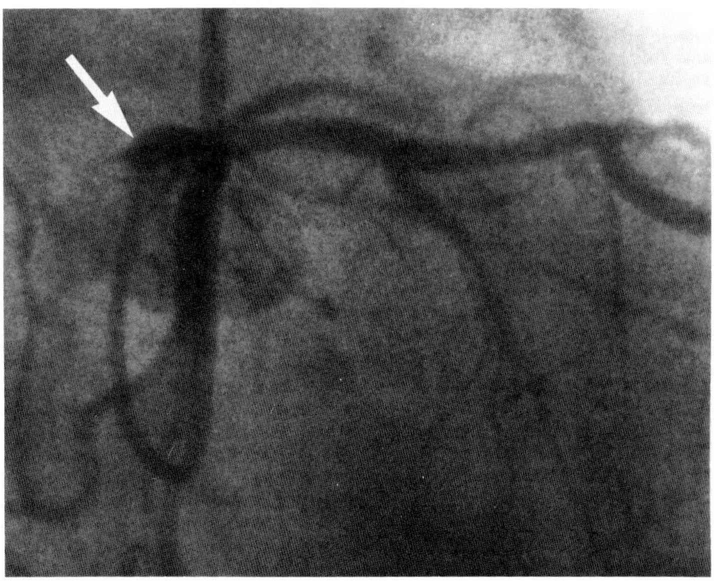

B

Figure 6-16 When the tip of the Sones catheter lies slightly below and posterior to the ostium of the left coronary artery *(a)*, injection of contrast material in the 30° right anterior oblique projection produces an artifact which resembles an ostial obstruction of the left main trunk (arrow). When the tip of the Sones catheter lies within the left main trunk *(b)*, the artifact is no longer present, and the ostium of the left main trunk is normal (arrow).

Before attempting to catheterize the left coronary artery, the angiographer should exclude a left main trunk obstruction by flushing the left sinus in the 35° LAO or LAO cranial projection. If an ostial obstruction is present, the angiographer should use the long-loop method and gently place the catheter tip at the ostium. If a distal left main trunk obstruction is present, the angiographer may use either the long-loop or short-loop method, but should avoid clockwise rotation of the catheter once it is in the left main trunk.

In people less than 5-foot 3-inches tall, the aortic root is often so narrow that the Sones type I catheter forms an excessively long loop in the left coronary sinus. In this case, the angiographer may switch to the Sones type II catheter. An unusually wide aortic root is often encountered in patients who are very tall or those with aortic valve diseases, hypertension, diffuse aortic atherosclerosis, or cystic medial necrosis of the ascending aorta. In these situations, the loop of the Sones catheter may be too short to reach the ostium of the left coronary artery. The angiographer may either preform a large loop by hand in the Sones type I catheter or use a catheter with a longer loop, such as a Sones catheter with a type A curve, a Shirey left atrial open tip catheter, or a Cordis brachial coronary catheter in which a long loop has been preformed in hot water.

When the catheterization is performed from the left brachial approach, the long-loop technique of coronary cannulation is preferred. When the tip of the catheter lies in the left sinus and the loop in the noncoronary sinus, sudden rapid withdrawal of the catheter with the left brachial approach usually results in downward displacement of the catheter tip, instead of the upward displacement which occurs with the right brachial approach. This makes the short-loop technique more difficult from the left arm.

CATHETERIZATION OF THE RIGHT CORONARY ARTERY

Catheterization of the right coronary artery is accomplished most easily during deep inspiration in the 45° LAO projection (Fig. 6-17). When the tip of the Sones catheter enters the right sinus, it usu-

Figure 6-17 Catheterization of the right coronary artery in the left anterior oblique projection. *(a)* Aim the tip of the catheter toward the sternum and advance it (1); when the catheter tip touches the right sinus, advance it and rotate clockwise (2); then withdraw the catheter slightly (3). *(Continued on p. 158)*

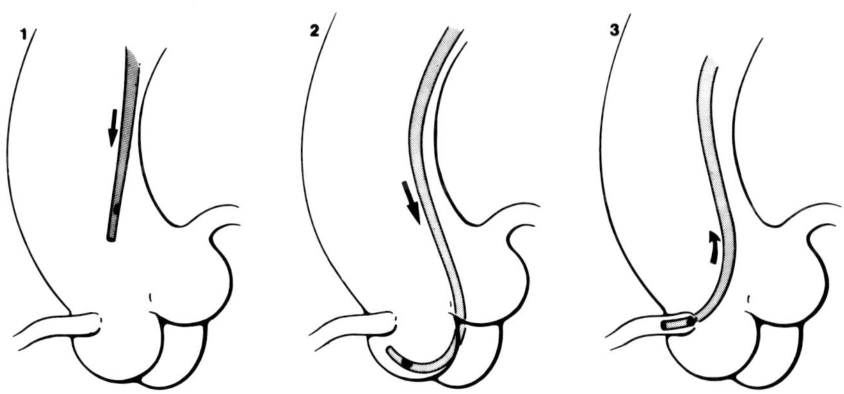

A

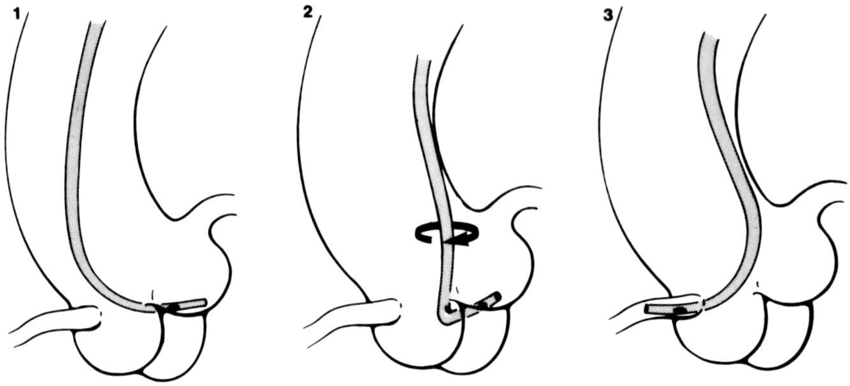

B

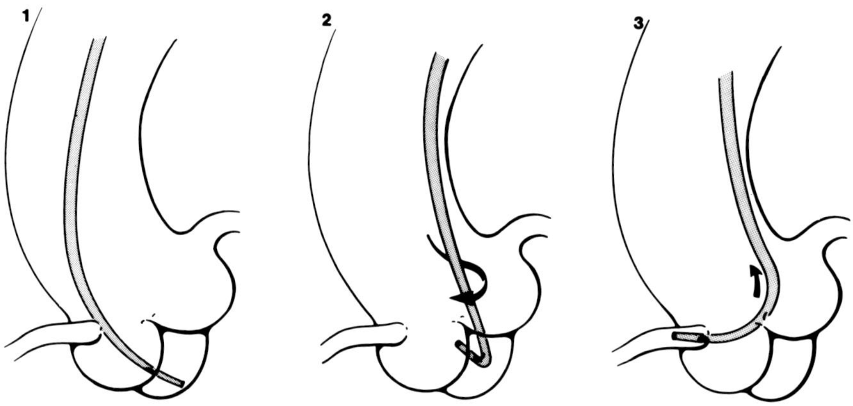

C

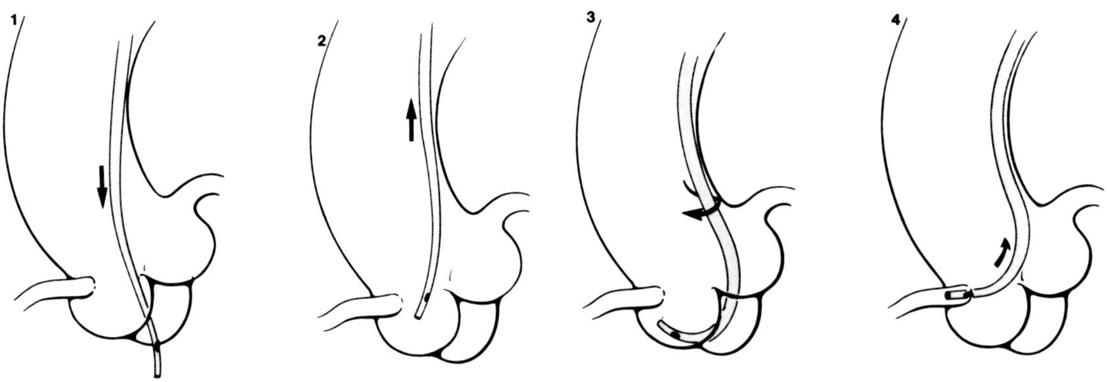

D

(Figure 6-17, continued)

(b) When the catheter tip lies in the left sinus (1), rotate it clockwise, keeping the distal 2 cm of the loop nearly horizontal, pointing slightly upward (2); after the catheter tip rotates into the right coronary artery (RCA) (3), apply slight counterclockwise torque to neutralize the remaining clockwise torque.

(c) When the catheter tip lies in the noncoronary sinus (1), advance the tip and rotate clockwise until it reaches the right sinus (2); then withdraw the catheter abruptly, and the tip will enter the RCA (3).

(d) When the catheter tip lies in the left ventricle, turn the tip clockwise until it points toward the sternum (1); then rapidly withdraw the catheter tip above the aortic valve (2) and immediately advance it into the right coronary sinus while rotating clockwise (3); then withdraw the catheter slightly (4).

ally falls into the ostium of the right coronary artery. If not, clockwise rotation will usually advance the tip into the artery. With the left brachial approach, it is more difficult to catheterize the right coronary artery. Therefore, the operator should attempt to enter the right coronary first, while the catheter is still "stiff." When it is impossible to enter the right coronary artery from the left arm with the Sones type I catheter, the angiographer should use a type II catheter.

CATHETERIZATION OF ANOMALOUS CORONARY ARTERIES

Separate Conus Artery

In approximately 50 percent of people, the conus artery arises from a separate origin in the right coronary sinus, slightly leftward and superior to the ostium of the right coronary artery.[5] Usually, it is not necessary to selectively catheterize this vessel. If no collaterals are visualized to a totally obstructed anterior descending or right coronary artery, the angiographer should attempt to selectively opacify the conus artery, since it may be a major source of collaterals. This artery may be entered by rotating the tip of the Sones catheter clockwise from the left into the right sinus or by slowly withdrawing the catheter from the right coronary artery and rotating it counterclockwise.

Separate Anterior Descending and Circumflex Arteries from the Left Sinus

When the anterior descending and circumflex arteries arise from separate origins in the left coronary sinus (0.5 percent of patients) the ostia are usually immediately adjacent, with the anterior descending lying slightly anterior and superior to the circumflex artery.[6] The initial portion of the anterior descending artery is usually angulated slightly superiorly and anteriorly. Therefore, the most effective approach is to aim the tip of the Sones catheter superiorly, briskly pull the catheter tip upward, and then rotate slightly clockwise. The circumflex artery usually arises more nearly perpendicular to the sinus and posteriorly. Therefore, this artery should be approached with a shorter loop after rotating the catheter extremely counterclockwise in the left sinus.

Separate Origin of the Circumflex Artery from the Right Sinus

The circumflex artery arises from either the right coronary artery or a separate origin in the right coronary sinus in 0.5 percent of patients.[6] When it arises from a separate origin, the ostium is located adjacent, but slightly posterior, inferior, and to the right of the ostium of the right coronary artery. The anomalous circumflex artery may be entered by gradually withdrawing the Sones catheter from the ostium of the right coronary artery, rotating clockwise, and directing the tip inferiorly during inspiration.

Origin of the Right Coronary Artery from the Ascending Aorta

When the right coronary artery arises from neither the left nor the right sinus, it usually arises from the ascending aorta (0.2 percent of patients), just above and between the right and left sinuses.[6] The anomalous vessel may be entered by rotating the Sones catheter clockwise out of the left coronary sinus with a large loop and then moving the catheter tip slowly up and down along the anterior wall of the aorta until the tip engages in the ostium.

Origin of the Left Coronary Artery from the Ascending Aorta

If the left coronary artery arises from neither the right nor the left coronary sinus, it probably arises from the aorta immediately above the left sinus. Such a vessel can be entered by forming a long loop in the noncoronary sinus and rotating clockwise while moving the catheter tip slowly up and down above the left sinus.

CATHETERIZATION OF AORTOCORONARY BYPASS GRAFTS

In our institution, the ostia of aortocoronary bypass grafts are usually located in a characteristic pattern in the ascending aorta (Fig. 6-18). Proceeding in

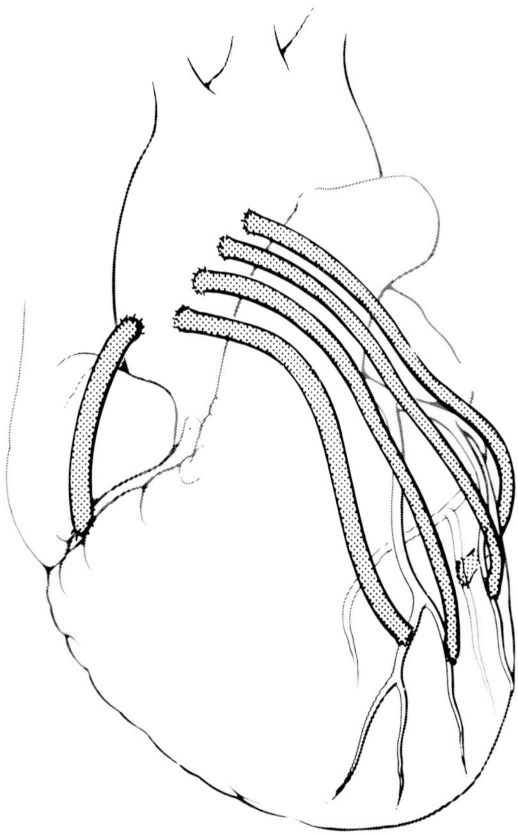

Figure 6-18 Typical locations of saphenous vein grafts to coronary arteries. The proximal anastomosis sites of the saphenous vein grafts lies in a characteristic "stepladder fashion," with the graft to the right coronary artery the lowest, and the grafts to the left coronary artery progressively higher and more posterior.

counterclockwise direction to the left and superiorly, the sequence of graft locations is as follows: right coronary artery, anterior descending, second diagonal, first diagonal, high lateral circumflex, lateral circumflex, and posterolateral circumflex.

Before attempting to selectively catheterize aortocoronary bypass grafts, the angiographer should know the coronary anatomy on the preoperative catheterization and the operative procedure which was performed. Since it is usually necessary to maintain a long, stiff loop to enter saphenous vein grafts, the angiographer may wish to catheterize them first, before the catheter becomes soft. Even when a saphenous vein graft has become totally occluded, selective catheterization is usually possible because a small stump of the proximal anastomosis site remains patent.

The technique for catheterization of the saphenous vein graft to the right coronary artery is demonstrated in Fig. 6-19. The technique for catheterization of a graft to the left coronary artery is illustrated in Fig. 6-20. To obtain optimal visualization of a saphenous vein graft, the angiographer should insert the catheter well into the graft and inject with sufficient pressure to produce homogeneous opacification (Fig. 6-21).

CATHETERIZATION OF INTERNAL MAMMARY ARTERY BYPASS GRAFTS

Catheterization of internal mammary artery bypass grafts is accomplished with a polyurethane Cordis brachial coronary catheter, which can be preformed in hot water. Since the left internal mammary artery is more commonly employed for bypass grafts, we usually perform the entire procedure from the left arm. After routine coronary arteriography and left ventriculography, the Sones catheter is withdrawn to the subclavian artery, where contrast material is injected to visualize the origin of the internal mammary artery (Fig. 6-22). The Cordis catheter is preformed to correspond to the arterial anatomy with a sterile paper clip inserted into the catheter tip. This tip is submerged in boiling water for 30 s and then cooled in sterile water for 10 s. After the paper clip is removed, the catheter retains the same curve which was preformed. This catheter is then advanced retrograde into the internal mammary artery (Fig. 6-22).

PREPARATION FOR INJECTION OF CORONARY ARTERIES AND BYPASS GRAFTS

Before injecting contrast material into a coronary artery or bypass graft, the angiographer must (1) eliminate air from the catheter-manifold-syringe system; (2) choose appropriate image intensifier angulation; (3) have the patient inspire deeply; and

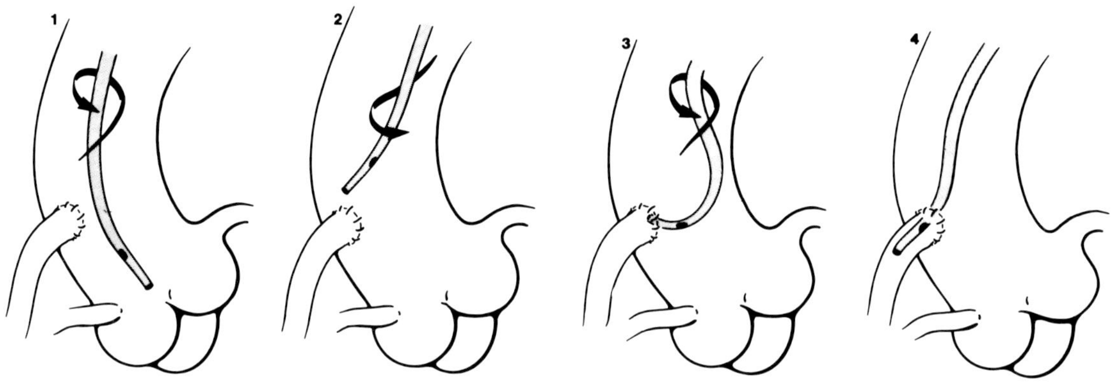

Figure 6-19 Catheterization of an aortocoronary saphenous vein graft to the right coronary artery in the 60° left anterior oblique projection. When the catheter tip lies just above the noncoronary sinus, it is pulled back into the ascending aorta and rotated counterclockwise (1). Once the catheter tip is proximal to the ostium of the graft, it is then advanced with counterclockwise rotation (2) until it impinges on the ostium of the graft. At this point, very gradual withdrawal of the catheter, with counterclockwise (sometimes clockwise) rotation (3), will advance the catheter tip into the graft (4).

(4) evaluate the catheter tip pressure wave. Before the first injection, the operator should clear the air from the catheter-manifold-syringe system by aspirating until blood returns into the syringe, then injecting enough contrast material to fill the catheter. This maneuver should be repeated if either the catheter or syringe becomes loosened from the manifold at any time during the procedure. The syringe should be loaded with enough contrast material (usually 6 to 8 mL) to permit adequate coronary visualization.

The choice of appropriate image intensifier angulation is the subject of Chap. 9. As a rule, the coronary arteries should be visualized in angles which minimize overlap with the spine, and each artery should be visualized in the LAO and RAO

Figure 6-20 Catheterization of an aortocoronary saphenous vein graft to the left coronary artery in the 60° left anterior oblique projection. The long loop of the Sones catheter is directed toward the greater curvature of the ascending aorta and then lifted upward and counterclockwise (1). When the catheter tip impinges on the ostium of the graft (2), it is directed nearly perpendicular to the long axis of the graft, and therefore the catheter should be rotated counterclockwise. After the counterclockwise rotation, the catheter tip lies well within the graft (3), and this permits optimal visualization of the graft.

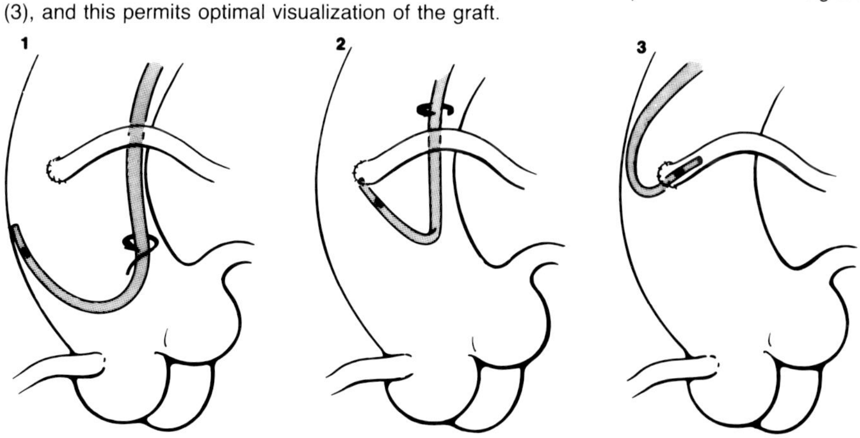

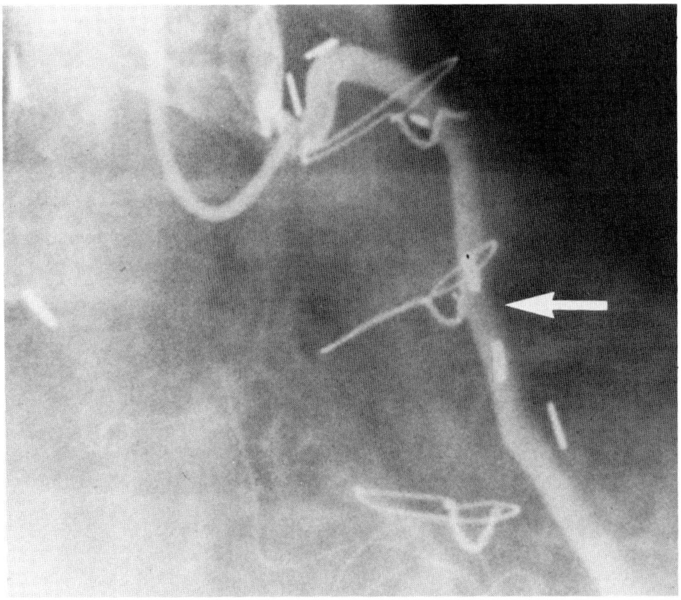

A

Figure 6-21 Aortocoronary bypass graft to the circumflex artery in the right anterior oblique projection, proximal *(a)* and distal *(b)* portions. The injection was made with the tip of the catheter at the ostium of the vein graft *(a)*, which resulted in hazy opacification of one wall of the graft (long arrow) and faint opacification of the lateral branch (short arrow) *(a, b)*. When the catheter tip was rotated counterclockwise into the saphenous vein graft *(c)*, injection of contrast material into the graft *(c, d)* produced excellent opacification of both the graft (long arrow) and the circumflex artery (short arrow).

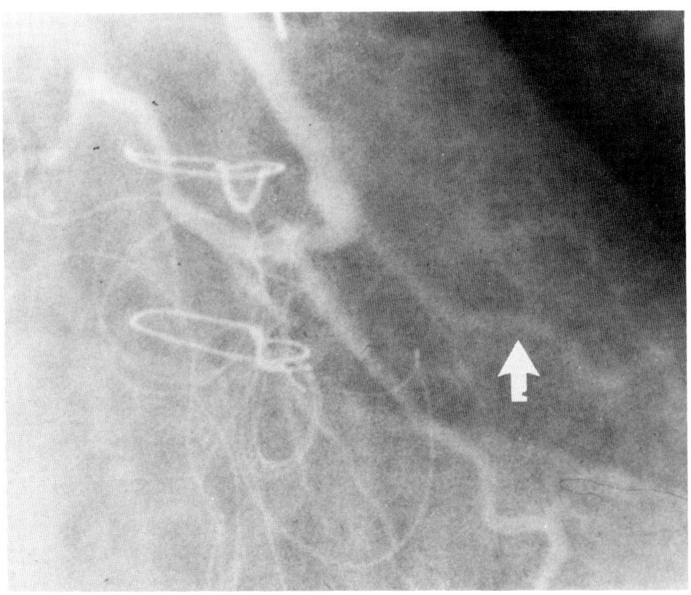

B

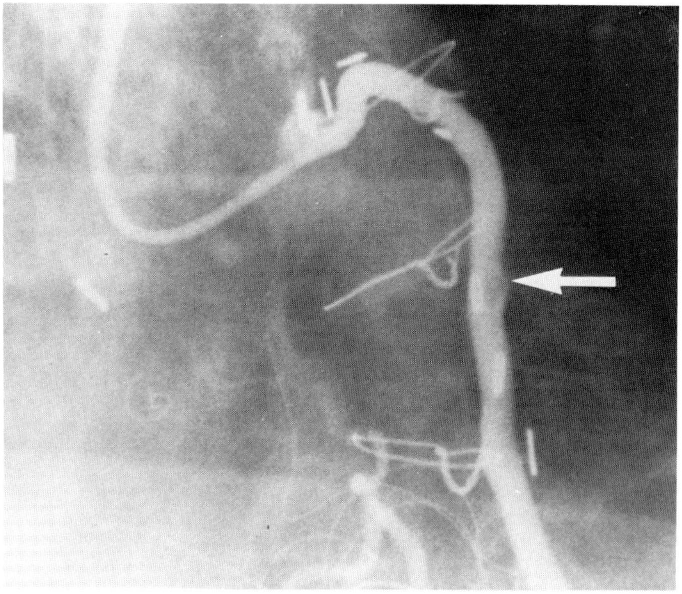

C

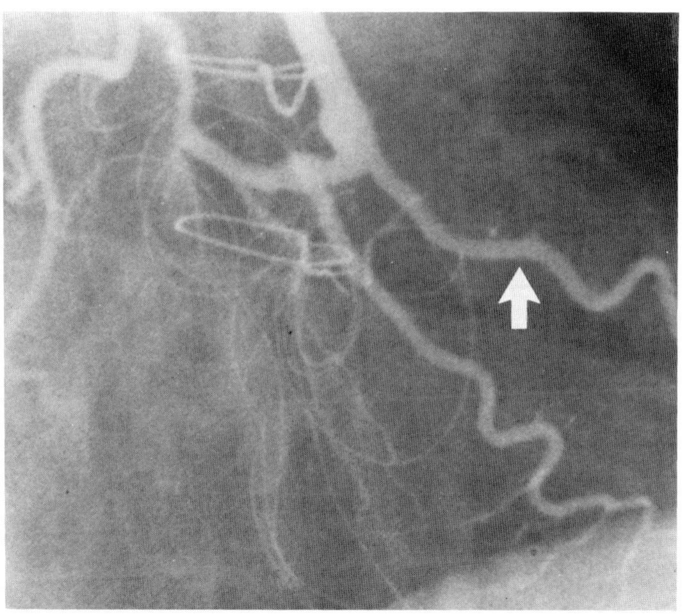

D

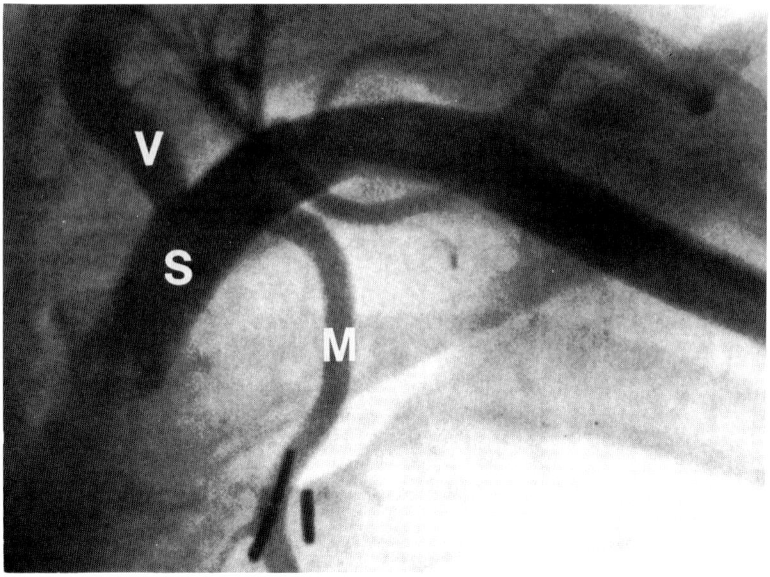

A

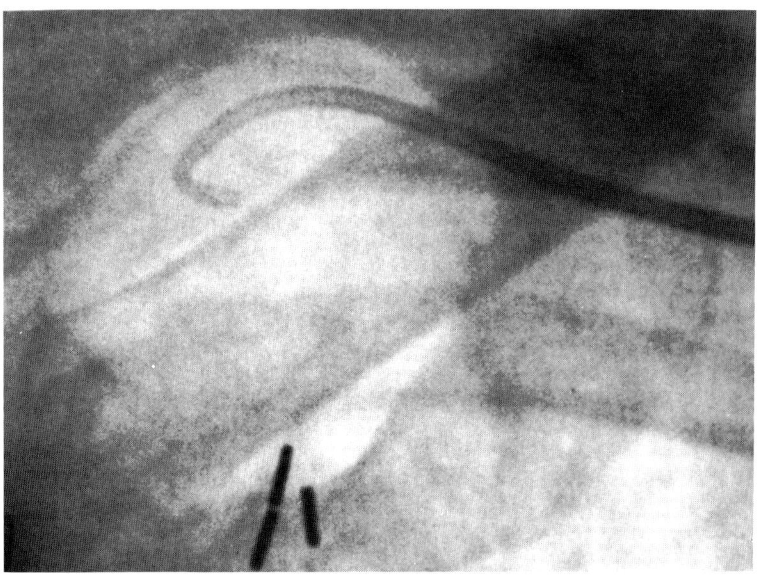

B

Figure 6-22 Injection of contrast material into the left subclavian artery in the posteroanterior projection *(a)* demonstrated the subclavian (S), vertebral (V), and internal mammary (M) arteries. After the Cordis brachial coronary catheter was preformed to correspond to the arterial anatomy, it was passed into the subclavian artery *(b)* until it reached the internal mammary artery, where selective injection produced dense opacification *(c)* of the internal mammary artery.

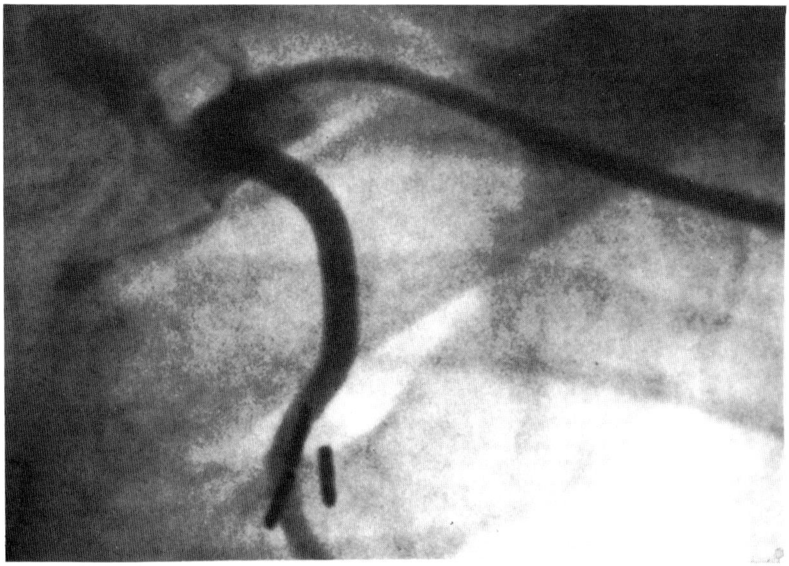

C

projections. The image intensifier should be positioned close to the patient's chest wall during cineangiography (Fig. 6-23).

Deep inspiration causes the diaphragm to be displaced inferiorly, and this permits better visualization of the vessels on the diaphragmatic wall of the heart (Fig. 6-24). During inspiration, the catheter should be advanced 1 to 2 cm under fluoroscopy to maintain catheter position, and during expiration it should be withdrawn the same distance.

The pressure fluctuations recorded from the tip of the Sones catheter should be observed up to and including the deep inspiration which precedes contrast injection into the left coronary arteries. Sudden damping of pressure (Fig. 6-25) after the catheter enters a coronary artery may occur because the catheter tip (1) slid beyond an obstructing plaque; (2) advanced into a small artery or branch; or (3) produced a dissection in the artery. Occasionally, a coronary artery may be so small that it is impossible for a catheter tip to enter it without damping of pressure. In this case, 1 or 2 mL of contrast material may be injected under low pressure, followed by immediate withdrawal of the catheter. Damping of pressure when the tip of the Sones catheter is in the left main trunk is important. If it is due to dissection, injection of contrast material could produce a sudden catastrophe by extending the dissection. When damping of pressure occurs with the catheter tip in a coronary artery, the safest course is to slowly withdraw the catheter until damping is no longer present and then make a small test injection at the ostium of the artery to determine why it occurred.

TECHNIQUE OF INJECTION AND FRAMING

The optimal quantity and force of injection of contrast material vary directly with the size of the coronary artery and the rate of coronary flow. Both "streaming" and "washout" of contrast material may occur when an injection is made with inadequate force (Fig. 6-26). Streaming, which is due to laminar flow, occurs when contrast material flows along one side of the arterial wall and the other side is not visualized due to nonopacified blood. Streaming may produce the false appearance of severe coronary artery narrowing. Washout occurs

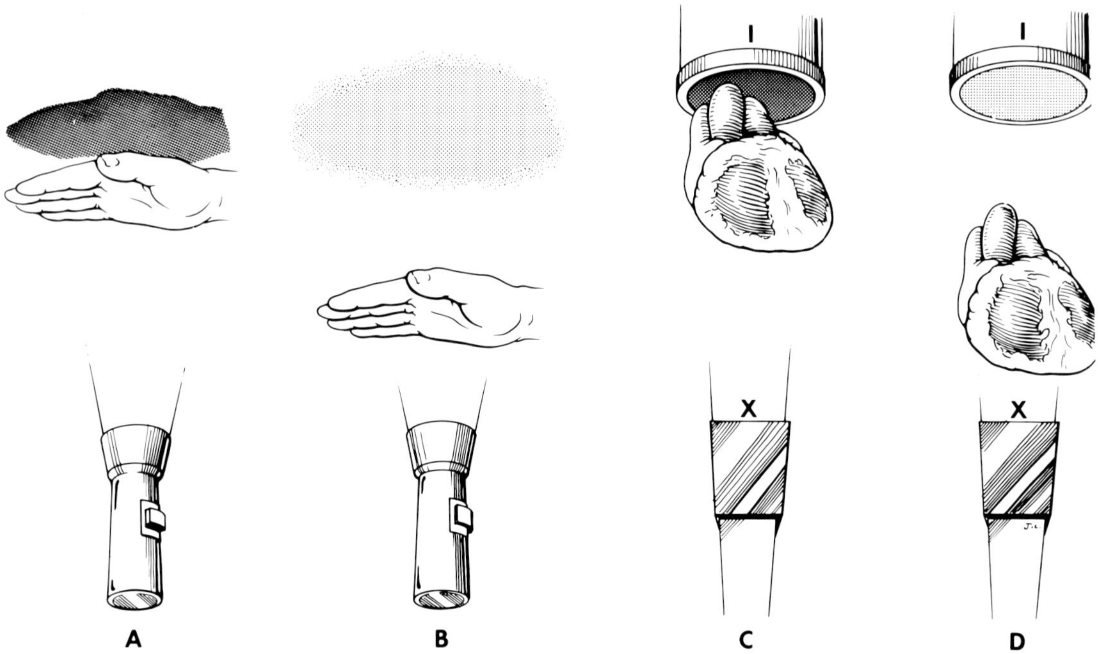

Figure 6-23 Effect of amplifier distance on image quality. *(a)* When a hand is held close to the surface on which the shadow falls, the image is sharp. *(b)* The farther the hand moves from this surface, the larger and "fuzzier" the image becomes. *(c)* When the image intensifier (I) is close to the chest wall and the heart, the image obtained is sharp. *(d)* When the heart lies farther from the image intensifier and closer to the x-ray source (X), the image is magnified but poorly defined and "hazy". Increased source-to-image distances also require more kilovoltage, thereby degrading the image (see Chap. 14).

when contrast material is replaced by nonopacified blood during diastole, as coronary blood flow increases transiently. This results in intermittent filling and a "hazy" appearance of the coronary arteries.

When the coronary arteries are large and coronary flow is rapid, as in left ventricular hypertrophy, the angiographer may need to inject with increased force and volume. When a coronary artery is less than $1\frac{1}{2}$ mm in diameter, such as a small right coronary artery might be, the force of injection should be low. Excessively high-pressure injections produce a dramatic myocardial "blush" and heavy opacification of cardiac veins (Fig. 6-27). This is associated with an increased incidence of arrhythmias.

The angiographer should inject enough contrast material to opacify the coronary arteries for at least three cardiac cycles. Thus, if there is intermittent overlap of vessels during the cardiac cycle, the angiographer will obtain multiple glimpses of the arteries during the phase when there is no overlap. After the three cycles, the angiographer should move the amplifier to the distal artery and discontinue injection of contrast material. A nondominant right coronary artery may require no more than 2 mL of contrast material. A dominant left coronary artery in a patient with chronic aortic regurgitation may require 8 to 10 mL. The average amount of contrast material is about 4 mL for a dominant right coronary artery and 6 mL for a left coronary artery. Once the operator has started the cine camera, at least two systoles should pass before injection of the contrast material because (1) it requires a fraction of a second for the kilovolts or milliamperes of the x-ray tube to adjust; (2) the operator can adjust the catheter and amplifier positions before injections; and (3) the operator can observe the earliest entry of contrast material into the artery.

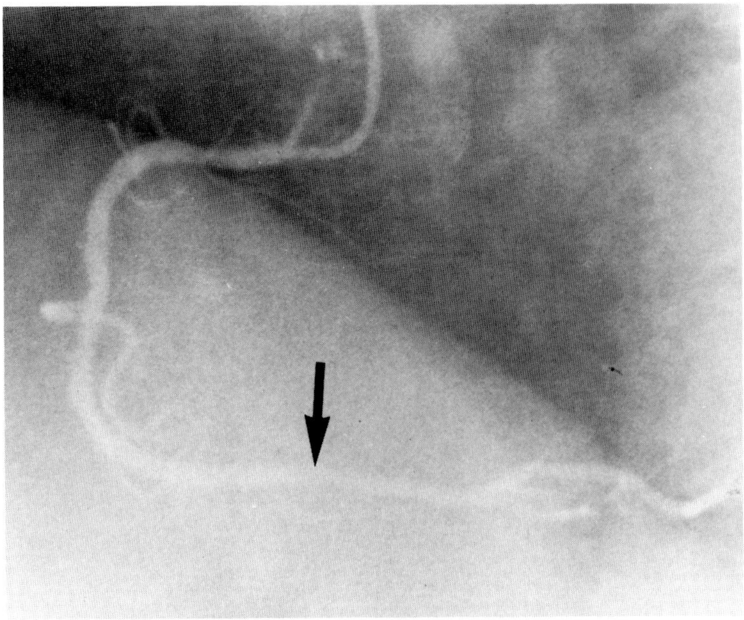

A

Figure 6-24 Right coronary artery in the left anterior oblique projection. Before deep inspiration *(a)*, the severe obstruction (arrow) in the distal right coronary artery was poorly visualized due to overlap of the diaphragm. During deep inspiration *(b)*, the severe obstruction (arrow) in the distal right coronary artery was clearly demonstrated.

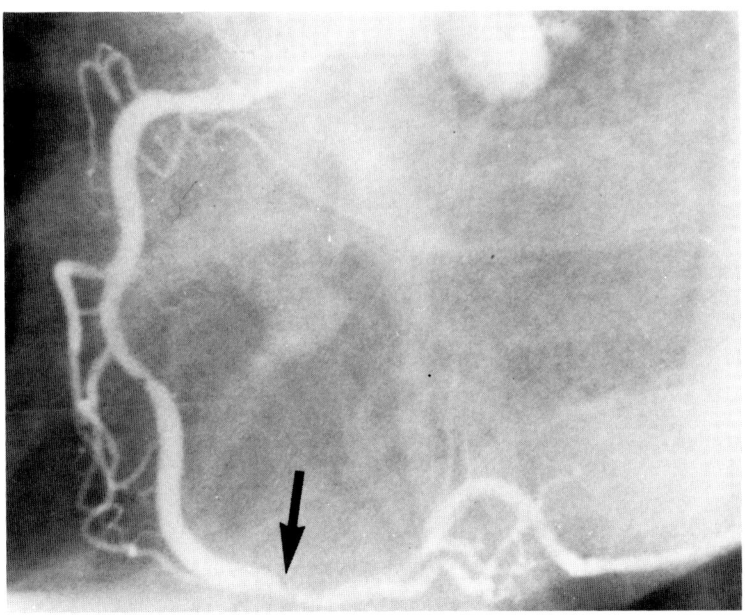

B

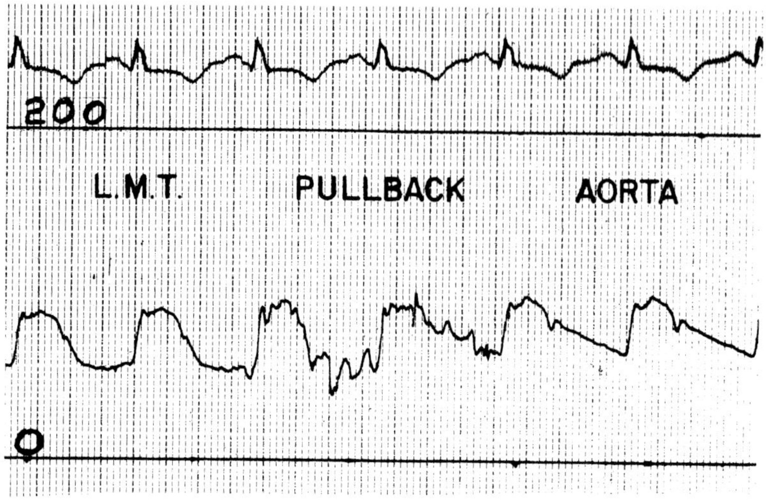

A

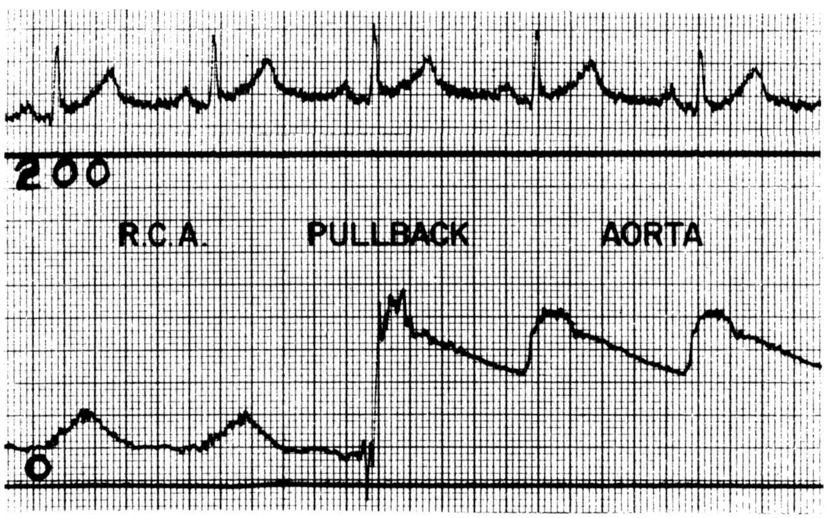

B

Figure 6-25 Damping of pressure at the catheter tip during coronary catheterization. *(a)* Mild damping of pressure during diastole occurred as the catheter tip crossed a 60 percent ostial obstruction of the left main trunk (LMT). After pull-back into the aorta, the pressure wave normalized. *(b)* Severe damping of pressure occurred as the catheter became wedged in the right coronary artery (RCA), and the pressure became normal after the catheter was withdrawn.

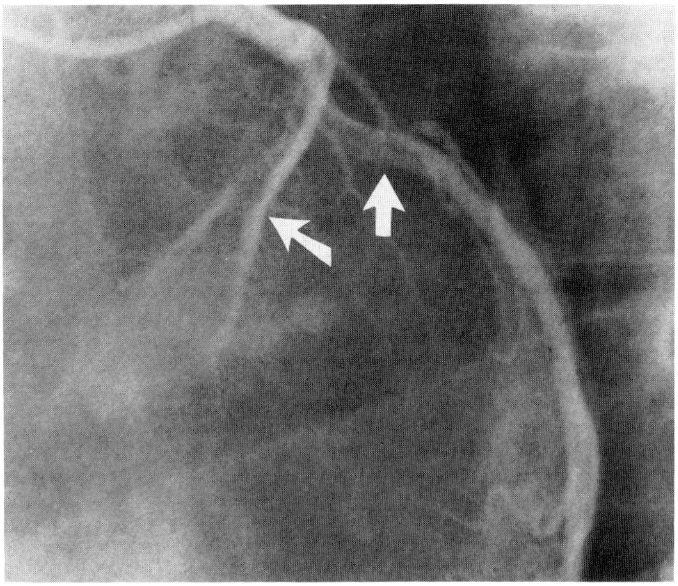

A

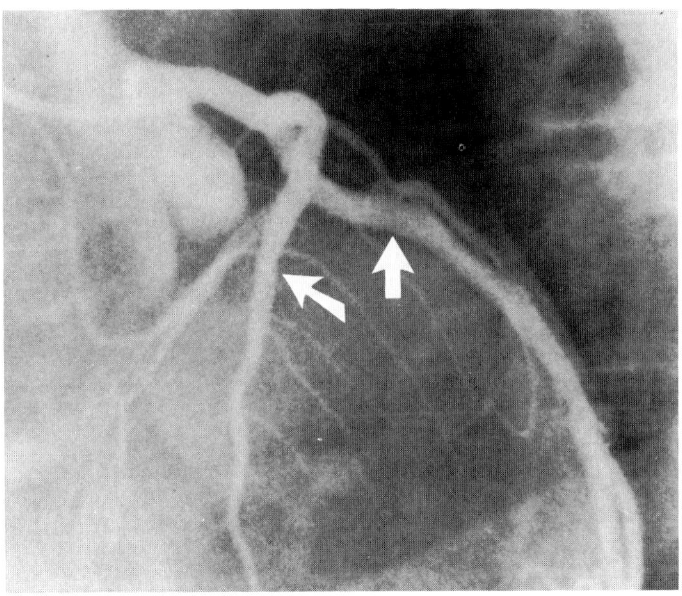

B

Figure 6-26 Left coronary artery in the left anterior oblique projection. *(a)* Inadequate pressure of injection in the left coronary artery produced streaming of contrast material in the anterior descending artery (thin arrow) and intermittent washout of contrast material in the circumflex artery (wide arrow). *(b)* Forceful injection of contrast material into the left coronary artery produced excellent opacification of both arteries.

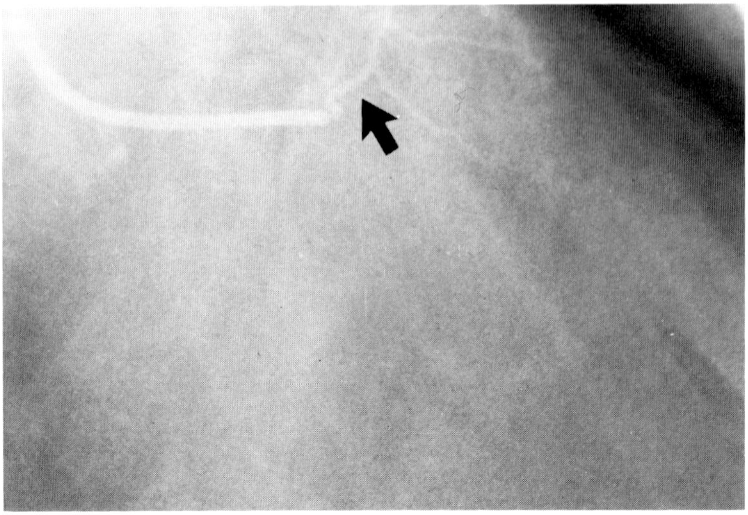

A

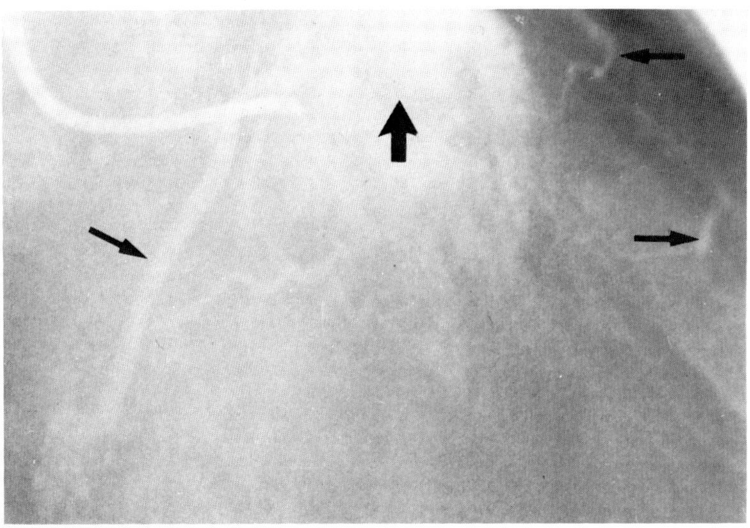

B

Figure 6-27 Subselective injection into the conus branch in the right anterior oblique projection. In the early phase *(a)*, the tiny conus branch (arrow) was visualized. Later *(b)*, a heavy myocardial blush (wide arrow) appeared, followed by heavy opacification of right ventricular veins (thin arrows) which drained into the right atrium and into the anterior cardiac vein.

Proper "framing" and "panning" are important in coronary arteriography. Framing refers to the initial position of the amplifier with respect to the opacified arteries. Panning refers to the subsequent movements of the amplifier as the contrast material passes into the distal artery. Panning is usually not necessary with a 9-inch amplifier, but it is almost always necessary with a 6-inch amplifier.

Proper framing of the opacified images requires positioning of the amplifier so as to obtain maximal information on the film. To accomplish this, two coordinates should be selected for each view. The superior coordinate is the same for each view: position the upper border of the amplifier so that the tip of the catheter appears on the fluoroscopy screen 1 cm below the upper edge. The lateral coordinate differs for each view (Fig. 6-28). Regardless of the view, the amplifier should always be positioned to minimize the amount of lung tissue on the screen.

Panning permits the visualization of (1) distal branches of the coronary artery which was injected; (2) collaterals to the contralateral artery; (3) the proximal part of the injected artery after the contrast material has cleared; and (4) the position of the catheter tip at the end of the injection. The usual patterns for panning are demonstrated in Fig. 6-28. When the amplifier is returned to its original position at the end of the cine period, the angiographer should look for persistence of contrast material in the proximal part of the artery, which may occur for several reasons: (1) tortuous or dilated arteries; (2) coronary artery aneurysm; (3) slow "runoff" into the tiny vessels proximal to a total obstruction; and (4) subintimal dissection of the coronary artery.

It is not necessary to remove the Sones catheter

Figure 6-28 "Panning" technique during coronary arteriography.
(a) Right coronary artery in the left anterior oblique projection. The amplifier is positioned over the proximal right coronary artery (1), then the distal right coronary artery (2), then the lateral wall of the left ventricle (3), and finally back to the proximal right coronary artery.
(b) Right coronary artery in the right anterior oblique projection. The amplifier is positioned over the proximal right coronary artery (1), then the distal right coronary artery (2), then the distal anterior wall and apex (3), and finally back to the proximal right coronary artery. *(Continued on p. 172)*

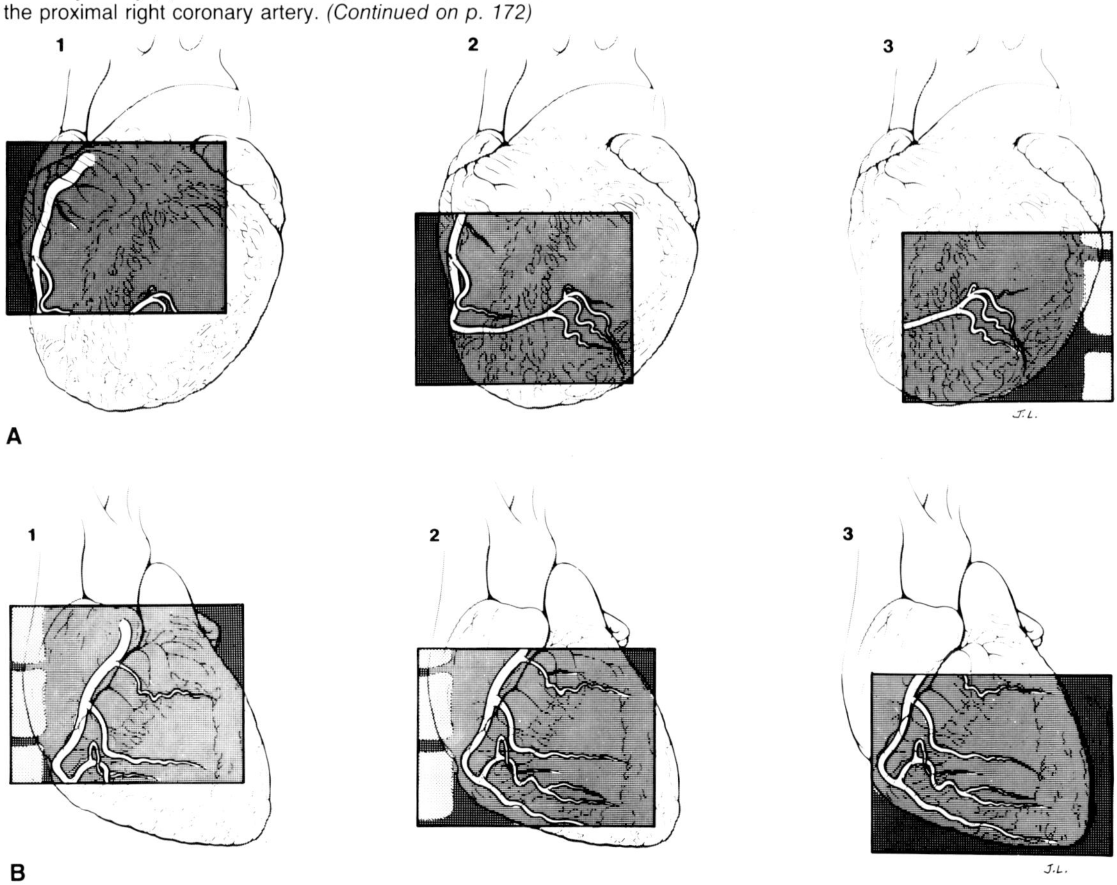

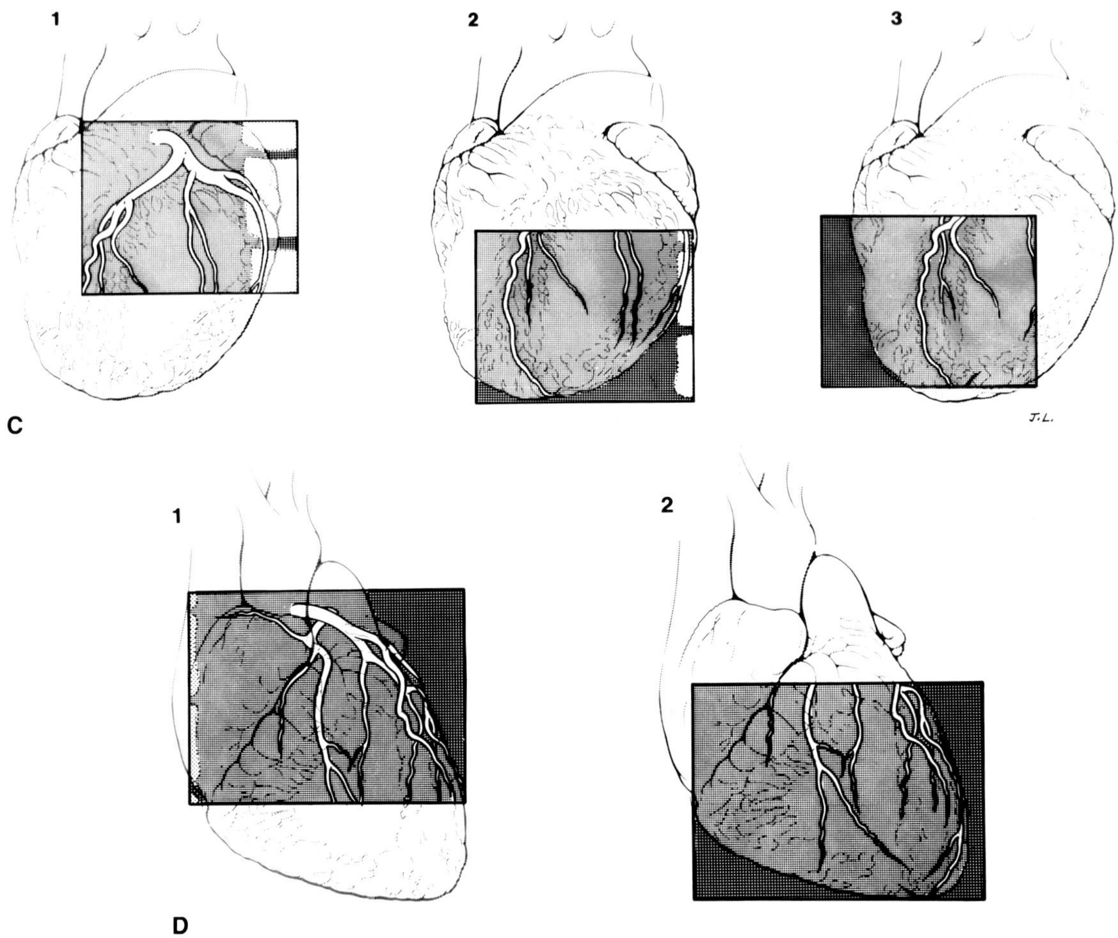

(Figure 6-28, continued)

(c) Left coronary artery in the left anterior oblique projection. The amplifier is positioned over the proximal left coronary artery (1), then the distal left coronary artery (2), then the distal right coronary artery (3), and finally back to the proximal left coronary artery.

(d) Left coronary artery in the right anterior oblique projection. The amplifier is positioned over the proximal left coronary artery (1), then it is moved diagonally downward to the right over the apex (2), and finally back to the proximal left coronary artery.

from the coronary artery after each injection. However, when a severe left main trunk obstruction is present, the catheter should be removed after each injection to prevent trauma at the site of the obstruction.

LEFT VENTRICULOGRAPHY

The Sones type I coronary catheter is suitable for ventriculography in most patients. After this catheter has been passed into the left ventricle in the 45° LAO projection, it should be rotated until the tip is pointing toward the apex. Ideally, the catheter tip should not touch either the septum or the free wall of the left ventricle, because this produces ventricular tachycardia during the ventriculogram (Fig. 6-29). A test injection of contrast material should be made in the LAO projection to verify the catheter position. Catheter position should then be checked in the 35° RAO projection (Fig. 6-30).

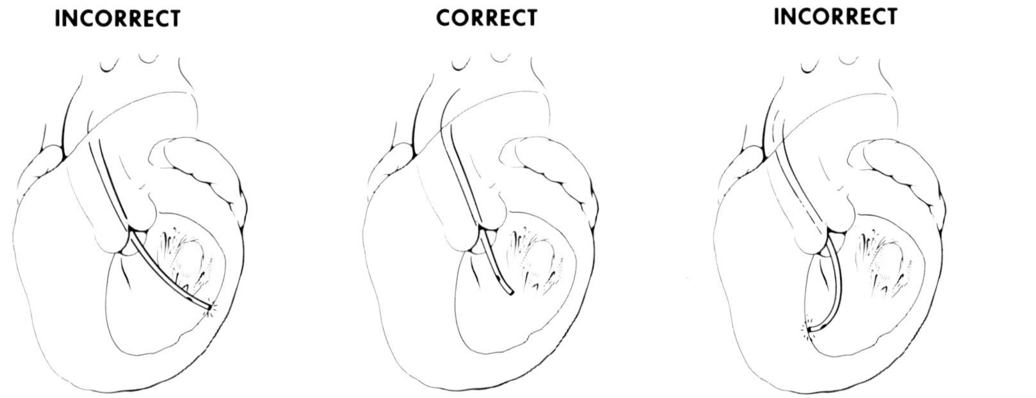

Figure 6-29 Catheterization of the left ventricle in the 45° left anterior oblique projection. When positioned correctly *(center),* the catheter tip should be lying free in the left ventricular cavity, aiming toward the amplifier. If the catheter tip is touching the inferolateral wall *(left),* it should be rotated clockwise, and if it is touching the septum *(right),* it should be rotated counterclockwise.

The tip of the catheter should be positioned near the papillary muscles. If it lies in the left ventricular outflow tract, the left ventricle will be poorly opacified and the catheter tip will tend to recoil into the ascending aorta.

The volume of contrast material required for left ventriculography is 25 to 30 mL if the ventricle is normal and 40 mL or more if it is dilated. A volume-controlled power injector should be set to deliver 10 to 15 mL/s, depending on the size of the ventricle. A pressure-controlled injector will deliver approximately 10 mL/s through a Sones catheter if set at 250 psi.

After attaching a power injector to the catheter, the angiographer grasps the portion of the catheter which emerges from the artery in the right hand and maneuvers the control handle for the image intensifier with the left hand. The image intensifier should be positioned to obtain a maximum amount of the left ventricle on the fluoroscopy screen.

Usually, the left ventricle is best evaluated in the 35° RAO and 45° LAO projections. Since the

Figure 6-30 Catheterization of the left ventricle in the 35° right anterior oblique projection. When positioned correctly *(center),* the catheter tip should be near the tip of the papillary muscles, aiming toward the apex. If it is touching the inferior or inferolateral wall *(left),* it should be rotated clockwise. If it is touching the anteroseptal wall *(right),* it should be rotated counterclockwise.

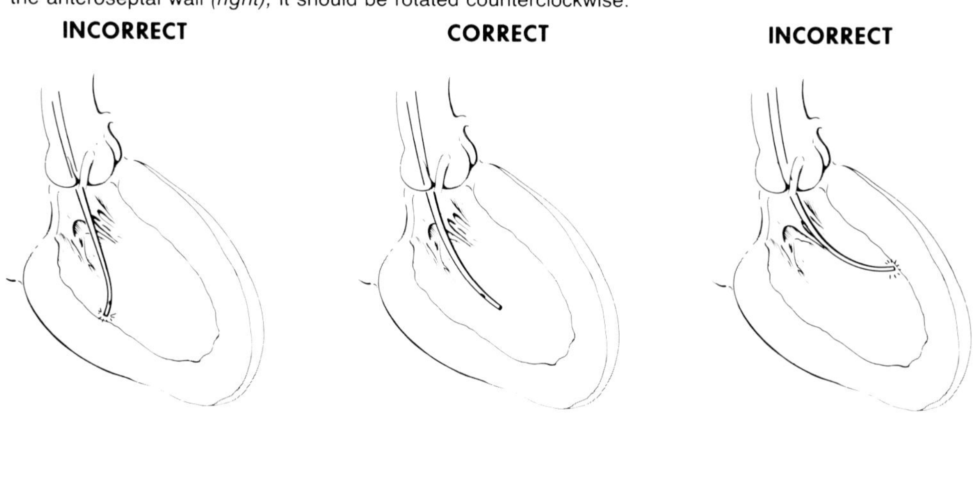

left ventricle appears foreshortened in the LAO view, 20° to 30° of cranial angulation may permit better separation of the basal and apical portions. The advantages of this angulated view must be weighed against the disadvantage of increased overlap of the left ventricle with the diaphragm.

When injection of contrast material into the left ventricle begins, the catheter may have to be withdrawn 1 or 2 cm if frequent premature ventricular contractions (PVCs) occur. Catheter withdrawal tends to prevent intramyocardial injection of contrast material and minimize premature beats. The catheter should not be advanced during injection, since this markedly increases the risk of intramyocardial injection.

COMPLICATIONS OF CORONARY ARTERIOGRAPHY

The complications associated with coronary arteriography are the subject of Chapters 5 and 11. However, those complications which are related to the Sones technique will be reviewed in this chapter. Recently, the Society for Cardiac Angiography formed a registry which collected data on 53,581 patients from 66 laboratories between October, 1979, and December, 1980.[7,8] No statistically significant difference was found in the mortality of coronary arteriography by the Sones technique (0.10 percent) versus the Judkins technique (0.12 percent).

Coronary arteriography is associated with a variety of complications which require prompt recognition and treatment in order to prevent or minimize permanent sequelae. Listed below are some of the most important complications encountered in the catheterization laboratory.

Median Nerve Injury

This injury is a rare complication of the Sones technique. When the median nerve is contacted during arteriotomy, patients complain of a severe electric shock sensation in the hand. Severe or repeated trauma to the median nerve during a cutdown may produce residual neurologic sequelae, which include numbness and painful dysesthesias in the hand and weakness of the flexors of the hand. Over a period of 3 to 12 months, the weakness improves in most patients, but the dysesthesias tend to persist. Management consists of physical therapy and symptomatic treatment for pain. Median nerve injury is usually a result of traction or compression, not transection. If transection occurs, paralysis of the flexor muscles is complete and permanent. In this case, the patient should be evaluated by a neurosurgeon for reanastomosis of the severed nerve.

Subintimal Dissection of the Subclavian Artery

This dissection is most likely to occur when this artery is tortuous or elongated. This complication does not usually produce pain or any permanent sequelae. The angiographer should suspect a subclavian dissection if the catheter tip repeatedly meets an obstruction which is not due to a side branch and if there is damping of pressure. The dissection can be verified by injection of 1 mL of contrast material. After the catheter tip has entered a subintimal dissection, it should be withdrawn a few centimeters, and further attempts to advance the catheter should be made only after a J-spring guidewire has been passed beyond the point of dissection. Occasionally, the guidewire loop will repeatedly enter the subintimal dissection, in which case the catheter should be withdrawn and the catheterization procedure should be performed from the other arm. Perforation of the subclavian artery is a very rare and serious complication, which is associated with pain and massive swelling in the clavicular area. The angiographer should apply local pressure and obtain immediate consultation with a vascular surgeon.

Coronary Artery Dissection

Coronary artery dissection is a serious complication which can usually be prevented if the angiographer avoids stiff catheters, forceful insertion of the catheter, and injection while the pressure is damped. The angiographer should suspect subintimal coronary dissection when contrast material "hangs up" in the artery proximally, near the tip of the catheter, after completion of the coronary injection (Figs. 6-31 and 6-32). The dissection may vary in length from 1 mm to more than 1 cm. The contrast ma-

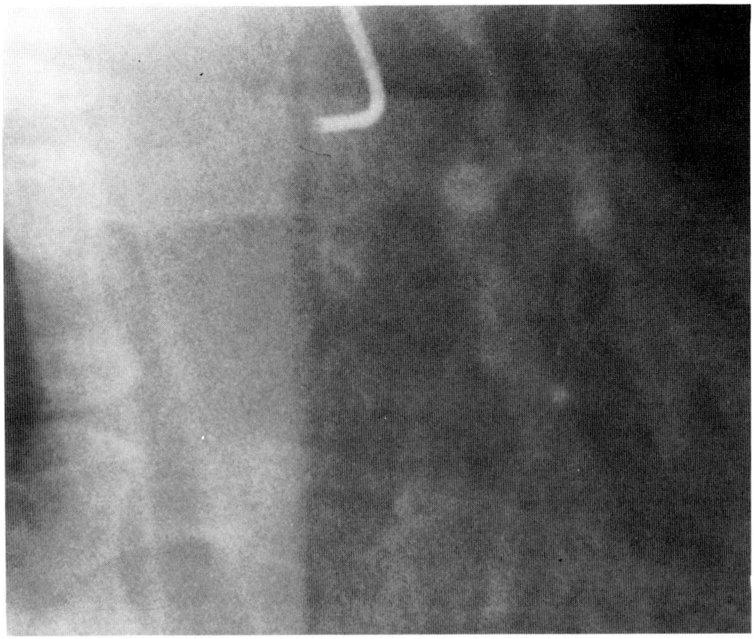

A

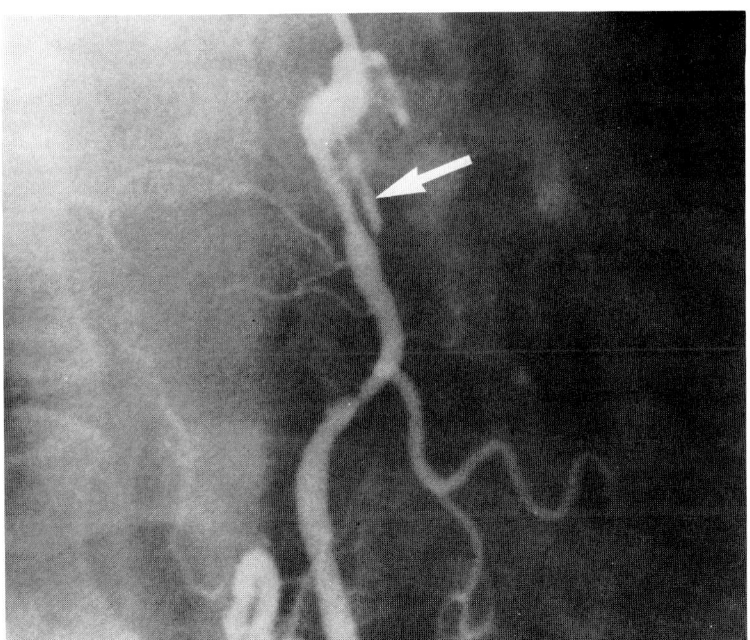

B

Figure 6-31 Right coronary artery in right anterior oblique projection. *(a)* The catheter lies in the proximal right coronary artery before injection of contrast material. *(b)* During injection, contrast material (arrow) enters a subintimal dissection and is separated from the true lumen by a thick subintimal flap. *(c)* After completion of injection, contrast material (arrow) persists in the dissected flap.

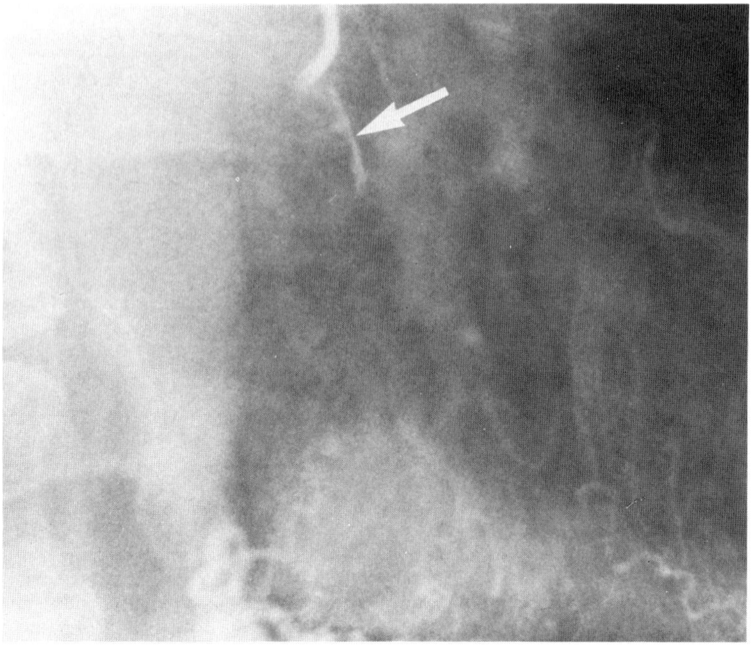

C *(Figure 6-31, continued)*

terial in a small subintimal dissection may be washed out by nonopacified blood within 10 s, and therefore the angiographer should move the intensifier back up to observe the proximal portion of the coronary artery immediately after completion of the injection and before turning off the cine. Once the dissection has been recognized, the catheter tip should not be replaced in the vicinity of the dissection because repeat injections there may extend the dissection. Repeat injections may be made cautiously with the catheter at the ostium of the artery or in the sinus. Coronary artery dissection may precipitate angina or an acute myocardial infarction. If the patient suffers angina at the time of the dissection and if the dissected artery is suitable for grafting, immediate surgical consultation should be obtained for possible emergency coronary bypass surgery. If no angina or electrocardiographic changes occur, and if the patient is not otherwise a candidate for coronary surgery, the patient may be observed for a few days and then discharged if no symptoms or ECG changes occur.

Myocardial Ischemia

The patient who develops myocardial ischemia, with or without angina, during coronary arteriography must be treated before any more coronary injections are made, especially if left main trunk or multiple vessel disease or severe left ventricular dysfunction is present. If the patient has normal or mildly abnormal coronary arteries, it is usually preferable to visualize the coronary arteries during chest pain before giving nitroglycerin in order to see if coronary spasm has occurred. If the patient develops angina or acute ischemic changes on the ECG during catheterization, the angiographer should check the left ventricular end-diastolic pressure, which is usually elevated during acute myocardial ischemia (Fig. 6-33). Injection of 0.4 mg of nitroglycerin solution directly into the left ventricle produces a dramatic drop in left ventricular end-diastolic pressure and reverses the ischemia in most patients within several minutes. Extremely unstable patients may require several milligrams or more

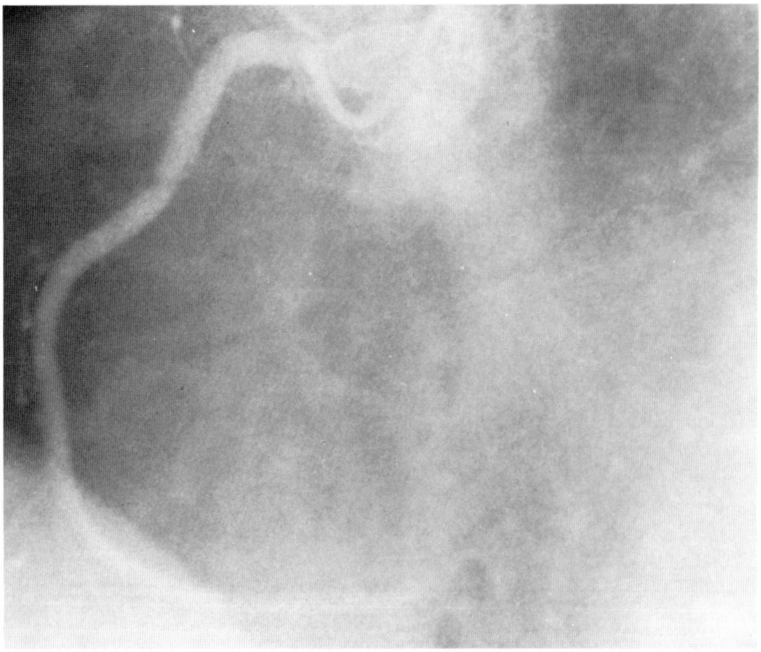

A

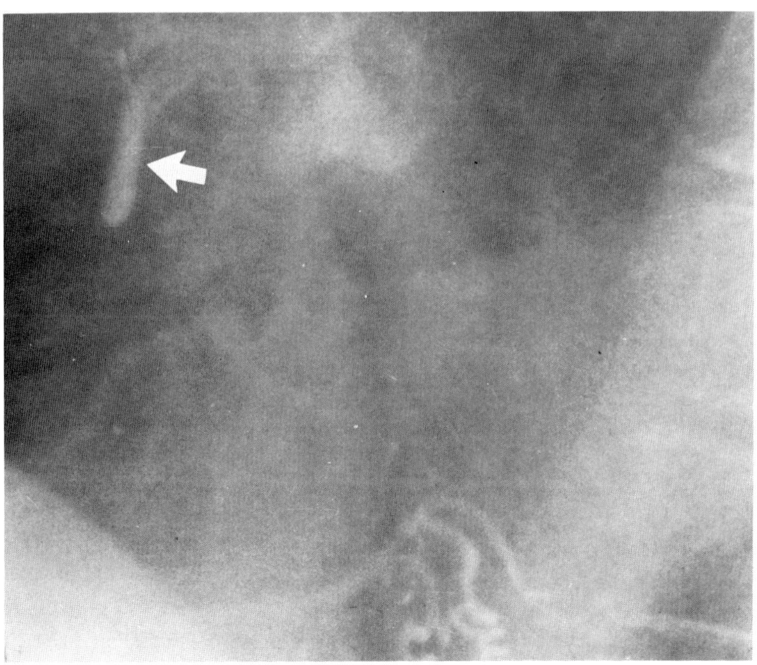

B

Figure 6-32 Right coronary artery in left anterior oblique projection. *(a)* Injection into the right coronary artery demonstrates mild narrowing in the proximal third. *(b)* After the injection, contrast material persists in a subintimal dissection although no discrete intimal flap is detected.

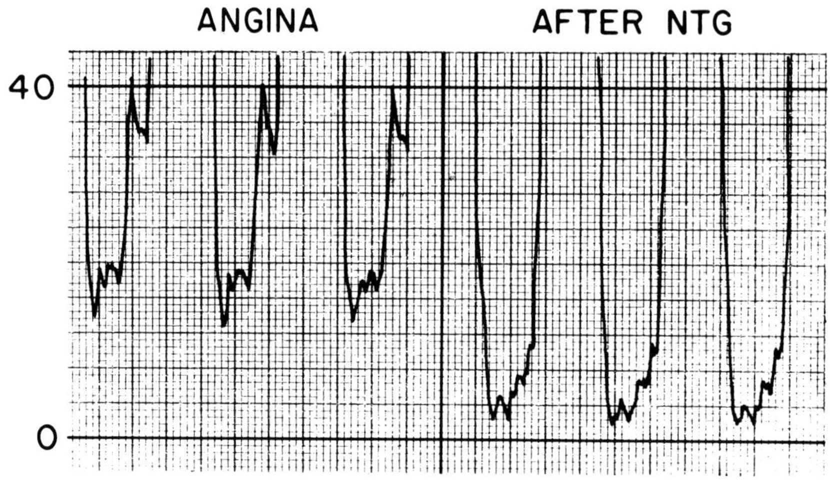

Figure 6-33 During angina *(left),* the left ventricular mid-diastolic pressure rose to 18 mmHg, and the end-diastolic pressure to 34 mmHg. Three minutes later *(right),* after 0.4 mg nitroglycerin (NTG), the mid- and end-diastolic pressures fell to 4 and 10 mmHg, respectively.

of nitroglycerin acutely for relief of angina. If angina persists, repeat coronary arteriograms should be obtained to look for coronary dissection.

Severe global myocardial ischemia may result in electromechanical dissociation. Characteristically, this occurs in the patient with severe left main trunk or triple vessel disease, and it may be precipitated by superimposed coronary spasm or dissection. If it is due to spasm, immediate injection of 0.4 mg of nitroglycerin solution into the coronary arteries will usually reverse the spasm rapidly and produce an increase in pulse pressure and blood pressure.

Since ventriculography produces a stress on the left ventricle, it may further aggravate myocardial ischemia and precipitate angina, or it may produce increases in the left ventricular end-diastolic pressure sufficient to produce pulmonary edema. For this reason, if the left ventricular end-diastolic pressure is markedly elevated (e.g., more than 30 mmHg), it is safer to treat the patient with nitroglycerin before proceeding with ventriculography.

Intramyocardial Injections

Intramyocardial injections of contrast material produce a characteristic endocardial "stain," which usually clears spontaneously in a few minutes (Fig. 6-34). This complication can usually be avoided by careful positioning of the catheter and gradual withdrawal of the catheter tip during ventriculography. Most intramyocardial injections are small and produce no symptoms or ECG changes, although they may produce PVCs, T-wave changes, and rarely chest pain.

Perforation of the Left Ventricle

Perforation by a catheter is extremely rare. It is most likely to occur with excessively vigorous retrograde catheterization of the left atrium. Ventricular perforation can be recognized by an immediate drop in pressure, and it can be confirmed by injection of a small amount of contrast material. Unlike perforation of the low-pressure right ventricle, perforation of the left ventricle is likely to result in cardiac tamponade. If the tip of the catheter is lying in the pericardial cavity, it should be left there while emergency surgical consultation is obtained. Meanwhile, a right heart catheter should be inserted for measurement of venous pressure. If tamponade occurs while the left heart catheter is still in the pericardium, blood can be aspirated through the catheter to relieve the tamponade. If the patient

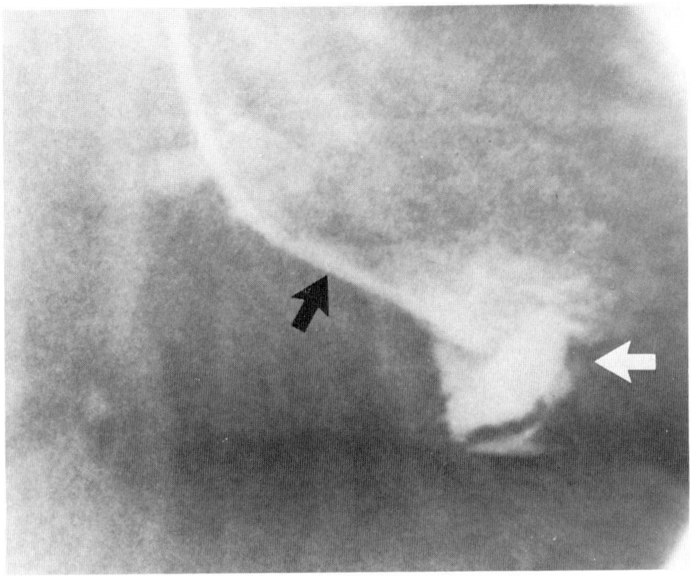

A

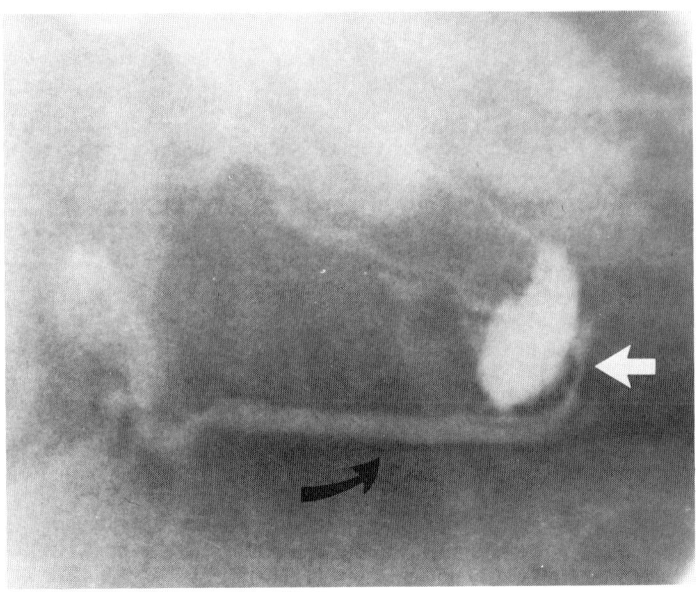

B

Figure 6-34 Intramyocardial injection during left ventriculography. *(a)* Early in the injection, the catheter tip (dark arrow) recoils against the diaphragmatic wall, producing a large "myocardial stain" (white arrow) of contrast material. *(b)* Later, the contrast material enters a coronary vein (black arrow) which then empties into the coronary sinus.

remains hemodynamically stable, the left heart catheter is withdrawn, and the patient can be transferred to an intensive care unit for observation.

Complete Heart Block

Sudden complete heart block during left ventricular catheterization is rare and usually occurs in patients with preexisting conduction tissue disease. The heart block is usually precipitated during ventriculography by sudden recoil of the tip of the Sones catheter against the basal portion of the interventricular septum, which produces mechanical trauma to the conduction tissue. In the patient with bifascicular block and a history of syncope, merely introducing the Sones catheter into the left ventricle may be sufficient to provoke complete heart block. In this case, the angiographer may insert a temporary transvenous pacemaker prophylactically before catheterization of the left side of the heart. When heart block occurs during the ventriculogram, the left ventricle enters a prolonged "diastole" during which it becomes progressively dilated. In this situation, the catheter should not be withdrawn from the left ventricle. If heart block persists, the Sones catheter may be used to mechanically stimulate the left ventricular endocardium. In this manner, the blood pressure may be maintained while another physician inserts a temporary pacemaker catheter from the leg or the opposite arm.

Brachial Artery Occlusion

Brachial artery occlusion occurs in approximately 2 to 3 percent of patients catheterized by the Sones technique.[9] The angiographer should check for this complication after the arteriotomy is closed. If the radial pulse is not palpable, the problem may be either thrombosis or spasm of the artery. If there was good arterial flow from both ends of the arteriotomy before closure, and if the closure appeared adequate, the angiographer may close the skin and wait for an hour to see if the pulse returns as the spasm subsides. Total occlusion of the brachial artery may produce numbness, coldness, and rest pain in the fingers when ischemia is very severe, and claudication when ischemia is less severe. The angiographer should be notified immediately if any of these symptoms occur following catheterization. Brachial artery occlusion is usually obvious within the first 4 hours after arterial closure. Occasionally, it may be delayed for a day or more. Because of the rich collateral supply around the elbow, total occlusion of the brachial artery often produces no symptoms. However, we generally recommend repair of a brachial artery occlusion even when it produces no symptoms.

False Aneurysm of the Brachial Artery

False aneurysm of the brachial artery is a rare complication of brachial arteriotomy.[10] The aneurysm may not become obvious for weeks or months after the catheterization. It must be differentiated from the common seroma, a collection of sterile fluid beneath the skin incision. A seroma may appear to pulsate if it overlies an artery and if it is pressed against the artery; however, only an aneurysm will also pulsate laterally when grasped between the thumb and index finger. Because a false aneurysm has a tendency to rupture, any patient with this complication should be evaluated by a vascular surgeon.

ACKNOWLEDGMENT

I am grateful to Dr. William Sheldon for his review of the manuscript, to Patricia Durnwald for preparing the manuscript, and to Jeff Loerch for his excellent artwork.

REFERENCES

1 Sones FM Jr, Shirey EK: Cine coronary arteriography. Mod Concepts Cardiovasc Dis, 31:735–738, 1962.
2 Balter S, Sones FM Jr, Brancato R: Radiation exposure to the operator performing cardiac angiography with U-arm systems. Circulation, 58:925–932, 1978.
3 Shirey EK, Sones FM Jr: Retrograde transaortic and mitral valve catheterization. Am J Cardiol, 18:745–753, 1966.

4 McAlpine WA: *Heart and Coronary Arteries*. Springer-Verlag, New York, 1975.

5 Schlesinger MJ, Zoll PM, Wessler S: The conus artery: A third coronary artery. Am Heart J, 38:823–836, 1949.

6 Hobbs RE, Millit HD, Raghavan PV, Moodie DS, Sheldon WC: Congenital coronary artery anomalies: Clinical and therapeutic implications, in Vidt DG (ed): *Cardiovascular Therapy 12/2, Cardiovascular Clinics*. Davis, Philadelphia, 1982, pp 43–58.

7 Kennedy JW: Complications associated with cardiac catheterization and angiography. Cathet Cardiovasc Diagn, 8:5–11, 1982.

8 Kennedy JW, Baxley WA, Bunnel IL, Gensini GG, Messer JV, Mudd JG, Noto TJ, Paulin S, Pichard AD, Sheldon WC, Cohen M: Mortality related to cardiac catheterization and angiography. Cathet Cardiovasc Diagn, 8:323–350, 1982.

9 Sheldon WC: Techniques for coronary arteriography. Cathet Cardiovasc Diagn, 5:191, 1979.

10 Adams DF, Fraser DB, Abrams HL: The complications of coronary arteriography. Circulation, 48:609–618, 1973.

Chapter 7

Coronary Arteriography and Left Ventriculography: Judkins Technique

Part I: The Judkins Technique

Melvin P. Judkins, M.D.
Eileen Judkins, R.N., N.P.

Selective coronary arteriography is the gold standard for identification and evaluation of ischemic heart disease despite the introduction of multiple noninvasive modalities for diagnosis. The precise depiction of coronary anatomy and left ventricular function makes it possible for the clinician to direct definitive therapy to the pathology of the individual patient.

HISTORY OF DEVELOPMENT

Early in the sixties I learned the technique of selective coronary arteriography by observing Mason Sones and Earl Shirey at the Cleveland Clinic. Using this method, I performed coronary arteriography in the cardiovascular laboratory of the University of Oregon department of radiology (Charles T. Dotter, professor and chairman), where I was a faculty member. In our institution Albert Starr was developing his prosthesis for the treatment of mitral and aortic valvular disease. He noted that many aortic prosthesis patients were succumbing to unsuspected coexisting coronary artery disease. Coronary arteriography became routine in the preoperative evaluation of aortic valvular replacement candidates over age 50. Selective left coronary arteriography from the brachial approach was often quite difficult in these patients who had enlarged aortic roots.

As a vascular radiologist trained in percutaneous transfemoral insertion and manipulation of catheters for visceral angiography, my search for a solution to the problem of consistent selective catheterization of the coronaries involved using techniques most familiar to me. At that time a technique for doing consistent selective transfemoral coronary arteriograms had not been developed.*

Vascular catheterization techniques evolved under the influence of two basic but different approaches. One system, then most often identified with the cardiologist, utilized basically straight woven catheters (initially ureteral) for cardiac physiological studies and selective chamber visualization. The catheter, usually introduced via vascular cutdown of the brachial artery, was deformed on normal intravascular structure and manipulated into the desired cardiac chamber or vascular orifice. The other system, identified with the vascular radiologist, employed preformed moldable catheters designed for percutaneous insertion and for catheterization of branches of the great vessels. In this system, the catheter was preshaped to the anticipated anatomy, inserted, and subsequently manipulated into the desired vessel.

Working with patients needing coronary arteriography promptly taught me that conventional concepts of vascular catheter curvature were unsatisfactory for the coronary vessels. Animal models were not used in the development of the technique because they were unsuitable for application of the concept of tailoring catheter configuration to aortic size.

Principles traditional to transfemoral selective visceral angiography were modified to conform to the anatomy of the aortic root. Knowledge of catheter mechanics and of the properties of vascular catheter material lead to the development of a left "coronary seeking" catheter. The then unique configuration was preshaped to conform to the usual arch and orifice anatomy; it was unconventional to the thinking of the day. The same basic principles were applied in developing a companion right coronary catheter technique. Despite the long entrance-to-objective distance, the coronary arteries were selectively catheterized with astonishing ease.[1] The aortic arch, which has been considered an obstacle to successful transfemoral catheterization, was used to assist an appropriately preshaped catheter into the target orifice.

* Two different techniques of quality nonselective transfemoral coronary arteriography had been developed. Sven Paulin of Gothenburg, Sweden, used a coiled aortic catheter. Bjorn Nordenström of Stockholm used increased intrabronchial pressure.

CATHETER MATERIAL AND DESIGN

Consistent safe catheterization of the coronary arteries from a femoral artery requires a catheter with *sensitive positive rotary control*, preferably fabricated from a low-temperature thermoplastic with inherent pliability and elasticity. The original catheters were made from polyurethane with internal braided stainless steel wire, which provides torque control without compromising pliability. Barium salts gave dense radiopacity.[2] Several companies, using different materials, have tried to produce catheters patterned after the originals with varying degrees of success. The most common error in material selection is lack of pliability and increase in stiffness. Polyurethane is kind to the vascular wall, and I prefer catheters made from this thermoplastic.

The tip of the catheters was designed with a thinned, blunt "bullet nose" to reduce the chance of intimal injury or lumen obstruction. The catheters had only an end hole for accurate monitoring of tip pressure.

The original catheter was a no. 8 French with a tip thinned to 1.8 mm in diameter and 18 mm in length; the catheter body was 100 cm long and 2.7 mm in diameter. Now both no. 7 and no. 8 French catheters are commonly used. Thin-walled versions are also available. Even smaller diameter catheters sometimes may be appropriate. The coronary catheter selected for a particular patient should be as small in diameter as practical. However, in diameter selection there should be a balance between facilitating speed and convenience of coronary visualization and reducing the size of the arterial puncture. A no. 8 French is preferable when catheterizing the coronaries of a patient whose aorta is dilated, tortuous, or uncoiled.

CATHETER CONFIGURATION

A properly shaped catheter is the key to success (Figs. 7I-1 and 7I-2). A correct concept of cardiovascular anatomic relationships as well as knowledge and understanding of vascular catheter mechanics is essential to mastery of the Judkins technique of coronary arteriography. The catheters are preshaped by the manufacturer to conform to the usual arch and coronary vessel anatomy and to the usual anatomic relation of the ostia to the sinus of Valsalva and to the aortic arch.

At first glance, the configurations of the left and right catheters appear to be radically different; they are really quite similar. Because the relationship of the arch to the right orifice differs from that to the left, the configuration of the left catheter was modified for catheterizing the right coronary vessel. Each catheter has a primary, secondary, and tertiary bend (Fig. 7I-3). The primary, or tip, curve of each approximates 90°. The major difference is in the secondary bend. The left catheter has a curve that approaches 180°; the right has a more gentle curve of about 30°. The tertiary, or arch, curves are reversed. In the right catheter, excessive tertiary bend interferes with proper rotation and de-

Figure 7I-1 Left coronary catheters. (*a*) no. 3.5L; (*b*) no. 4L; (*c*) no. 5L; (*d*) no. 6L.

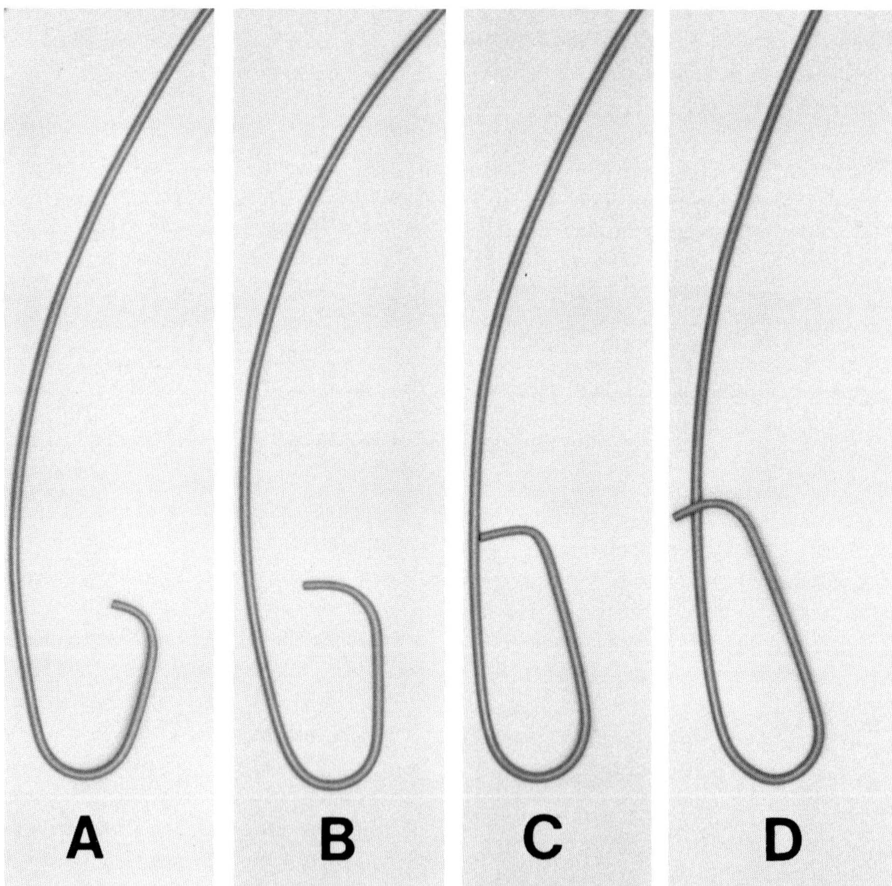

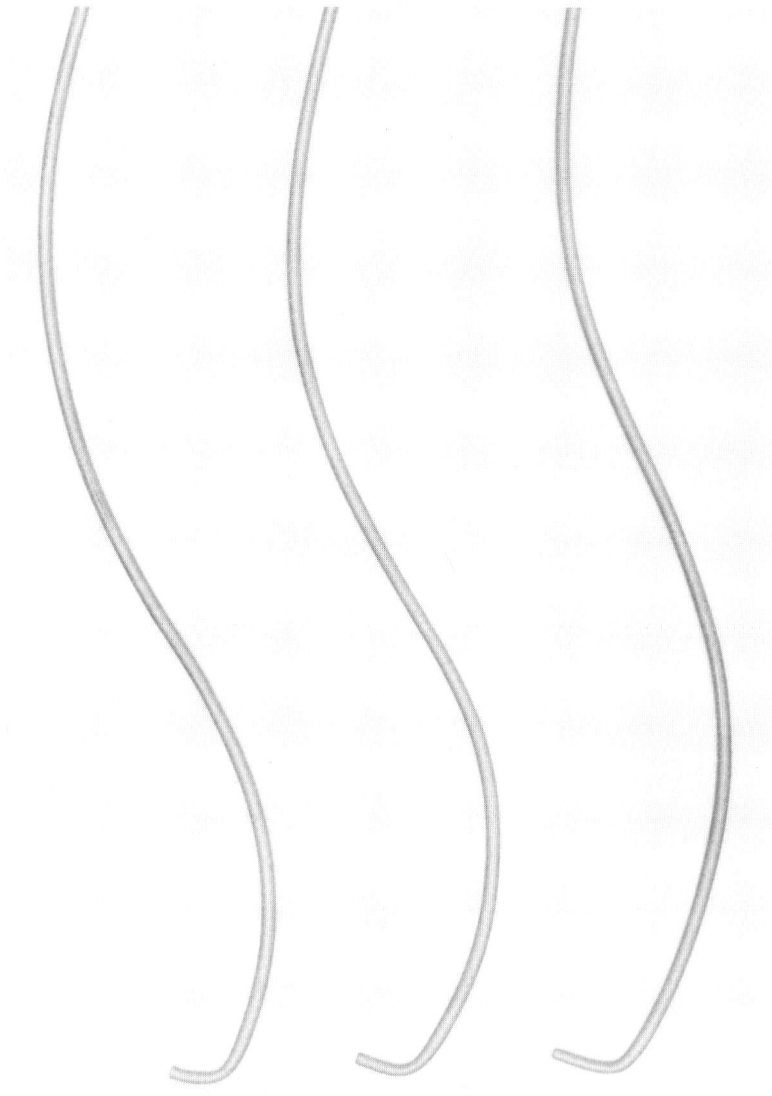

A B C

Figure 7I-2 Right coronary catheters. (*a*) no. 3.5R; (*b*) no. 4R; (*c*) no. 5R.

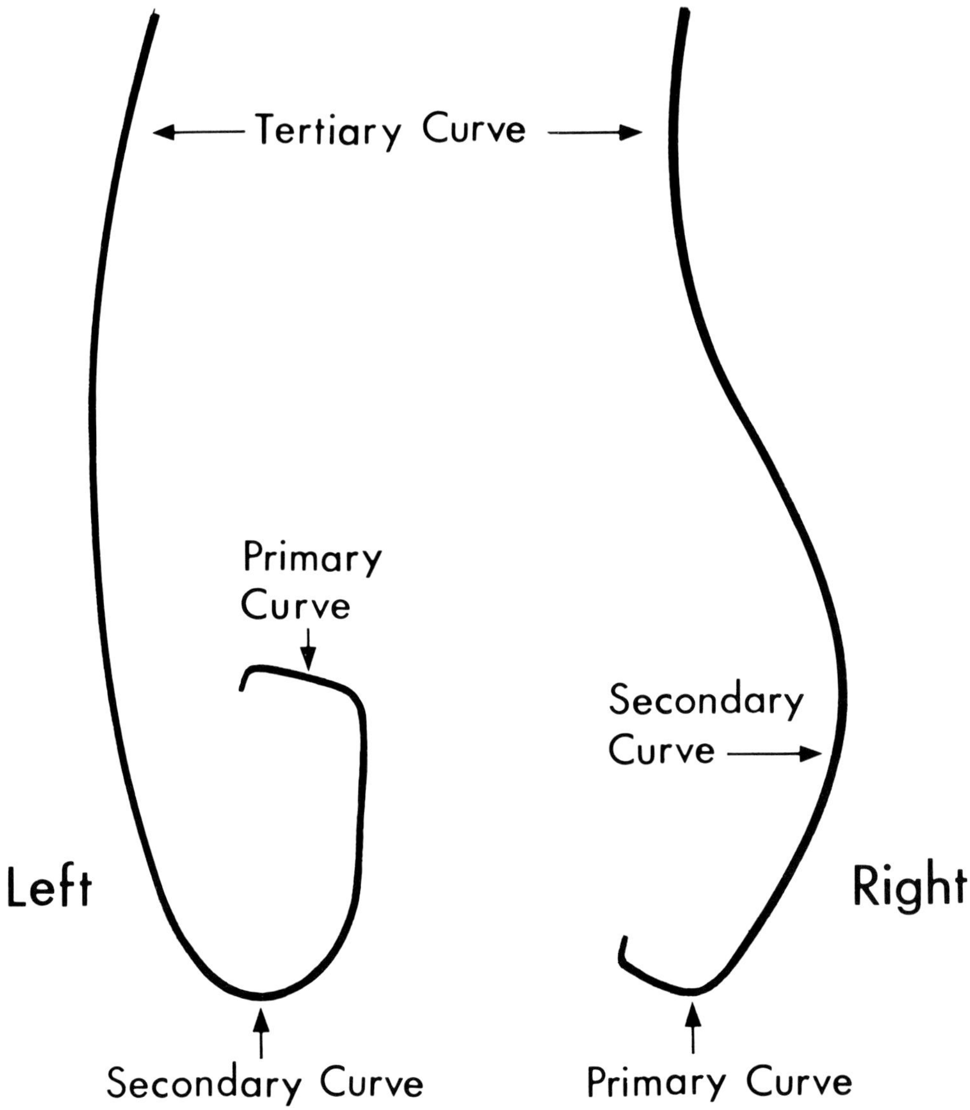

Figure 7I-3 Shaping wires for no. 4 coronary catheters.

scent. In the case of the left catheter, absent or inadequate tertiary bend may cause the catheter to rotate out of the plane of the coronary orifice.

Left Configuration

The orifice of the left main coronary artery is usually within 15° of the plane of the ascending aorta and the proximal portion of the aortic arch. A vascular catheter inserted retrogradely over the arch into the ascending aorta will rest on the right lateral aortic wall, a stable fix point. The anatomic relationship of the left orifice and the arch and the associated mechanics of transfemoral catheterization were combined and used to advantage in the design and configuration of the left catheter. These same factors minimize the need for operator manipulation. In fact, attempted operator manipulation is the most common cause of unsuccessful left coronary catheterization. The catheter *knows* where to go if not thwarted by the operator.

The exaggerated secondary curve designed into the preshaped left catheter provides the "spring" that holds the tip in place. Once correctly positioned, the catheter is secure, the tip in the orifice and the secondary bend braced on a stable fix point, the right aortic wall.

Right Configuration

The right coronary artery usually arises 120° to 130° anterior and to the right of the plane of the aortic arch and the position of the left orifice. In order to catheterize the right orifice, the configuration must facilitate establishment of a relatively stable fix point opposite the right coronary orifice. A satisfactory secondary stable fix point for the preshaped right catheter is on the left posterior aortic wall. The catheter must be rotated into this position from a primary, more stable right lateral wall rest.

CATHETERIZATION TECHNIQUE

The catheter configurations which conform to the arch anatomy effectively seek the appropriate orifice because of the dynamics of shape and motion. The technique is based on the interrelated dynamics of catheter memory, aortic pulsation, and sensitive positive rotary control of the catheters. The majority who use these catheters do not understand the basic principles of the Judkins technique. They are reasonably successful because when the catheters assume their preformed configuration in the aorta, *they know where to go unless thwarted by the operator*. Excessive manipulation is one of the greatest deterrents to successful selective catheterization. The catheters do better on their own than when an operator tries to "guide" them. The more an operator manipulates, the more the problems increase.

Percutaneous entry of the common femoral artery is accomplished with a no. 18 thin-walled arterial needle. A 145-cm 0.038-inch Teflon-coated safety guidewire is threaded through the iliac artery to a point above the aortic bifurcation *before* the needle is removed.[3,4] A dilator or short segment of no. 7 French Teflon catheter is inserted into the artery over the guidewire and then removed. This maneuver creates a pathway, through the fascia and vessel wall, for the soft tip of the catheter.

Left Coronary

The guidewire and catheter are quickly eased up the aorta until the tip of the guidewire reaches the distal part of the aortic arch. The guidewire is then held stationary while the left catheter is advanced to a relaxed position in the arch (Fig. 7I-4*a*). While in this position, the catheter is cleared, flushed with heparin-saline solution, and then filled with contrast agent.

The left catheter should be advanced slowly down the medial wall of the ascending aorta (Fig. 7I-4*b*) until it rotates slightly and the tip drops into the left coronary orifice (Fig. 7I-4*c*). When the catheter enters the orifice, it should be advanced a few millimeters to take up the slack. Once correctly positioned, the catheter is fixed in place—the tip in the orifice and the secondary bend resting on the right aortic wall (Fig. 7I-4*c*). Following a small test injection to verify satisfactory tip alignment, hand injection of 6 to 10 mL of a suitable contrast agent, delivered at a rate of 2 to 4 mL/s (depending on the size or rate of flow in the coronary system), should be imaged in multiple projections such as right anterior oblique 20°, caudocranial left anterior oblique, lateral, and other projections dictated by existing anatomy, pathology, and patient habitus. The lateral projection is one of the most diagnostically valuable but is frequently omitted.

Right Coronary

The right coronary catheter is introduced in a manner similar to the left, then cleared and filled with contrast agent while the leading end is in the descending thoracic aorta. The catheter is advanced into the ascending aorta to the neutral starting position, 1 to 2 cm above the left orifice, or approx-

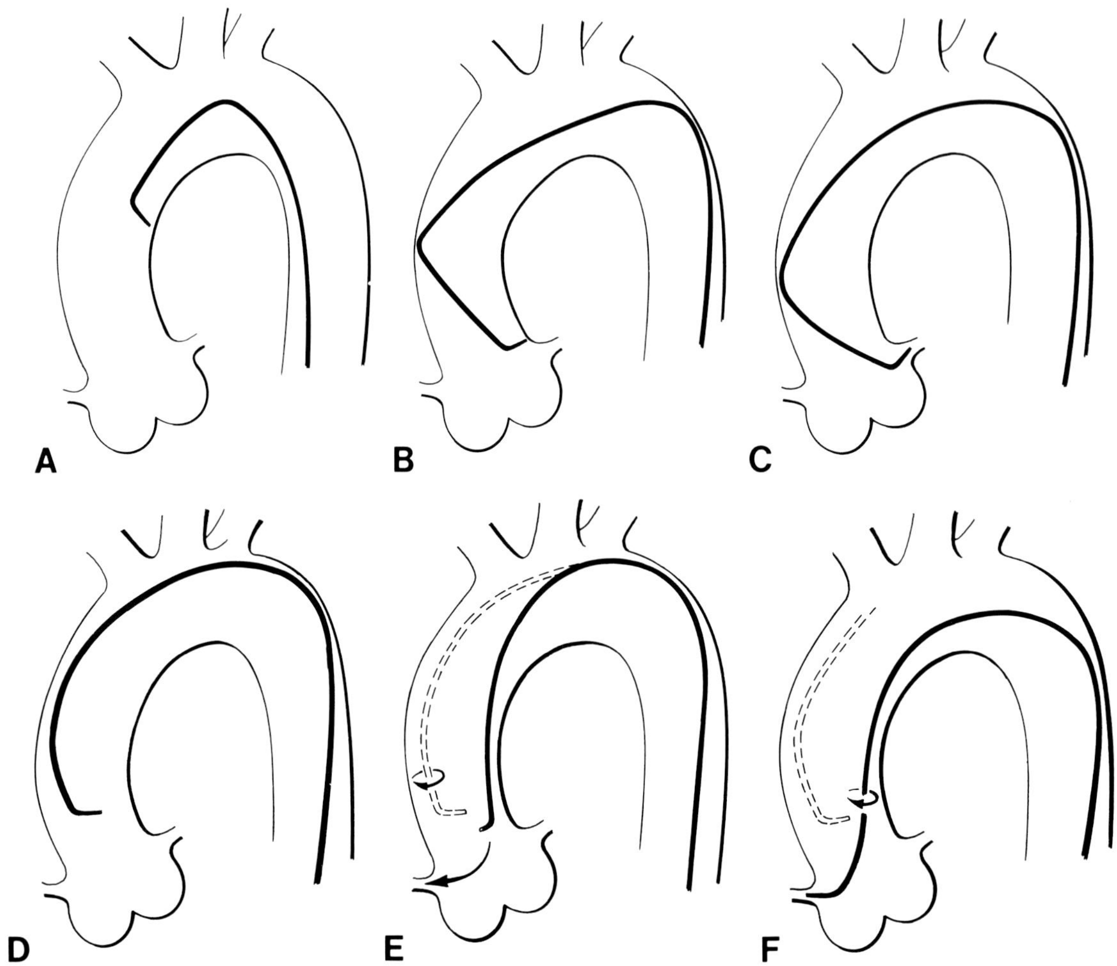

Figure 7I-4 Diagrammatic illustrations of coronary catheterization. (*a–c*) Left coronary catheterization. (*d–f*) Right coronary catheterization. (See text.)

imately 2 to 4 cm above the valve (Fig. 7I-4*d*). The catheter should be rotated *very slowly clockwise*. During this maneuver, before the rotation has reached 60°, the catheter tip will spontaneously descend about 3 cm into the right sinus of Valsalva (Fig. 7I-4*e*). Continue *slow* rotation of the catheter, anterior and to the right (clockwise catheter hub rotation); the tip will visibly drop into the right coronary orifice (Fig. 7I-4*f*).

The most common error in right coronary catheterization is failure of the operator to allow the mechanism of slow catheter rotation combined with the pulsation of the aorta to accomplish the rotation and descent sequence described. A common operator error is rotating the catheter like an eggbeater.

Following test injection to verify satisfactory tip alignment, hand injections of 6 to 10 mL of contrast delivered at 2 to 4 mL/s should be imaged in multiple projections tailored to existing anatomy, pathology, and patient habitus.

SELECTION OF CONFIGURATION SIZE

The most common initial technical error is selection of a catheter with a size configuration inappropriate for the patient to be studied. Aortic roots differ in width and configuration, a reflection of patient habitus, age, or disease. These are the primary factors affecting aortic root size.

Selective catheterization of the coronaries or any other branch of the aorta requires a catheter of suitable configuration and an effective diameter of curvature somewhat greater than the span of the aorta. Three common variations of aortic root size and shape are considered: the "normal" aorta, the unfolded or "rounded" aorta, and the poststenotic aorta (Fig. 7I-5).

Left Catheter

The configuration of the left catheter within the ascending aorta automatically aligns the primary and secondary curves in the plane of the left main coronary. The only significant variable is aortic root width. A preprocedural chest radiograph (posteroanterior) should be used to estimate aortic size. If this film demonstrates a normal-appearing aortic arch (Fig.7I-5*a*), as is common in coronary disease, select a left catheter with a 4.2-cm arm (the segment between primary and secondary curves), a no. 4 left catheter (Fig. 7I-1*b*). This size will accommodate 80 percent of the patients examined.

A 5.2-cm arm catheter, a no. 5 left catheter (Fig. 7I-l*c*), should be selected if the posteroanterior (PA) chest film shows a rounded, unfolded thoracic aorta with aortic shadow protruding on both sides of the cardiac silhouette. This variation occurs primarily in patients with hypertension or advanced age. When there is unfolding of the arch, the distance between the "fix point" of the secondary bend of the catheter and the coronary orifice is increased, even if the transverse diameter of the aorta is not dilated (Fig. 7I-5*b*). A no. 5 left catheter may also be useful in patients with modest poststenotic dilatation of the aorta.

A 6-cm arm catheter, a no. 6 (Fig. 7I-l*d*), should be selected if there is a history or findings of aortic stenosis and radiographic evidence of poststenotic dilatation of the aorta (Fig. 7I-5*c*). On rare occasions, catheters with arms as long as 9 cm (severe aortic dilatation) or as short as 3 cm (infant) may be needed.

The length of the arm is only moderately critical. The position of the secondary curvature in the ascending aorta and inherent spring of the "overbent" secondary curve will usually accommodate to aortic width variance of 1 cm. However, if the arm is too short, the catheter will double back on itself in the aorta. If the arm is too long, the catheter will assume a relatively vertical position in the aorta; the arm will rest on the lip of the sinus of Valsalva, thereby preventing the tip from reaching the orifice high and deep in the sinus.

If the initial catheter size selection is incorrect, prompt recognition of the error by the operator and expeditious catheter change will avoid futile manipulation and procedural delay.

Right Catheter

Three sizes of right coronary catheters are used to accommodate for variance in aortic width and configuration. They are designated nos. 3.5, 4, and 5 (Fig.7I-2). The size reflects the distance in centimeters from the primary curve to the midpoint of the secondary curve (Fig. 7I-3). The right catheters are used in anatomic situations equivalent to their left numerical counterparts.

The right catheter is more flexible in its adjustment to the aortic width than the left. A no. 4 right (no. 4R) commonly will satisfactorily catheterize the right coronary artery arising from a moderately wide aorta (Fig. 7I-5*e*). The no. 5 right is most useful in the widened aorta with an elongated arch or when there is poststenotic dilatation of the aorta (Fig. 7I-5*f*). A no. 4R with a flattened tip bend (110°) will work equally well. The original no. 6 right configuration could be abandoned.

CORONARY CATHETERIZATION TECHNICAL TIPS

The coronary ostia, located superior to the aortic valve, should be approached with a minimum of manipulation directly from the tubular aorta. If this technique is correctly performed, the coronary catheters will remain above the valvular leaflets or a prosthetic valve of usual configuration. Valvular function is unimpaired and injury secondary to ma-

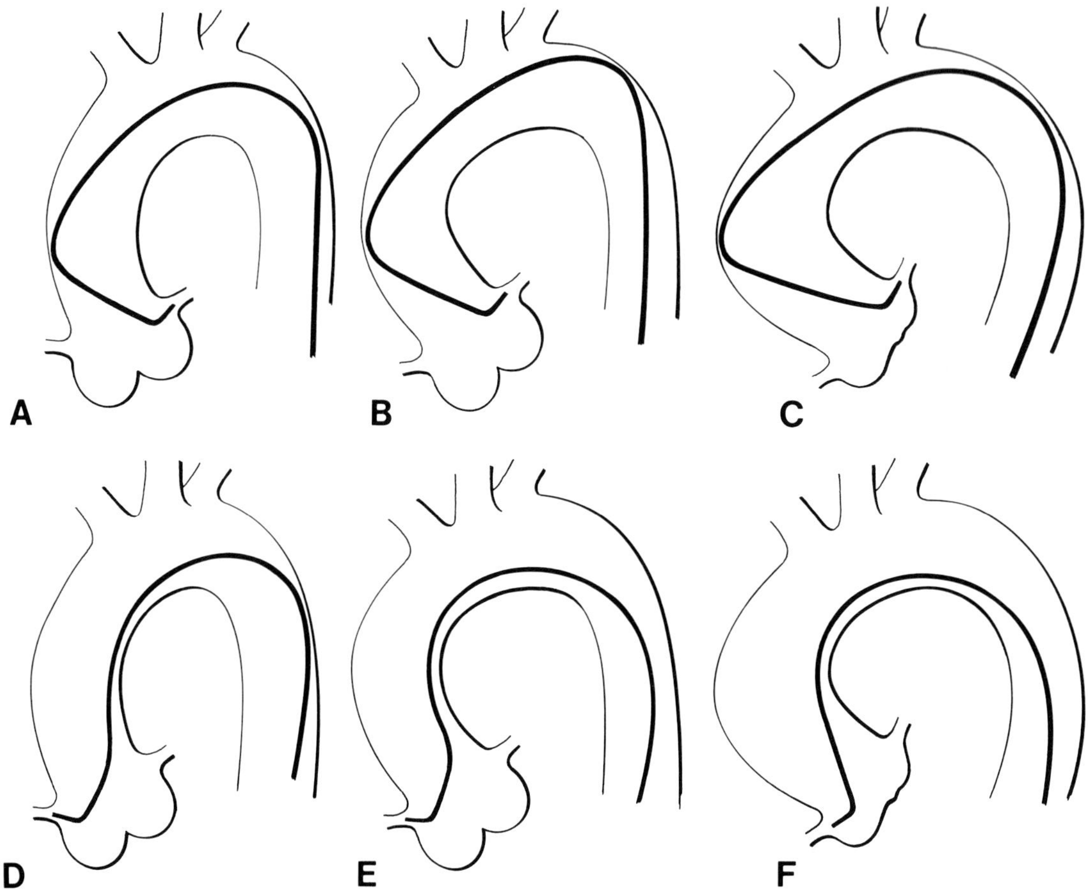

Figure 7I-5 Catheter mechanics for variations in aortic size and configuration. (*a–c*) Left coronary. (*d–f*) Right coronary. (*a*, *d*) Normal or usual aorta. (*b*, *e*) Unfolded aorta. (*c*, *f*) Poststenotic aorta.

nipulation or repeated catheter slapping is eliminated. Presence of a prosthetic valve requires no technical modifications; properly manipulated coronary catheters will not touch the prosthesis.

Anyone who attempts to cross the aortic valve or to perform ventriculography with a coronary catheter courts complications. These catheters were *never* intended for this purpose, and such use is contraindicated. The pigtail catheter is used for crossing the valve and performing ventriculography.

Left System

When catheterizing the left coronary, the catheter should be advanced at moderate speed down the ascending aorta. When the tip passes over the aortic "lip," it will rotate and drop into the orifice. This maneuver is quite automatic and does *not* require rotary manipulation by the operator. As previously stated, *the catheter knows where to go if not thwarted by the operator!*

If the operator advances the catheter too rapidly, or if the configuration size is too large, the catheter may pass over the orifice and come to rest in the sinus. If this occurs, the catheter should be withdrawn to the arch and *without* applied torque again advanced down the ascending aorta. If the initial missed catheterization was the result of too rapid advancement, the catheter will now enter the coronary orifice. If the tip again passes over the orifice, it is probable that the size configuration is too large, e.g., no. 5L being used rather than a needed no. 4L. The remedy is a catheter change to the appropriate configuration size.

If on opacification of the left system, a single vessel is visualized, there may be a very short left main, and subselective catheterization may have been achieved. Withdrawal of the catheter to the orifice of the left main and contrast visualization will identify this circumstance. Subselective catheterization of the anterior descending and circumflex arteries may be necessary. Alternatively, contrast injection at the orifice of the left main may be satisfactory. If there is a very short left main or separate orifices, the two vessels can be opacified and imaged separately. If only one left branch can be readily identified, suspect that the "missing" branch may be originating from the right coronary or the right sinus of Valsalva.

Both left and right coronary catheters readily enter the coronary ostia and should be advanced slightly. In fact, the neophyte may be surprised to find the left catheter has sought the orifice quite on its own. The operator should exercise care lest the catheter is inadvertently advanced too deeply into the left orifice.

If the left catheter is overinserted or the secondary arm is too short, there is risk of subintimal injection and/or poor vessel filling. A tip position near 90° to the vessel wall in two planes is not acceptable (Fig. 7I-6*b*). If the secondary arm is too long, the tip of the catheter will tend to jump over the orifice and lie in the sinus. Selective injection is missed. The position and relationship of the tip to the left main orifice should be evaluated by an initial test injection. If indicated, alignment should be adjusted or catheter exchange made and satisfactory tip position confirmed by another small-volume test injection (Fig. 7I-6*a*).

Right System

If rotation of the right coronary catheter is initiated too near the valve (common error of a novice), the catheter will not descend as previously described, but will descend only a short distance (1 cm or so) deep into the right sinus of Valsalva or will prolapse

Figure 7I-6 Left catheter position. (*a*) Correct alignment. (*b*) Incorrect position and overinsertion.

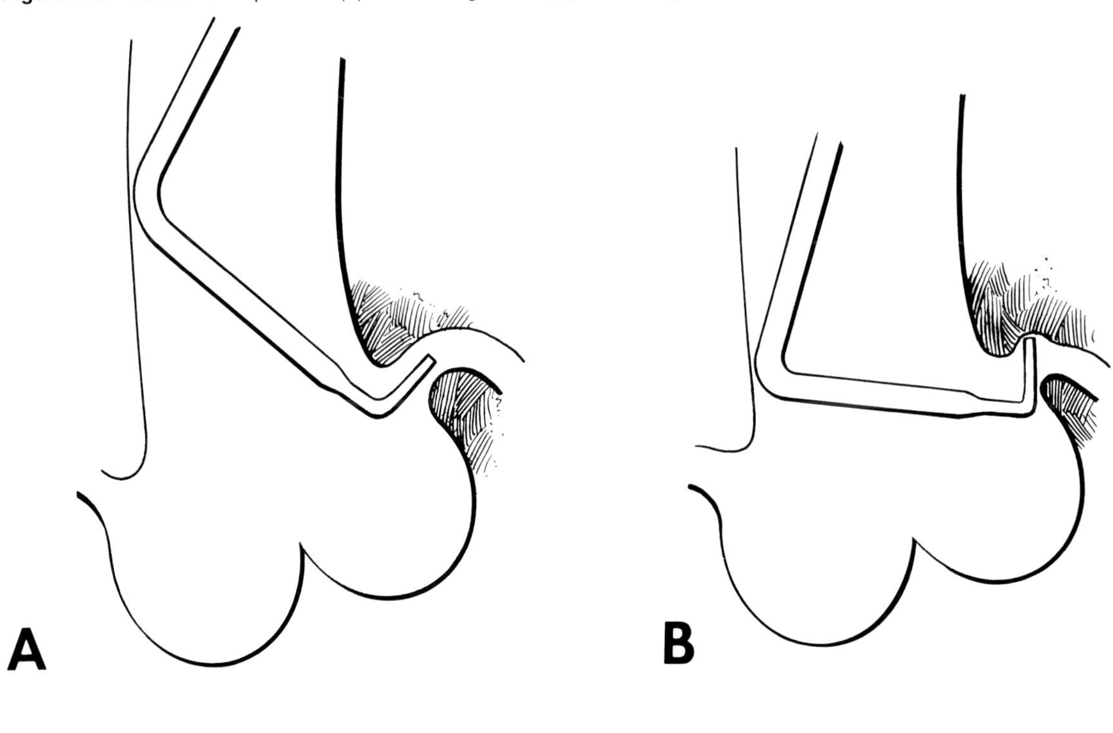

across the aortic valve. If rotation is initiated too high above the valve, the catheter will not descend, but will rotate tip cephalad in the ascending aorta. If a patient has a *very* high or tortuous arch, the normal descent mechanism will not occur. Catheter descent must then be accomplished by advancing the catheter during rotation.

Avoid introduction of excessive torque in the catheter during rotation. The angiographer should allow the pulsation in the aorta to assist in the slow, deliberate rotation. It is the mastery of this maneuver that separates the expert from the novice. Initial excessive application of torque can be reduced by slight reversal of torque as the tip rotates into the right coronary orifice. If torque is not excessive, the catheter is quite stable and will require a definite tug to remove it from the orifice (Fig. 7I-7*a*).

When the catheter enters the right orifice, if there is pressure damping, a small contrast test injection should be made; this will identify the reason for damping. One of three situations may exist. The conus branch of the right system may have been subselectively catheterized (Fig. 7I-7*b*). There may be a proximal stenosis of the right vessel (Fig. 7I-7*c*). The tip of the catheter may be against the lateral wall of the right coronary (Fig. 7I-7*d*).

Conus branches may arise from the right coronary or directly from the aorta. A large conus branch with a separate aortic orifice may be selectively catheterized. A conus branch may arise in such a position in the superior proximal right vessel that the catheter may repeatedly subselectively catheterize this branch. Occasionally it is necessary to increase the primary curve of the right catheter to 110° (from 90°) to bypass this branch orifice. If the catheter has entered the conus artery (Fig. 7I-7*b*), the contrast injection will reveal the opacified vessel. The catheter should be removed and the right vessel recatheterized. If the conus branch is again intubated, do one of two things: (1) straighten the tip of the right catheter, or (2) replace the catheter with a larger size configuration, e.g., use a no. 5R rather than a no. 4R.

The catheter may wedge in the narrowed orifice of a diseased or nondominant right vessel (Fig. 7I-7*c*). If there is repeated wedging during several attempts to satisfactorily position the catheter, I suggest proceeding as follows: Position the patient for filming, insert the catheter in the right orifice, film, and immediately remove the catheter. The elapsed time from catheter insertion to removal should be less than 10 s. This procedure can be repeated until the required imaging is accomplished.

If the catheter is found to damp on the lateral wall of the vessel (Fig. 7I-7*d*), the tip is too long. The catheter should be replaced with one with a shorter tip. The tip length of the right coronary catheter should be about 5 or 6 mm. Several manufacturers use a longer tip. The right main is extremely short in its transverse portion, and the catheter tip may need to be straightened and/or shortened. Shortening the tip about 0.1 cm is occasionally helpful both in obviating false damping in a short right coronary stem and in avoiding subselective catheterization of the conus branch.

Catheter Modification

This technique owes consistency of selective catheterization to the use of catheters preshaped to the usual vascular anatomy. If anatomy varies significantly from the usual, successful catheterization may require modified configurations. My experience indicates that such variance is unusual.

Because of occasional need, a laboratory should have the capability for procedural modification of catheters. Configuration of a polyurethane catheter may be altered by inserting a shaping wire (Fig. 7I-3) with the desired modification and immersing catheter and wire in boiling water for 2 minutes. Immediate subsequent immersion of catheter and wire in cold water sets the new memory. The modified configuration re-forms when the shaping wire is removed.

Anatomical Variations

The right coronary orifice classically originates from the right sinus of Valsalva. The variations in origin from the right sinus are much more common than the left, but the variation usually causes little procedural difficulty if the angiographer remembers

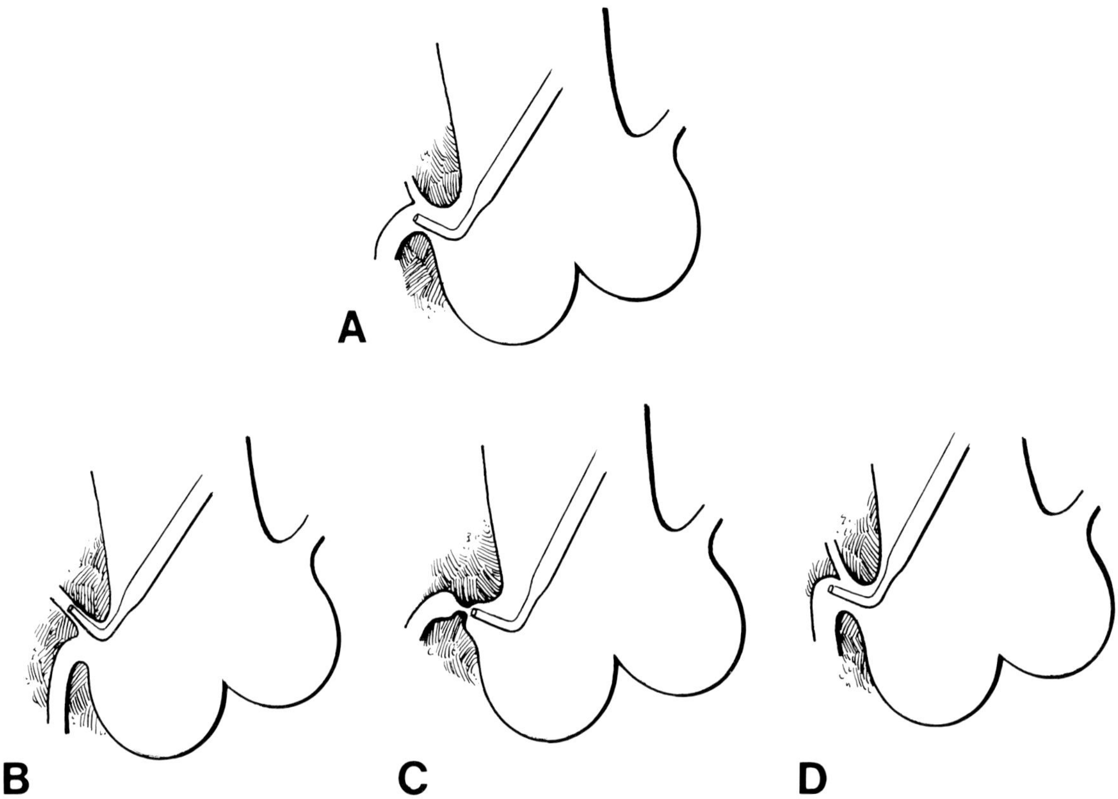

Figure 7I-7 Right catheter position. (*a*) Correct alignment. (*b*) Tip subselectively in conus artery. (*c*) Tip wedged in proximal stenosis. (*d*) Tip impinging on lateral vessel wall.

that the orifice may lie somewhat superior in the sinus of Valsalva or even above the lip of the sinus.

The two most frequently encountered variations from normal are these: (1) A nondominant right coronary may originate in the superior part of the sinus or in the tubular aorta. The small size may increase the difficulty of locating the orifice. (2) Either the left or right vessel or one of their major branches may originate in the superior part of the right sinus or in the tubular aorta.

Catheterization may be more difficult because of the absence of the normal "funnel" leading to the orifice. An operator who recognizes the anatomic situation can readily catheterize the orifice by simply probing the superior portion of the sinus of Valsalva or lower tubular aorta. If the ostium arises in the tubular aorta, manipulation of the right coronary catheter will have to start from the more superior position with more precise control of the catheter.

SELECTIVE BYPASS GRAFT CATHETERIZATION

In the mid 1960s our surgical colleagues developed techniques to directly revascularize obstructed coronary arteries. Two basic methods were utilized: anastomosis of the internal mammary to a coronary vessel, and end-to-end and then end-to-side anastomosis of saphenous vein bypass grafts. Postoperative evaluation is frequently indicated to establish patency or to assess the presence of disease or the site of obstruction. Graft catheterizing is facilitated from a time standpoint if the thoracic surgeon places a small metal clip or ring at the graft orifice.

Aortocoronary bypass grafts are usually attached to the aorta beginning 2 or 3 cm cephalad of the native right orifice, and along a line extending obliquely superior and medial to the native right coronary orifice, following a course dictated by the anatomy.

Coronary bypass grafts can be selectively catheterized with consistency by an expert angiographer who uses suitably preshaped catheters of appropriate design.

Grafts to the Right Coronary

A graft to the right vessel is usually best catheterized by using a catheter of the configuration shown in Fig. 7I-8*a*. This right graft catheter is similar to a Judkins right except that the primary (tip) bend is 110° to 120°. The primary bend prevents excessive caudal travel down the graft. A catheter with a relatively straight primary bend would intubate most grafts; however, nothing would prevent the tip from traveling to the diaphragmatic level.

A right graft usually originates from the aorta and courses obliquely in a caudal direction. To engage the graft orifice, it is best to rotate the graft catheter in a similar fashion to the right coronary catheter, but at a level more cephalad, until the tip is superior to the probable site of the graft orifice. Then advance the catheter down the aortic wall to the graft orifice. If the graft catheter inadvertently engages the native right orifice, it is usually not appropriate to attempt to slide the catheter cephalad from the natural to the graft orifice. The proper technique is to make the approach by advancing the catheter down the aorta to the graft orifice.

Grafts to the Anterior Descending System

A graft to the anterior descending artery and its branches is usually best catheterized by using a catheter of the configuration shown in Fig. 7I-8*b*. This graft catheter differs in configuration from the right coronary catheter in that the primary bend is approximately 90° and the secondary bend is approximately 70°. The center of curvature of the secondary bend is similar to that of the no. 3.5 right coronary catheter.

Most commonly an anterior descending graft originates superior and to the left of the usual position of the right graft or native right ostium. The graft orifice can be readily engaged by the left graft catheter if the catheter is rotated anteriorly at the appropriate height until it visibly passes the midpoint of the ascending aorta and stabilizes with the tip pointed toward the left.

Grafts to the Circumflex System

A graft to the circumflex system usually originates superior and to the left of the position of an anterior descending graft orifice. The catheter and the maneuver for catheterizing a graft to the circumflex system are virtually identical to those for catheterizing an anterior descending graft.

An aortic root flush is inadequate for evaluation of revascularization. There are too many false positives and false negatives. Widely patent grafts are frequently missed, and failure to visualize is not evidence of closure.

Internal Mammary Catheterization

The internal mammary artery is usually best catheterized by using a catheter of the configuration shown in Fig. 7I-8*c*.

The operator should be aware that the internal mammary artery originates from the anterior inferior side of the subclavian artery after it curves toward the extremity. The internal mammary is readily engaged by the tip of the internal mammary catheter (Fig. 7I-8*c*).

Note that the internal mammary catheter is similar to the Judkins right catheter with the following important differences: (1) the primary (tip) curve is less than 90° (approximately 80° to 85°). (2) The tip length is 1.5 to 2 cm. The wider the subclavian artery, the longer the tip length needs to be.

Personally I dislike doing an internal mammary artery visualization. This vessel supplies the muscle of the chest wall, and injecting contrast is quite painful to a patient. Additional sedation is indicated.

VENTRICULOGRAPHY

Angiographic examination of the coronary arteries is incomplete without evaluation of left ventricular

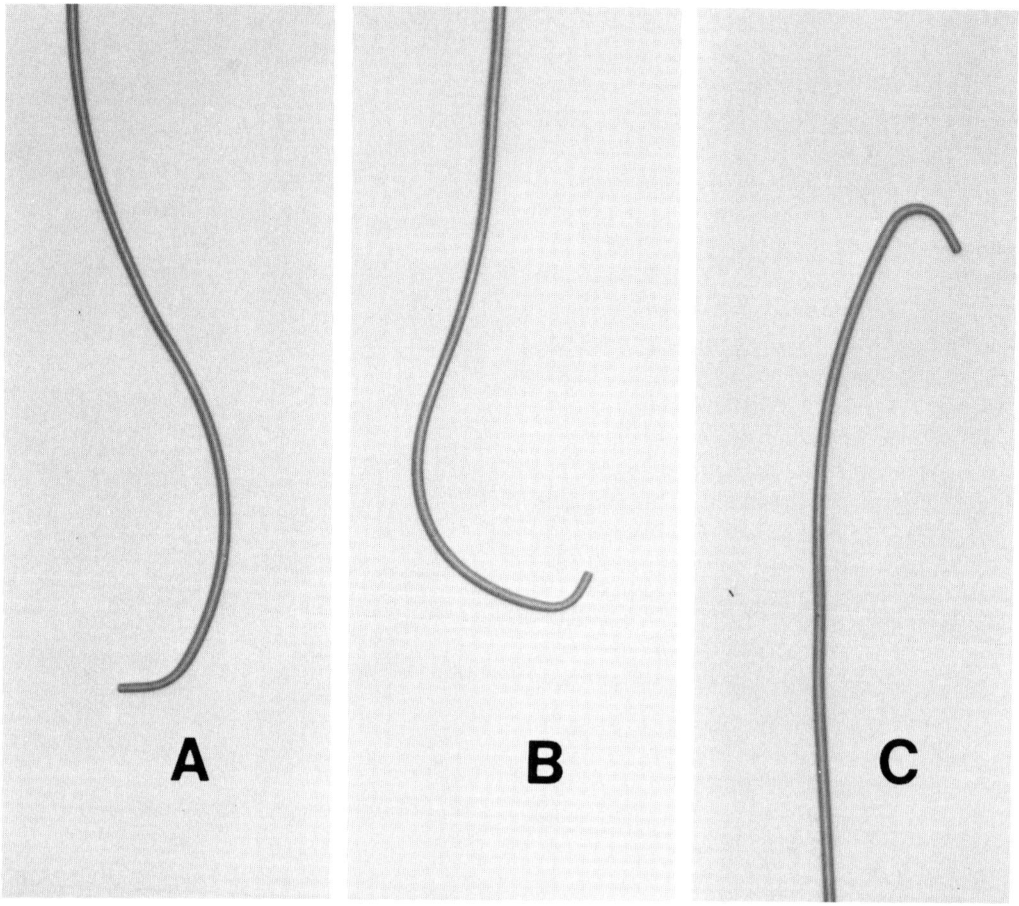

Figure 7I-8 Bypass graft catheters. (*a*) Right bypass catheter. (*b*) Left bypass catheter. (*c*) Internal mammary catheter.

function. This is best assessed by observation of the contrast-filled functioning ventricle, measurement of left ventricular end-diastolic pressure, and calculation of ejection fraction. Depicting ventricular anatomy requires the ability to detect abnormalities within the ventricular cavity and of the cardiac valves. Depicting ventricular function calls for the ability to assess both global and segmental wall motion.

By visual inspection of cineangiographic film an experienced observer can make a clinically useful assessment of ventricular performance. Quantitative measurement from a single plane study is reasonably accurate and useful. However, in the presence of regional or extensive generalized wall motion dysfunction, visualization of only a portion of the ten recognized contractile segments of the ellipsoid left ventricle may not give a true picture of contractility. Two-plane or biplane ventriculography offers visualization of all segments (five best seen in the right anterior oblique and five in the left anterior oblique projection) and facilitates more accurate evaluation.[5]

The Pigtail Catheter

A companion ventriculography catheter constructed of the same polyurethane material as the coronary catheters was designed. The curled tip suggested the "pigtail" designation.[2] The shaft is straight and the elongated, 5-cm, thinned terminal segment is curled into a tight loop; it has four side holes (Fig. 7I-9). Although the tip has an end hole, it functions similar to a closed-end catheter and has the added advantage of a soft, round leading end.

The introduction of the pigtail catheter as part of the Judkins technique of percutaneous transfemoral coronary arteriography provided a method of accomplishing ventriculography consistently and with ease without the hazard of myocardial injury. Manipulation in normal or significantly diseased major vessels and the cardiac chambers is straightforward. The atraumatic leading end virtually eliminates inadvertent penetration of a vessel or cardiac chamber; subendocardial injection is virtually a nonexistent hazard. The catheter is stable and does not whip during pressure injection. Consistent, high-quality ventriculography can be performed with safety and without precipitation of premature ventricular contractions (PCVs).

Left Ventriculography with the Pigtail Catheter

To assess ventricular function optimally, the ventricle should be visualized in two planes during normal sinus rhythm. Assessment of both global and segmental function requires ventriculography free of PVCs. A cardiac angiographer should learn to position the pigtail in the inflow tract of the ventricle near the mitral valve, where there is considerably less likelihood of contrast injection initiating PVCs.

The technique for advancing the pigtail from the aorta into the ventricle and properly positioning the catheter for ventriculography is as follows: With the patient either supine or in shallow 15° right anterior oblique (RAO) position, advance the soft, rounded tip of the pigtail catheter from its initial position in the ascending aorta (Fig. 7I-10*a*) onto the valve assembly. Using firm, gentle pressure, roll up the catheter on the valve to the position shown in Fig. 7I-10*b*, with the loop on the medial side of the tubular aorta, position 1. Take care not to advance the catheter beyond the first 2 to 3 cm of the tubular aorta. A momentary pause with the catheter in this position allows the operator to prepare for the next carefully timed maneuver. Slowly

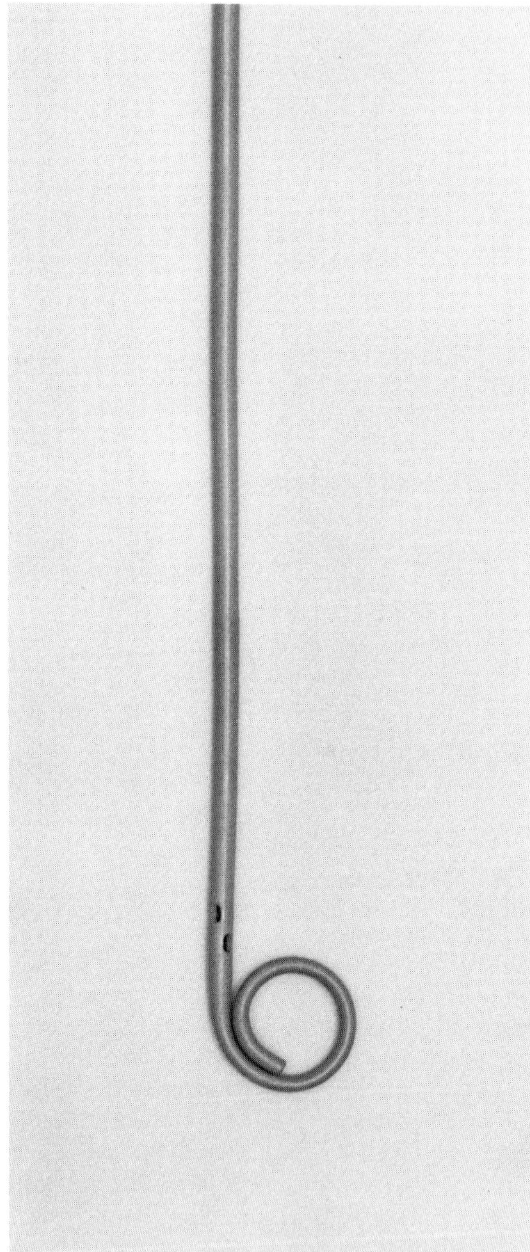

Figure 7I-9 Pigtail catheter for ventriculography and other mainstream injections.

withdraw the catheter (Fig. 7I-10*b*, maneuver 2) until the leading end drops to a near transverse position in the sinus of Valsalva as shown in Fig. 7I-10*c*. As part of a continuous single motion, withdraw the catheter 1 or 2 cm and advance it across the open valve as the coiled tip flips caudally (Fig. 7I-10*c*). This coordinated maneuver, bringing the catheter to a transverse position in the sinus of Valsalva, imparts a certain amount of spring to the shaft, and withdrawal allows the catheter to flick across the valve. A near simultaneous advancing maneuver places the catheter in the ventricular cavity (Fig 7I-10*c*, maneuvers 3 and 4).

At least half of the time, before the previously described sequence is completed, the pigtail catheter will have spontaneously prolapsed across the valve. Nevertheless, the operator should become familiar with the proper sequence of crossing the valve. After a little practice, an operator will find this easy to accomplish.

In the ventricle, the catheter will assume a natural resting position with the coiled tip directed superiorly and rotated from 0° to 30° anteriorly. The catheter is withdrawn slowly until it assumes a more vertical position in the base of the ventricle (Fig. 7I-10*d*).

In preparation for ventriculography, place the patient in the RAO position for the next series of maneuvers, illustrated in Fig. 7I-10*e*. The pigtail catheter will be in position 1 after crossing the aortic valve. Withdraw the catheter 2 or 3 cm and rotate it 70° to 90° counterclockwise as shown in maneuver 2. This will place the coiled loop in the inflow tract of the mitral valve as shown in position 3. If the catheter moves excessively in this position, advance it somewhat until it is stable (Fig. 7I-10*e*, position 4), but the loop should be above the base of the ventricle to obviate occurrence of PVCs during injection.

The maneuver of placing the catheter in the inflow tract near the mitral valve provides good mixing of contrast material and nonopacified blood entering from the mitral valve. Good opacification of the entire ventricular cavity can be accomplished with a relatively small volume of contrast medium, obviating blind spots in the ventricle created by the presence of nonopacified blood. Correct position of the pigtail provides even opacification and a "quiet" ventriculogram (without PVCs). It is amazing how many cardiac angiographers do not understand or use this simple maneuver.

Slow injection of the contrast bolus is desirable. A properly placed pigtail will *not* cause PVCs when contrast is injected at a moderate rate of 10 to 12 mL/s for 4 to 5 s. During pressure injection with desirable flow rates, the coiled tip straightens into a J-shape configuration. A large portion of the injected contrast is dissipated laterally in a fountain-like configuration through the side holes. Contrast flow from the side holes tends to stabilize the catheter laterally. Contrast flow from the end hole reduces recoil and tends to counteract the retrograde forces of the pressure injection.

It may be useful, but is not essential, to visualize ventricular motion during a premature contraction. An angiographer can develop the skill, when using a pigtail catheter, of obtaining a quiet ventriculogram during the first few contractions after ven-

Figure 7I-10 (*a–e*) Diagrammatic illustrations of catheterizing the left ventricle with the pigtail catheter (see text).

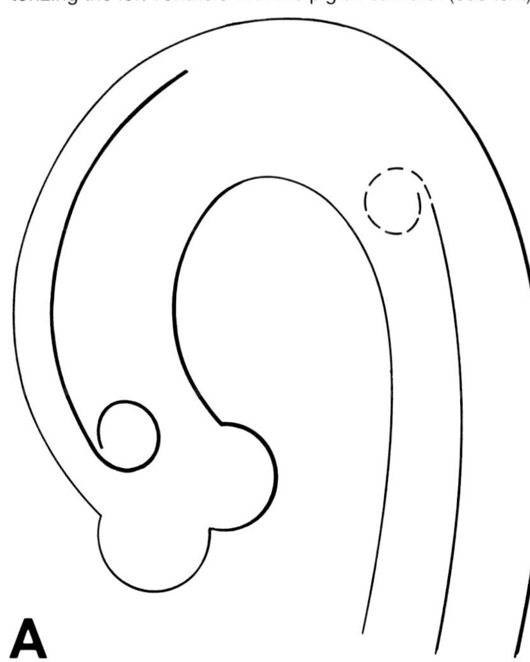

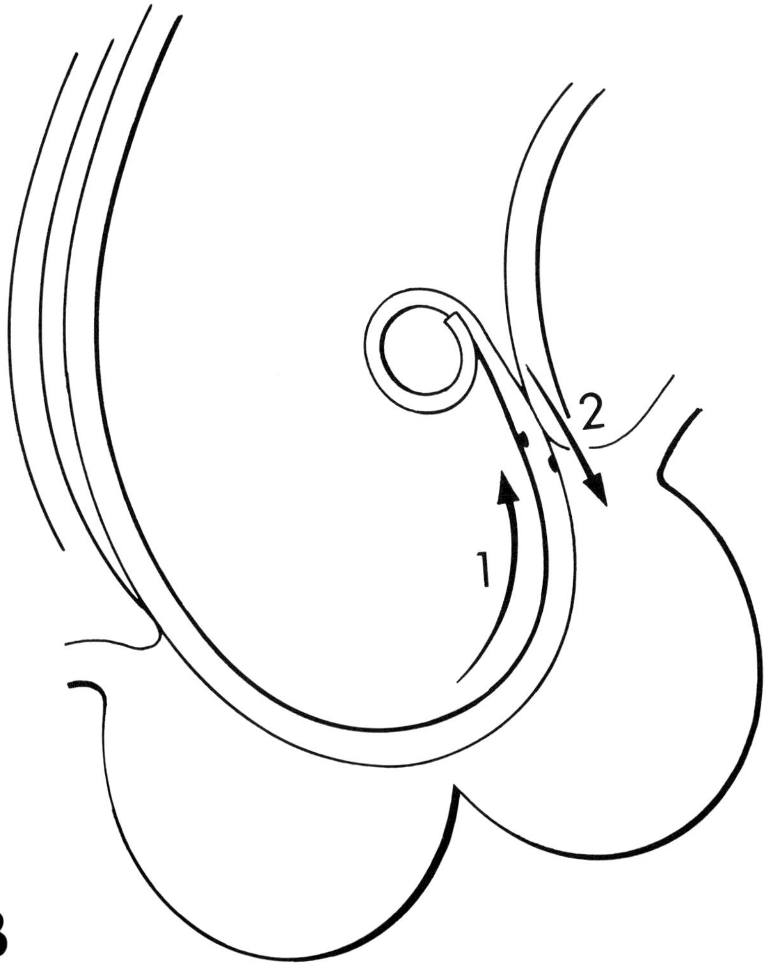

B
(Figure 7I-10, continued)

tricular filling and then stimulating a premature contraction by manipulating the catheter against the ventricular wall while the injection progresses.

Occasionally, a quiet position for the pigtail catheter in the inflow tract of a hyperdynamic ventricle cannot be established. Under this circumstance, it may be desirable to make the injection directly into the left atrium. The pigtail catheter is readily maneuvered into the left atrium from the ventriculography injection position just described.

LEFT ATRIAL CATHETERIZATION WITH THE PIGTAIL

The configuration of a pigtail catheter was modified to facilitate crossing the mitral valve from the left ventricle.[4] To cross the mitral valve from the left ventricle use a pigtail catheter in which a 30° or more angle has been preshaped in the distal 5 to 10 cm. This angle can be in the form of a gentle curve or sharp angulation as shown in Fig. 7I-11*a* and *b*. The 30° angle usually works quite satisfac-

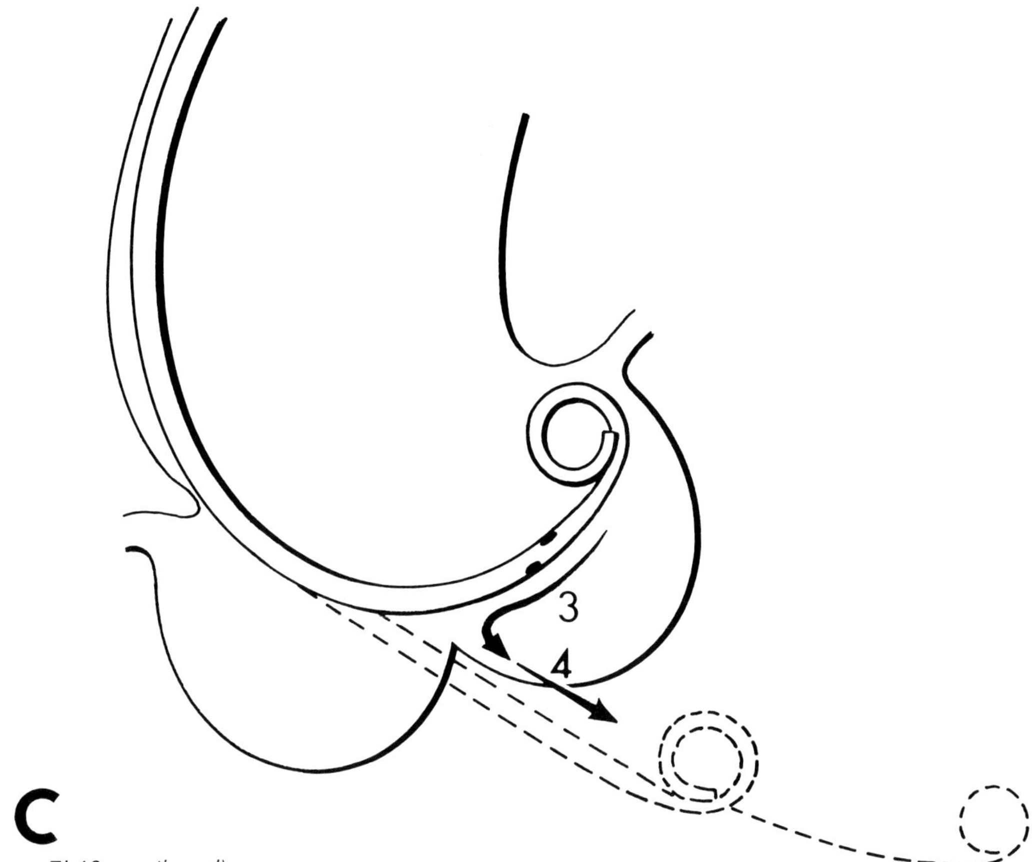

(Figure 7I-10, continued)

torily. However, when structures are small or anatomy is atypical, the angle may be increased to near 180°.

This technique uses usual anatomy to direct the catheter consistently into the left atrium. Once positioned, the catheter will remain in place without recoil during contrast injection. Contrast opacification or direct pressure measurements can be obtained. Contrast injection into the left atrium should be made at a rate of 15 mL/s for 3 to 4 s.

CROSSING A STENOTIC AORTIC VALVE WITH THE PIGTAIL CATHETER

If the aortic valve is stenotic or deformed, the operator will need to use a spring guidewire to initially traverse the stenotic canal. A *tight* pigtail loop (Fig. 7I-9) is essential to successful crossing of a stenotic valve. The valve usually lies in a near transverse plane.

The coiled configuration of tight loop pigtail is used to manipulate the tip of a flexible guidewire across the stenotic valve. The orifice is usually in a plane almost 90° from the long axis of the patient. Under fluoroscopic control, the tip of the guidewire is directed toward the central portion of the valve, into the stenotic canal, and through the orifice. The channel through the orifice may be somewhat angled in relationship to the valve plane. The trick is to maneuver the guide across the domed valve by directing the tip of the guidewire to the center of the dome, remembering that the tightly stenotic

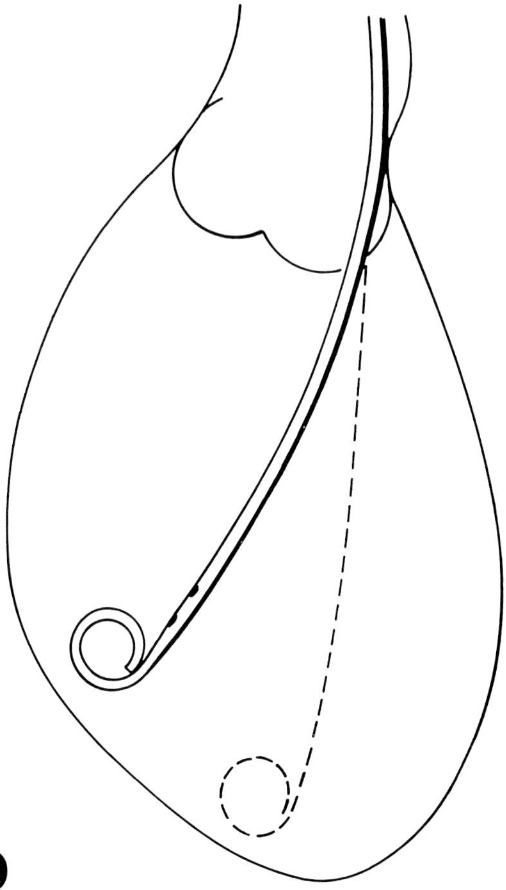

(Figure 7I-10, continued)

orifice is almost 90° from the long axis of the patient. Once the guidewire enters the channel, it can be maneuvered into the ventricle while advancing the catheter over the guidewire. The catheter should not be advanced over the guidewire until the straight portion of the guide has traversed the stenotic channel. Experience has taught me that calcium in the valve tends to be somewhat inferior to the stenotic orifice (0.5 cm on average). The calcium serves as a landmark, alerting the angiographer that the orifice is a few millimeters superior to the calcium.

Because of the distorted anatomic relationships and the variability between manufacturer's angiographic tools, I have found that certain products are easier to use. The Cook* 0.038 inch guidewire used through a tight Cordis† pigtail provides me the most satisfactory combination of tools for crossing the aortic stenosis associated with a dilated aortic root. In addition to controlling the guide angle by the length of the guidewire that protrudes from the uncoiled pigtail, it may be necessary to slightly angulate the guidewire 5 to 7 cm from its tip to cross the valve. In markedly dilated aortas, it may be necessary to use a movable core guidewire.

An operator who uses a catheter and guidewires of different material and structure than those mentioned will have to learn the combination of tools personally most suitable. Nevertheless, the maneuvers are basically the same.

Some associates of mine have found it advantageous and time-saving to use biplane fluoroscopy in directing the guidewire across the valve. If biplane fluoroscopy is available, I urge developing this skill.

Once an operator has mastered the concept of maneuvering the coiled pigtail and the flexible tip of the guidewire, crossing the valve can be accomplished in over 95 percent of patients with aortic stenosis. Because structural relationship varies with patient anatomy, achieving 95 percent success is predicated on operator skill and experience and procedural modification of tools as necessary.

PROCEDURAL SAFETY

The ease of performance of this technique induces many to undertake it with scarcely any grounding in the transfemoral approach or the use of preformed catheters. The potential for misadventure should give pause to an operator undertaking coronary arteriography unprepared.

Operator obsession to overmanipulate the catheter into a coronary ostium is counterproductive and invites complications. As stated several times, *the catheters know where to go if not thwarted by the operator!*

* Cook, Inc., P.O. Box 489, Bloomington, Indiana, 47401.
† Cordis Corp., P.O. Box 525700, Miami, Florida, 33152.

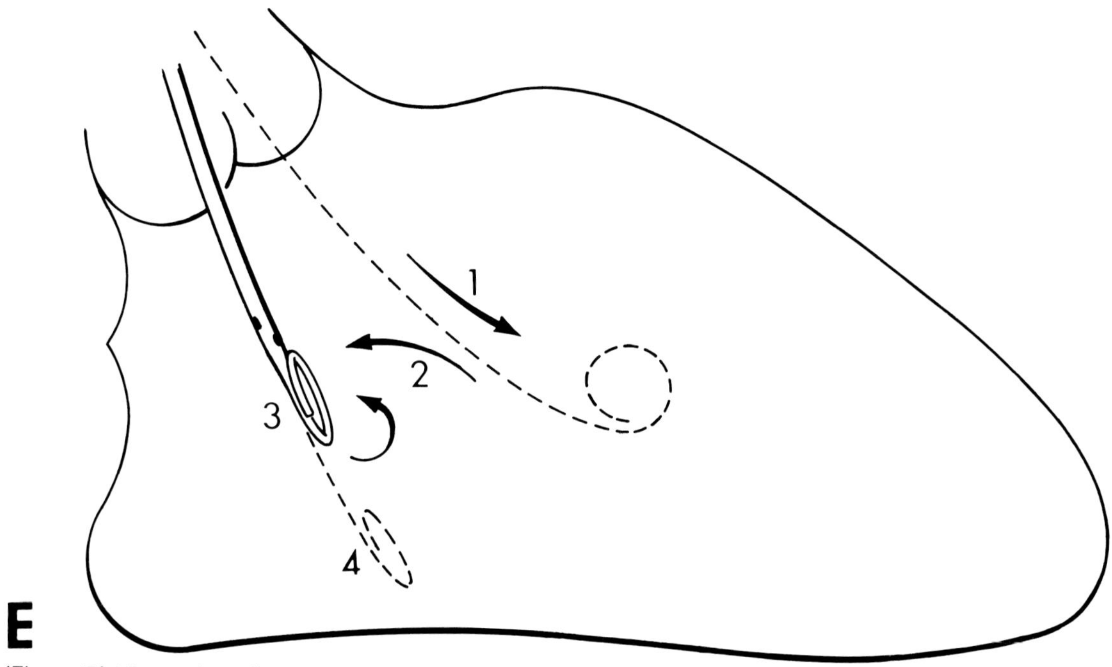

(Figure 7I-10, continued)

Consistent procedural safety is of prime importance and demands a no-compromise approach. Team effort by professional and technical laboratory staff is essential to safety and quality of examination. Meticulous attention to good procedural and catheter technique is of utmost importance. Studies should be carried out expeditiously and with purpose. Procedure time should be kept as short as possible consistent with retrieval of radiographic and physiological data essential to therapeutic decision making. It is attention to details that counts.[6]

Operators who perform both coronary arteriography and therapeutic techniques such as percutaneous transluminal coronary angioplasty (PTCA) should carefully separate these studies in their thinking and in their technical approach. Coronary arteriography requires meticulous care. Transluminal angioplasty is controlled trauma. The acceptable mishap rates are vastly different. Recognizable intimal injury during diagnostic studies should be very rare; intimal injury during PTCA is a necessary part of the procedure.

Guidewires

Teflon-coated safety guidewires can be inserted or withdrawn through polyurethane catheters with ease. This effortless handling markedly reduces the chance of damaging the guidewire and shortens procedure time. Use of coated guides is an integral part of the no-compromise-for-safety approach of this technique.[2]

Safe, consistent selective transfemoral coronary catheterization requires operator ability to effectively traverse tortuous atherosclerotic iliac vessels without intimal injury. The safety-J guidewire with its flexible, broadly rounded leading end, provides such a lumen-following device. If the operator encounters resistence to passage of a conventional guidewire on entrance into the iliac artery, a J guidewire should be used.[2,7] If the J-spring guidewire will not advance after brief gentle manipulation, *forget it*! Abandon the attempt and choose another entry vessel. If a catheter is never inserted until a guidewire is passed to the bifurcation, the only penalty will be an arterial needle puncture and

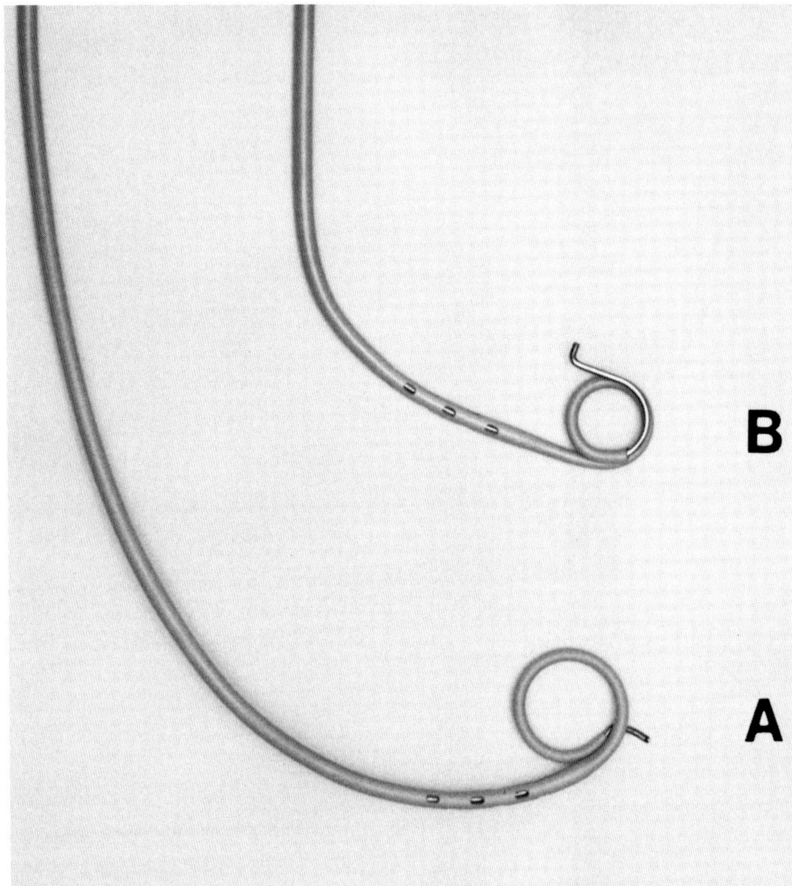

Figure 7I-11 Left atrial catheters with (*a*) gentle curve and (*b*) sharp angulation.

a short procedural delay. True, some tortuous iliac vessels can be traversed by further manipulation, but the only reward for your effort will be an uncontrollable catheter and high incidence of complications. *Most iliofemoral complications are the direct result of recognized or unrecognized arterial injury!*

Catheter Side Holes

Coronary catheters *should not* have side holes! Side holes in a coronary catheter predispose to increased clotting, obscure and do not prevent subintimal tip placement, and invalidate tip pressure monitoring (Fig. 7I-12).

A pigtail catheter should have no more than four side holes.* This number facilitates good contrast delivery; the volume is equal from all side ports. Volume flow from the side ports decreases as the number of side holes increases. A large amount exits from the first few side holes, and flow from those more distal is negligible (Fig. 7I-13). The extra ports serve no purpose and provide sites for accumulation of formed blood elements.

* The original design of the pigtail called for four side holes. Manufacturers thought that if four holes were good, twelve would be better. Tests clearly show that only the first few side holes are functional. I do not believe that catheters with twelve holes should be used for cardiac angiography.

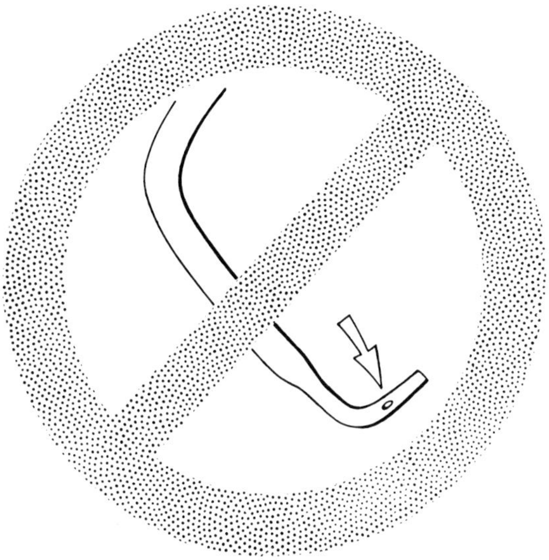

Figure 7I-12 Coronary catheters should not have side holes.

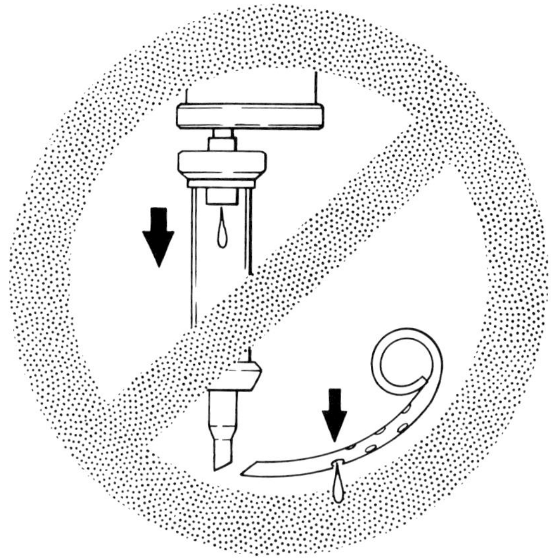

Figure 7I-13 A constant drip should not be used.

General Principles

Before a coronary catheter is advanced to the coronary orifice, it should be filled with contrast and should remain filled throughout catheterization and filming. Frequent contrast injection for filming, every 1 or 2 minutes, normally keeps the catheter tip free of blood and attendant clotting. If there is procedural delay for any reason, the catheter should be withdrawn from the orifice and frequently flushed with heparin-saline. Although the catheter tip may be safely left in place much longer than required for filming, it should not be left in the artery a moment longer than needed.

There should be a simple, effective closed system for delivery of fluids. The angiographer by appropriate manipulation of the manifold can selectively monitor pressure or inject fluids. Periodic flushing is required. A constant drip *should not* be used since the fluid exits the first available side hole (Fig. 7I-13). This complicates the system and increases the chance of thrombotic accident.

Careful, continuous catheter tip pressure monitoring is mandatory for procedural safety. *Constant, vigilant monitoring will ensure instantaneous recognition of damping.* Fluid injection should not be made if there is damping of catheter tip pressure. *If there is any damping or slowed washout on test contrast injection, the catheter should be withdrawn* and repositioned. Electrocardiographic changes lag hopelessly behind regional myocardial ischemia produced by catheter malposition. The angiographer who depends on ECG changes to reflect catheter obstruction has waited too long. The result will be only a record of an iatrogenic complication. Electrocardiography is used to monitor cardiac rhythm, or over time, evidence of myocardial injury. With currently available contrast agents, typical ECG changes occur after each injection. A physician or appropriately trained member of the technical staff should be assigned to monitor pressure and the electrocardiogram throughout the procedure.

Arrhythmias are considered by some a hazard of selective coronary arteriography. Atrial pacing and even a standby anesthesiologist have been advocated. In some areas a temporary pacing catheter is inserted routinely. None of these measures is indicated. Routine prophylactic placement of a temporary pacemaker for selective coronary arteriography cannot be justified.

Significant arrhythmias occur as a result of myocardial anoxia or contrast medium "toxicity." True contrast agent reactions or toxicity are rare. A vasovagal reaction is frequently interpreted as a contrast reaction and inappropriately treated. Ventricular fibrillation most often occurs directly or indirectly as the result of myocardial anoxia. Anoxia should be scrupulously avoided by careful catheter tip pressure monitoring and by refraining from making contrast injections into a vessel in which rapid washout is impeded by catheter position.

Selection of a suitable contrast agent will minimize arrhythmias. The opaque agent should be satisfactory from the standpoint of its effect on cardiac rhythm and contractility and its radiodensity; viscosity must not limit the speed of injection through a catheter. Sodium content is of particular concern. There is evidence that methylglucamine salts are less toxic than sodium salts. In my experience meglumine diatrizoate 76 percent has a wide margin of safety; I believe it is currently the medium of choice. More dilute concentrations, i.e., 60 percent, increase rather than decrease incidence of arrhythmias.

Patient peripheral pulses should be checked before and after the procedure and before hospital discharge.

The patient should be well-hydrated prior to coronary arteriography.

Single dose total body heparinization should be accomplished unless specifically contraindicated.

Catheter exchange should be done in the descending thoracic aorta. The guidewire should not be withdrawn below the aortic bifurcation during catheter exchange.

Careful compression of the femoral artery puncture site requires monitoring of peripheral pulses. Mechanical puncture site compression devices are mindless and should not be used (Fig. 7I-14). There is no substitute for the skillful, sensitive fingers of the angiographer in regulating the amount and method of pressure application. Pressure should be applied at least 10 minutes *by the clock*.

Meticulous postangiographic observation of the patient is important in detecting bleeding from the puncture site.

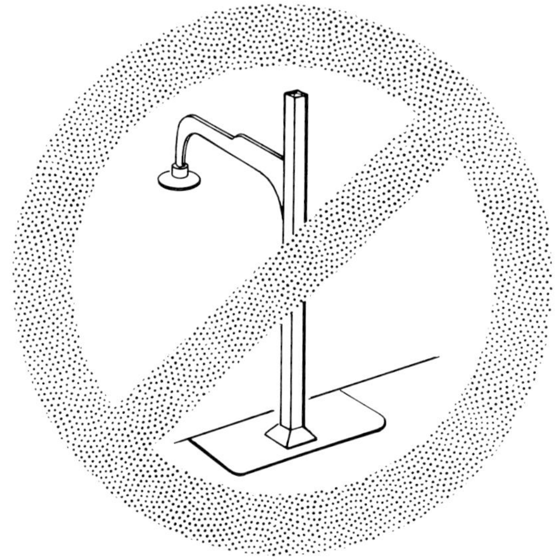

Figure 7I-14 Mechanical compression devices should not be used.

Catheter Reuse

Polyurethane coronary and pigtail catheters come from the manufacturer in sterile packages. The label indicates that the catheter is not to be reused. Extensive experience for many years in my laboratories has demonstrated that these catheters may be reused safely if properly cleaned and reprocessed. It is my opinion that multiple use is feasible in a *high-volume* laboratory that has the tools and commitment and a technical staff capable of remanufacturing the catheters with scrupulous care. Other experienced angiographers concur with this opinion.[8] If reuse is elected, the entire procedure is the responsibility of the laboratory director. The number of times a catheter may be reused will vary with catheter material and procedural handling; catheters should be replaced on the basis of appropriate inspection. After repeated reuse they lose resilience, memory, and torque control, jeopardizing the success of catheterization. It has been my practice not to reuse a catheter more than four times. If a laboratory director elects reuse, I recommend following the protocol outlined by a professional organization of cardiac angiographers.[9]

IMAGING

At least one member of the laboratory team should be thoroughly versed in the complexities of function and the limitations of the radiological equipment in an angiocardiographic laboratory as well as the applicable Bureau of Radiological Health standards.[10]

Patient Respiration

The role of patient respiration in cardiac imaging cannot be overemphasized. Appropriate synchronization of proper inspiration by the patient and of filming by the angiographer will improve cardiac imaging more than any other single factor, including hundreds of thousands of dollars worth of radiographic equipment.

When taking an x-ray of thoracic structures, a radiographic technologist waits to initiate exposure until the patient nears full inspiration. The average cardiac angiographer tells a patient to take a deep breath and hold it. When a patient responds to the command, ''Hold it!'' the diaphragm rises, obscuring a portion of the cardiac structures. This dooms the radiographic image to mediocrity. Always initiate a cardiac angiographic image series while the patient is inspiring.

Because the duration of the desired inspiration is 4 or 5 s, a patient must be instructed and rehearsed *prior to angiography*. An appropriately trained technical team member should be designated to do this teaching. The patient should be taught to take in a deep breath and to keep inspiring more fully without interruption; the patient should keep drawing in breath until the imaging run is completed. Every patient brought to the laboratory requires careful instruction and needs time to practice coordinating breathing with appropriate commands such as, ''Slowly take in a deep breath,'' ''Keep pulling!'' ''Keep pulling!'' ''Keep pulling!'' ''Breathe.'' (A patient can be instructed to breathe when the camera stops.) During the stress of the procedure, instructions are often forgotten and need to be reinforced.

The cardiac angiographer should practice in order to understand how to keep increasing inspiration without pause for 4 to 5 s. The mechanics of coordinating proper patient breathing with filming should also be practiced.

Image Recording

At the present time, cineradiography is the unquestioned primary imaging modality for angiocardiography. Cineangiography affords optimal dynamic studies. The most economically feasible high-quality laboratory handling a moderate volume is the single plane cineangiographic facility. Biplane imaging is useful only for ventriculography and has no role in coronary imaging except for research. Other methods of image recording are supplementary or complementary and are unneeded in the great majority of cardiac catheterization laboratories.[11]

The anatomy of the coronary tree should be clearly depicted in multiple planes without obscuring overlap (Fig. 7I-15). Contrast should completely replace blood for 3 to 4 s while high-resolution images are recorded in multiple projections (Fig. 7I-16). Diagnostic accuracy is improved with the use of angled views designed to profile all aspects of the coronary arterial system (Figure 7I-17). (See also Chapter 9.)

In most patients left ventricular function can be optimally assessed with two-plane ventriculography. Ventricular function imaged by alternately firing biplane equipment obviates two contrast injections and the consequent load in patients with marginal ventricular function. It is desirable but not necessary to have the capability for biplane ventriculography. The additional cost of fluoroscopic and cineangiographic capability in the second plane is considerable.

SUMMARY

The Judkins technique, true coronary intubation, takes advantage of the ease and speed of transfem-

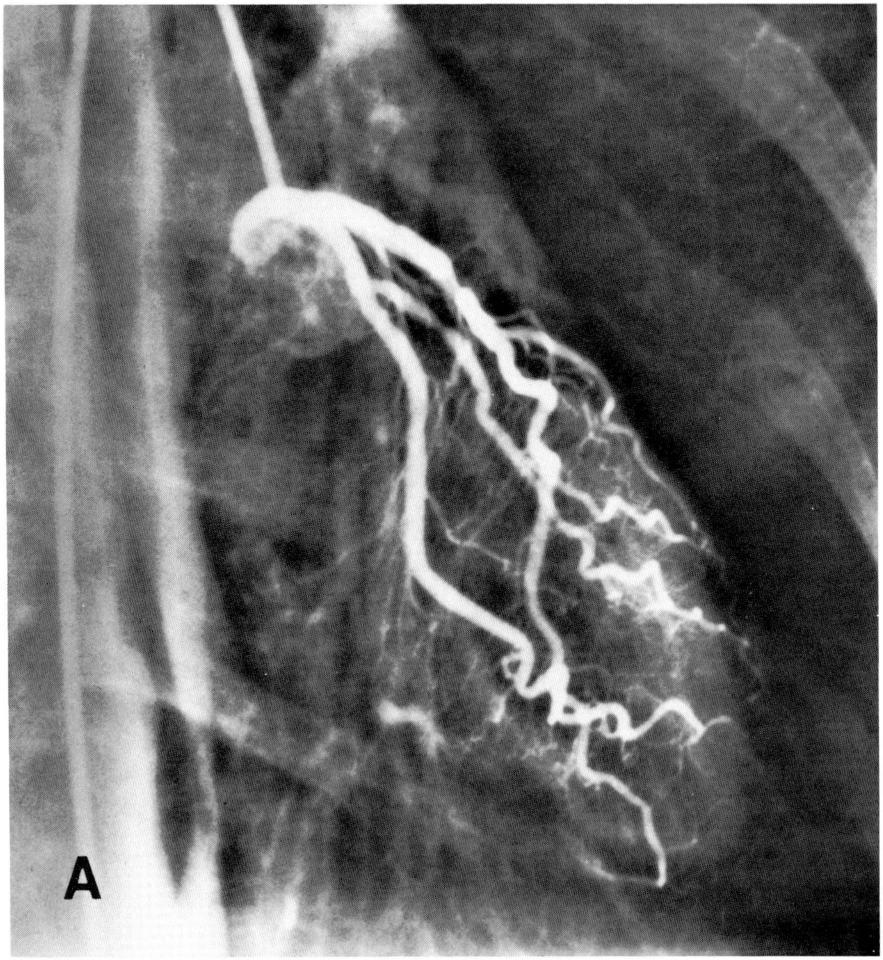

Figure 7I-15 Selective left coronary arteriogram. (*a*) Right anterior oblique projection. (*b*) Left anterior oblique projection. (*c*) Lateral projection.

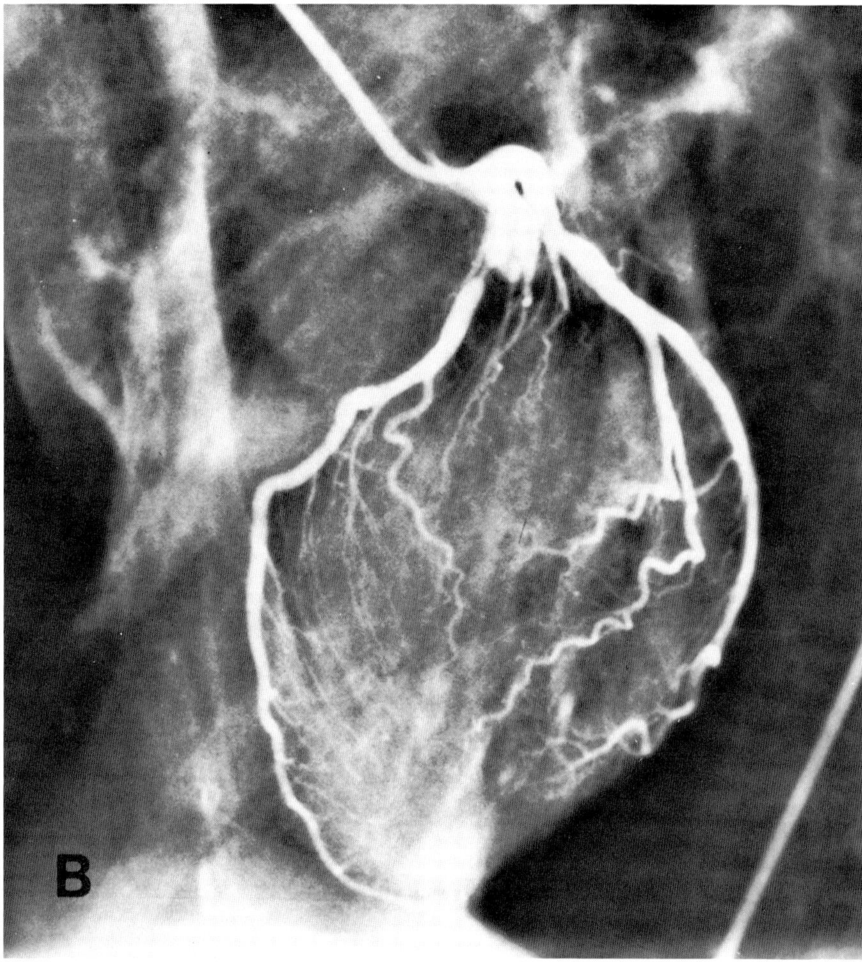

(Figure 7I-15, continued)

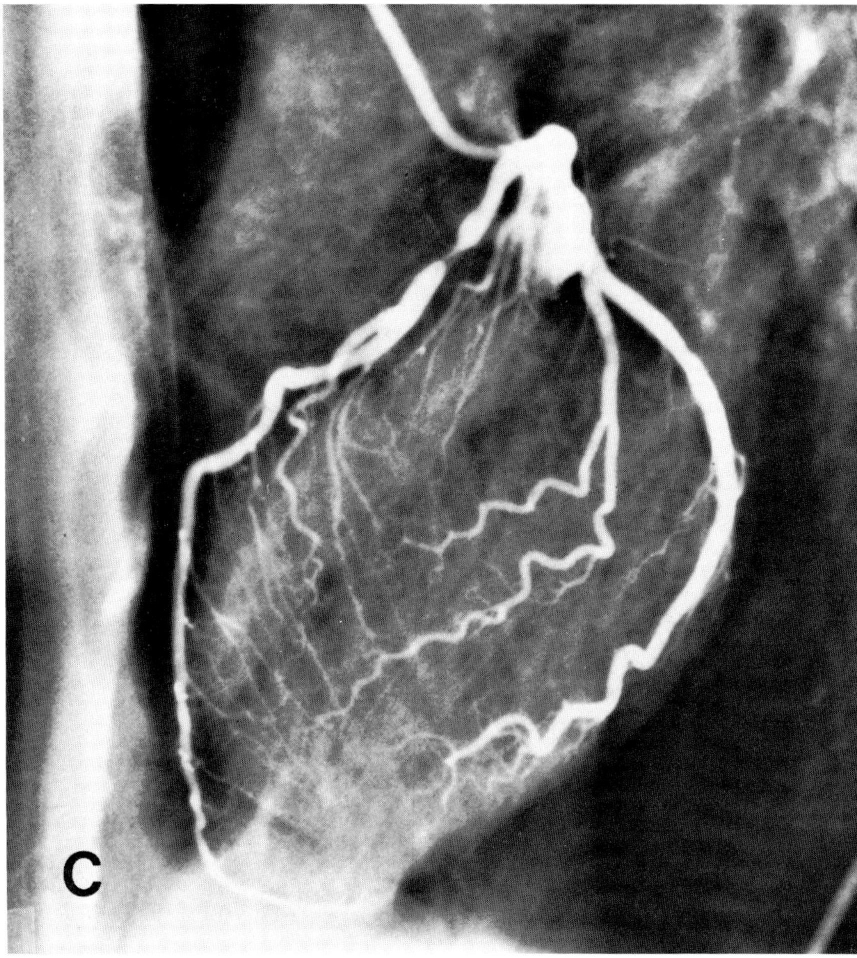

(Figure 7I-15, continued)

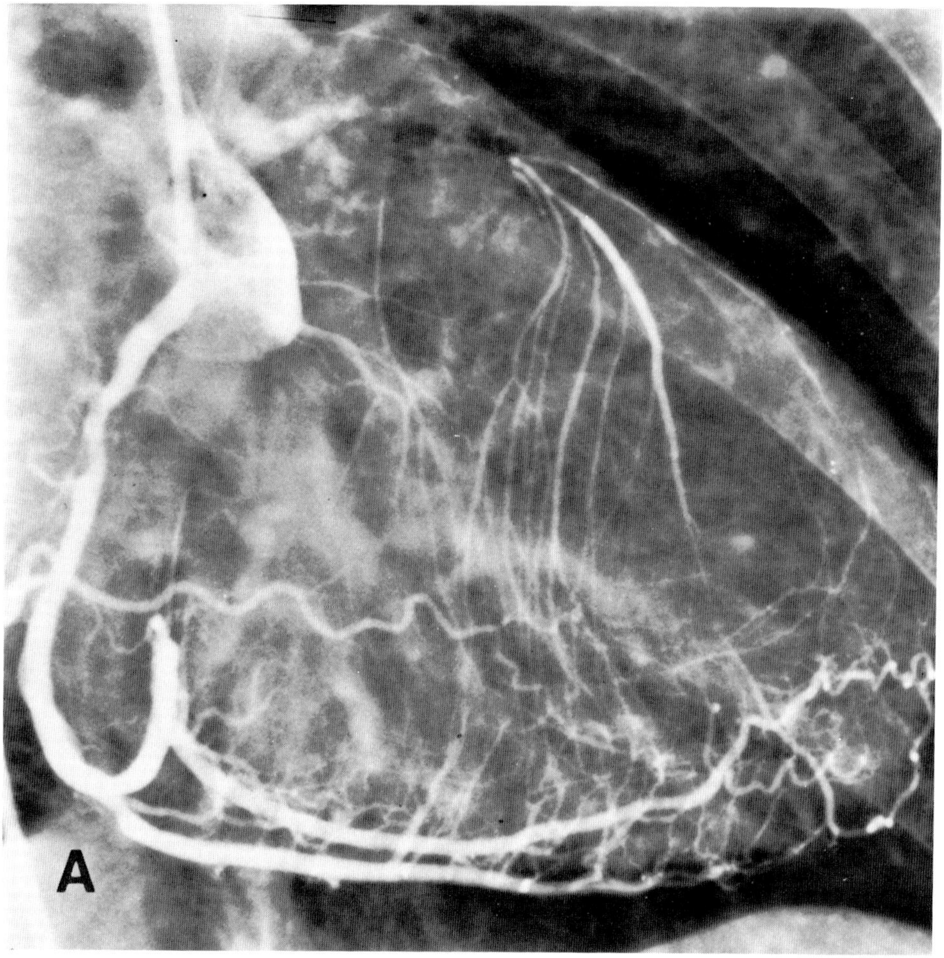

Figure 7I-16 Selective right coronary arteriogram. Patient 1. (*a*) Right anterior oblique projection. (*b*, *c*) Lateral projections. Note how different phases of the cardiac cycle may show the anatomy of a given segment more clearly. Patient 2. (*d*) Right anterior oblique projection. (*e*) Left anterior oblique projection.

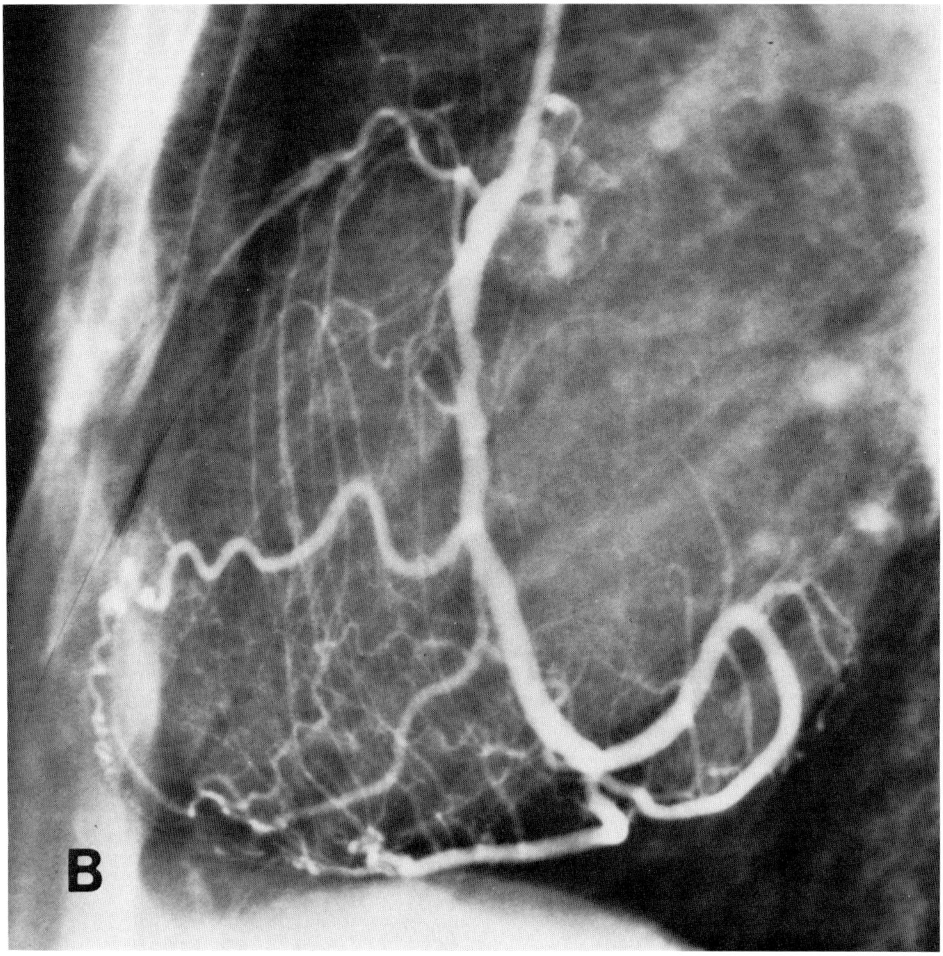

(Figure 7I-16, continued) Patient 1.

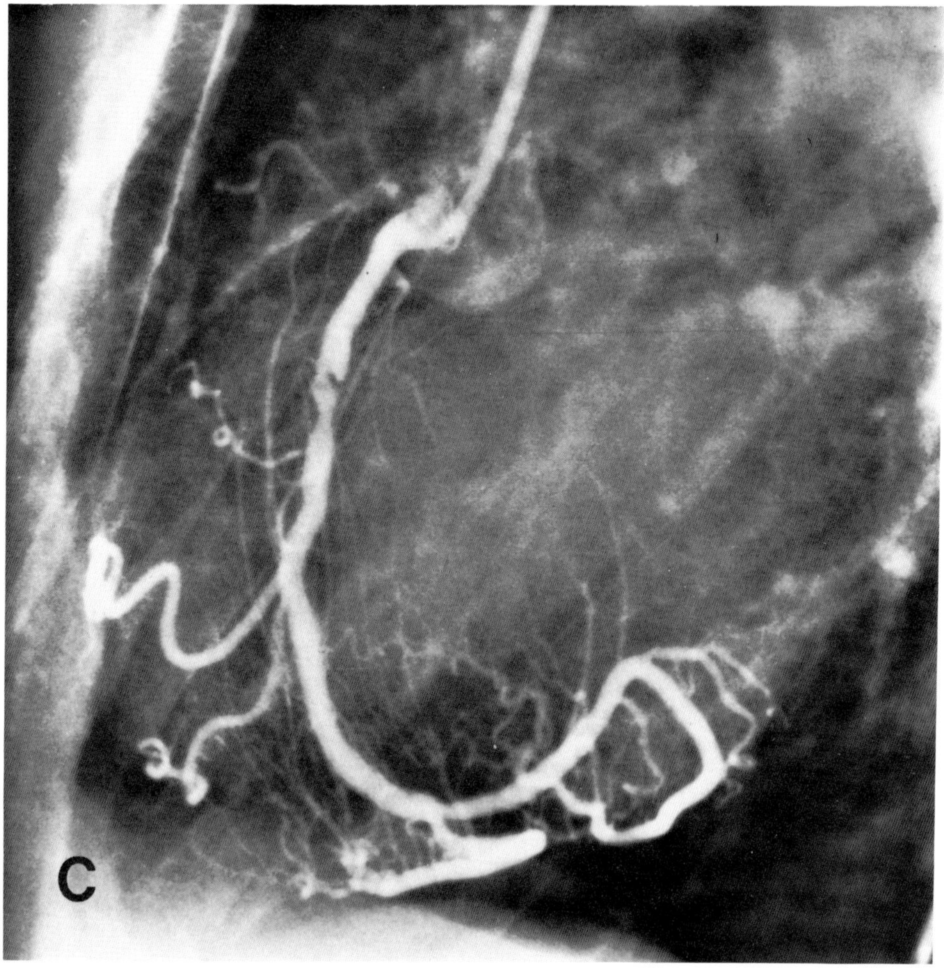

(Figure 7I-16, continued) Patient 1.

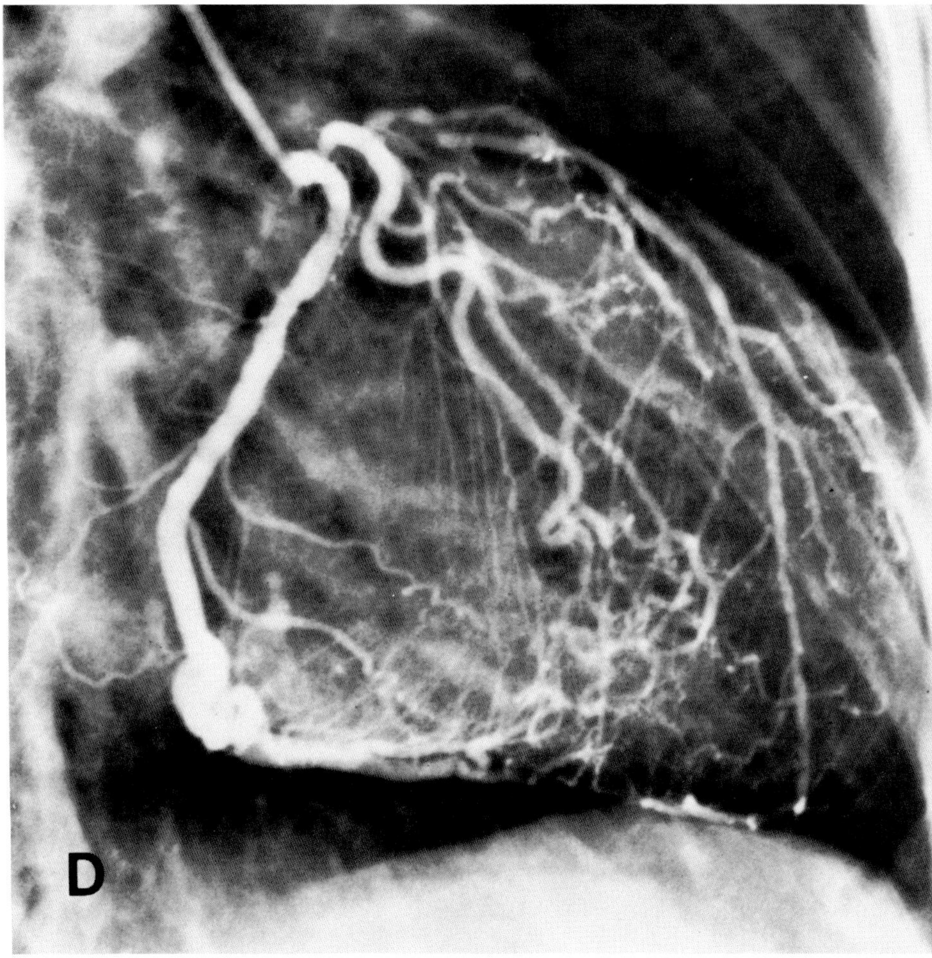

(Figure 7I-16, continued) Patient 2.

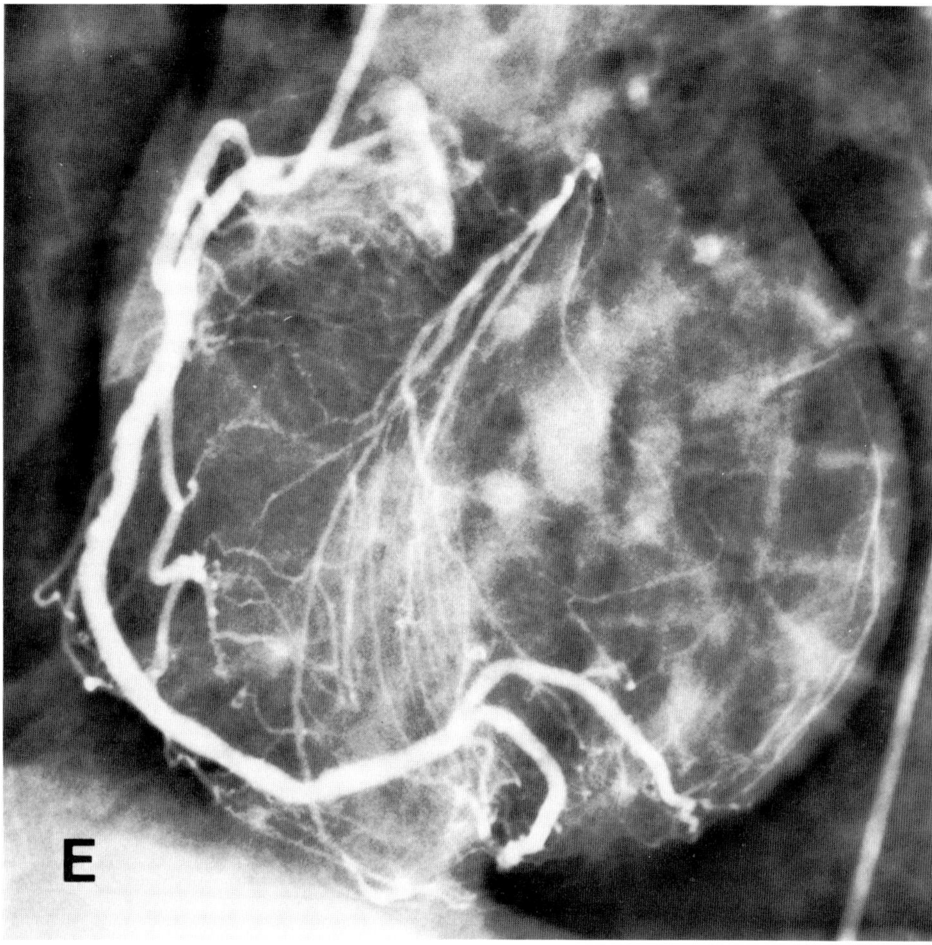

(Figure 7I-16, continued) Patient 2.

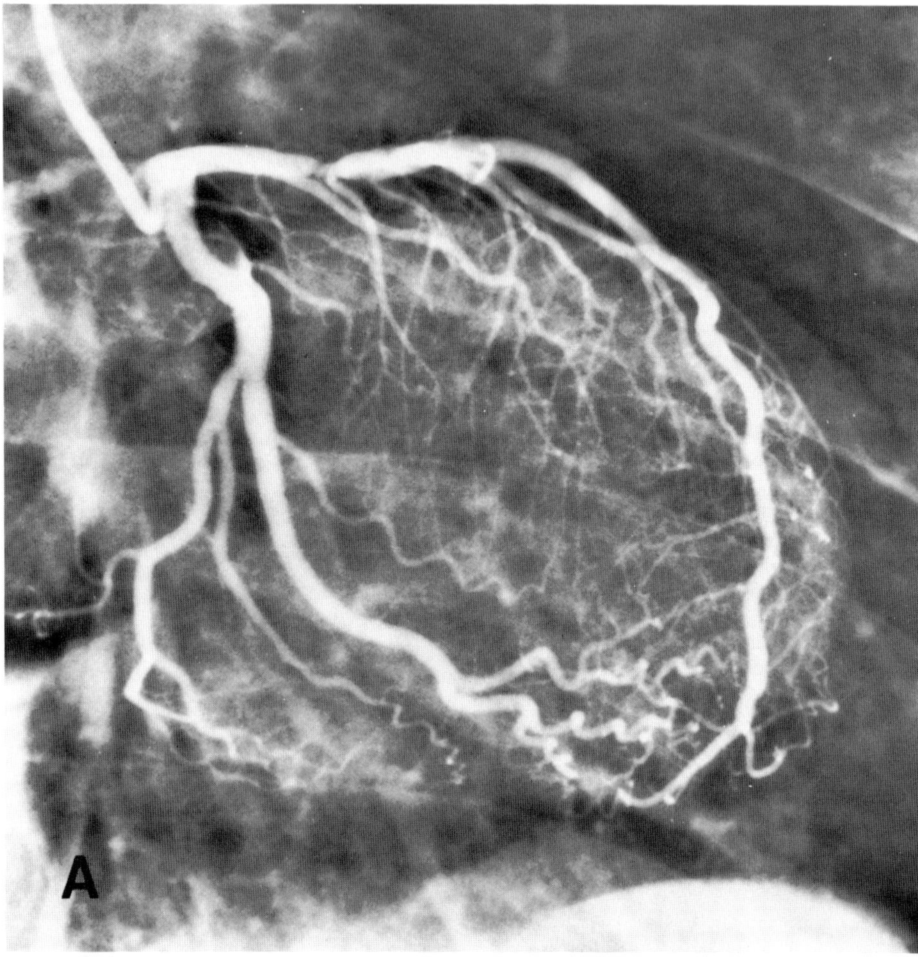

Figure 7I-17 Selective left coronary arteriogram. (*a*) Right anterior oblique projection. (*b*) Left anterior oblique projection with cranial angulation. (*c*) Lateral projection.

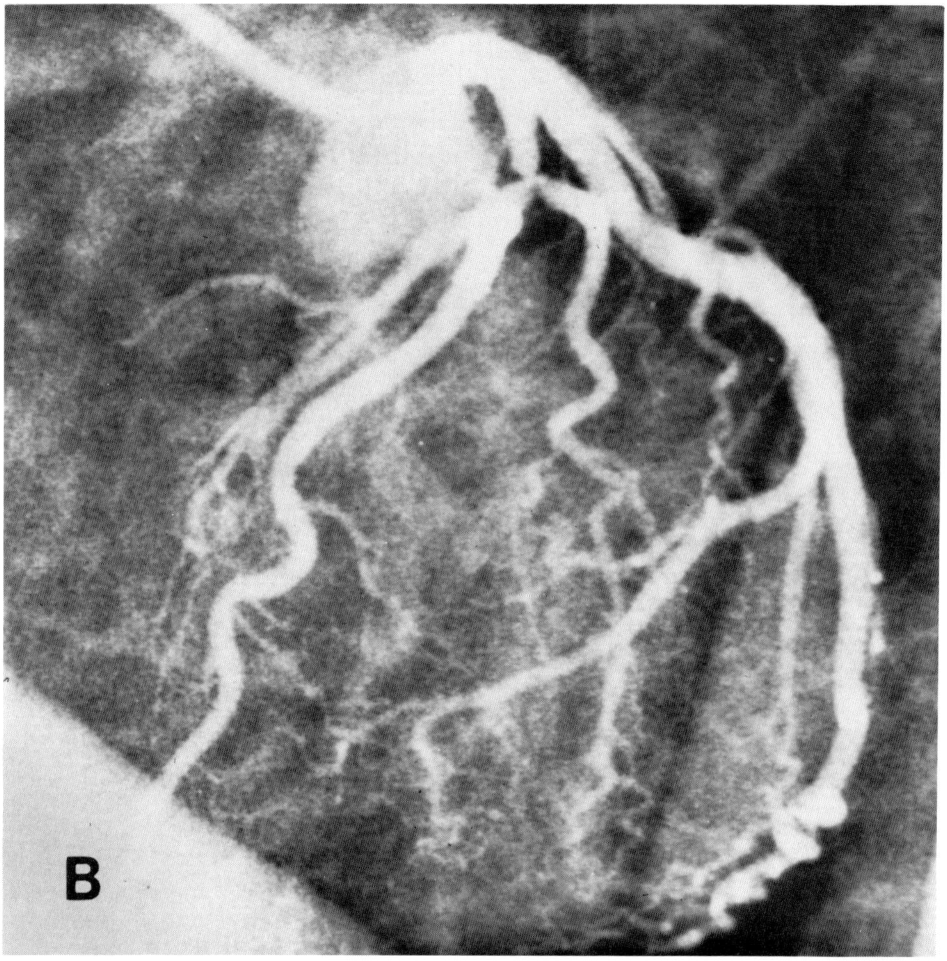

(Figure 7I-17, continued)

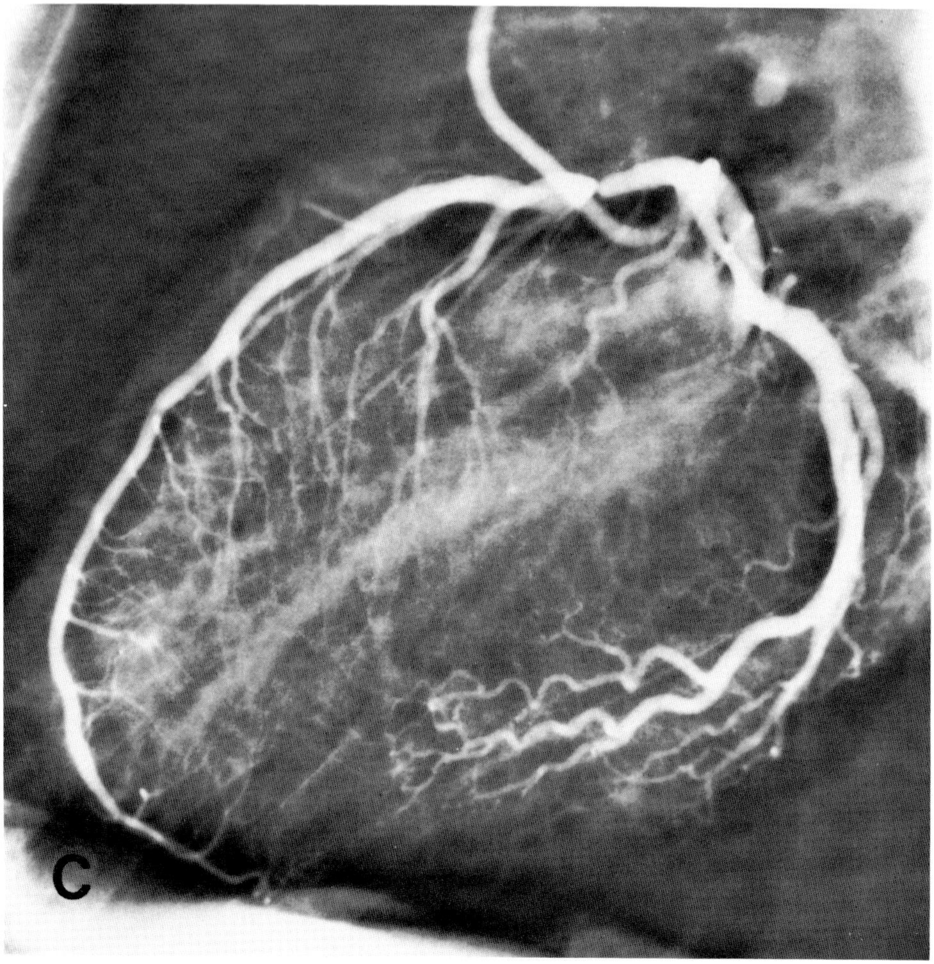

(Figure 7I-17, continued)

oral insertion and facilitates swift, consistent selective catheterization with minimal manipulation and an enviable freedom from hazard. However, the degree of experience of the operator directly relates to quality of images, technical skills, and the procedural complication rate.[6] Stability of catheter placement provides opportunity for selection of imaging projections and filming techniques that speaks for itself.

The femoral and brachial techniques for coronary arteriography are as different as day and night; the catheter mechanics are entirely different. Correct brachial technique maneuvers are inappropriate and may be hazardous to the patient when applied in the femoral approach. Both approaches are excellent, but the cardiac angiographer should elect to become proficient in *one*. *Select one technique, become proficient,* and *stay with that technique*. Patient safety, laboratory team skill and efficiency, as well as the skill and diagnostic acumen of an angiographer are enhanced by the "one technique" concept. Equipment selection, particularly the patient support, should reflect the coronary arteriographic technique projected for use in a facility. Important compromises with quality and safety are inevitable in a laboratory where multiple angiographers randomly schedule studies from both the brachial and femoral approaches. An angiographer who claims equal proficiency in femoral and brachial techniques is a *master of neither*.

ACKNOWLEDGMENT

I wish to give special thanks to Robert Knabenbauer, Loma Linda University medical illustrator, for his superb art work.

REFERENCES (Part I)

1 Judkins MP: Selective coronary arteriography: A percutaneous transfemoral technic. Radiology 89: 815–824, November 1967.

2 Judkins MP: Percutaneous transfemoral selective coronary arteriography. Radiol Clin North Am, 6:467–492, December 1968.

3 Dotter CT, Judkins MD, Frische LH: Safety guide-spring for percutaneous cardiovascular catheterization. Am J Roentgenol, 98:975–980, December 1966.

4 Judkins MP, Hinck VC, Dotter CT: Teflon-coated safety guides: An adjunct to the use of polyurethane catheters. Am J Roentgenol, 104:223–224, September 1968.

5 Principal investigators of CASS and their associates: National Heart, Lung, and Blood Institute Coronary Artery Surgery Study (CASS): Coronary Artery Surgery Study. Circulation, 63(suppl I): I-1–I-81, June 1981.

6 Judkins MP, Gander M: Prevention of complications of coronary arteriography. Circulation, 49 (4): 599–602, April 1974 (editorial).

7 Judkins MP, Kidd HJ, Frische LH, Dotter CT: Lumen-following safety-J guide for catheterization of tortuous vessels. Radiology, 88:1127–1130, June 1967.

8 The Society for Cardiac Angiography: "Reuse of catheters labeled 'for single use only,' " adopted by the Board of Trustees, November 14, 1982. The Society for Cardiac Angiography, 9500 Euclid Ave., Cleveland, OH 44106.

9 The Society for Cardiac Angiography: "Protocol for the reuse of cardiac catheters," adopted by the Board of Trustees, May 11, 1983. The Society for Cardiac Angiography, 9500 Euclid Ave., Cleveland, OH 44106.

10 Report of Inter-Society Commission for Heart Disease Resources: Optimal resources for examination of the heart and lungs: Cardiac catheterization and radiographic facilities. Examination of the Chest and Cardiovascular System Study Group, Friesinger GC (chairman), Adams DG, Bourassa MG, Carlsson E, Elliott LP, Gessner IH, Greenspan, RH, Grossman W, Judkins MP, Kennedy JW, Sheldon WC (members). Circulation, 68:891A–930A, October 1983.

11 Judkins MP: Angiographic equipment: The cardiac catheterization angiography laboratory, in Abrams HL (ed): *Coronary Arteriography: A Practical Approach*. Little, Brown, Boston, 1983.

Part II: Modification of Judkins Catheters and Similar Methods

William H. Willis, Jr., M.D.

Since 1967, when the Judkins technique of coronary arteriography was introduced,[1,2] there have been no major modifications of the technique other than those made by Dr. Judkins in subsequent years. These new aspects of the Judkins technique have been practiced frequently by Dr. Judkins and his colleagues in the Cardiac Catheterization Laboratories of Loma Linda University Medical Center. This section is intended to give a concise description of the cardiac and coronary catheters which are currently used to provide consistently high-quality cardiac angiography of some unusual and potentially difficult anatomic variations. The standard Judkins technique has been discussed in Part I of this chapter.

Judkins catheters are designed for selective entry into the coronary arteries. To obtain films of high diagnostic quality, an end-hole catheter must be selectively positioned in the vessel. If the catheter is only close to the artery, there may be incomplete filling of the vessel, usually resulting in poor visualization. Incomplete studies may be worse than none at all, especially if an incorrect decision is made from the information. With the development of coronary angioplasty[3] the principles of selective coronary catheterization have become even more important as their application will provide stable guiding catheter positions.

Standard Judkins coronary catheters are usually constructed with polyurethane. Polyurethane gradually loses its memory at the boiling temperature of water. An electric hot plate with a pot of water may be very valuable in reshaping catheters in the cardiac catheterization laboratory. The tip of a polyurethane catheter may be reshaped by immersion in boiling water and then immediate immersion into a cold scrub water basin as previously described. More proximal portions of the catheter may require up to 5 minutes of submersion in boiling water for reshaping. The polyurethane catheters are best reshaped with the use of stainless steel shaping wires (Fig. 7II-1). To shape Teflon-lined angioplasty guiding catheters, higher temperatures are required. This must be accomplished with a heat gun.

UNUSUAL OR ECTOPIC CORONARY ORIGINS

A short or absent left coronary mainstem is encountered in about 2 percent of angiographic studies.[4] This leads to selective catheterization of either the circumflex or left anterior descending arteries (Fig. 7II-2*a*). Oftentimes one vessel may fill selectively, but with a forceful injection the other vessel will fill indirectly by overflow. This may provide adequate opacification of both vessels, but often it will not. To selectively catheterize the other artery two maneuvers may be used. The first is to place the patient in a 60° left anterior oblique (LAO) projection and withdraw the catheter from the orifice of the left coronary. If the catheter is to go into the anterior descending, then rotate the tip slightly anterior or torque the catheter clockwise and reengage the coronary. If it is to go into the circumflex, rotate the tip slightly posterior or counterclockwise. If this maneuver isn't successful, note the size of the Judkins catheter and which artery was selectively catheterized. If a 4.2-cm secondary curve (no. 4) Judkins was used and it entered the left anterior descending, then select a 5.2-cm (no.

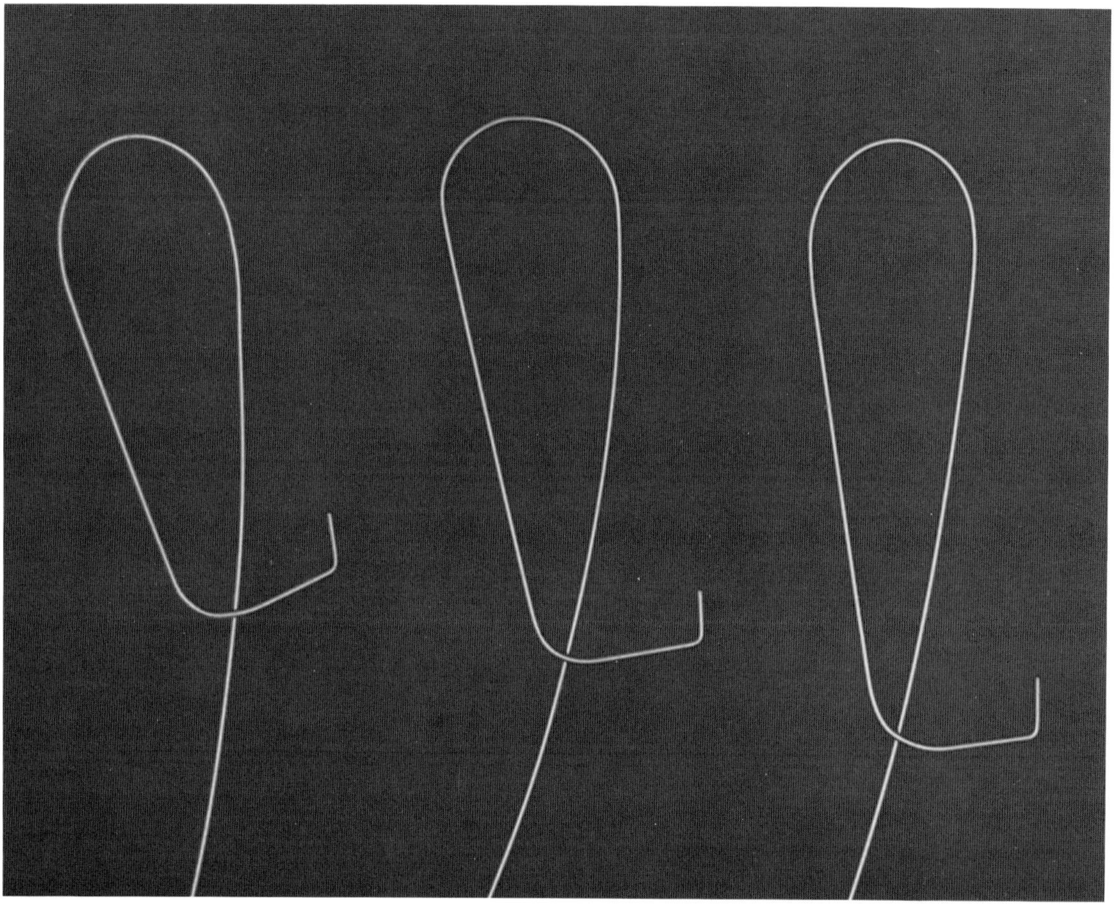

Figure 7II-1 Stainless steel shaping wires to reshape left coronary catheters to sizes nos. 6, 7, and 8.

5) Judkins, and it will almost always enter the circumflex (Fig. 7II-3). If the no. 4 Judkins enters the circumflex, select a 3.5-cm (no. 3.5) left Judkins for the left anterior descending. This same method may be used for guiding catheter selections for coronary angioplasty when selectively guiding balloons into the circumflex or left anterior descending coronary arteries.

Another difficult, although not rare, left coronary takeoff is the superiorly oriented left coronary artery origin.[5] The origin may be located high in the left coronary sinus and oftentimes at or near the junction of the tubular portion of the aorta (Fig. 7II-4*a*). This situation requires slightly less distance across the aorta, that is, a shorter secondary length and a more superiorly angled distal tip. This may be achieved by selecting either a smaller size 3.5-cm (no. 3.5 Judkins) catheter for a normal aortic root or a no. 4 Judkins if the root is larger (Fig. 7II-4*b* and 7II-5). When a smaller size Judkins is selected, there is a tendency for the catheter to curl up in the root. This may be overcome by carefully passing the catheter over a guidewire down into the coronary sinus region, being careful not to enter the artery. Careful attention must be directed to keeping guidewire times short and to proper flushing of the catheter prior to entering the coronary ostia. Another method of achieving the same re-

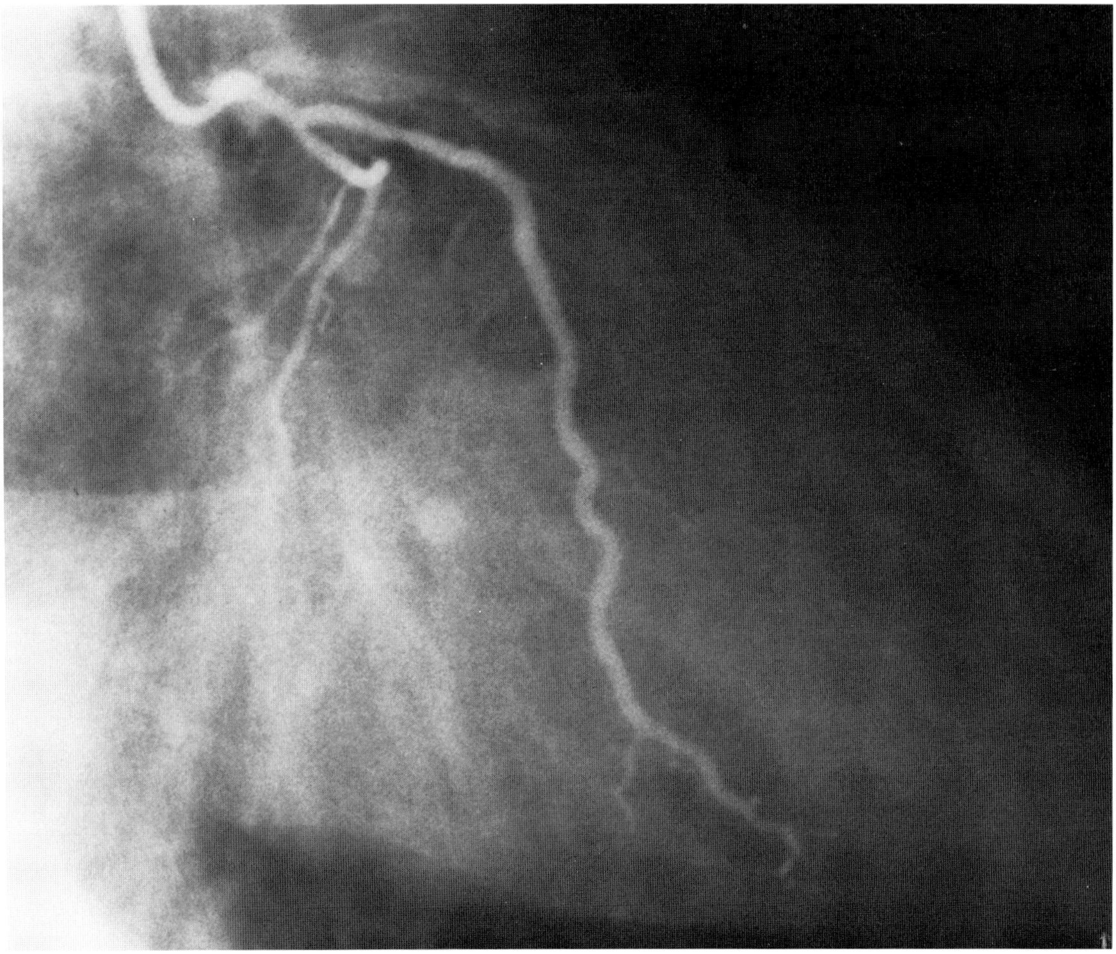

Figure 7II-2 The circumflex is selectively catheterized in the RAO position with a no. 5 Judkins catheter in a patient with separate anterior descending and circumflex origins.

sults would be to reshape the catheter in boiling water. The newly shaped catheter would have less secondary length across the aorta and a longer tip pointing superiorly. When there is additionally an anterior or posterior ectopic position, an A2 multipurpose catheter might be used to reach superiorly.[6]

The dilated or aneurysmal aortic root is initially approached by using a no. 5 or 6 Judkins catheter. If these are not of sufficient reach to span the aorta, then the catheter may be modified by lengthening the secondary curve, as determined by the aortic width using shaping wires with progressively longer secondary curve lengths (Fig. 7II-1). In unusual cases such as an ascending aortic aneurysm with aortic insufficiency we have reshaped catheters with up to 9-cm secondary curves for the left coronary. The right coronary artery catheterization is much less affected, and usually a standard size no. 4 or 5 right coronary catheter will be adequate in the presence of an aneurysmal aorta.

The right coronary artery origin, however, has its own special set of problems. Perhaps the most common is a superiorly directed takeoff, or shep-

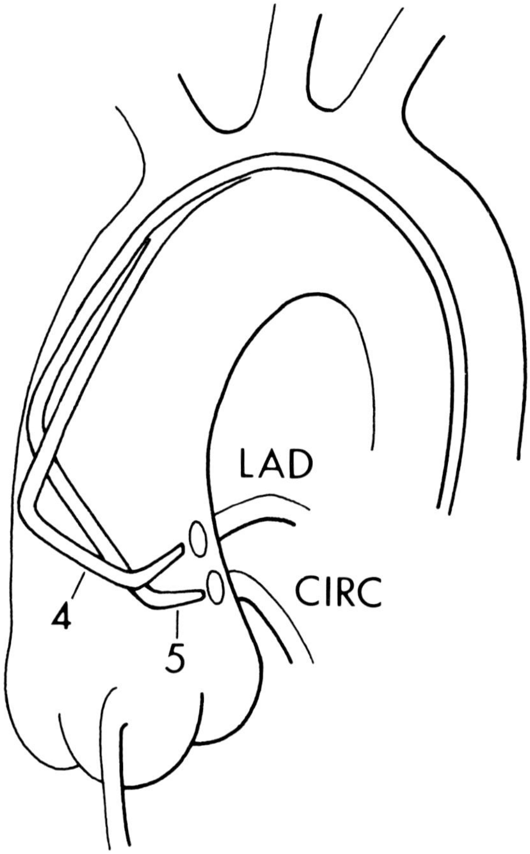

Figure 7II-3 Absent left main with separate origins of left anterior descending (LAD) and circumflex (Circ) arteries. The no. 4 left catheterizes the LAD and the no. 5 catheterizes the circumflex.

herd's crook, right coronary artery. If the artery arises from the usual location in the right coronary cusp it is visualized well with the standard no. 4 right catheter. However, if it is more superiorly located in the cusp on the tubular aorta, the right coronary tip will need to point upward. This may be accomplished by reshaping the right coronary catheter tip superiorly or by selecting a left coronary bypass catheter (Fig. 7II-6). This catheter was developed to catheterize superiorly oriented left bypass grafts from the upper ascending aorta. Its upward tip allows for selective catheterization of the superior right coronary as well. We have found this configuration also to provide stable support for angioplasty of the shepherd's crook right coronary artery.

The right coronary artery occasionally arises not only superiorly from the tubular aorta, but anteriorly.[7] This is the most difficult of all right coronary origins to selectively catheterize. It can usually be recognized by placing the patient in the left anterior oblique position or right anterior oblique projections and making aortic root injections near the coronary origin. After the situation is recognized, a three-dimensional catheter with an anterior bend is shaped (Fig. 7II-7). This usually permits selective catheterization of the coronary artery. This uncommon right coronary origin is likely to result in an incomplete study unless recognized.

When the right coronary artery heads inferiorly, it can usually be visualized well with a 4-cm right catheter. If there is difficulty, the catheter tip may be straightened, but we frequently use a right venous bypass catheter with less of an angle at the tip (Fig. 7II-8).

The pulmonary conus branch in 50 percent of patients arises separately from the right coronary artery.[4] Occasionally this branch rather than the main right is entered repeatedly. Usually, by withdrawal and readvancement with additional clockwise rotation, this can be avoided. However, if conus catheterization repeatedly occurs, a right venous bypass catheter may be selected.

Ectopic origins of the circumflex from the right coronary artery or right coronary sinus occur in about 0.5 percent of patients studied.[8,9] The right venous bypass graft catheter may be used also for visualizing these ectopic origins of the circumflex from the right coronary artery. Also, an A2 multipurpose catheter may give good visualization of the ectopic circumflex.

Though we currently feel that Judkins catheters most consistently give the best opacification of the coronary arteries, there are a couple of special situations in which they may not be the catheters of choice. When there is a right coronary ostial stenosis or when there is a proximal right coronary catheter–induced spasm, the Judkins catheters may

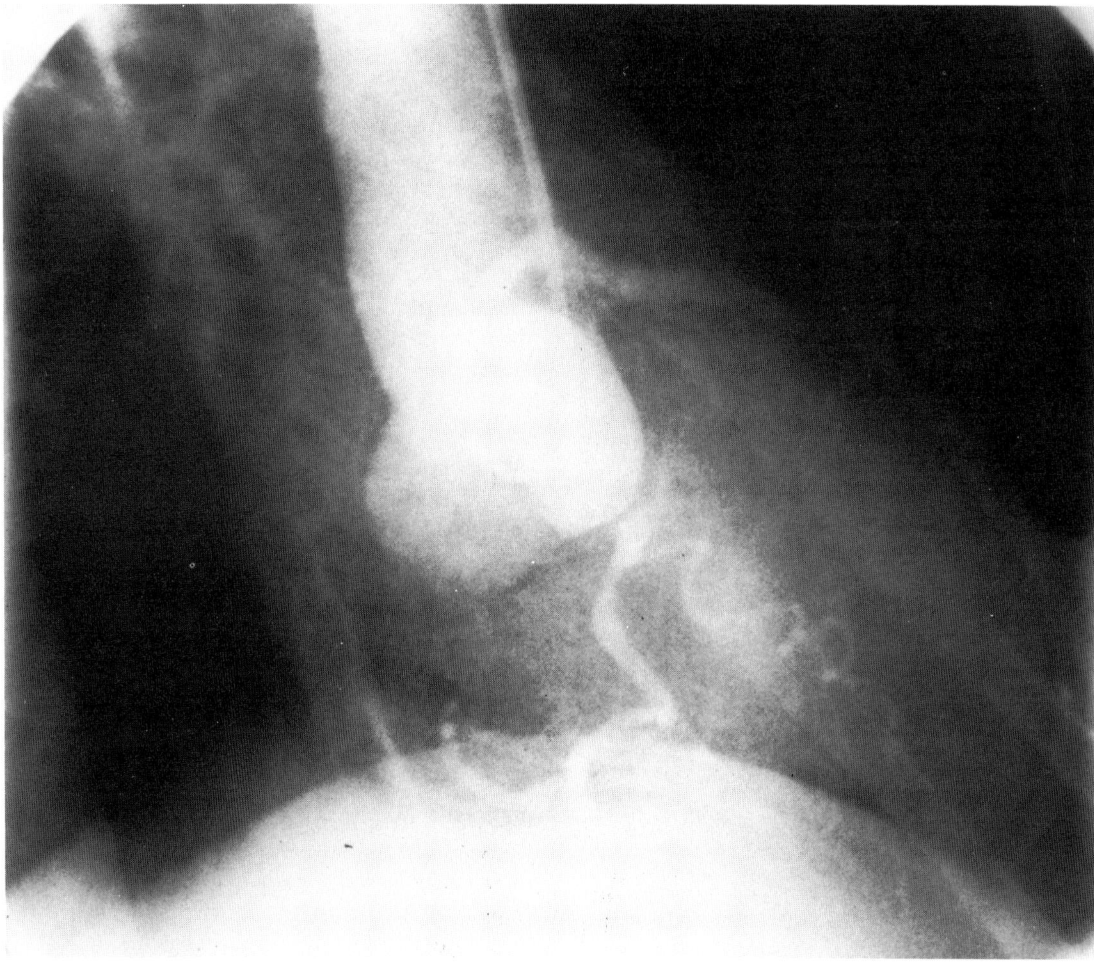

A

Figure 7II-4 (*a*) An aortic root injection in the RAO projection shows the superior origin of the left coronary artery. (*b*) A left size no. 3.5 Judkins catheter and shaping wire are shown.

be less than ideal. This is because they are meant to enter the ostium selectively rather than be positioned next to it for a cusp injection of the right coronary ostium. If an adequate cusp injection is not obtained with the right Judkins, then a multipurpose catheter often provides good cusp opacification due to its side holes. Catheter-induced spasm of the left coronary artery or proximal left anterior descending is less common. It can, however, be evoked by the left catheter being too far into the left coronary artery. Intracoronary nitroglycerin and a left cusp injection should be given to avoid this potential dilemma.

CORONARY BYPASS GRAFT CATHETERS

Though coronary artery bypass grafts are very frequently encountered by the coronary angiographer, it is surprising how few are aware of the full spectrum of graft catheters which are available for use with the Judkins technique. The best known and most frequently used is the right venous bypass

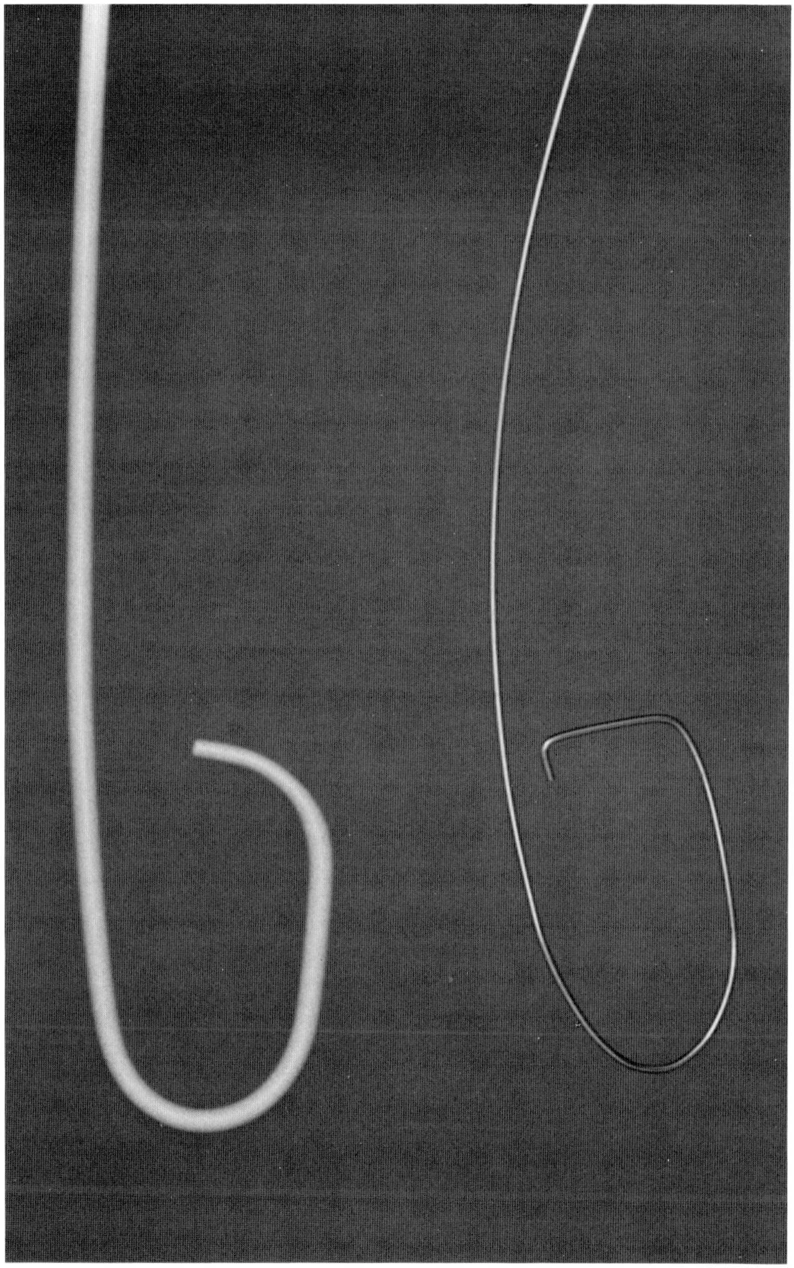

B

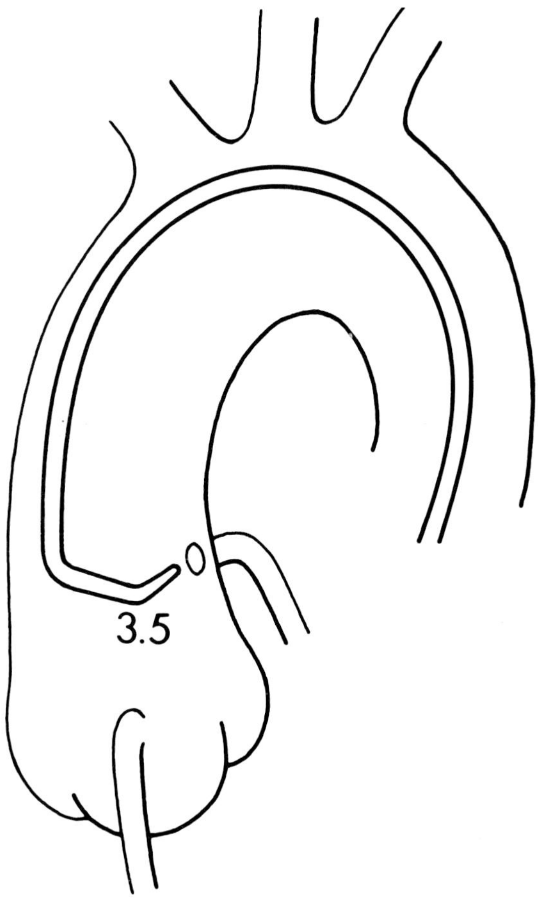

Figure 7II-5 A size no. 3.5 Judkins catheter is shown entering a left coronary with a superior origin.

catheter, commonly referred to as the RVB (Fig. 7II-8). This catheter is used in our laboratory as one of the routine catheter choices for any patient who is undergoing diagnostic angiography after bypass surgery. After the native left system is visualized, the RVB catheter is used to inject the native right coronary artery and the right coronary bypass graft when one is present. To catheterize a right coronary graft the patient is usually placed in a 60° LAO projection. The catheter is positioned just above the site of the native coronary origin and just below the anticipated origin of the graft. The catheter is slowly withdrawn and rotated counterclockwise to bring it to the outer margin of the aorta (Fig. 7II-9). If it rises above the graft and doesn't enter it, a clockwise motion with advancement is recommended. This catheter rarely fails to catheterize a right coronary graft. The RVB catheter also catheterizes any left coronary grafts which have a fairly horizontal takeoff from the aorta.

To catheterize left coronary vein grafts, the patient is initially positioned in a 20° to 30° RAO position, and the catheter is advanced from the upper portion of the aorta inferiorly as it is rotated clockwise. Should the RVB catheter fail to engage any of the left coronary saphenous vein grafts, the catheter should be exchanged for a left venous bypass graft catheter (LVB) (Fig. 7II-6). This catheter, as was previously mentioned, has a superior orientation to its tip and is especially good for the left circumflex and anterior descending coronary grafts which course initially upward. The patient is placed in a 20° to 30° RAO projection, and the catheter is advanced with a clockwise motion to cause its tip to move along the inner portion of the aorta (Figs. 7II-10 and 7II-11). We have noticed that patients who have been bypassed in our own institution, where the surgeons attach the left grafts so that they arise from the left anterior aorta, are most easily catheterized in the RAO projection. However, some patients who have received their operations elsewhere are best positioned in the 60° LAO projection for localization of the left vein grafts. Because of these findings each angiographer should become familiar with the usual locations of the different vein grafts implanted by a particular group of surgeons.

Internal mammary artery grafts are often not as easily catheterized from the groin. The internal mammary graft catheter is most often introduced into the left subclavian by the use of a soft guidewire. The patient is in an anteroposterior position, and the left subclavian is entered with a guidewire extending 2 to 3 cm beyond the catheter. The catheter and guidewire are passed distal to the internal mammary origin (Figs. 7II-12 and 7II-13). Reno-

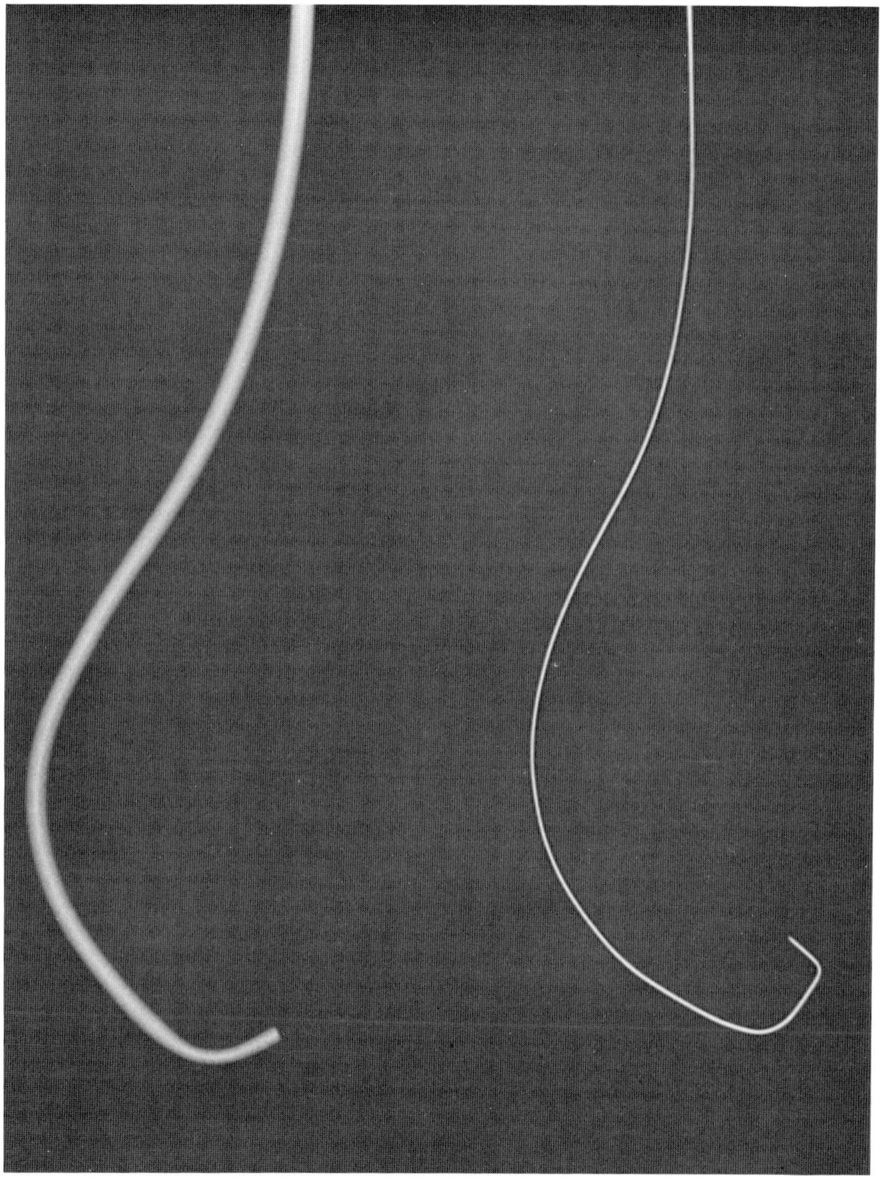

Figure 7II-6 A left venous bypass catheter and shaping wire are shown.

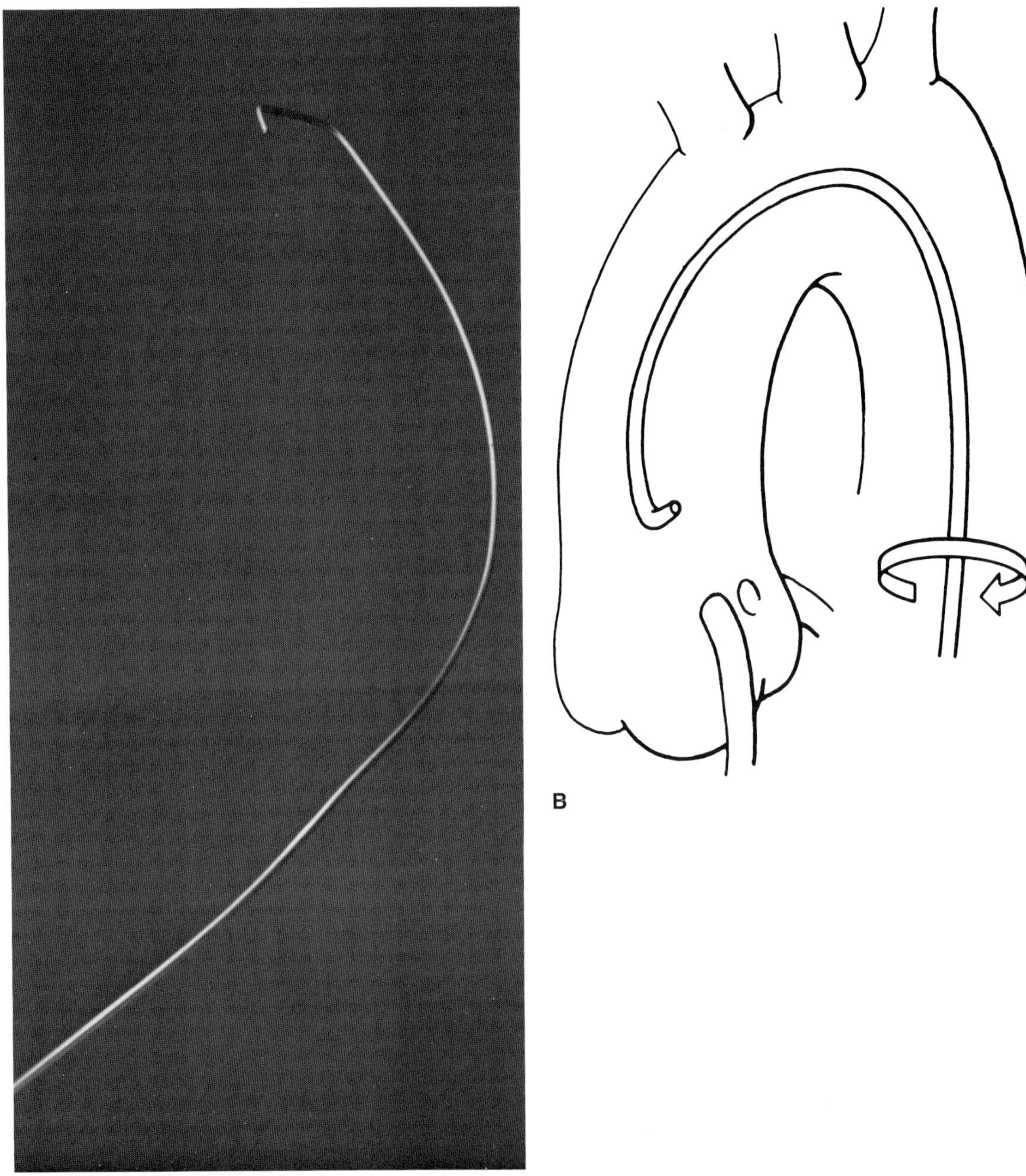

Figure 7II-7 (*a*) Right coronary shaping wire with an anterior bend. (*b*) Superior and anterior origin of right coronary artery with reshaped right catheter in a LAO projection. (*c*) Angiogram of vein graft injection using the anterior bend catheter.

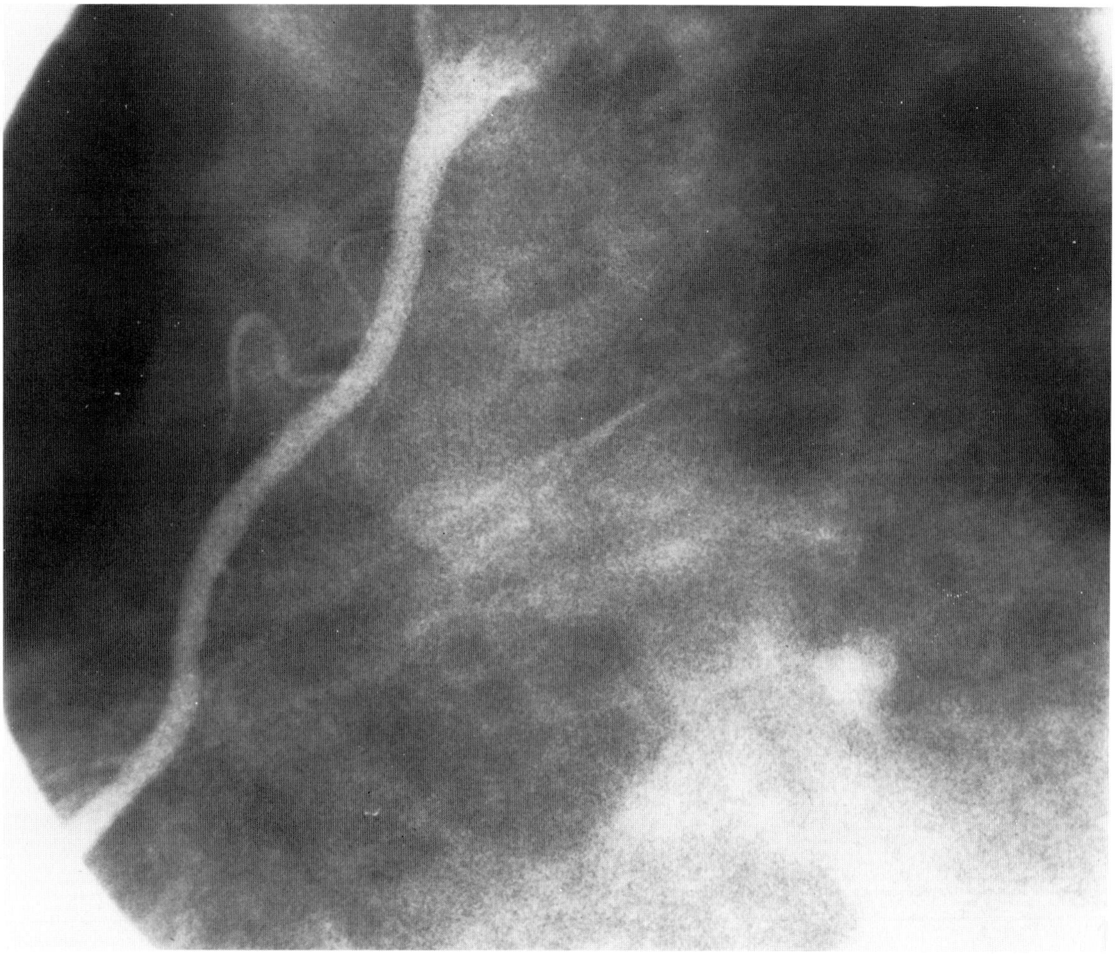

C

grafin 76 is diluted by 50 percent to reduce any noxious side effects should it incidentally be injected into the cerebral circulation. This may also help reduce the burning sensation with the internal mammary injection. Selective small tests are made in the left subclavian as the catheter is slowly withdrawn. If the internal mammary cannot be selectively catheterized, then a soft guidewire may be again passed into the left subclavian and into the internal mammary so the catheter can be passed into the internal mammary origin. A light test injection with good opacification and nondamped pressures should be made before a full injection is performed.

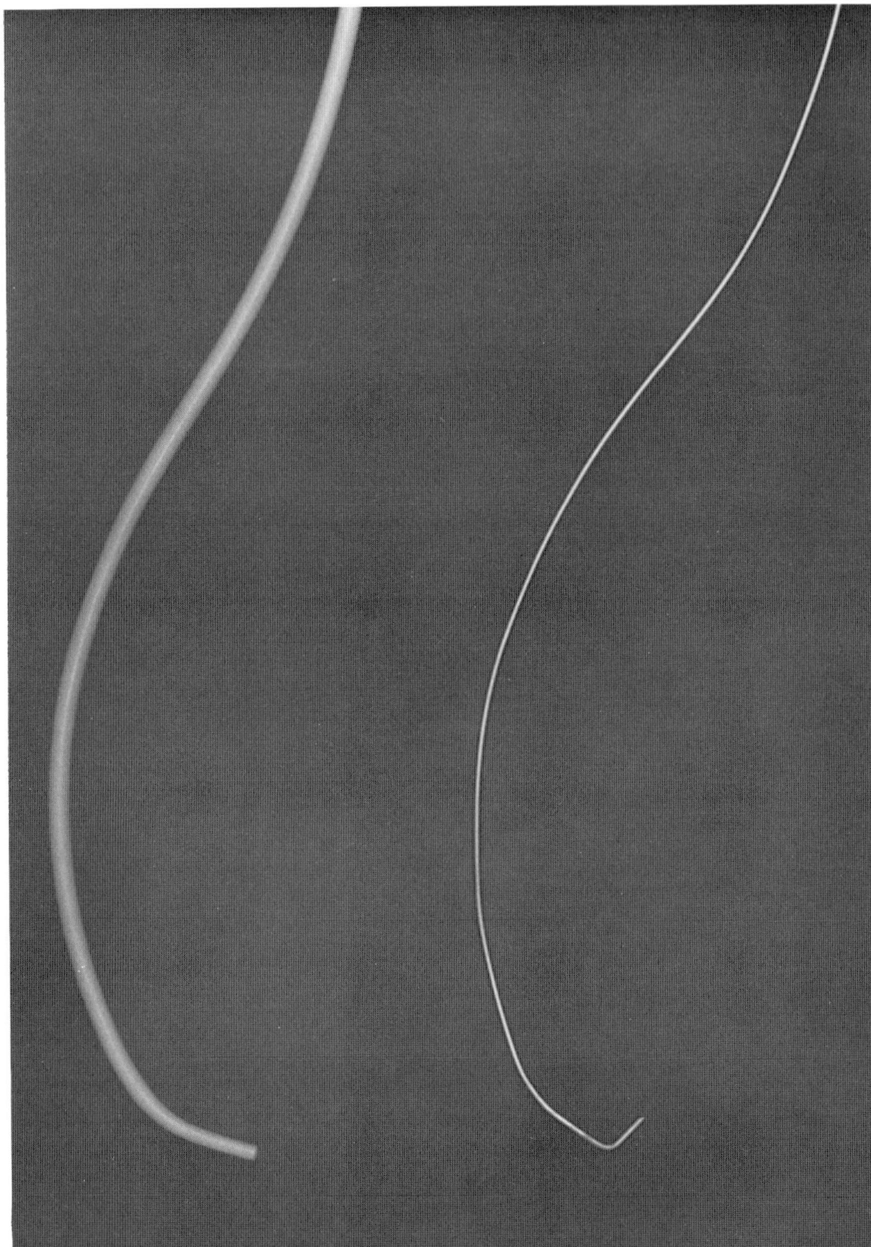

Figure 7II-8 Right venous bypass graft catheter with shaping wire.

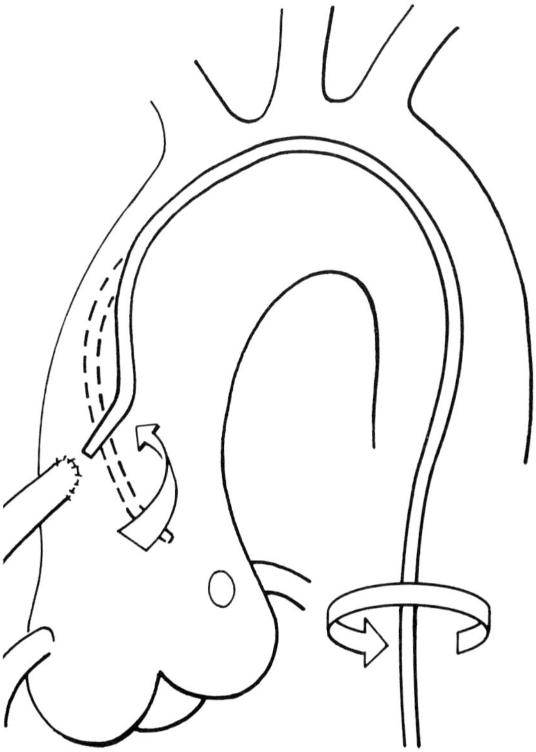

Figure 7II-9 The right venous bypass catheter is shown in the LAO projection entering a right saphenous vein graft. The catheter is rotated counterclockwise and slowly withdrawn.

Figure 7II-10 The left venous bypass graft catheter is rotated clockwise and advanced into the left coronary vein graft in the RAO projection.

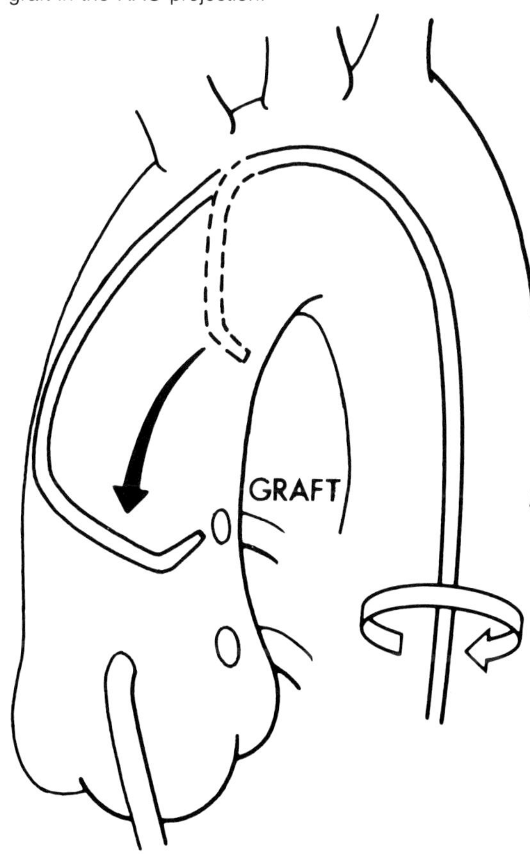

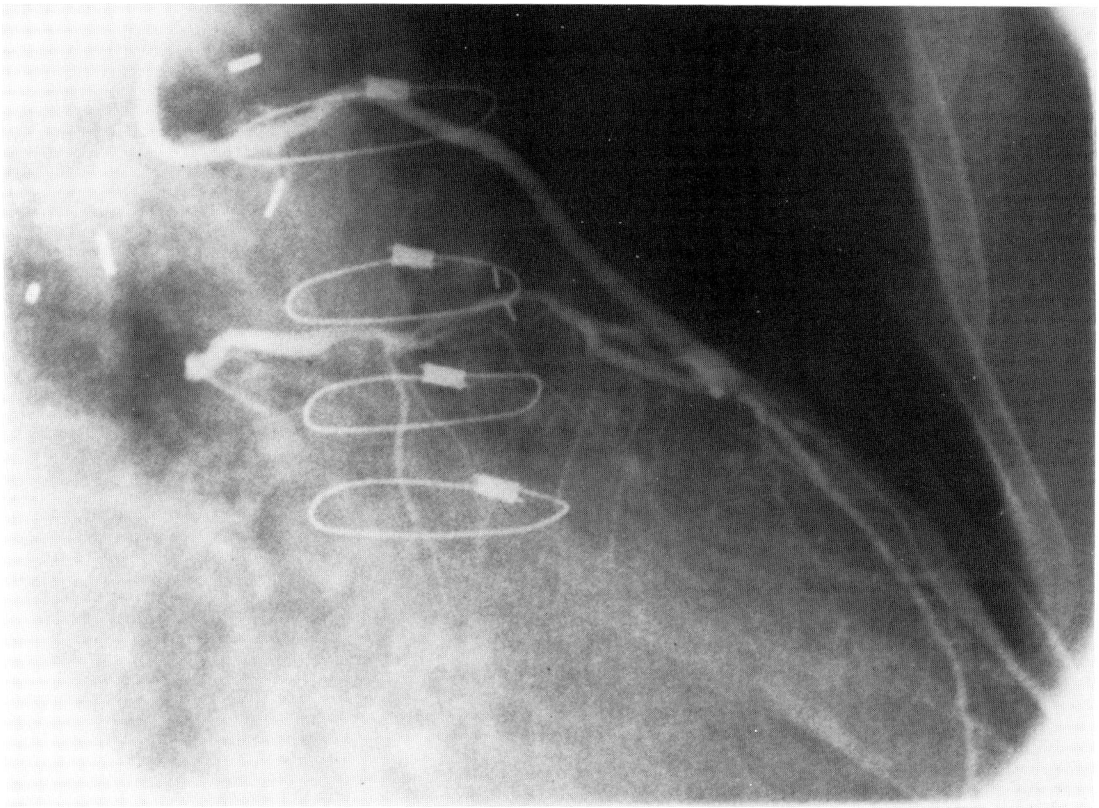

Figure 7II-11 A left venous bypass graft catheter is positioned in a superiorly oriented left anterior descending vein graft.

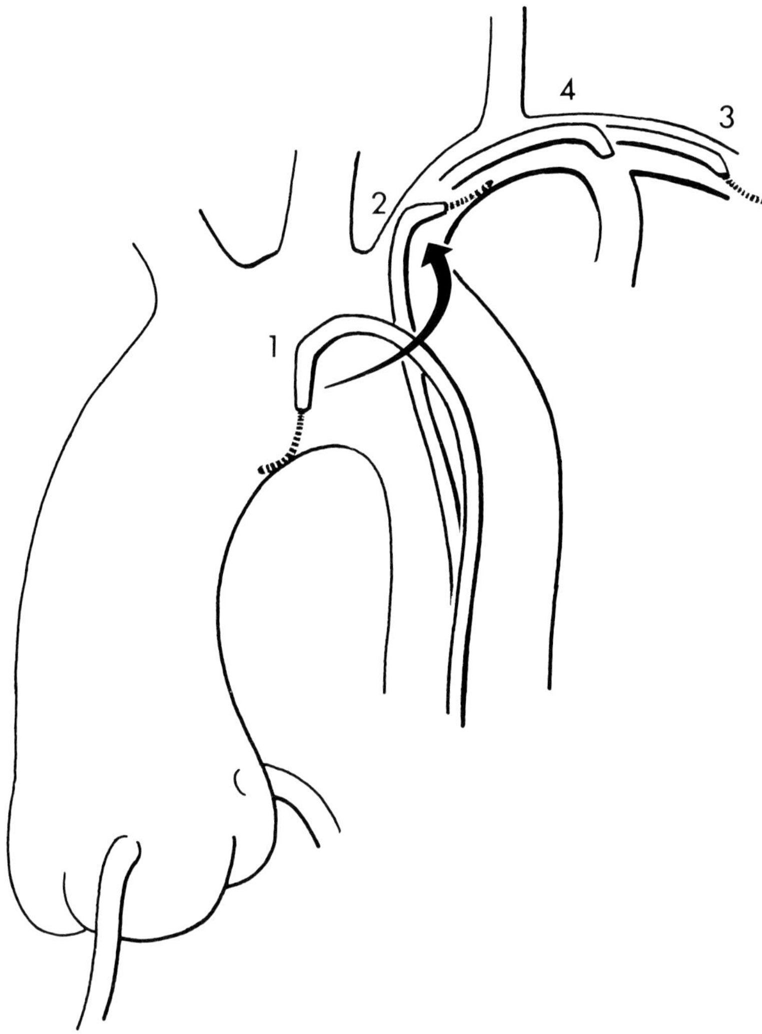

Figure 7II-12 A guidewire is inserted in the internal mammary graft catheter until it is passed into the left subclavian. It is removed and withdrawn into the internal mammary artery.

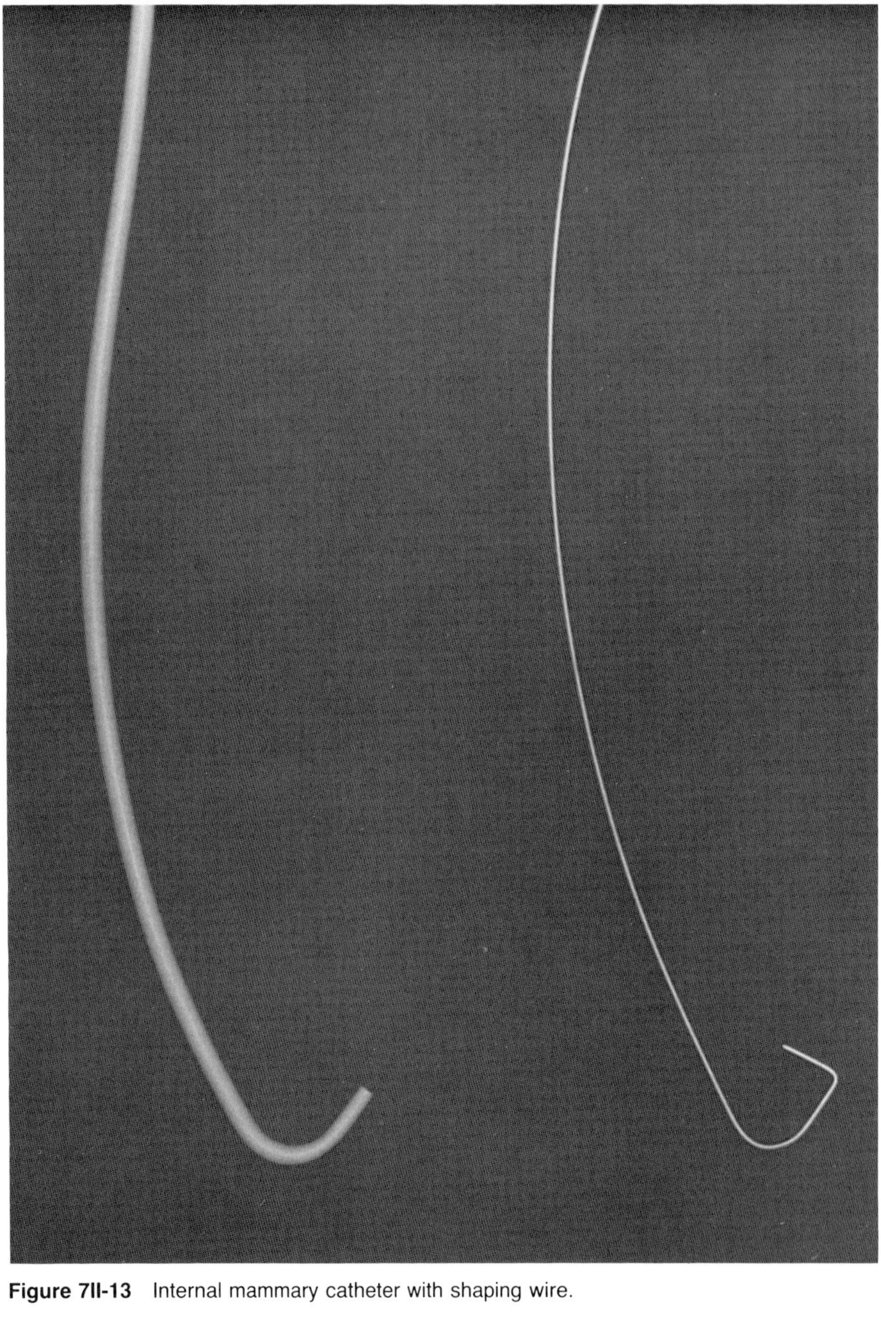

Figure 7II-13 Internal mammary catheter with shaping wire.

PIGTAIL CATHETER MODIFICATIONS

In most patients without aortic stenosis the pigtail catheter easily enters the left ventricle and allows for nontraumatic left ventricular injections. The most commonly used pigtail catheters come in sizes no. 7 or 8 French and have 12 side holes just before the curled tip. However, in patients with a horizontal and ectatic proximal aorta, especially if there is aortic stenosis, it becomes more difficult to cross the aortic valve. To help compensate for this the loop or curl on the pigtail is tightened into what is called an aortic stenosis pigtail or tight loop pigtail (Fig. 7II-14). This may give a better angle to the guidewire in the aortic root and facilitates crossing these abnormal aortic valves. Some companies have not only tightened the loop but have angled the distal catheter for a few centimeters before the loop. Also, by placing a 45° angle on the last 2 to 3 cm of the guidewire, the guidewire may be directed more into the central aortic lumen. When difficulty is encountered crossing the aortic valve, biplane fluoroscopy is used with or without test injections into the aortic root. By using the above technique of left ventricular catheterization in patients with aortic stenosis at our institution, we rarely need to perform transseptal catheterization of the left ventricle.

The 12-side-hole pigtail creates the necessity for forceful flushes and has the potential of additional sites for emboli. Persistent cerebral events after cardiac catheterization were reported to occur in only 0.07 percent of over 50,000 patients in the Society for Cardiac Angioplasty Registry.[10] Theoretically, if the number of side holes were reduced, this might further lessen the occurrence of these uncommon events. We have tested six-side-hole and four-side-hole pigtail catheters and find they deliver contrast adequately for left ventriculography in both the no. 7 and 8 French sizes. The six- and four-side-hole pigtail catheters are an advantage in the no. 7 French high-flow catheters because there will be less kinking when curling the catheter in the aortic root before crossing the aortic valve. An ideal left ventriculography pigtail catheter therefore would be no. 7 or 8 French. It would have only four side holes with a tight loop to facilitate crossing abnormal aortic valves. (Fig. 7II-15).

Pigtail catheters may also be modified for right ventriculography or pulmonary angiography by making a Grollman curve[11] (reverse 60° bend) (Fig. 7II-16). These catheters should also have a tight loop and four or six side holes as near to the loop as possible so as not to produce factitious tricuspid regurgitation with right ventricular injections. In a patient with idiopathic hypertrophic subaortic stenosis use of a right ventricular catheter and a left ventricular catheter with simultaneous injections of contrast into both ventricles and cranial and oblique projections will clearly show the anatomic pathology of septal hypertrophy and abnormal mitral valve motion (Fig. 7II-17). The total contrast injection can be limited to 70 mL or less.

The use of the above mentioned pigtail catheters should provide less trauma, good opacification, and reduced arrhythmias to assist in the production of consistently good ventriculography.

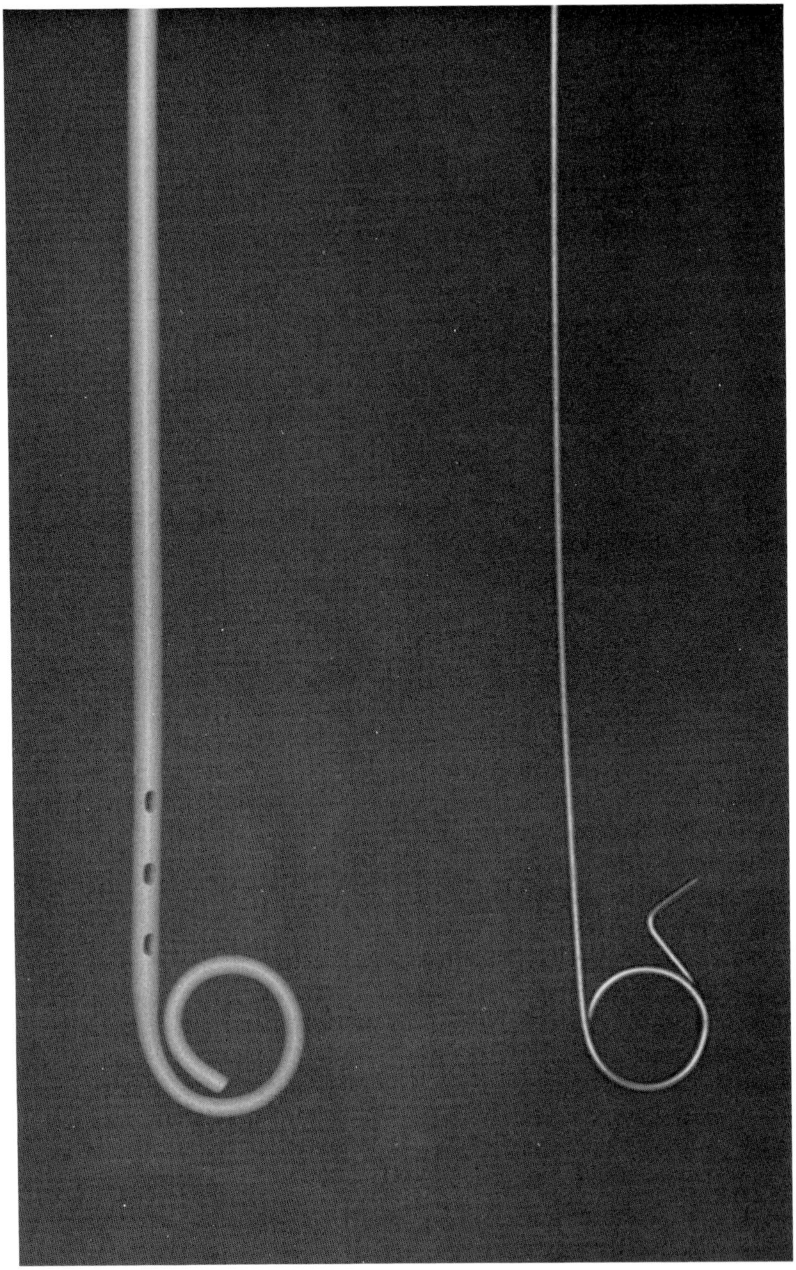

Figure 7II-14 A tight loop pigtail catheter size no. 8F with 12 side holes and a tight loop shaping wire.

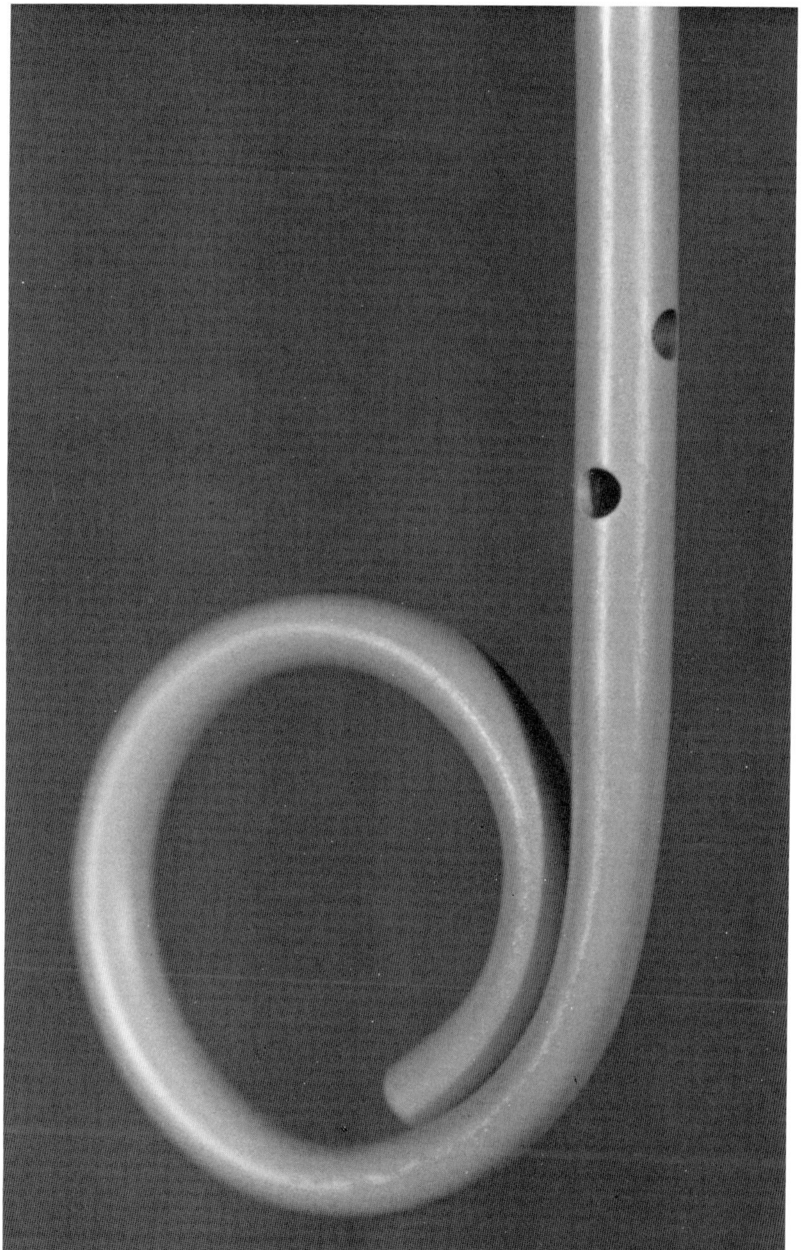

Figure 7II-15 Pigtail catheter size no. 8F with four side holes.

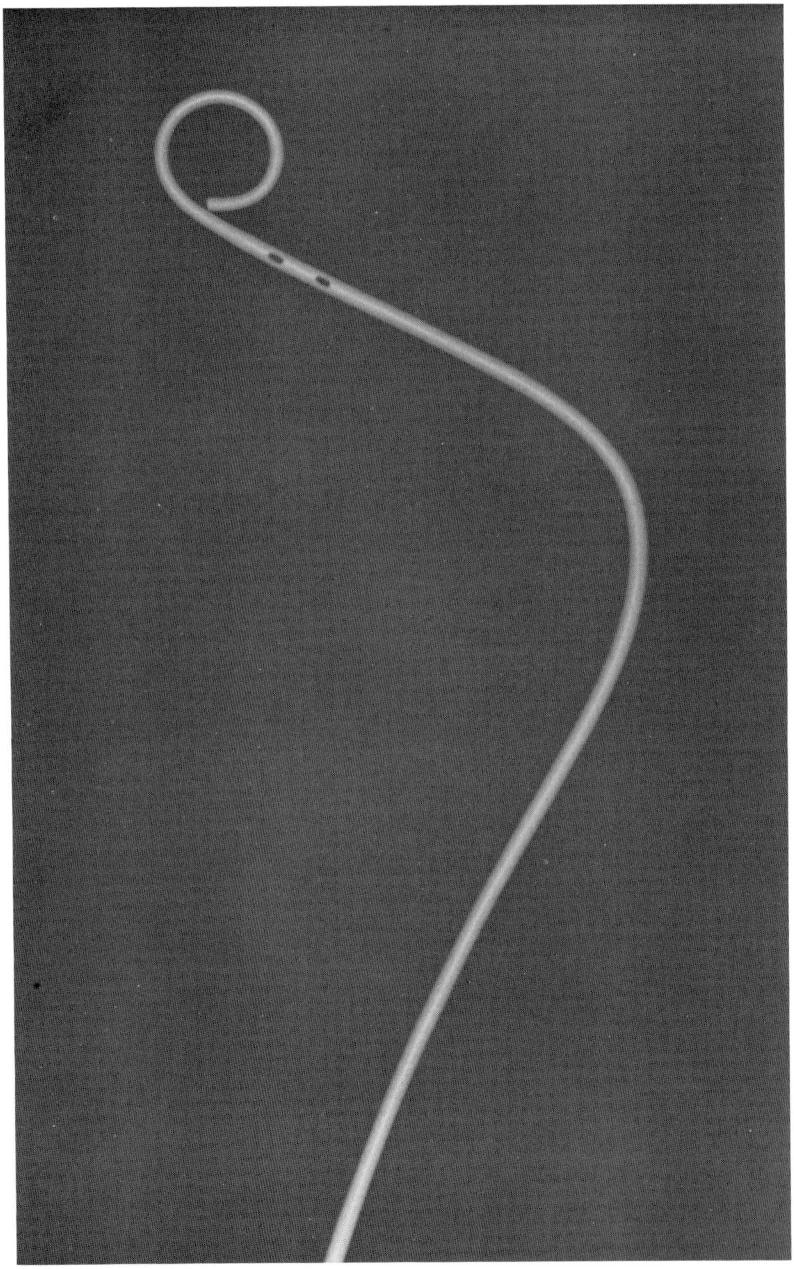

Figure 7II-16 Pigtail catheter size no. 7F with six side holes and a Grollman curve for right ventriculography.

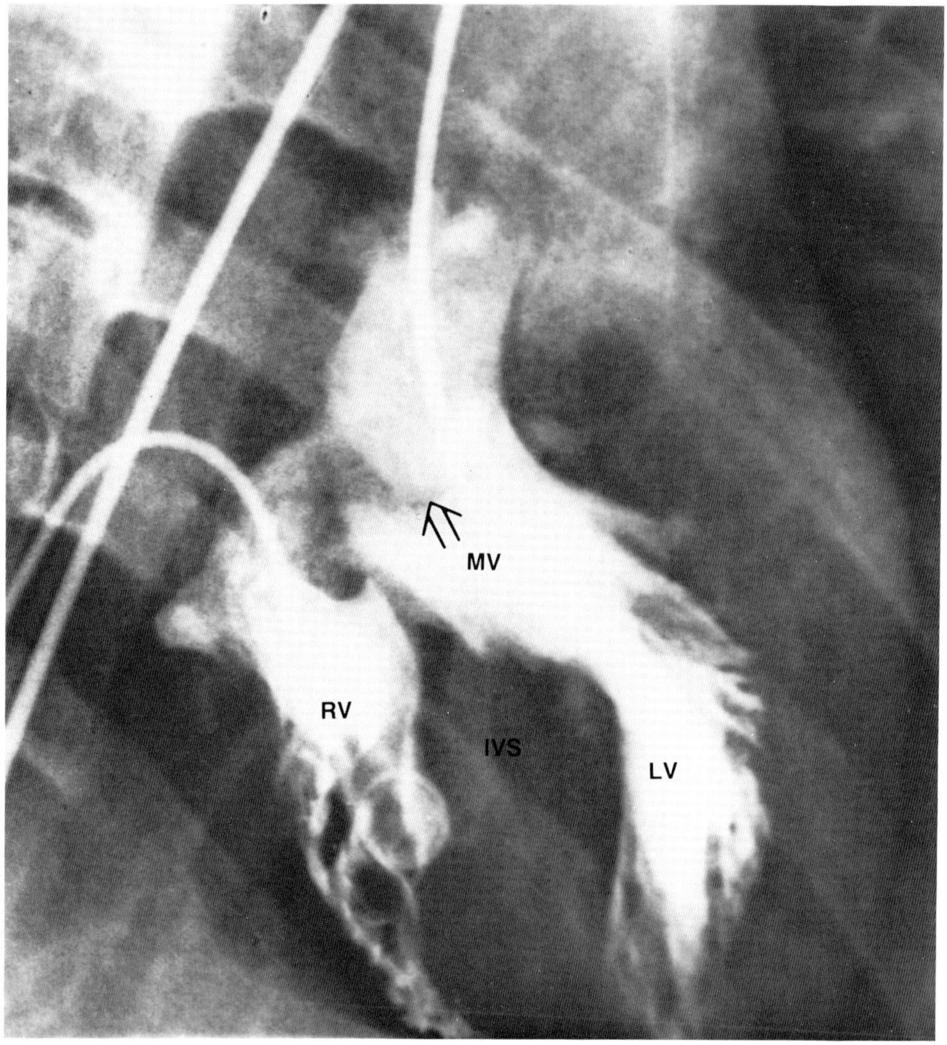

Figure 7II-17 A simultaneous biventricular injection filmed in a cranial RAO projection in a patient with idiopathic hypertrophic subaortic stenosis (IHSS). The mitral valve (MV) with anterior motion, interventricular septum (IVS), and both left ventricle (LV) and right ventricle (RV) are seen.

ACKNOWLEDGMENTS

The author would like to acknowledge the assistance of John Durkos, Roxie Poser, Judy Saunders, and Robert Marsa, M.D., in the preparation of this manuscript. The photography of Robert Rearick, Jim Simmons, and the artwork of Robert Knabenbauer and Wayne Harlow are much appreciated. This discussion was made possible by Dr. Melvin Judkins, whose outstanding teaching communicated the techniques of using the catheters which he ingeniously developed.

REFERENCES (Part II)

1 Judkins MP: Selective coronary arteriography: I. A percutaneous transfemoral technique. Radiology, 89:815, 1967.
2 Judkins MP: Percutaneous transfemoral selective coronary arteriography. Radiol Clin North Am, 6:467, 1968.
3 Gruentzig AR, Senning A, Seigenthaler WE: Non-operative dilation of coronary-artery stenosis. N Engl J Med, 301:61, 1979.
4 James TN: *Anatomy of the Coronary Arteries*. Harper and Row, New York, 1961, pp 38–41.
5 Ogden JA: Congenital anomalies of the coronary arteries. Am J Cardiol, 25:474, 1970.
6 Schoonmaker FW, King SB: Coronary arteriography by the single catheter percutaneous femoral technique. Circulation, 50:735, 1974.
7 Paulin S: *Normal Coronary Anatomy, Coronary Arteriography*. Little, Brown, Boston, 1983, p 138.
8 Page HL, Engel HI, et al: Anomalous origin of the left circumflex coronary artery. Circulation, 50:768, 1974.
9 Chaitman BR, Lesperance J, et al: Clinical, angiographic and hemodynamic findings in patients with anomalous origins of the coronary arteries. Circulation, 53:122, 1976.
10 Kennedy JW, et al: Complications associated with cardiac catheterization and angiography. Cathet Cardiovasc Diagn, 8:5, 1982.
11 Grollman JH, Gyepes MT, Helmer E: Transfemoral selective bilateral pulmonary arteriography with a pulmonary artery seeking catheter. Radiology, 96:202, 1970.

Chapter 8

Coronary Arteriography and Left Ventriculography: Multipurpose Technique

Spencer B. King III, M.D.
John S. Douglas, Jr., M.D.

In this chapter, we will describe the techniques of coronary arteriography using the percutaneous transfemoral approach and a single multipurpose catheter as described by Schoonmaker and King[1] in 1974 and as practiced and taught at Emory University Hospital.

PREPARATION OF THE PATIENT

Most patients have considerable anxiety concerning coronary arteriography, both from the prospect of discomfort and potential risk from the procedure itself and from the concern over what the procedure may reveal. Following admission to the hospital, the patient is visited by the catheterization team, including the physician who will be performing the procedure. The primary nurse responsible for the patient is also extremely important in this first patient contact and through extensive knowledge of the catheterization procedure can do much to reassure the patient. All members of the team caring for the patient should strive to be consistent in the instructions given and the description of the events to take place. It is helpful to have prepared educational materials which describe the procedure and potential risks and benefits in a realistic yet nonthreatening way. Regardless of the amount of time spent describing the events surrounding catheterization, an illustrated booklet gives the patient the chance to reflect on the procedure at leisure and can clear up questions the patient is unwilling to ask.

The physician performing the procedure must take the ultimate responsibility for ensuring that the patient understands what is to happen and the potential risks and alternatives to the procedure. Most states require written informed consent, and all require some consent from the patient. It is important, however, in fulfilling this responsibility to the patient not to lose sight of the fear and anxiety that must be alleviated. It is necessary to go into great detail in describing the procedure and risks to some patients, while others would rather not dwell on these aspects. The astute physician can discern these needs and meet them. Communication between physician and nurse can prevent further misunderstandings a patient might have while awaiting catheterization.

A review of current medications is made. Usually all cardiac medications can be continued through the period of catheterization without interruption. Food and drink are withheld for at least 4 hours prior to the procedure. Patients who will be catheterized in the morning are held without food or drink after midnight the night before. If the catheterization is to be done in the afternoon, a liquid breakfast is allowed. When patients are dehydrated, water by mouth can be continued up until 1 to 2 hours prior to the procedure. If avoidance of dehydration is more crucial, an intravenous line can be inserted for administration of appropriate fluids. This is especially important in patients who must maintain good renal output, such as those with renal dysfunction or myeloma.

PATIENT EVALUATION

Evaluation of the patient prior to the procedure includes a review of all medical problems previously identified through a history and physical examination, laboratory tests, x-ray, and ECG. Items which will modify the procedure are identified. Several examples are as follows: (1) Insulin-dependent diabetes: patients with this problem should have catheterization early in the morning with insulin and breakfast held until after the procedure. (2) Coagulation abnormalities (most commonly use of oral anticoagulants): if the prothrombin time is greater than 1.6 times control, we would usually administer vitamin K_1 the evening prior to the catheterization to avoid excess bleeding from the femoral puncture site. (3) Severe hypertension: systolic blood pressure greater than 200 mmHg may cause significant difficulty with postcatheterization hemostasis and should be controlled prior to catheterization. (4) Leg claudication or abnormal peripheral pulses: femoral pulses are necessary for reasonable success in performing the catheterization from the femoral artery. Absent peripheral leg pulses or claudication confined to the calf of the leg do not preclude successful femoral catheterization. Hip claudication, however, signals disease in the iliac artery. Previous aortoiliac surgery is not a contraindication to the femoral approach. If a graft has been placed into the femoral artery, the arm approach is usually preferred. (5) History of transient ischemic attacks or carotid artery bruits: patients with such history should be considered for study of the carotid circulation. In some laboratories, cineangiograms or cut film studies of the extracranial carotid arteries are done at the same time as the coronary arteriogram. In other laboratories, the patient is referred to other colleagues involved with neuroradiology for either digital subtraction angiography or direct carotid arteriography.

We prefer not to use premedications prior to moving to the catheterization laboratory but instead rely on reassurance of the patient that the procedure will not cause significant discomfort. On arrival in the laboratory, technicians and nurses take over the job of comforting and reassuring the patient. A professional yet cheerful manner usually puts the patient at ease. An intravenous line is started to provide a port for administration of medications. ECG monitor leads are attached which provide for both frontal plane and V_5 precordial lead observation and recording. The area over the femoral artery to be catheterized is shaved widely and prepped. Sterile drapes are applied. We find that the disposable drapes which have an opening bounded by adhesive provide the best sterile field and eliminate the chance of the drape slipping or the patient's hand entering the sterile field.

CONTRAST MEDIUM ALLERGIES

If the patient describes a previous allergy to contrast medium, this must be carefully investigated.

Usually the reaction the patient is concerned about is simply nausea or some discomfort, not a true allergy. If, however, the patient experienced extensive hives, wheezing, or a drop in blood pressure with the previous use of an iodine-containing contrast medium, then premedication with 50 mg diphenhydramine hydrochloride and 100 mg hydrocortisone should be given intravenously prior to the start of the catheterization.

Premedications in the laboratory are 0.6-mg atropine IV and diazepam in 2.5- to 5-mg increments to maintain relaxation without significant sedation. Atropine is withheld in patients who are very unstable and in whom a rapid heart rate is to be avoided and in patients in whom ergonovine provocation for spasm is contemplated.

CATHETERIZATION LABORATORY EQUIPMENT

The types of x-ray and physiological monitoring equipment will be described in Chapter 14. A sterile tray setup includes all items necessary for entering the femoral artery by the Seldinger approach and performing coronary arteriography (Fig. 8-1).

The Catheter

Various catheters have been used in an attempt to perform coronary arteriography from the femoral approach. The Sones Positrol USCI (U. S. Catheter Inc.) catheter, although excellent from the brachial approach, did not have the 1:1 torque response needed for positioning the tip after the 180° turn of the aortic arch is made. A polyurethane catheter with wire reinforcement gives excellent torquing capabilities even when passed 180° around the aortic arch as is done with the femoral approach. The tip must be flexible enough to allow it to be deformed off the aortic cusp but to maintain enough memory so its curve can be utilized for right coronary artery and vein graft cannulation. The multipurpose A2 catheter from Cordis has served this purpose for years. Recently developed woven Dacron catheters with somewhat different characteristics from USCI are also used (Fig. 8-2).

THE SELDINGER TECHNIQUE OF FEMORAL PUNCTURE

Percutaneous arterial catheterization was described by Seldinger[2] in 1953 and was used to study the coronary arteries by Rickets and Abrams in 1962[3] and later by Amplatz[5] and Judkins.[6]

The inguinal ligament, which runs from the anterior superior spine of the ilium to the pubis, is palpated. One identifies the point of maximal pulsation of the femoral artery as it crosses the ligament (Fig. 8-3*a*). The operator places the middle finger on this spot with the index finger palpating the artery just below the ligament (Fig. 8-3*b*). If the right femoral artery is entered, this maneuver is performed with the left hand. If the left femoral artery is used, the procedure is reversed, and the right middle and index fingers are used to palpate the artery. The point for entry of the needle into the skin is approximately one-half fingers breadth below the index finger and directly over the artery. Lidocaine 2% is used to anesthetize the skin in this area (Fig. 8-3*c*). The left hand is then moved so that the index and middle fingers now straddle the artery just below the ligament so that equal pulsations can be perceived on each finger. This identifies the point between the fingers as the center of the artery. Lidocaine is injected on either side of the artery below the palpating fingers using $1\frac{1}{4}$-inch no. 21 needle. A stab incision is made in the skin with a no. 11 blade at the needle entry site (Fig. 8-3*d*). One then holds the Seldinger needle in the right hand between the index and middle fingers so that the thumb can press on the hub of the needle and advance it into the artery (Fig. 8-3*e*).

The needle is advanced at an angle of 30° to 45° from the horizontal directly at the center of the femoral pulse being palpated by the fingers of the left hand. A steeper approach, greater than 45°, will make catheter manipulation difficult and should be avoided. As the needle is advanced, one can often feel a pop as the femoral artery is entered. A bit of blood on the end of the hollow stylus also signals entry into the artery (Fig. 8-3*f*). Once the artery has been entered, the stylus is removed, al-

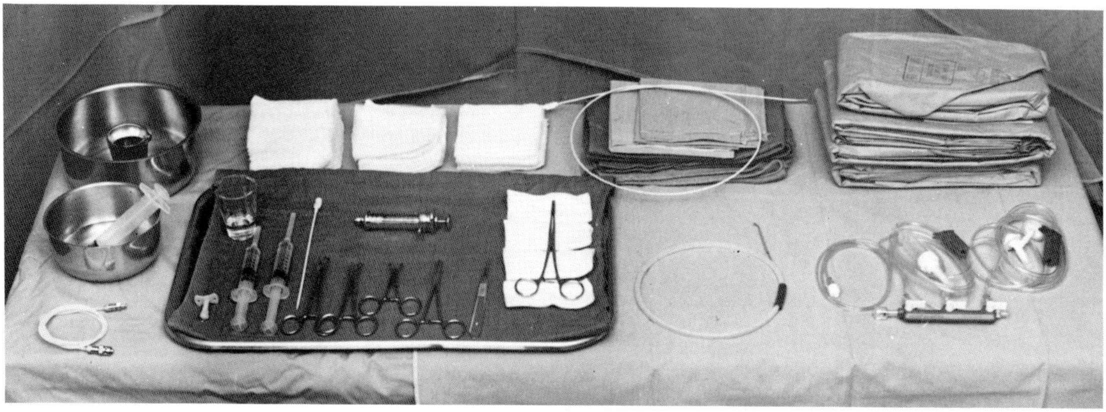

A

Figure 8-1 (*a*) Setup used in performing coronary arteriography. Reading counterclockwise from lower left-hand corner: A high-pressure connector, the tray containing a disposable Seldinger needle, a cup of 2% xylocaine, two syringes (one with a short no. 25 needle and one with a longer no. 20 needle), a vascular dilator, towel clips, a surgical clamp, a no. 11 blade and handle, sterile sponges and a sponge forcep, and a Swiss syringe. Next a 0.038-inch safety J-spring guidewire; the manifold with connecting tubing, drapes, the angiographic catheter, 4 × 4 inch sponges, a basin with povidone-iodine solution for prepping and for discarding flush solutions, and a basin with sterile heparinized saline with a 10-mL flush syringe. (*b*) Syringe and manifold arrangement used in coronary arteriography. A metal and glass Swiss syringe is connected to the rear of a three side port manifold with a rotator attached to its distal end. The catheter is attached to the rotator. (A) Line for contrast medium, (B) line for saline flush, (C) connector for pressure monitoring.

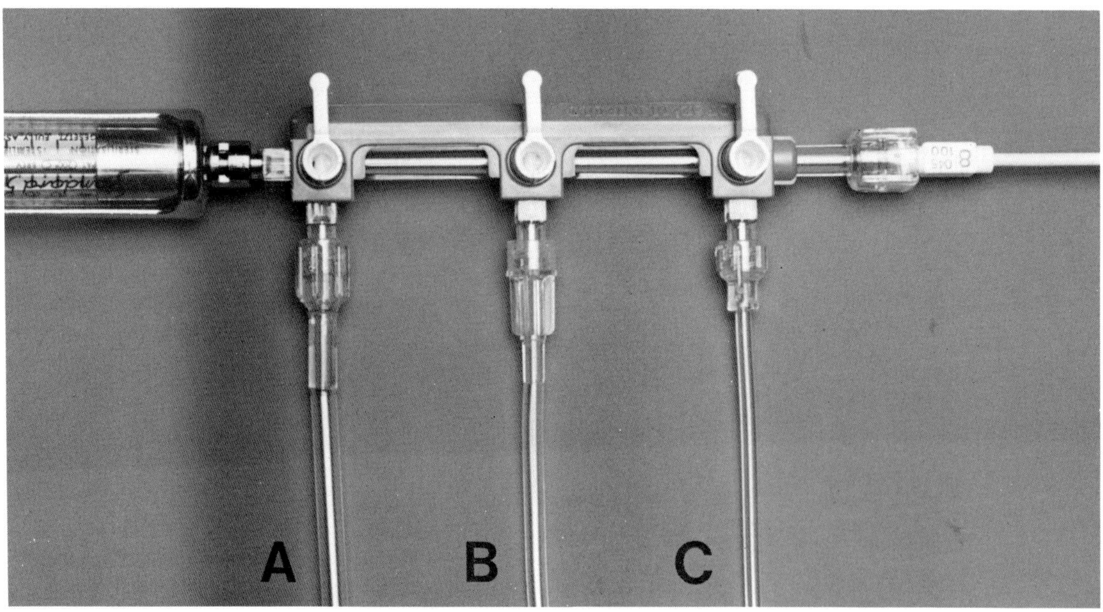

B

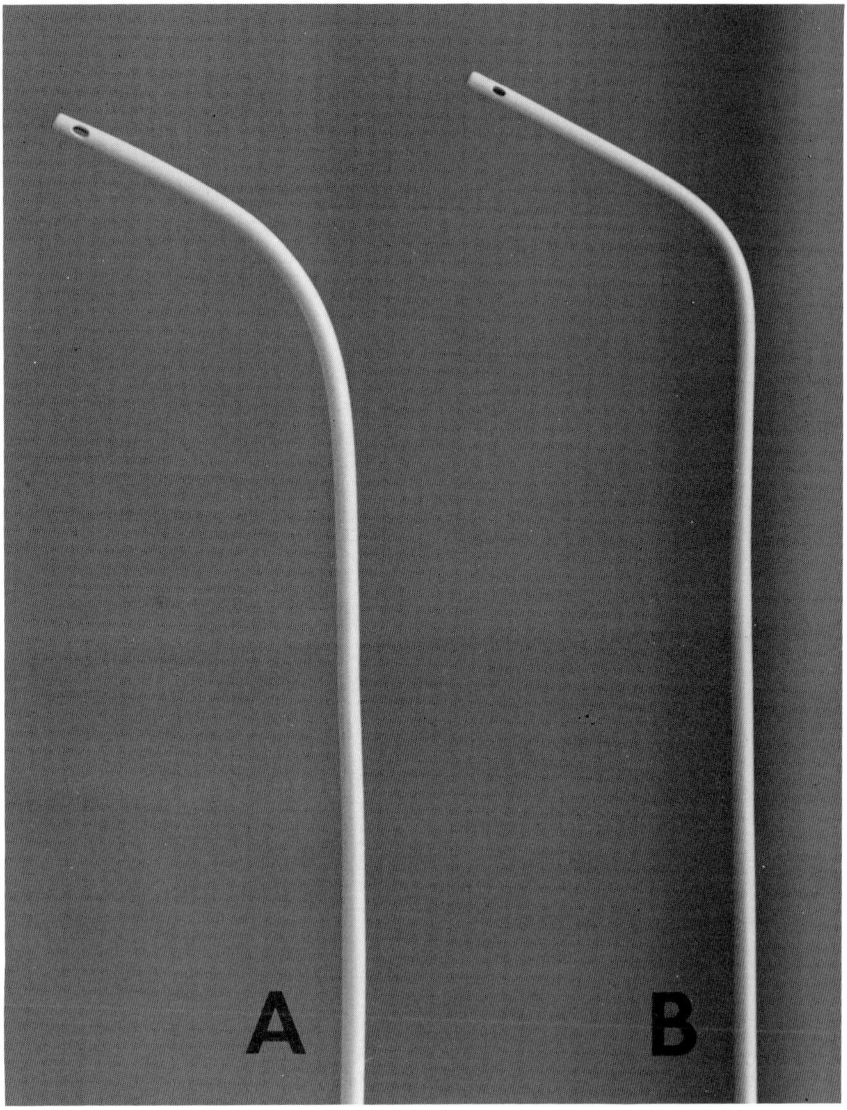

Figure 8-2 Catheters used for multipurpose technique. (*a*) Cordis multipurpose A2 catheter of extruded polyurethane with wire reinforcement. (*b*) A new catheter manufactured by USCI of woven Dacron with wire reinforcement.

lowing free flow of blood through the needle (Fig. 8-3*g*). If both walls of the artery have been punctured, no backflow will be seen. After the stylus is removed, a gradual withdrawal of the needle will produce brisk back bleeding when it enters the artery (Fig. 8-3*h*).

A 0.035-inch or 0.038-inch safety J-spring guidewire is then inserted through the needle for 15 to 20 cm into the artery if the guidewire travels easily (Fig. 8-3*i*). The needle can then be withdrawn over the guidewire and pressure applied over the artery to prevent hematoma formation (Fig. 8-

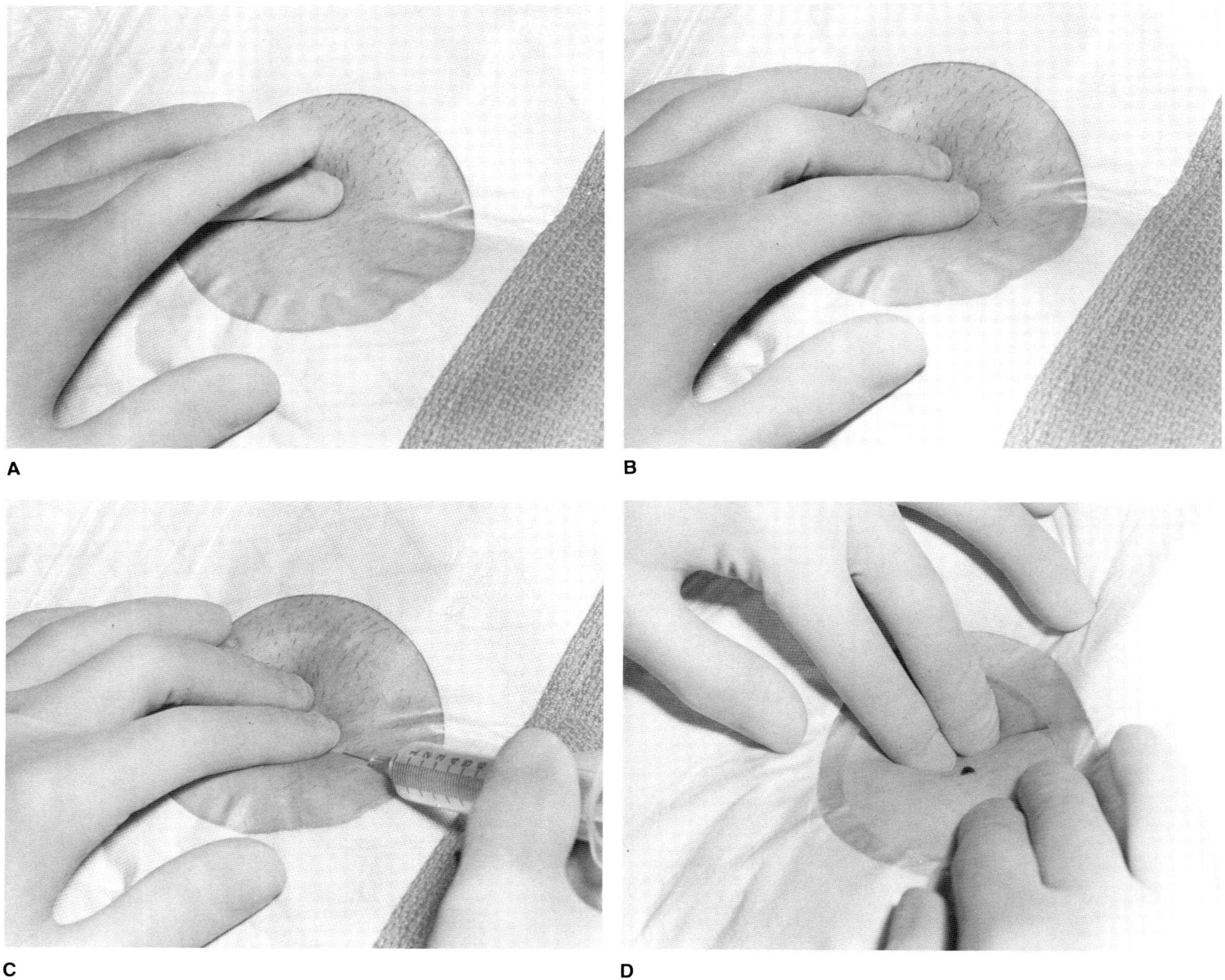

Figure 8-3 (*a–l*) Technique for identifying the femoral pulse performing Seldinger puncture of the artery and inserting the catheter. See text for description of the technique.

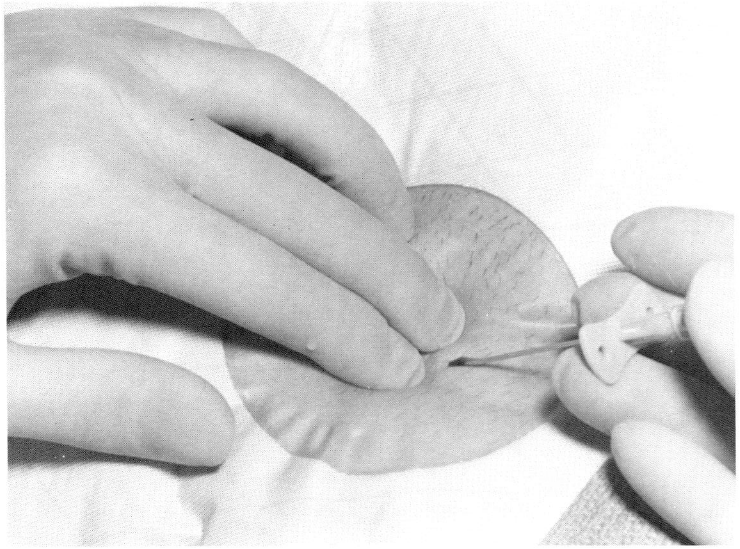
E

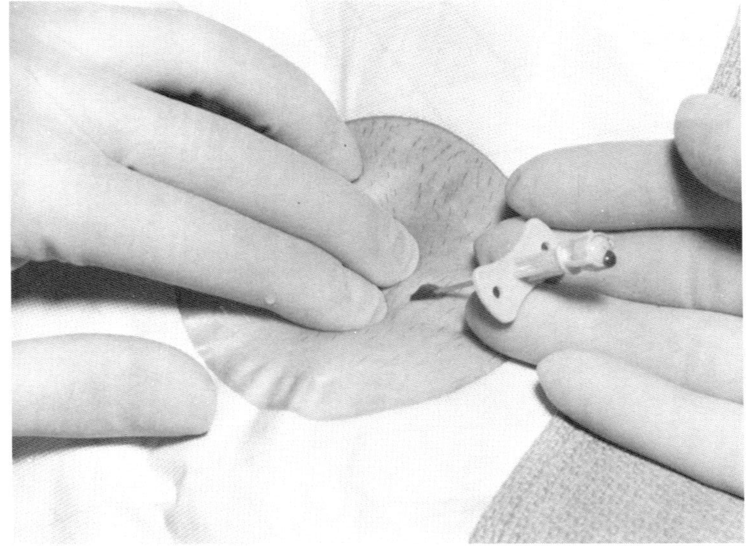
F

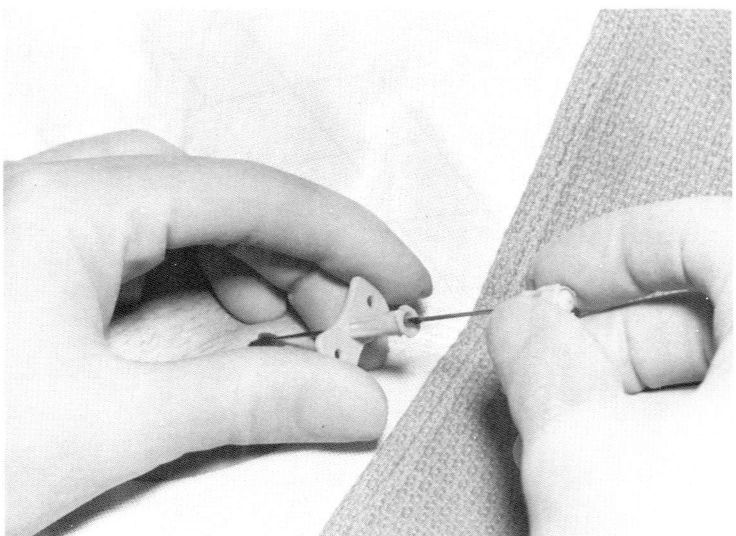
G

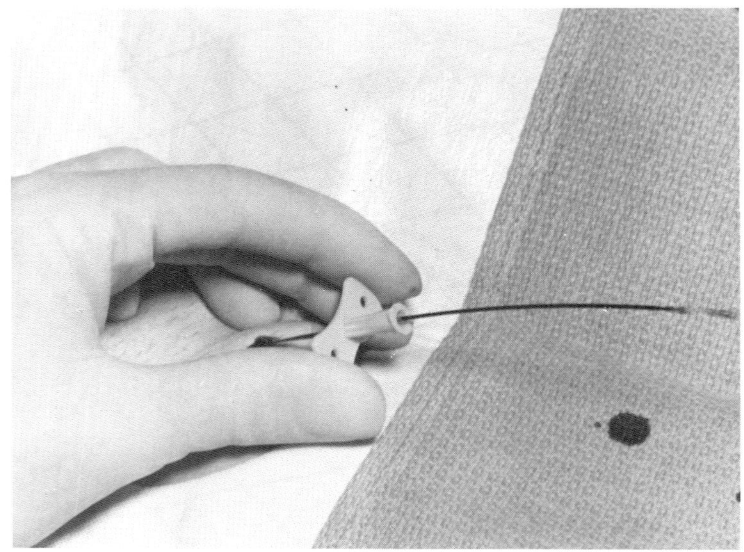
H

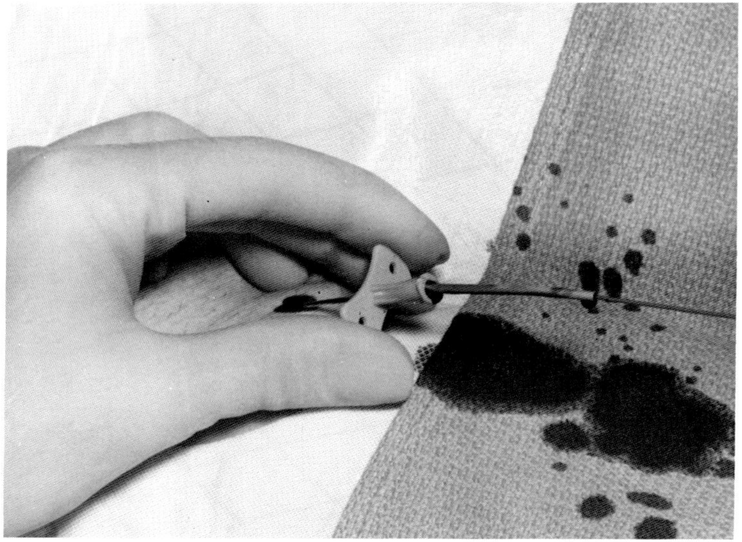

I

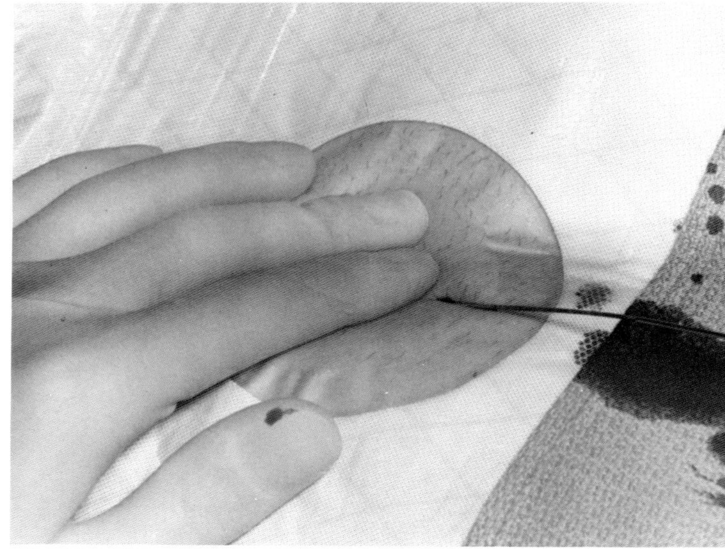

J

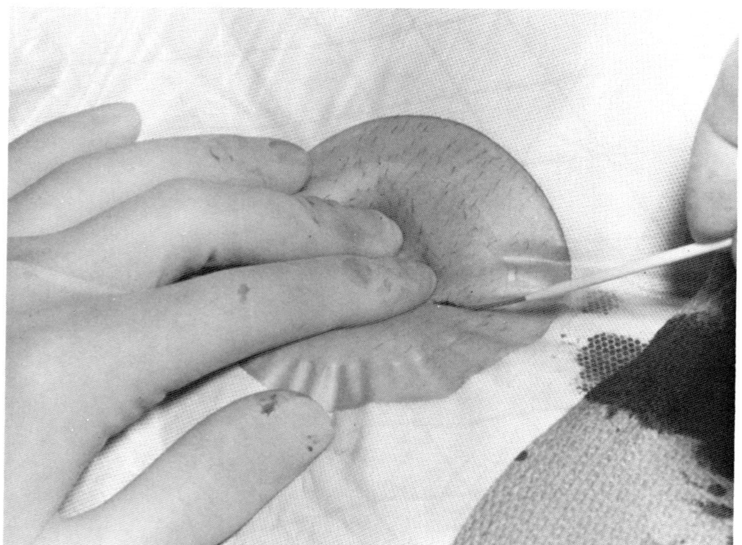

K

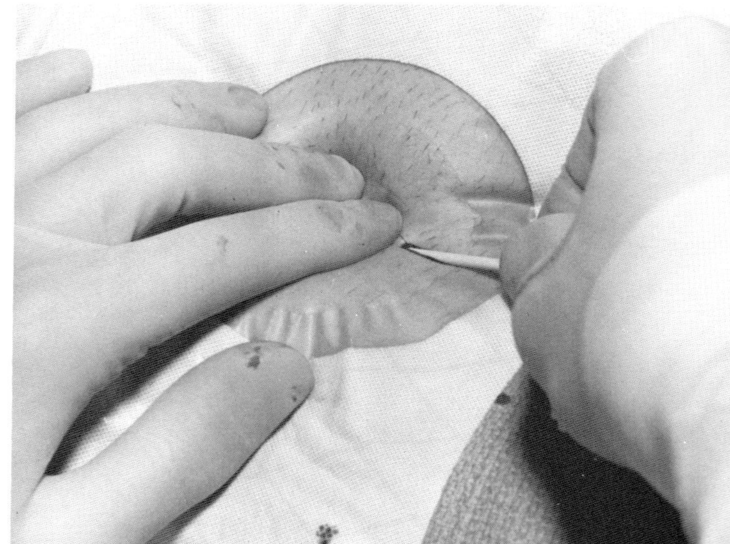

L

(*Figure 8-3, continued*)

3*j*). The nurse assistant cleans the guidewire with sterile saline, and a no. 8 French vascular dilator is advanced over the guidewire with a rotating motion into the femoral artery (Fig. 8-3*k*). Easy entry into the artery is achieved by maintaining compression over the artery with the left hand while inserting the dilator in a rotating motion with the right hand. The dilator is removed and the guidewire once again cleaned. The assistant advances a no. 8 multipurpose catheter over the guidewire and again with the clockwise rotating motion the operator advances the catheter into the femoral artery (Fig. 8-3*l*). The catheter is passed over the guidewire until it reaches the level in the descending aorta just below the renal arteries, at which point the guidewire is removed and the catheter flushed vigorously to dislodge any particulate matter that may have been picked up on entry into the femoral artery. The steps for entering the femoral artery by the Seldinger technique are illustrated in Fig. 8-4.

When a catheter is inserted into the artery over the guidewire, the potential for picking up thrombus material, plaque, or platelet thrombi is ever-present even if the patients are anticoagulated. Because of this potential risk, we feel the catheter should be vigorously debrided by flushing technique in the abdominal aorta prior to crossing the aortic arch.[4] Once the flush has been accomplished, the catheter can then be advanced up the aorta and around the aortic arch without the use of the guidewire. However, if there is any hold-up of the catheter or evidence of significant plaque formation in the aortic arch, the guidewire can be reinserted and the catheter passed over it around the aortic arch and into the ascending aorta.

If an incision is made too low, the superficial femoral artery rather than the common femoral will be entered. This may create no problem, but in patients with small arteries, it could produce a high risk of occlusion of the vessel. An additional problem is the takeoff of branches from the superficial femoral which may entrap the guidewire, thereby preventing passage into the common femoral and iliac vessels. If this situation occurs, the needle should be removed and puncture site made higher so that the common femoral artery can be entered.

Occasionally the safety guidewire will not pass easily through the iliac artery into the aorta. When this occurs, one should make certain that the guidewire is indeed in the femoral artery by removing it temporarily and watching vigorous backflow through the needle. If backflow is seen, then the wire can be reinserted to the point of obstruction. The artery is then dilated with the vascular dilator and the multipurpose catheter advanced over the guidewire gently to the level of the obstruction. The wire is removed. A flush injection of contrast medium into the iliac artery will demonstrate the anatomy and the difficulty encountered in passing the catheter. Usually with this knowledge the catheter tip can be rotated and the guidewire used to move through the obstruction and into the aorta. Sometimes it is necessary to exchange for a movable core safety spring guidewire which has a straight tip. This allows for entering very small obstructed areas much in the same manner as for crossing a narrowed aortic valve. When the artery is extremely tortuous, a Judkins right coronary catheter can be employed as the guiding device for traversing heavily obstructed iliac vessels in conjunction with a movable core J-spring guidewire. This is a step-by-step procedure in which the wire is passed to the point of obstruction. The catheter is then advanced near that point. Flush injection shows the direction flow is coming from. Rotation of the catheter tip can then point to that inflow point. Then by reinserting the straight guidewire, the stenosis can be crossed (Fig. 8-5). It may take several such maneuvers to cross a severely tortuous and diseased iliac artery. The important point for safety is to avoid advancing the wire or catheter against a significant resistance.

ENTERING THE LEFT VENTRICLE

Once the catheter has been successfully positioned above the aortic valve, the 30° right oblique view is obtained either by rotating the patient or by rotating the x-ray beam, depending on the type of system that is being used. In this right oblique view, the left coronary cusp appears on the screen to the operator's right. The catheter tip is oriented

A

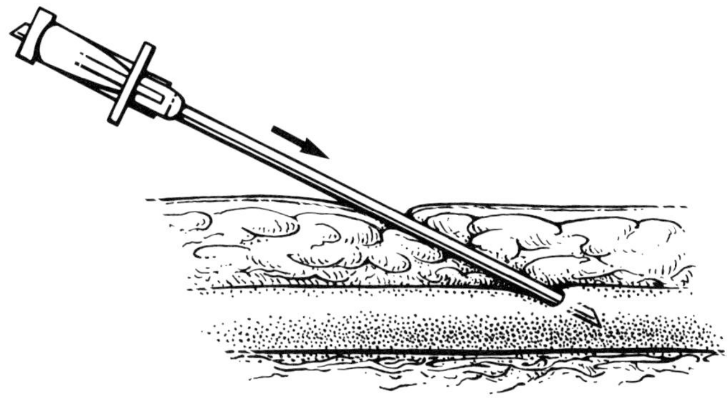

Figure 8-4 Technique for inserting the catheter by Seldinger approach. (*a*) The Seldinger needle is inserted into the femoral artery at the point of maximum impulse between the two palpating fingers. An attempt is made to puncture only the anterior wall of the artery. (*b*) A guidewire is passed through the needle into the artery. (*c*) The needle is removed over the guidewire. (*d*) A vascular dilator is advanced over the guidewire and into the artery with a rotating motion. (*e*) The dilator is removed and compression is held over the puncture site to avoid back bleeding. (*f*) The catheter selected is then advanced over the guidewire and into the artery again with a rotating motion.

B

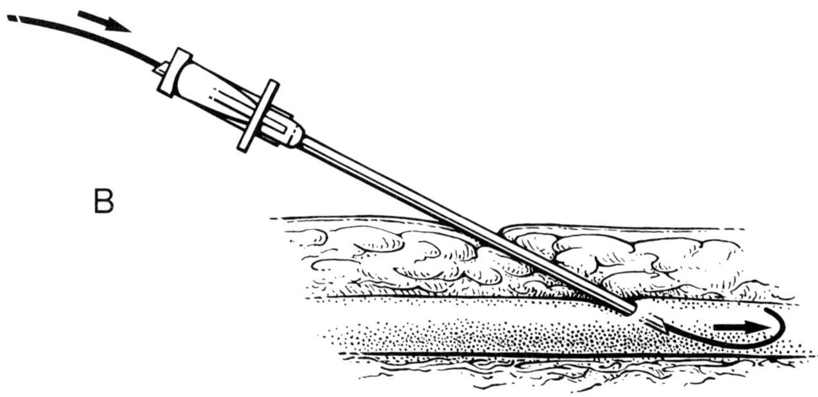

C

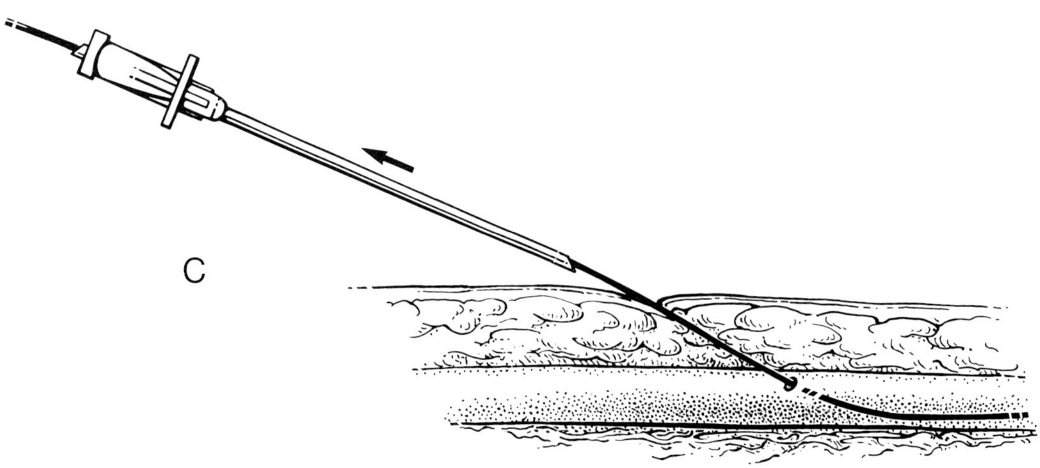

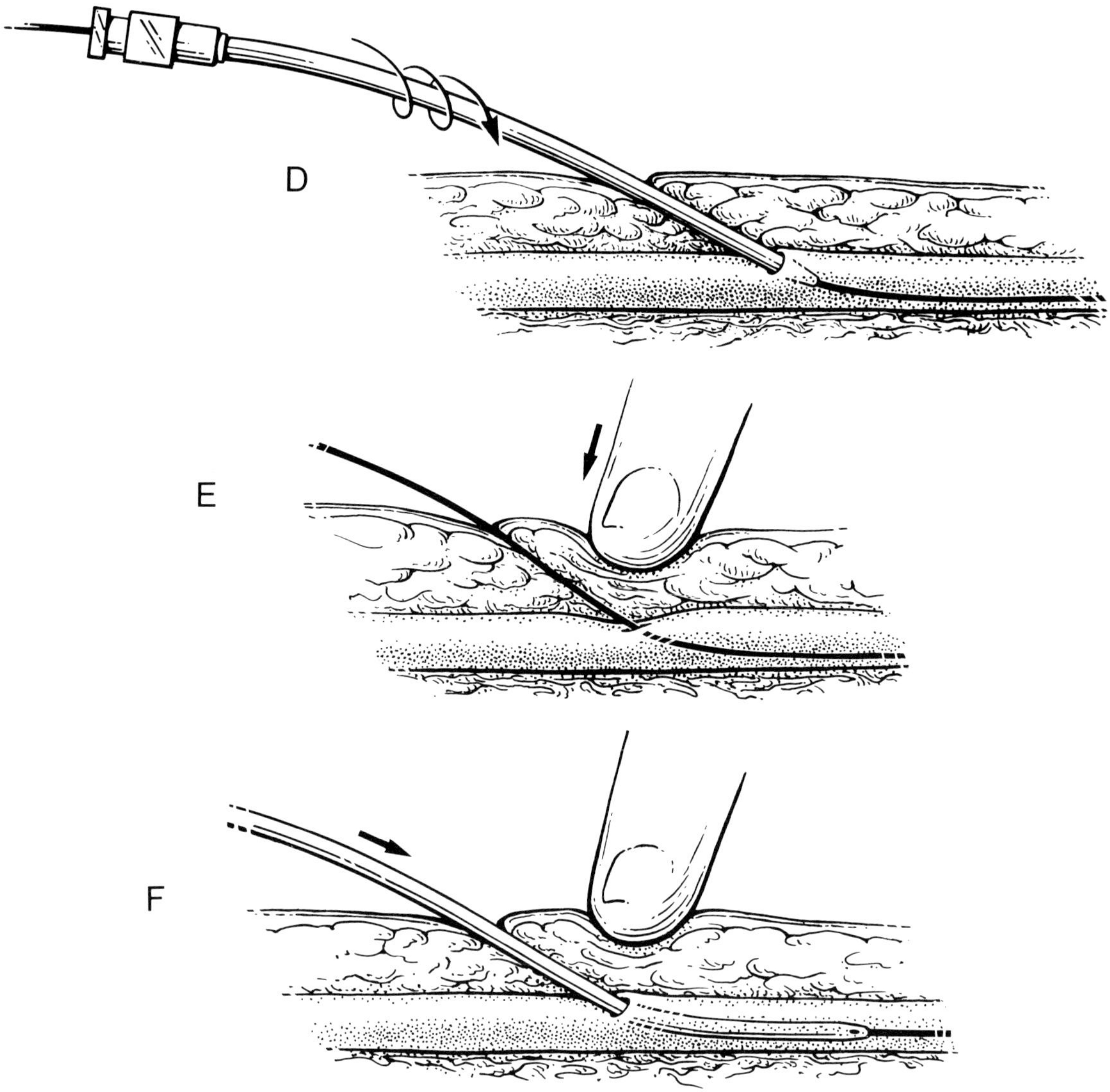

so it lies on the left coronary cusp and the curve of the multipurpose catheter points in the direction of the long axis of the left ventricle. Gentle pressure will result in formation of a loop, and then the catheter will pop through the aortic valve into the left ventricle. It is sometimes necessary to withdraw slightly as the catheter may migrate towards the apex. The ideal position for the catheter is lying in the left ventricle with the tip pointed slightly posterior toward the anterior leaflet of the mitral valve at the midventricular level (Fig. 8-6). In this position there is little chance for ectopic activity or intramyocardial injections and the curve of the multipurpose catheter is very smooth around the aortic arch through the valve and into the left ventricle. This position is essential to avoid recoil once the left ventricular injection is made. If biplane fluoroscopy is available, catheter tip positioning is made easier. With single plane systems, however, experience quickly teaches the operator the correct

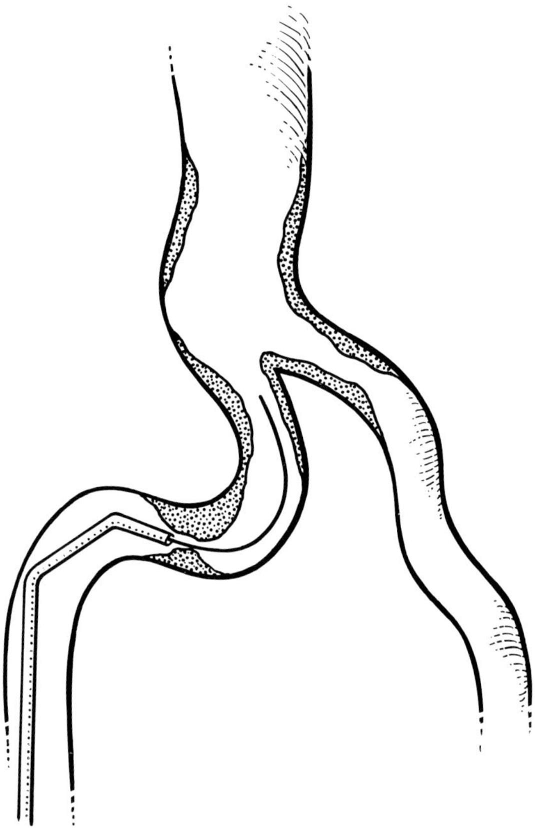

Figure 8-5 Technique for crossing tortuous and stenotic iliac arteries using the right Judkins catheter. Using frequent flush injections, the tip of the catheter can be pointed at stenotic areas and a movable core floppy J-spring guidewire is then advanced through the area of obstruction and on to the next point of blockage. Once the wire has advanced up the artery, the Judkins catheter can safely be advanced over it and additional contrast injections made until the unobstructed portion of the aorta is reached.

position for bringing the catheter tip to the proper place in the long axis of the left ventricle pointed slightly posterior toward the anterior leaflet of the mitral valve. Once a stable position is obtained, left ventricular pressures are measured with the patient supine.

LEFT VENTRICULOGRAM

Following these measurements, the 30° right oblique view is again obtained and the catheter is attached via a high-pressure connector to an automatic injector for performance of the left ventriculogram. Our experience indicates that a flow rate of approximately 10 mL/s is the maximum that can be used in order to avoid recoil of the catheter into the aorta. This injection rate is continued for 4 s giving a total volume of 40 mL into the left ventricle. Small patients can usually be adequately imaged using 8 mL/s for 4 s.

Several points of caution are observed before and during the left ventriculogram. Small-volume testing of the injection is made in order to ensure that the catheter tip is not lying against the myocardium. The test injection should be made under the same conditions as the actual injection: that is, if deep inspiration is needed, then the test should also be done with deep inspiration to be sure there is no change in the catheter tip position during injections. During the left ventricular injection, the assistant holding the injector button should watch the fluoroscopic screen at all times. If any myocardial staining occurs, then injection is immediately terminated. Likewise, the operator holds the catheter during the injection being prepared to withdraw the catheter immediately should any staining of the myocardium appear. Although the multipurpose catheter has an end hole which delivers the greatest portion of the flow, it is extremely rare to have any staining of the left ventricular myocardium with this technique if proper testing of the position of the catheter is made prior to injection. If, however, the catheter is positioned against the lateral wall of the left ventricle, then it is possible to deliver the entire 40 mL into the left ventricular myocardium or into the pericardial space. This should always be avoided with test injections.

Once the left ventriculogram has been accomplished, the patient is returned to a supine position for measurement of left ventricular pressure which is obtained 2 minutes following left ventriculogram, then a pull-back is accomplished from left ventricle to aorta to establish whether an aortic valve gradient is present.

LEFT CORONARY ARTERY CANNULATION

The left coronary artery orifice is located at variable distances above the left coronary cusp ranging from

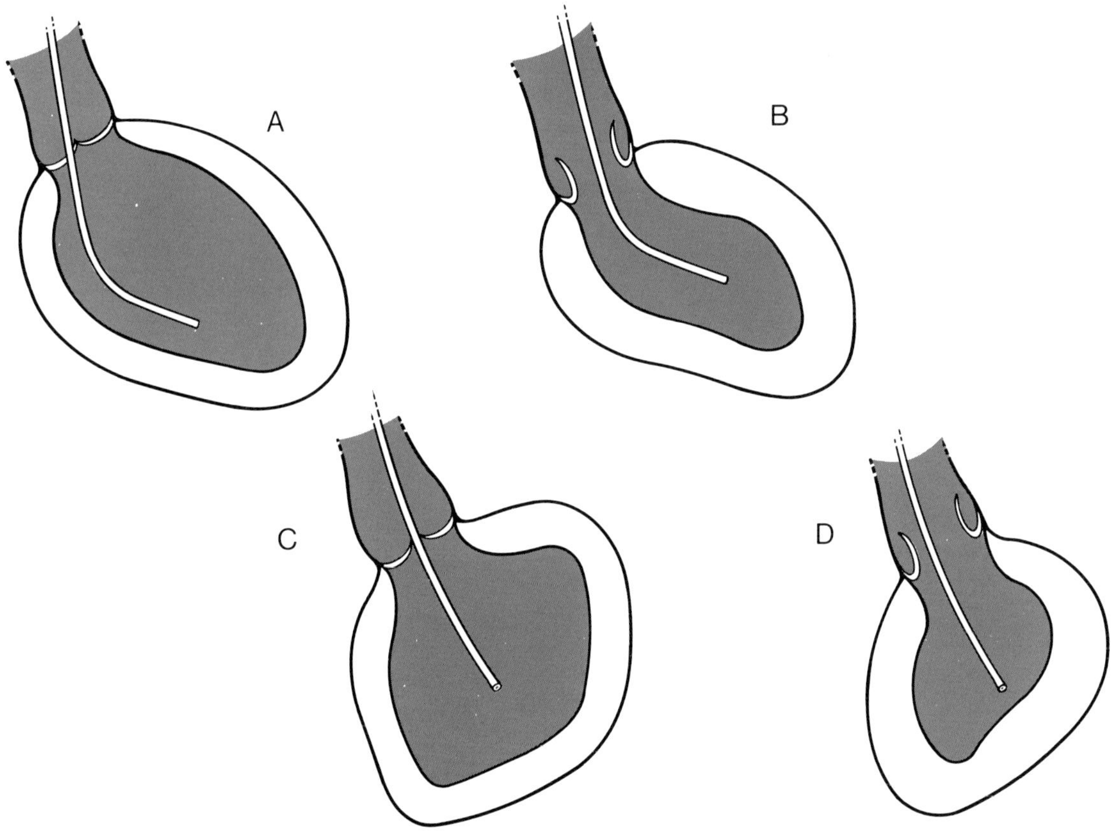

Figure 8-6 (*a*) Right anterior oblique view of left ventricle at end diastole with catheter tip in the mid ventricle. (*b*) Right anterior oblique view of left ventricle at end systole. (*c*) Left anterior oblique view of left ventricle at end diastole with the catheter tip pointed slightly posterior and away from the interventricular septum. (*d*) Left anterior oblique view of left ventricle at end systole. (*e*) Initial portion of left ventricular injection showing catheter position.

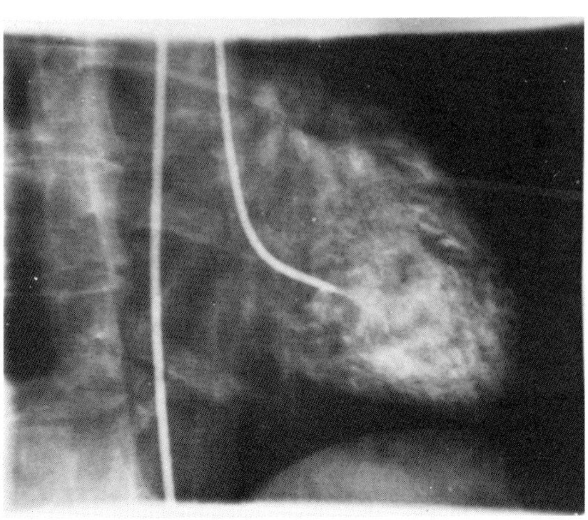

E

just above the leaflets to high adjacent to the sinotubular ridge where the left aortic sinus joins the tubular portion of the ascending aorta. The most successful method of cannulating the left coronary orifice with the multipurpose catheter is first to form a loop with the tip lying in the left coronary cusp and then to advance the catheter up into the orifice. This is accomplished by first positioning the patient in the x-ray beam so that the right anterior oblique view is obtained. The degree of obliquity that is most useful will vary but is usually approximately 30° right oblique. The multipurpose catheter is rotated counterclockwise so that it points toward the spine or in a posterior direction so that it will, when advanced, engage the noncoronary cusp (Fig. 8-7*a*). The catheter is then advanced

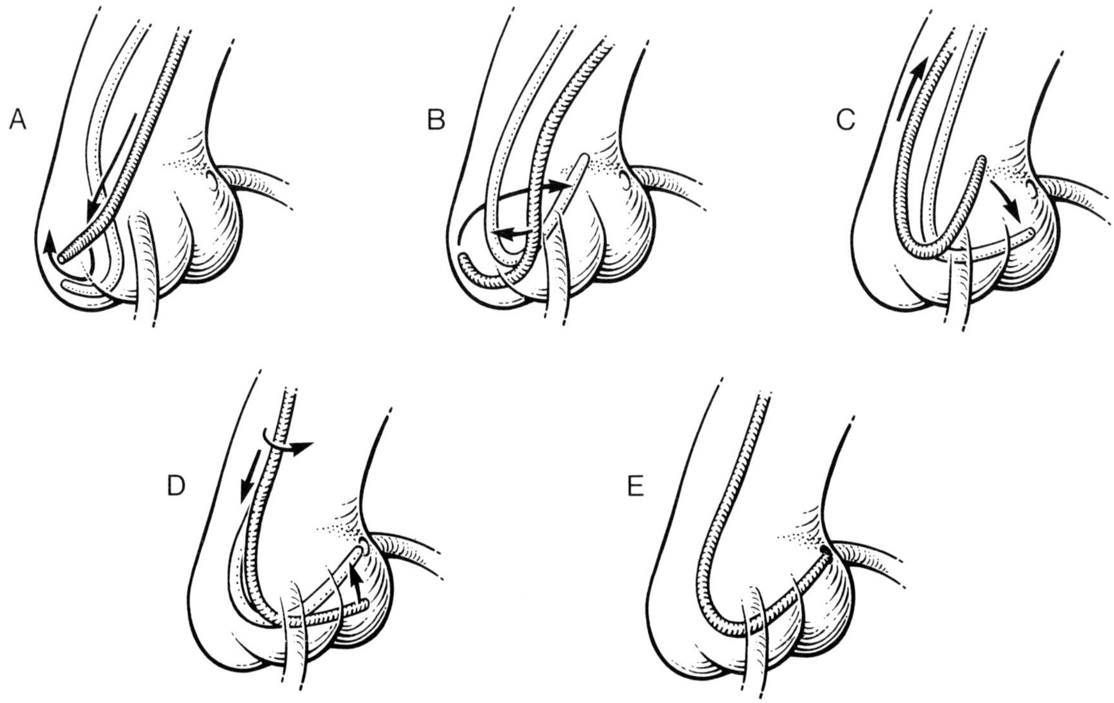

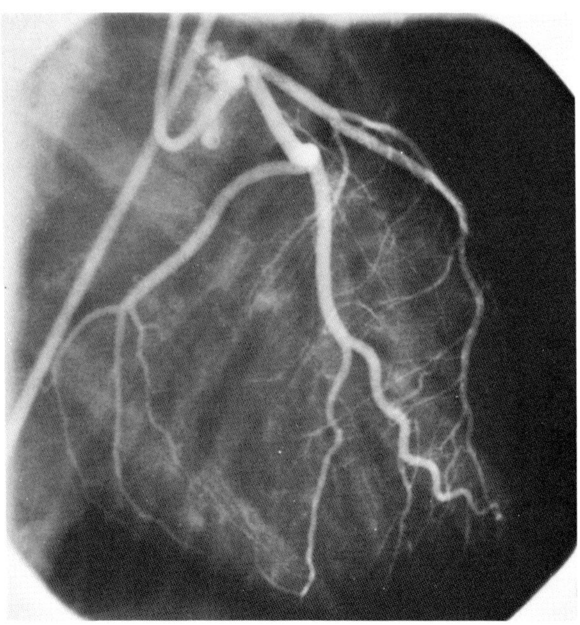

F

Figure 8-7 Technique for catheterizing the left coronary artery in the right anterior oblique view using the multipurpose catheter. (*a*) Catheter tip is advanced into the noncoronary cusp and rotated slightly clockwise while advancing continues. (*b*) When the catheter flips upward, the body is rapidly withdrawn a short distance. (*c*) If the tip remains above the left coronary orifice, the catheter is withdrawn slightly until the tip falls down into the left coronary sinus. (*d*) The body of the catheter is then rotated counterclockwise and advanced gradually until the tip rises to enter the left coronary ostium as illustrated in *e*. (*e*) Injection into left coronary artery. Note reflux of contrast medium into aorta. The catheter does not enter the left orifice deeply.

into the noncoronary cusp so that the tip is held there and the heel of the catheter begins to buckle toward the left cusp or toward the right of the operator positioned looking toward the television screen. The catheter is advanced and a slight clockwise rotation is applied, usually consisting of only a one-quarter to one-half turn. As the catheter is advanced further, the tip will flip from the noncoronary cusp superior toward the left coronary cusp, and the heel of the catheter will swing in the opposite direction toward the right or noncoronary cusp (Fig. 8-7*b*).

Frequently this continued advancing of the catheter and the flipping of the tip will result in prolapse of the catheter into the left ventricle. In order to counter this, the operator must anticipate the point at which the catheter has reached its maximum deformity without flipping and then at that point advance the catheter forward a very short distance and immediately pull back a short distance. One cannot observe the catheter tip and react to the flip of the catheter by pulling back and expect to form the proper loop. The motion is simply too fast, and the catheter will always fall into the ventricle. The trick for forming the loop is to anticipate the degree of deformity needed on the catheter, then advance so that the flipping motion will occur, and then pull back on the catheter immediately so that by the time the flip does occur, the downward pressure on the catheter tip has been relieved and there is no prolapse into the ventricle. One should realize that there is stored kinetic energy in the shaft of the catheter as it traverses the aorta. The slightly coiled tension tends to advance the catheter further than one would like, so the pulling-back maneuver simply relieves that kinetic energy from the portion of the catheter that lies throughout the length of the aorta.

This maneuver of flipping the catheter and pulling back simultaneously has been compared to the touch required for utilizing a fly rod in fishing. Once the tip has been flipped out of the noncoronary cusp and toward the left side of the aorta, it may come to rest in various positions. The tip may flip directly into the left coronary orifice, it may flip far anterior along the aorta near the junction of the left cusp and right cusp, or it may flip very high into the tubular portion of the aorta along the left side. If the tip flips into any position other than directly into the left coronary orifice, then the action required is to cause the tip to come to lie in the left sinus just above the valve. If the tip has gone into a high position, then carefully positioning the catheter tip with clockwise or counterclockwise rotation so that it lies directly above the left coronary orifice and pulling back on the shaft of the catheter will cause the tip to fall down on the left coronary cusp (Fig. 8-7*c*). This is another point at which the catheter may prolapse into the ventricle, so it is important, once the tip has fallen down on the left cusp, to advance the entire catheter slightly so that the tip will be held in the left sinus rather than passing through the valve into the left ventricle.

Once the tip is positioned deep in the left coronary sinus just above the valve, continued advancing of the catheter will cause the tip to rise in the left sinus. Puffs of contrast medium injected through the tip of the catheter will usually visualize the site of the orifice of the left coronary artery. If this orifice is located more posterior and superior, counterclockwise rotation is required prior to advancing the catheter so that as the tip rises in the aorta (Fig. 8-7*d*), it will come up just under the orifice and engage it (Fig. 8-7*e*).

When using the multipurpose catheter as opposed to the Sones or Judkins catheters, it is not necessary to enter the left coronary artery completely in order to have adequate visualization. The tip of the catheter is large and delivers a rapid flow rate giving quite adequate visualization of the left coronary system even if the tip is sitting just at the orifice and has not directly entered the artery. Since the tip is riding up off the left coronary sinus, it frequently enters the left coronary artery at a right angle and therefore entering the artery directly is unlikely. Once the artery has been contacted, however, pulling back on the catheter will orient the tip a bit more in the direction of the left coronary artery and give the best opportunity for complete visualization. Since the multipurpose catheter has side holes located just at the tip, there is little risk of wedging the catheter against the coronary wall and causing dissection of the artery. If the tip is against the wall, then much of the dye will be ejected through the side holes at the tip and may still result in adequate visualization of the artery.

If the loop just described is difficult to form and the catheter continues to prolapse into the left ventricle despite this anticipatory maneuver of fly fishing, then another approach must be entertained. At this point, it is worthwhile to turn the catheter in a clockwise direction so the tip points toward the left coronary cusp rather than toward the noncoronary cusp. By advancing the catheter, one can occasionally enter the left coronary cusp directly and then make the maneuver to advance the catheter causing the tip to rise along the left coronary sinus until it engages the orifice (Fig. 8-7*d*). More commonly, when this maneuver is tried, the tip is placed into the right coronary cusp. When the catheter is advanced, the heel will bend in a posterior direction necessitating a good deal of counterclockwise rotation to cause the tip to flip up and back toward the left coronary sinus. This maneuver can be thought of as something of a mirror image of the usual maneuver, flipping out of the noncoronary cusp. We have found this maneuver to be only occasionally helpful, and usually it is best to stick with the original maneuver described, namely flipping the catheter out of the noncoronary cusp up into the left coronary sinus.

Cannulation of the left coronary artery by these maneuvers is possible in almost all patients who have a normal-size aortic root. The greatest difficulty is encountered in women who have a very small aortic root. In this situation, the catheter tip is too long and has too much stiffness to be able to be deformed in the small root, and therefore a loop cannot be adequately formed or when formed, will not fall down on the left coronary sinus properly. Two alternatives are available in this situation. A catheter has been developed with a multipurpose shape which has a more tapered and flexible distal segment that is well-suited for this situation. This more flexible catheter will easily deform even in the smallest aortic root and a loop can be made to enter the orifice as described previously. The other alternative, of course, is to use a 4-cm left Judkins catheter for entering the left coronary artery.

The left Judkins catheter is an ingenious device which is built for one job, namely entering the left coronary orifice. This is ordinarily the catheter selected after the usual maneuvers with the multipurpose catheter have been exhausted. The time required to make this decision is only 2 to 3 minutes of trying by an experienced operator. It becomes obvious very quickly when the left coronary orifice arises so high in the aortic sinus that the multipurpose catheter cannot possibly reach it that it should be exchanged for a Judkins catheter. Inability to form the loop is a less common cause for failure with the multipurpose catheter, but again this can be established in a short time by an experienced operator.

Injection Techniques

After the coronary artery orifice has been entered with the multipurpose catheter, pressure measurements are made. Damping of the pressure curve from insertion of the multipurpose catheter into the left coronary artery is most unusual. If damping is noted, this indicates that the catheter tip is entrapped in the left coronary artery, and it should therefore be removed. If a ventricularized contour is obtained, that is, a pressure tracing in which the diastolic pressure falls dramatically, as in the left ventricular pressure tracing, then the catheter should also be removed. This condition most commonly results from wedging of the catheter into the coronary orifice so that the intramyocardial tension is reflected back into the coronary circulation and to the tip of the catheter. When either a damped or ventricularized pressure contour is obtained from the diagnostic catheter, prompt action must be taken as flow in the artery is impeded at that point. When the catheter is positioned at the orifice of the left coronary artery, a small test injection is made. This not only identifies that the catheter is adequately positioned in the orifice so that the artery will be filled correctly but also identifies obstruction of the artery if the catheter has inadvertently become wedged into the orifice. If there is not rapid clearing of the contrast medium from the artery, then wedging has most likely occurred. The catheter, of course, should be removed in this situation. When proper positioning of the catheter has been achieved and it has been confirmed that there is no damping of the pressure, then the coronary injections can be made.

The Swiss syringe on the end of the manifold which is connected to the catheter is held in the right hand with the plunger end of the syringe higher than the muzzle end in order to ensure that an air bubble will not be injected into the coronary artery. Attempts should be made to clear the syringe of air; however, the operator should assume that some air is present, and therefore during injections the final 1 to 2 mL of contrast medium are never injected; the injection is stopped short of that position. By holding the catheter with the muzzle end down, there is no chance to inject that small amount of air that may reside in the barrel of the syringe. Prior to each injection, a slight aspiration on the syringe will confirm that there is no air within the proximal part of the catheter or the manifold. Some operators prefer to maintain a meticulously controlled closed system and not aspirate at all on the syringe. Others prefer to check before each injection with a slight aspiration. It is not so important which system is used, only that it be confirmed in a systematic and routine fashion that no air is injected.

The rate of injection of coronary arteries is important. It is best to inject rapidly, filling the entire coronary tree within 2 s, and then terminate the injection, allowing the contrast medium to run off while visualizing the coronary artery on cinefluoroscopy. This provides the best opacification and the least ischemia. Prolonged low-flow injections produce streaming with the blood, making interpretation of the coronary arteriogram more difficult, and also extend the time of relative ischemia. We find that slowing of the heart rate is minimized by vigorous short injections into the coronary arteries. Following each injection, the operator should perform several checks: (1) Be assured that the catheter pressure is normal by immediately turning in to pressure. (2) Be assured that the contrast medium has begun to run out of the coronary tree as observed on cinefluoroscopy. (3) Immediately check the patient's heart rate for undue slowing. These items are all checked routinely and simultaneously at the end of each injection.

Filming the Injection

Filming is obtained with the 6- or 7-inch mode in most laboratories. In some cases, this allows for visualization of the entire coronary tree without panning. In other cases, some panning is required. If the field does not cover the entire coronary tree, then the operator should move the tabletop at the termination of each injection so that the distal ramifications of the artery will be seen. In some views, no change in respiratory pattern is needed, while in others deep inspiration is helpful in improving the quality of the images since the diaphragm can be removed from the field of view. When at all possible, the coronaries should be viewed against the lung fields since this reduces the penetration necessary and enables one to operate at a lower kilovolt level; thus improving the contrast and sharpness of the fluoroscopic image.

The instructions for a deep-held inspiration are often misinterpreted by patients. Many patients will breathe in and then perform a Valsalva maneuver which results in a higher diaphragm than even quiet respiration produces. In coaching the patient to remove the diaphragm from the field of view, instructions should be given to breathe in actively and continually during the time of the filming. The success of this maneuver can be improved by having the patient practice once or twice prior to filming the coronary arteries.

Following injection of the coronary arteries, certain physiological reactions are common. There is usually a transient decrease in blood pressure. If the contour of the pressure pulse remains normal and the pressure begins to rise after a few beats, the catheter may be left in place. If any damping or ventricularization of the contour occurs or if the pressure does not rise after a few seconds, then the catheter must be removed from the artery. The transient drop in blood pressure is secondary to direct myocardial depressant and vasodilatory effects of the contrast medium. The patient may experience a tight feeling and begin to cough. The coughing actually is usually beneficial since deep breaths and coughing seem to aid in the passage of contrast medium through the coronary circulation. There is frequently a sensation of discomfort in the chest with each coronary injection. We find no consistent diagnostic value in this discomfort, as some patients with coronary disease will experience a discomfort quite similar to their previous angina pectoris while others will feel entirely different types of pain. Many patients with no angina pectoris at all will have discomfort during injections and patients who have had previous angina but normal coronary arteries may also experience discomfort. We think, therefore, that little emphasis should be placed on the character of the brief discomfort that patients have during the coronary injections. The electrocardiogram frequently undergoes a shift in the ST-T segments during coronary injections. When the left coronary artery is injected, the ST segment will become depressed and the T wave inverted in lead I and the lateral precordial leads while with right coronary injections, the ST segment may become elevated with a peak T wave in the same leads. These changes will usually revert rapidly toward the baseline and should be improving by the time the next injection has been undertaken.

If there is no pain following injection, the heart rate and blood pressure are stable, and the ECG changes have shifted back toward the baseline, then the next coronary injection can be undertaken. It is usually quite satisfactory to wait only 15 to 20 s between injections if these criteria have been met.

RIGHT CORONARY ARTERY CANNULATION

In order to visualize the right coronary artery, the multipurpose catheter is brought into the aortic root in a left anterior oblique (LAO) view with its tip lying anterior and to the patient's left in the left coronary cusp. By rotating the shaft of the catheter clockwise, the tip may be brought anterior and rightward in a sweeping motion around the anterior portion of the aortic root (Fig. 8-8). This brings the shaft portion of the catheter lying in the aortic arch from the upper part of the arch toward the lower part of the arch, thereby causing the tip of the catheter to advance down toward the aortic valve. This downward motion of the tip will be observed even though no advancing of the catheter has taken place. In order to hold the tip at the same level in the aortic sinus, it is necessary, therefore, to withdraw slightly on the shaft of the catheter as the clockwise rotation is being accomplished. Small puffs of contrast medium will help identify the orifice of the right coronary artery during this rotation procedure. When the tip comes to lie just at the coronary orifice, a small test injection is made to identify whether an adequate amount of contrast medium is entering the right coronary artery. Ordinarily the multipurpose catheter does not enter the right coronary artery for any distance since this vessel usually takes off at a right angle or even with an upward turn while the tip of the multipur-

Figure 8-8 (*a*) Cannulation of the right coronary artery (RCA) in the left anterior oblique view. The catheter tip is rotated clockwise and withdrawn slightly until the tip enters the right coronary ostium. (*b*) RCA injection with orifice directly cannulated. (*c*) RCA injection with tip at orifice but not entering. Note adequate filling of the vessel.

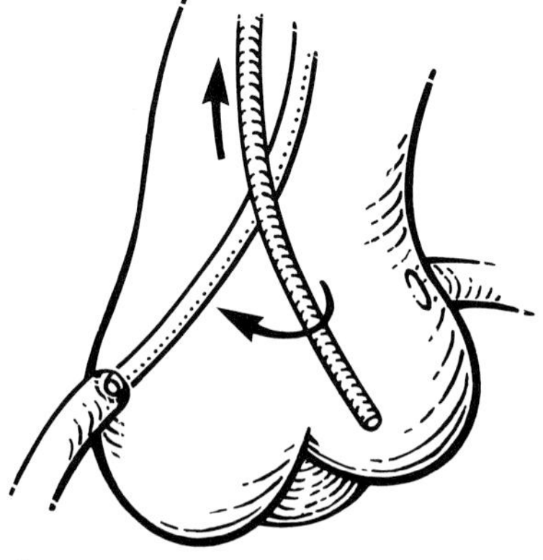

A

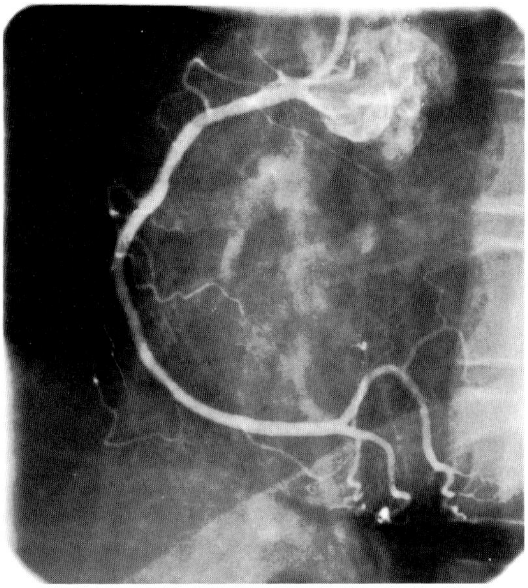

B

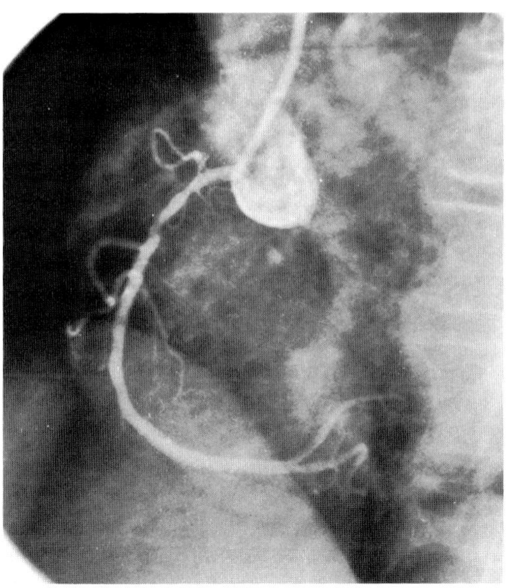

C

pose catheter has a definite downward orientation toward the valve. Occasionally the right coronary artery arises with the proximal portion coursing downward, and in this case the multipurpose catheter can enter the artery deeply. If the catheter does enter the artery and advance for one or more centimeters into the artery, then a slight withdrawal on the catheter will bring it into a more proximal location for injection. Pressures should be checked to rule out the possibility of entrapment of the catheter with resultant damping or ventricularization of the pressure curve and impedence of flow in the artery.

Sometimes it is impossible to achieve a position in the right coronary artery in which damping has not occurred. If that is the case, then the injection can be made rapidly and the catheter removed with no ill effects. It should be stressed, however, that if this occurs, the catheter must be removed between each injection. If the catheter tip is in the orifice and the injection is made with no damping and no impediment to flow, then it is not necessary to remove the catheter at the completion of each injection. The patient or the image intensifier is moved to the next position for injection while the coronary pressure is monitored.

Not infrequently the clockwise rotation and withdrawal of the tip of the right coronary catheter does not result in an adequate position at the orifice. If after several tries at this technique one is unsuccessful, then the maneuver of banking the catheter off the right coronary cusp is employed. With this approach, the catheter is brought by the same clockwise rotation over the right coronary cusp after which it is advanced into the cusp so that the tip will begin to curl in the cusp while the heel of the catheter prolapses over into the left coronary cusp (Fig. 8-9). If the aortic root is large enough, this maneuver will result in the tip riding up in the right coronary cusp gradually to the level of the orifice. When this maneuver is used, it is common for the tip to enter the right coronary orifice, whereupon slight withdrawal of the catheter will result in further travel of the tip down the coronary artery. If this happens, one should continue to withdraw the

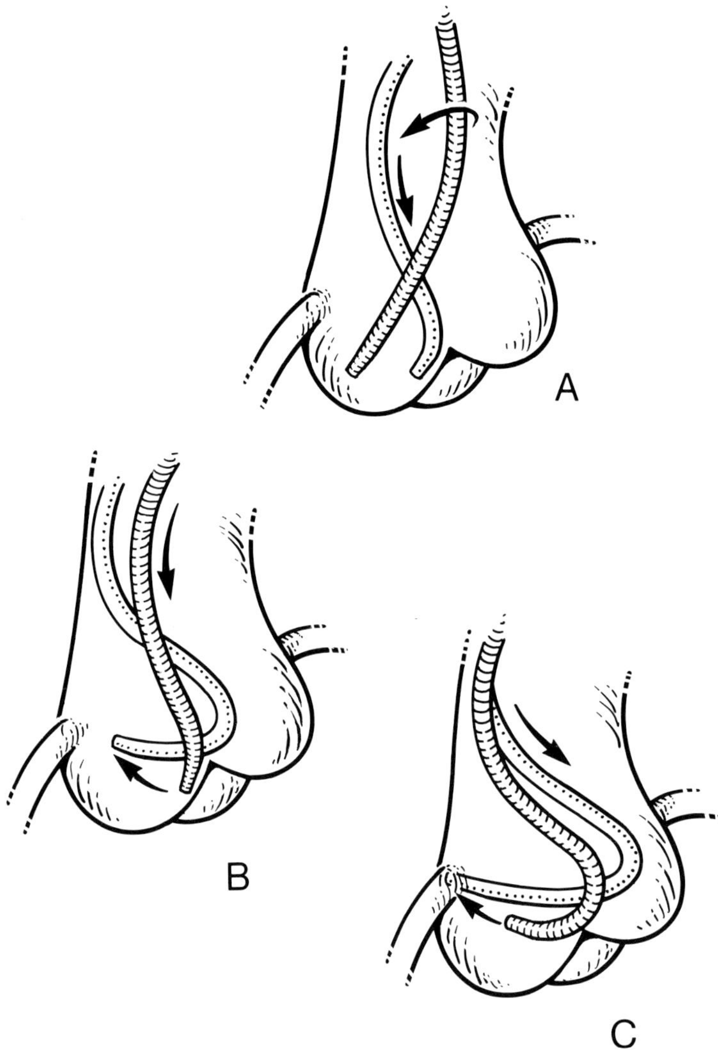

Figure 8-9 Cannulation of the right coronary artery in the left anterior oblique view. (*a*) The tip is rotated clockwise into the right coronary cusp and gradual advancement of the catheter is made until the tip begins to buckle. (*b*) The tip will then ride up in the right coronary cusp and (*c*) enter the orifice of the right coronary artery.

catheter until it lies in a proper position just inside the right coronary orifice. Small puff test injections will demonstrate whether there is any impediment to flow, and if there is not, the catheter can be maintained in a fairly deep position in the artery for a short time without fear of inducing ischemia.

Injection Techniques

If following any injection there is failure of the contrast medium to clear rapidly or if pressure measurements are damped or ventricularized, the catheter should be withdrawn. If these events do not occur, it is not necessary to withdraw the catheter, and in fact it may be safer to leave the catheter in the coronary artery between injections. With right coronary injections, it is important for the patient to perform deep inspirations, particularly in the left anterior oblique view so that the posterior descending and left ventricular branches of the artery can be seen free of the diaphragm. The size of the right coronary artery is so variable that it is impossible to predetermine the amount of contrast medium needed for adequate filling. It is therefore important to inject rapidly so that the artery is filled and to then terminate the injection promptly. Somewhere between 2 and 6 mL of contrast medium are usually required for the right coronary artery, and injections with a high flow rate over a short period of time are preferable to prolonged slow-flow injections in the right coronary artery for the same reasons as were enumerated for the left.

In our experience, the right coronary artery is somewhat more difficult to intubate than the left using the multipurpose technique. Approximately 10 percent of the patients cannot have adequate opacification of the right coronary artery using this catheter. After a brief trial of intubating the right coronary, an operator should change to a Judkins right coronary catheter.

PROBLEM AREAS IN PERFORMING CORONARY ARTERIOGRAPHY

Short Left Main or Separate Orifice for Left Anterior Descending and Circumflex Arteries

When the left main coronary artery is very short or there are actually separate orifices for the left anterior descending (LAD) and circumflex arteries, there may be difficulty filling both arteries from a single left coronary injection. There have been many examples of failure to study the LAD or circumflex coronary artery because of subselective cannulation of the other vessel and failure to recognize that the vessel had been missed. It is important to evaluate the left ventricle from the standpoint of the vessels needed to supply the total circulation. If these vessels are not seen and there is no hint of total occlusion or collateral filling, then an effort should be made to identify the missing orifice. With the multipurpose technique, it is unusual in the short left main situation or in separate orifices to totally miss the other vessels since subselective cannulation is unusual. It is, however, possible and if the catheter seems to enter the LAD, for instance, but does not enter the circumflex, then the circumflex should always be looked for in a more posterior location by rotating the catheter tip counterclockwise deep in the cusp prior to moving it upward toward the orifice. Similarly if the LAD has not been visualized, its takeoff will be anterior to the circumflex and can be best looked for by clockwise rotation prior to bringing the tip up out of the left coronary cusp.

In the absent left main situation when the left anterior descending orifice is superior and the circumflex orifice is inferior (toward the valve), the multipurpose catheter will enter the circumflex selectively. Sometimes it is impossible to maneuver the multipurpose catheter beyond this orifice from below. A Judkins catheter coming down from above will selectively enter the LAD, solving the problem (Fig. 8-10).

When the left coronary orifice is very high near the sinotubular ridge, it appears also to be very posterior because of the orientation of the aortic root (Fig. 8-11). This problem can often be solved by placing the catheter tip in the left coronary cusp through the usual maneuvers and then with severe counterclockwise rotation advancing the catheter so the tip will ride up very superior and posterior until it reaches the orifice of the left coronary artery. Posterior rotation sometimes has to be made so severely that the tip may flip out of the left coronary cusp. At the point just before it flips out of the cusp in a posterior direction, the catheter should be advanced up, engaging the orifice of the left coronary artery. Once the artery is engaged, a slight clockwise rotation and pulling back on the catheter will orient it so that it will hold in the left coronary orifice.

Anomalous Origin

The most common anomaly of the origin of the coronary arteries is the origin of the circumflex artery from the right coronary cusp or from the right coronary artery itself. If in studying the left coronary system it is discovered that the circumflex artery is not being filled and no explanation for that is found by injecting the right coronary artery, i.e.,

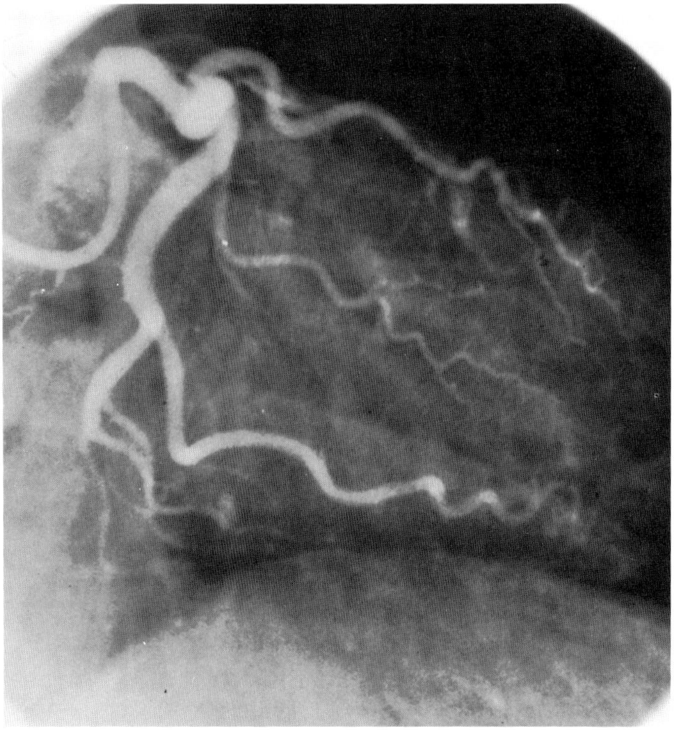

A

Figure 8-10 Selective cannulation of the left anterior descending artery (LAD) at the circumflex arteries because of a very short left main. (*a*) Right anterior oblique view (RAO) of left coronary with multipurpose catheter in the circumflex orifice. (*b*) Left anterior oblique view (LAO) of left circumflex injection showing LAD orifice slightly superior. (*From King SB III, Douglas JS: Coronary arteriography and left ventriculography, in Hurst JW (ed):* The Heart (4th ed). *McGraw-Hill, New York, 1978, p 403, fig 29D-2b.*) (*c*) RAO view of LAD injection, (*d*) LAO view of LAD injection. Note the Judkins catheter was necessary in order to adequately fill the LAD in this case.

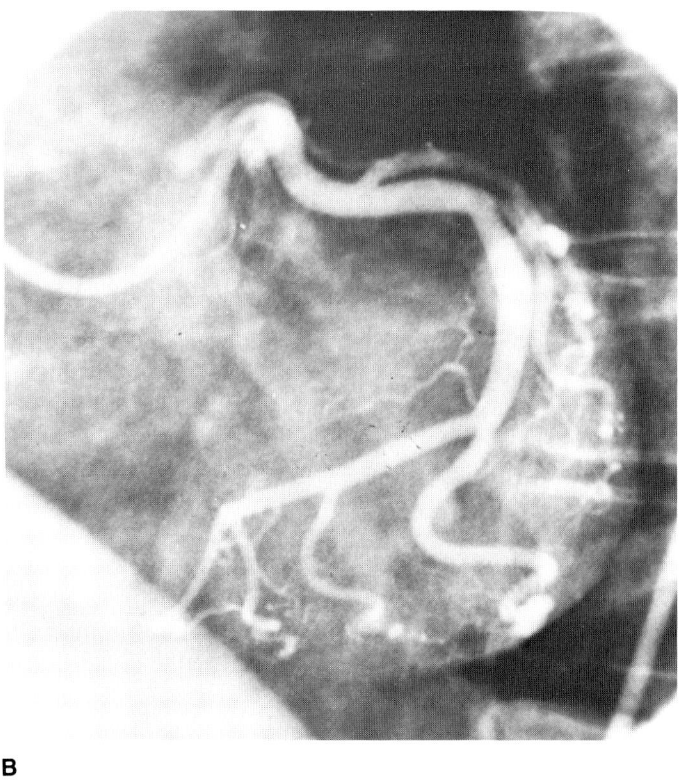

B

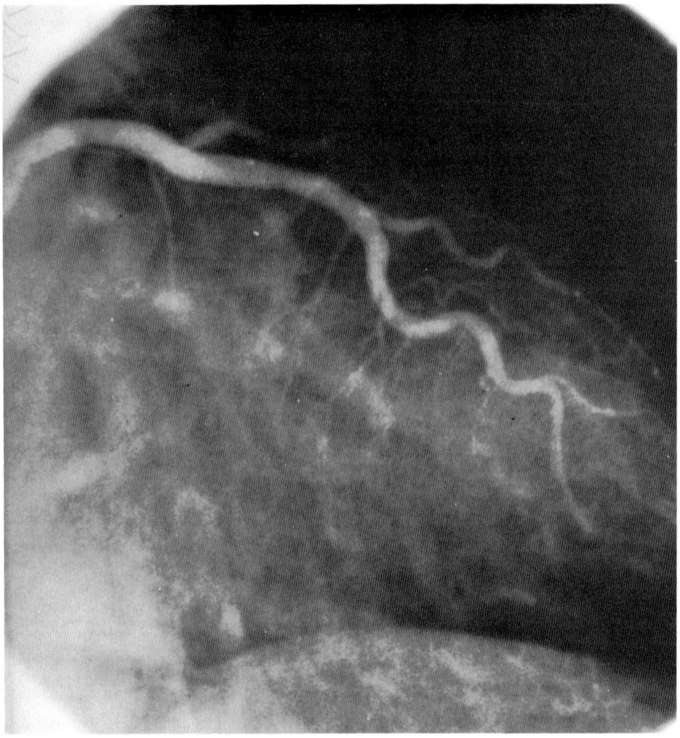

C

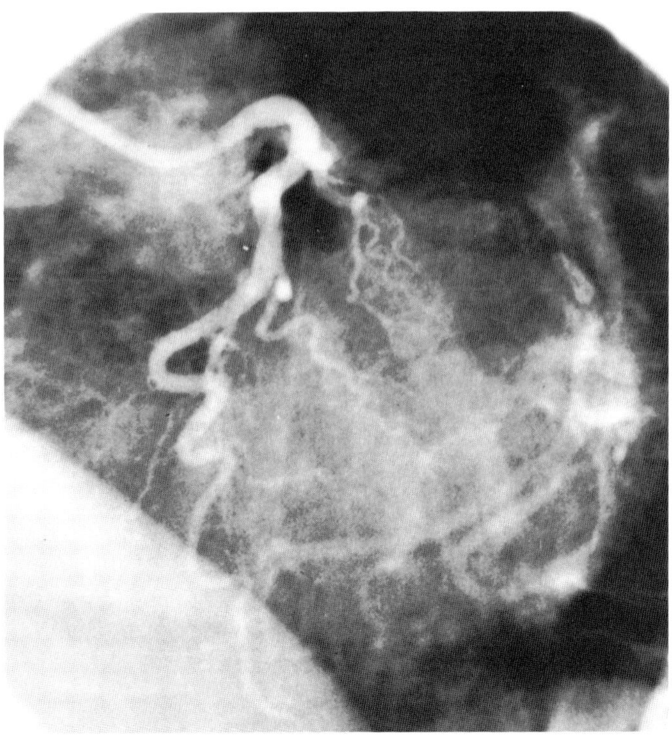

D

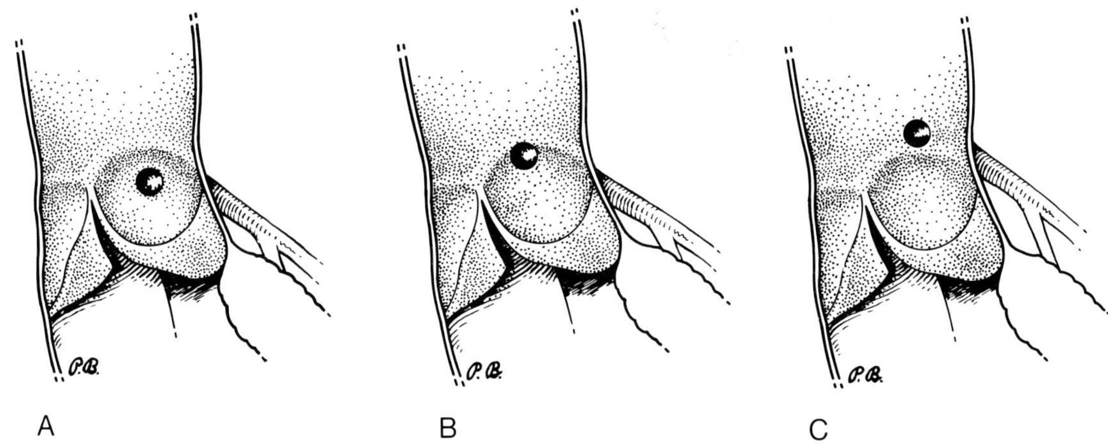

Figure 8-11 Location of left coronary orifice. (*a*) Mid-sinus location. (*b*) High position near the sinotubular ridge. (*c*) Extremely high position above the sinotabular ridge making cannulation with the multipurpose catheter unlikely.

the right artery does not continue past the crux and give very high left ventricular branches to take the place of the circumflex, then an anomalous origin of the circumflex should be looked for. With the multipurpose technique, it is usual that an injection of the right coronary artery will fill both the right and the anomalous circumflex. With other techniques, the right coronary artery may be entered deeply and the circumflex artery may be missed. If the catheter enters the anomalous circumflex artery, a note of caution should be issued. The circumflex always takes off at a sharp angle from the right aortic cusp and therefore any catheter entering it will be oriented perpendicular to the artery, so an injection should be made with caution since dissection of the circumflex artery is quite possible with this orientation (Fig. 8-12).

The entire left coronary artery may also arise from the right coronary cusp (see Chap. 3). The left coronary may arise from the right coronary artery or arise separately, usually anterior and leftward of the right coronary orifice. The angle between the left coronary artery and the wall of the aorta is quite acute, and therefore when the catheter enters, it has a tendency to impinge on the outer wall of the left coronary artery. Caution should be exercised when injecting in this position so as not to create a dissection of the left coronary artery.

Conus Branch

There are several problems related to catheterizing the right coronary artery which one should be aware of. As the catheter is rotated clockwise in an attempt to enter the right coronary artery, the conus branch may be entered. This will be seen as a small branch coursing over the right ventricular outflow tract. One may misinterpret the conus branch as being a nondominant right coronary artery and thus fail to catheterize and film the right coronary itself. When the conus branch does arise as a separate vessel, it is almost always anterior to the right coronary itself. Several attempts at passing the conus branch may be required in order to reach the right coronary artery.

When a nondominant right coronary artery is entered and injected, one sees early bifurcation of the vessel with two equal-sized vessels commonly arising within 1 to 3 cm of the orifice (Fig. 8-13). This appearance is usually quite different from a totally occluded right coronary artery which was previously large and supplied the posterior descending branch. If the left coronary has already been filmed, then it is clear that the posterior descending is arising from the circumflex branch if a true nondominant right artery exists. In many patients, however, there is a codominant posterior

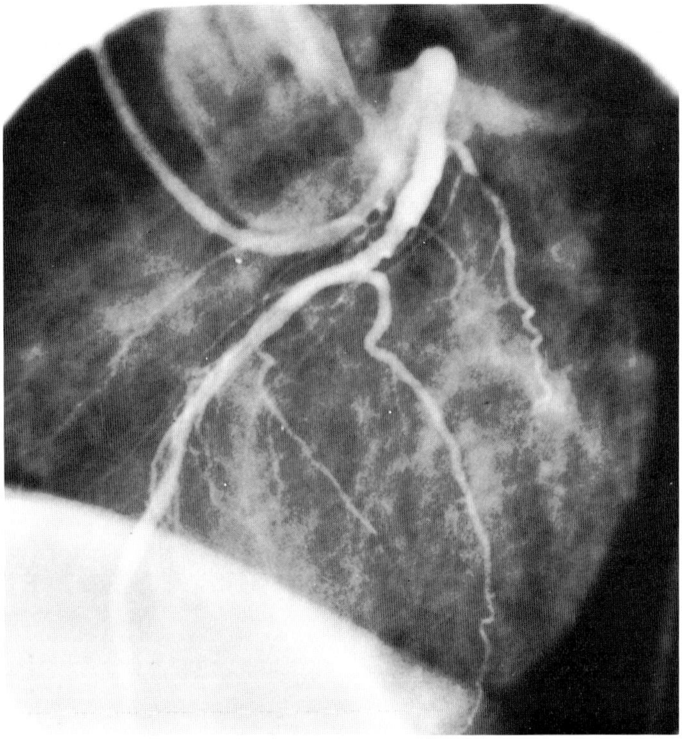

A

Figure 8-12 (*a*) Injection of left coronary artery fails to fill the circumflex in the left anterior oblique (LAO) view. (*b*) Right anterior oblique (RAO) view of left injection with contrast medium in cusp still failing to fill the circumflex artery. (*c*) LAO view of injection of anomalous circumflex artery arising beside right coronary orifice. (*d*) RAO view of circumflex injection. Note angulation of tip of catheter in the proximal circumflex and the posterior course of the circumflex behind the aorta. (*From King SB III, Douglas JS: Coronary arteriography and left ventriculography, in Hurst JW (ed)*: The Heart (4th ed). *McGraw-Hill, New York, 1978, p 404, fig 29D-3.*)

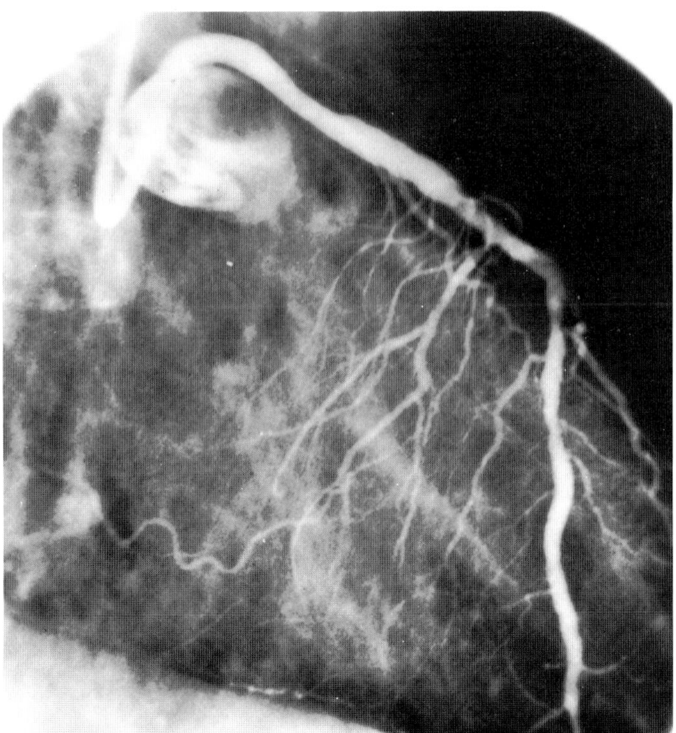

B

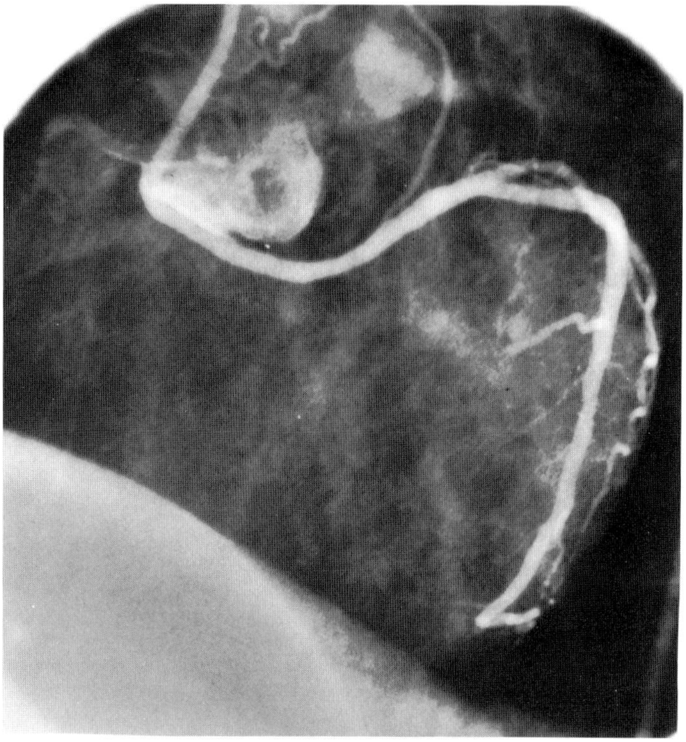

C

(Figure 8-12, continued)

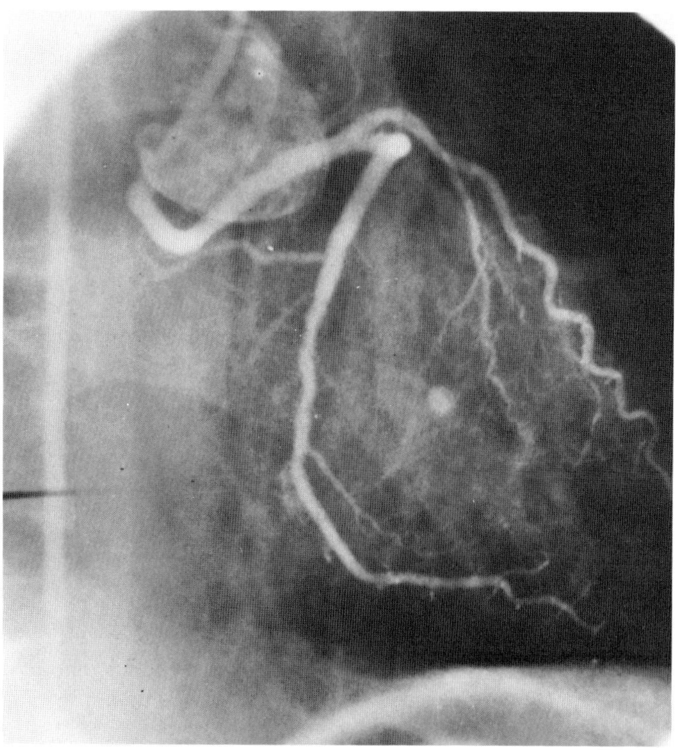

D

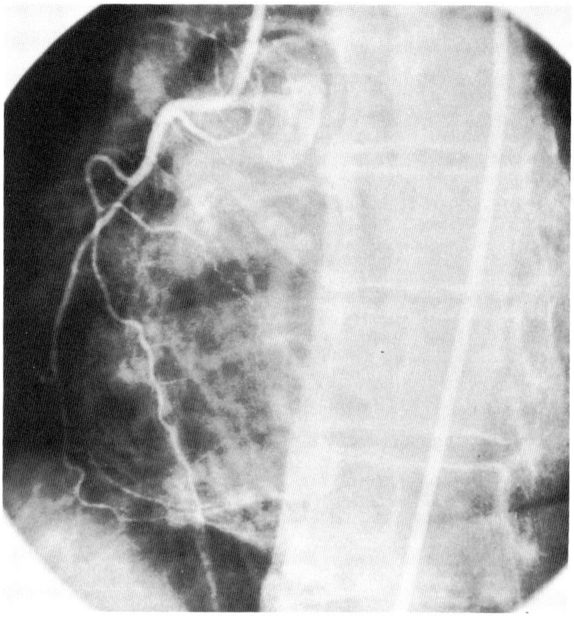

Figure 8-13 Left anterior oblique view of nondominant right coronary artery.

circulation in which posterior descending branches arise both from the left circumflex and from the right coronary artery. It is therefore important to recognize whether one has filmed a nondominant right, a conus branch, or a totally occluded right coronary artery.

Occasionally no artery can be seen arising from the right coronary cusp. In this case, the artery should be searched for in the left coronary cusp. When found there, it usually arises separately from the left coronary orifice. A clue to the right coronary artery's existence can be found on the aortic root injection or left ventriculogram.

The multipurpose catheter is well-suited for searching for these anomalous origins of coronary arteries since it can be easily rotated in a 360° pattern in the aortic root. Preformed catheters are designed for entering the left and right coronary arteries in their usual locations. They are not well-designed for the purpose of searching for anomalous vessels; they will frequently move only to the usual location and thus be unable to enter the anomalous branch.

Coronary Spasm

Coronary spasm occurring in the course of coronary arteriography is not an unusual finding. When it does occur, it is important for the arteriographer to identify that spasm is occurring so that nitroglycerin can be administered and the spasm relieved, otherwise the final interpretation of the film may be confusing and a lesion may be interpreted where none existed. Spasm most commonly occurs at the tip of the catheter especially when catheterizing the right coronary artery. The appearance is somewhat characteristic, with a smooth, hourglass shape, at both the inflow and outflow portions of the spastic segment. Despite that usual appearance, spasm is often confused with fixed coronary obstructions during the course of an arteriogram and therefore when any question arises, nitroglycerin should be administered and angiograms should be repeated several minutes following that administration in order to document that spasm has been cleared. If a segment of suspected spasm fails to clear with sublingual nitroglycerin, then intracoronary nitroglycerin should be administered and a repeat angiogram performed (Fig. 8-14).

Despite one's best intentions to give nitroglycerin when suspicious areas are seen during catheterization, occasionally arteriograms are performed and spasm goes undetected until the completion of the procedure. When one reviews the films, the points that favor coronary spasm as opposed to fixed lesion include a smooth, hourglass appearance of the defect and its occurrence at the tip of the arteriographic catheter. These findings can also occur in fixed coronary obstruction, and therefore the most reliable sign is a variation in the degree of stenosis between views. If there is a marked difference in the lumen diameter reduction seen in various views, then coronary spasm may be the explanation. Spontaneous spasm unrelated to the catheter stimulation and testing for spasm with ergot derivatives is discussed in Chap. 4.

Myocardial Bridging

The coronary arteries may dip beneath the myocardial surface and a bridge of myocardium may override the coronary artery (see Chap. 4). In this situation, systolic compression of the artery may be seen due to contraction of the overlying myocardium. This will leave the appearance of a defect in the coronary artery during systole, but the defect will be absent in diastole and should never be confused with a fixed coronary obstruction.

Catheterization of Saphenous Vein Bypass Grafts

The area of the aorta most accessible for placement of the proximal anastomosis of the saphenous vein bypass grafts is the anterior surface. For that reason, bypass grafts are located anteriorly, and frequently the anastomotic sites are one on top of the

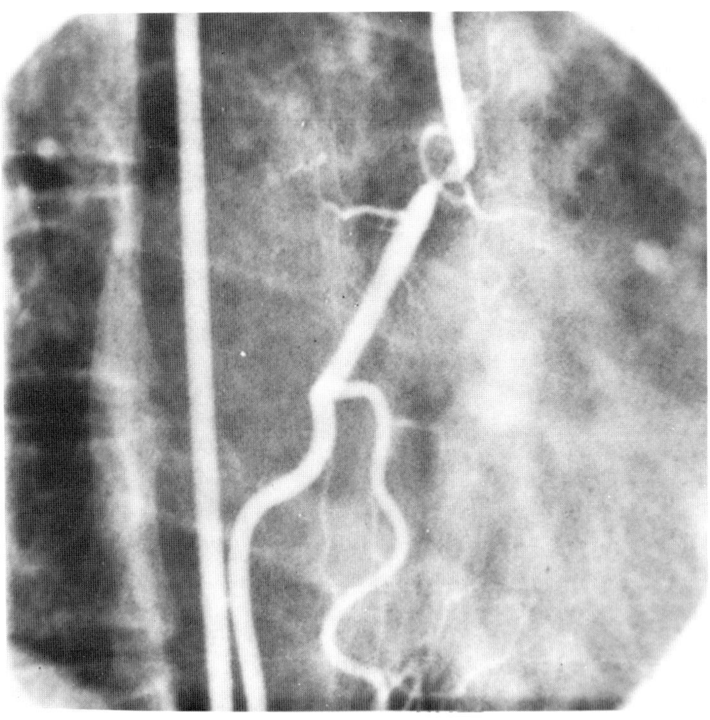

Figure 8-14 Right anterior oblique view of right coronary injection showing catheter tip spasm.

other starting in the tubular portion of the aorta. Some surgeons place the grafts one on top of the other in a vertically ascending position while others have some grafts more rightward and some more leftward but always on the anterior portion of the aorta. If the grafts are located anteriorly and slightly rightward or toward the outside curve of the aorta, then their position is quite similar to that of the right coronary orifice, only higher in the aortic root. When that is the location of the graft anastomosis, the multipurpose catheter can be rotated in the same manner as for cannulation of the right coronary artery (Fig. 8-15). Frequently, however, the orifice of the graft is more central or leftward, in which

Figure 8-15 Cannulation of the saphenous vein grafts using the multipurpose catheter. The catheter is rotated clockwise and withdrawn until it approximates the origin of each saphenous vein ostium. Once the ostium is contacted, slight advancement of the catheter will usually cause the heel of the catheter to buckle somewhat, thereby stabilizing the position for injections.

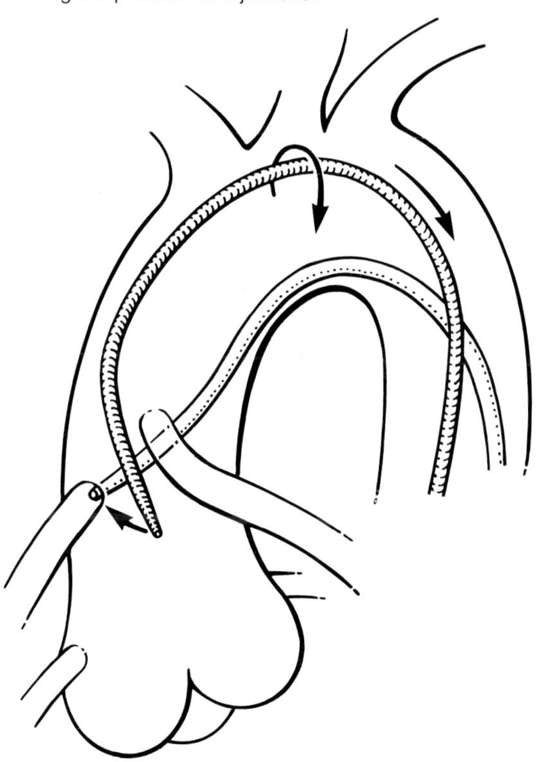

case the graft is encountered much more anterior and to the left than the usual right coronary artery location. The multipurpose catheter is quite good for reaching those locations. If the surgeon places some radiopaque material such as a small surgical washer or a silver clip at the site of each bypass graft, this facilitates location of the anastomotic site.

Sometimes the origin of the graft is so far anterior and leftward that it is on the inside or lesser curve of the aortic root. If that is the case, the usual maneuvers to engage the orifice are quite difficult. We find that by forming a more acute angle on the distal shaft of the multipurpose catheter leaving a long tip which will reach across the entire width of the aortic root at approximately a 90° angle, the vein orifice can be entered. This cannulation is frequently impossible with the standard right Judkins catheter and therefore the multipurpose or the modified multipurpose catheters with the 90° turn are quite beneficial. Newer multipurpose catheters with more pliable tips can be looped in the aorta so that pulling up under a graft site permits direct entrance into the graft. When the tip of the multipurpose catheter has reached the level of the vein bypass graft and made contact with its orifice, continued advancement of the catheter will sometimes result in an improved entry of the tip into the orifice of the graft. If the orientation of the vein is so superior that it is difficult to gain entry and proper opacification of the vein, then a further modification of the tip can be achieved by making a curve that exceeds 90° and comes around as something of a shepherd's crook resembling an Amplatz curve. These shapes can be easily achieved by the use of a shaping wire and a steam kettle in the laboratory. The catheter tip is heated by the steam emanating from the spout of the kettle and then the catheter is immersed in cold sterile water or saline to fix the curve in the position desired.

When the vein graft cannot be identified, several points are helpful in identifying that it is occluded. The site of an occluded vein graft often will consist of a small dimple in the aortic wall. The tip of the catheter can be placed in this area and an injection made in order to document the dimpling effect at the site. If a native coronary artery which had been grafted is seen to fill by antegrade flow or by collateral circulation, then the graft is either totally occluded or functionally occluded. If a graft were open with adequate circulation, there would be no opportunity for the artery to fill by collateral channels. Sometimes the vein graft will be seen to fill in a retrograde fashion during the native coronary injection. Continued filming after the injection will show runoff through the graft back into the native artery when the graft is present and functionally intact.

It is necessary to place the catheter tip at each vein graft site. Flush injections into the aorta have frequently resulted in inadequate filling of vein grafts and a false impression that the grafts are occluded when actually they may be present but simply did not fill by the flush technique.

Internal Mammary Injection

When the internal mammary artery has been chosen for bypass grafting, special techniques are necessary to opacify it. The most commonly used internal mammary artery is the left one, which arises from the subclavian artery a few centimeters distal to the takeoff of the left vertebral artery. This branch originates on the caudal and slightly anterior surface of the subclavian vessel. Although the multipurpose catheter can be directed into the subclavian artery, it is unusual to get direct cannulation of the internal mammary with that catheter. We prefer, therefore, to change to an internal mammary catheter which has a final tip curve greater than 90° facilitating entry into the vessel. By passing the catheter into the left subclavian artery with the tip pointed caudad, the subclavian artery may be entered 3 to 5 cm past the origin of the subclavian (Fig. 8-16). The internal mammary can be identified as a single branch passing directly caudal and parallel to the sternum. Sometimes one will pass the orifice of the mammary and go beyond it in the subclavian. In that case, the catheter can be withdrawn holding the tip in a caudal and slightly anterior position until it pops into the mammary orifice. The internal mammary catheter has a tip which we feel is slightly longer than it needs to be and for this reason it may enter the mammary artery for a greater distance than is desired. One should do careful test injections into the internal mammary artery before doing the actual angiogram because the tip may enter the artery deeply and dissection of the internal mammary artery may be possible from such a location. Injection of contrast medium into the subclavian artery predictably causes a significant amount of discomfort due to perfusion of some of the skeletal muscle branches of the artery in its upper portion or because of the splashover of dye into the subclavian and its proximal branches. The patient needs to be warned of this discomfort and injections need to be held to a minimum.

Although the left internal mammary artery is more commonly used, the right internal mammary artery is also used by a number of surgeons. The right mammary takes off the subclavian artery in a position just beyond the origin of the carotid artery and is entered in a manner similar to the left mammary artery. The preformed internal mammary catheter can usually be directed into both the left subclavian and the right innominate arteries without great difficulty if a counterclockwise rotation of the catheter is made just outside the orifice of those vessels. This brings the primary curve of the catheter away from its natural tendency to traverse the aortic arch and go down toward the aortic sinuses and directs it instead to the outside of the aortic arch so that it will enter the subclavian or innominate artery. Since the tip has a curve greater than 90°, it is occasionally difficult to enter these branches, and therefore a safety guidewire through the catheter will be required.

ADEQUACY OF VIEWS

Regardless of whether the native coronary circulation or the vein graft or internal mammary artery is opacified, it is critical that adequate views be taken to assess the vessel throughout its entire length so that each segment is seen without undue fore-

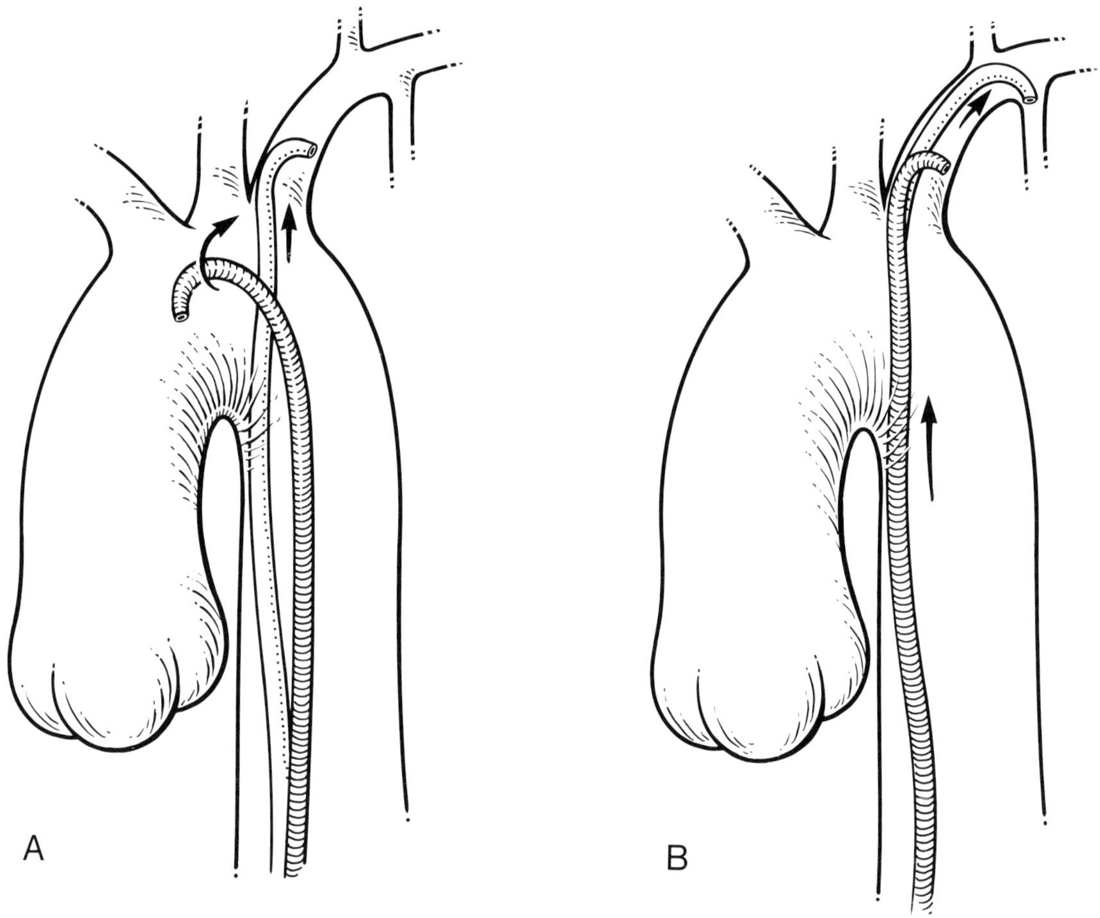

Figure 8-16 Cannulation of the internal mammary artery using an internal mammary catheter. (*a*) The catheter is positioned in the aortic arch and rotated counterclockwise until the tip pops into the subclavian artery. (*b*) The catheter is then advanced out the subclavian artery until it enters the internal mammary artery. Sometimes a slight anterior rotation of the tip is necessary in order to enter the artery.

shortening and without overlap from other vessels. These views will be described in detail in Chap. 9. A predetermined number of views is not important, rather it is important that at the time of arteriography, the operator carefully reviews each injection to determine that the goal of seeing each segment free of significant foreshortening and overlap has been achieved. When a lesion is being observed, extra attention must be paid to characterize that lesion as accurately as possible in multiple views keeping in mind the constraints of undue administration of contrast medium and the problem of inducing myocardial ischemia in patients with severe coronary disease.

REMOVAL OF CATHETER

When one is satisfied by the video replay that all necessary views of the coronary arteries and left ventriculogram have been obtained and the patient is in a stable situation, then the catheter can be removed. The removal is a simple procedure and does not require reinsertion of the guidewire. The catheter is pulled so that only approximately 20 to 30 cm remain inside the femoral artery. At that point, an assistant attaches a 20-mL syringe to the tip of the catheter. The operator grasps the catheter with the right hand near the femoral puncture site and places the left index and middle finger over the skin directly above the arterial entry site. While the assistant is applying negative pressure to the syringe, the operator withdraws the catheter briskly from the puncture site, allowing a gush of blood from the puncture site to occur momentarily, and then compresses the artery to obtain hemostasis (Fig. 8-17). This process of suction and flushing of the puncture site occasionally will dislodge some small thrombus that has occurred around the catheter or at the puncture site. Although no such thrombus is usually seen, this precautionary measure has proved effective in avoiding femoral thrombosis and distal embolization. Compression of the artery can usually be obtained with the two fingers of the left hand although in some patients with hypertension or considerable subcutaneous tissue, it is necessary to place the right hand on top of the compressing fingers of the left hand in order to gain adequate tamponade of the vessel. Compression adequate to prevent bleeding or hematoma formation is maintained but not so much compression as to totally eliminate the femoral pulse. Periodic monitoring of the pedal pulses is maintained throughout the time that the artery is being held in order to ensure adequate flow. This is important, especially in patients with very small femoral arteries and patients with low stroke volume such as those with cardiomyopathy or severe mitral stenosis. In such patients, undue compression can lead to femoral thrombosis.

Severe spasm of the femoral artery occluding the vessel is uncommon, and loss of pulse is more likely produced by thrombosis. In any case if spasm is suspected or if occlusion occurs very early after removal of the catheter, then an attempt at relieving spasm should be undertaken. If the catheter has not been removed, then 25 mg tolazoline can be injected through the catheter into the femoral artery just proximal to the puncture site. If the catheter has already been removed, a no. 20 needle can be inserted into the femoral artery just above the puncture site and again tolazoline can be injected. Rapid downstream vasodilatation will occur, producing a flushed appearance of the entire extremity if antegrade flow is achieved.

If the femoral artery is totally occluded, then the flushing will stop at the upper thigh showing a line of demarcation and indicating that there may be future problems with occlusion of the femoral artery. This maneuver has been used only rarely, and femoral occlusion requiring thrombectomy has occurred in only 0.04 percent of the patients catheterized in our laboratory. There has not been an example of the loss of an extremity in the cases catheterized to date. Management of complications of catheterization such as femoral occlusion and hematoma formation are discussed in Chap. 11.

Following removal of the catheter, compression of the artery as described is maintained for approximately 15 minutes or until hemostasis is ensured. The area around the puncture site should be observed closely for any swelling representing hematoma formation and then a tightly double-folded stack of three 4 × 4 inch gauze pads should be applied over the femoral puncture site and secured with elastic tape so as to provide mild compression during the ensuing several hours of bed rest. The patient is returned to bed and is kept in a near-supine position although some elevation of the head and shoulders can be accomplished without interfering with the puncture site. It is important that the patient not bend the hip joint since this will move the femoral artery and may lead to late bleeding. In order to aid the patient, a folded bed sheet is placed over the catheterized leg at the knee and tucked under the bed on either side in order to mildly restrain the leg and to remind the patient not to move the leg during the recovery period. Bed rest is usually recommended for 6 hours following catheterization after which time the nursing personnel can let the patient up, observe the femoral area for any late bleeding, and check for postural hypotension.

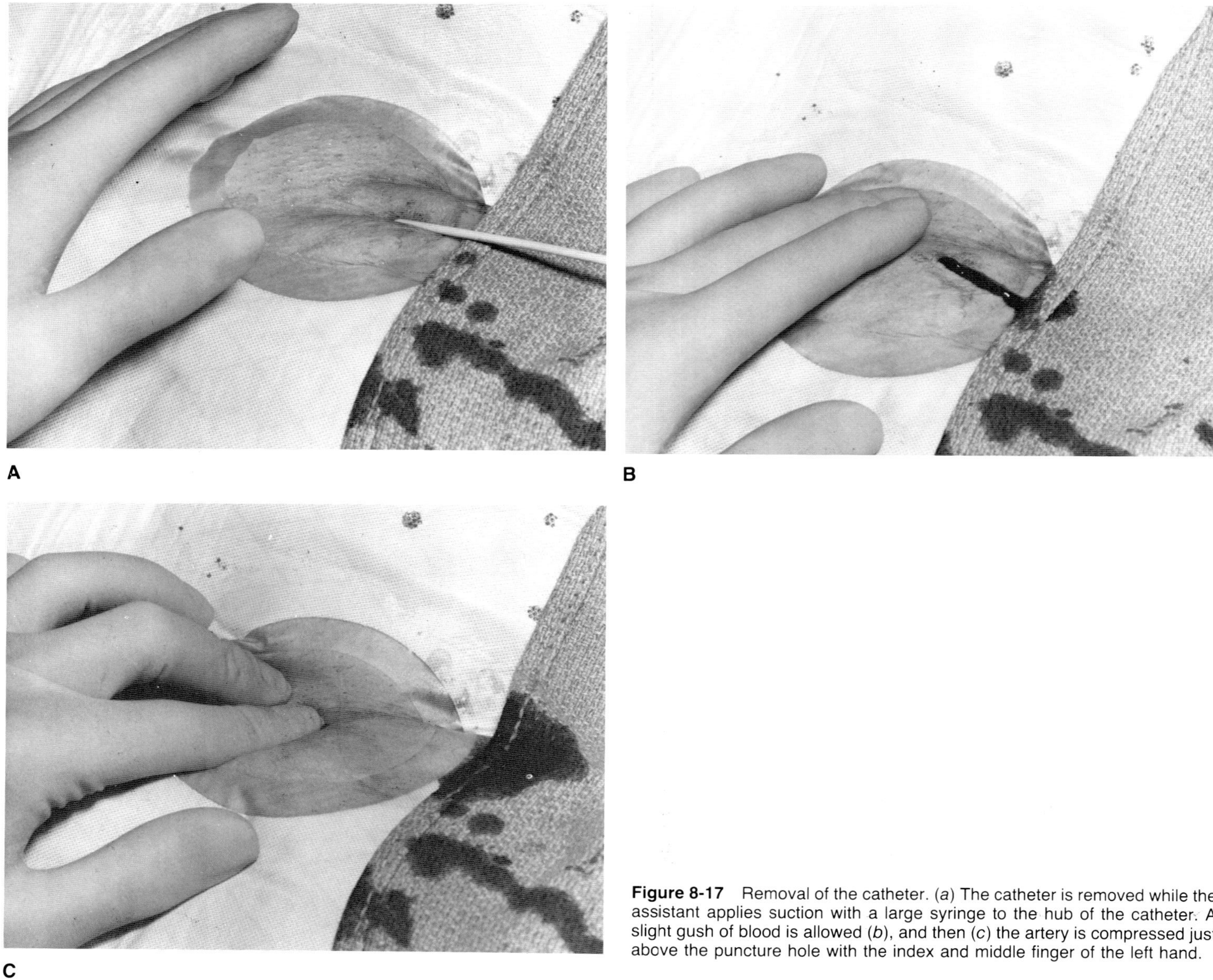

Figure 8-17 Removal of the catheter. (*a*) The catheter is removed while the assistant applies suction with a large syringe to the hub of the catheter. A slight gush of blood is allowed (*b*), and then (*c*) the artery is compressed just above the puncture hole with the index and middle finger of the left hand.

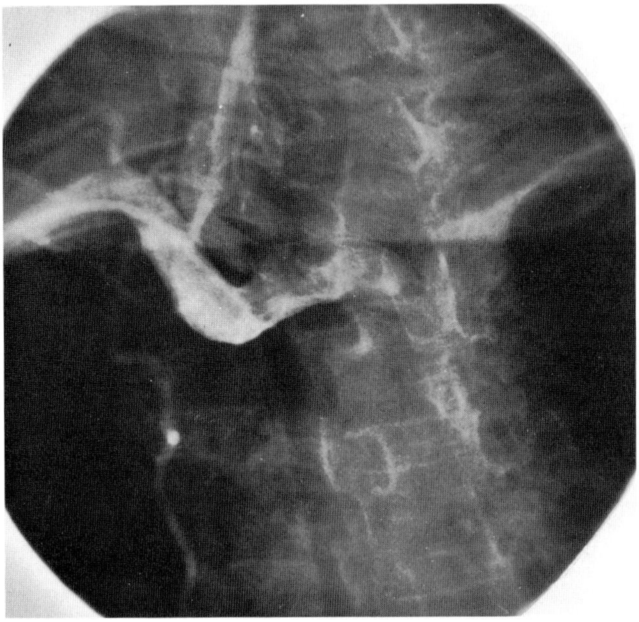

A

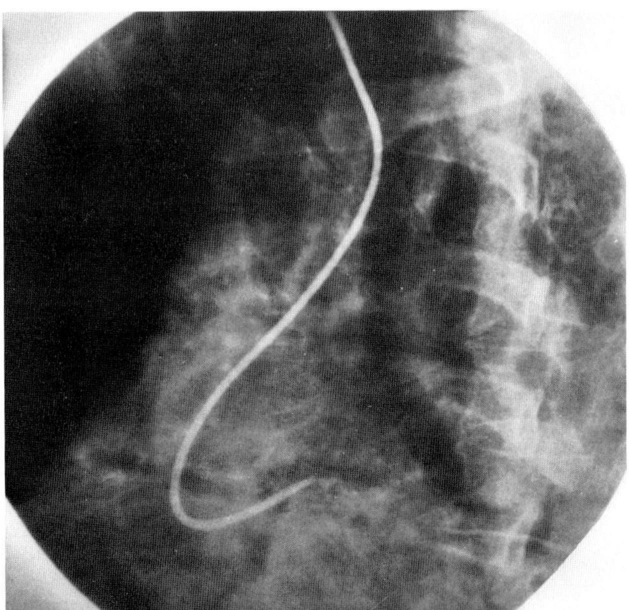

B

Figure 8-18 Percutaneous brachial artery catheterization. (*a*) The catheter is advanced from the brachial artery over a guidewire around the tortuous subclavian artery. (*b*) The tip is then advanced down into the aortic sinuses. (*c*) The tip is then maneuvered up through an approach similar to the femoral technique engaging the left coronary orifice. (*d*) Injecting the left coronary artery.

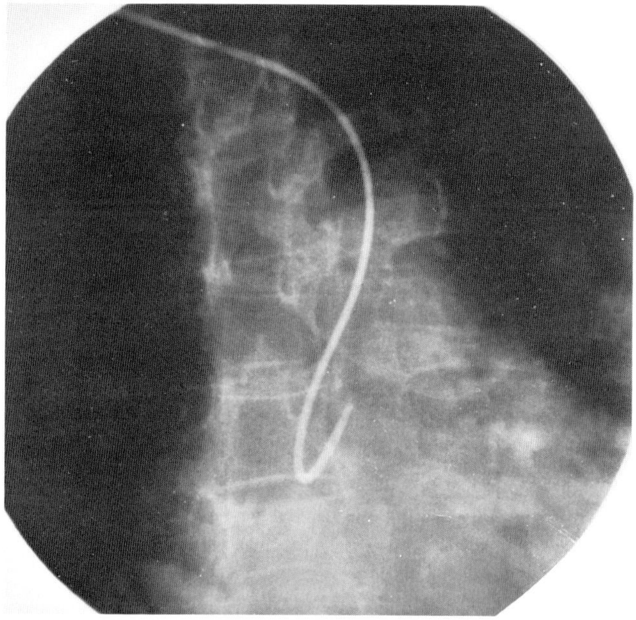

C

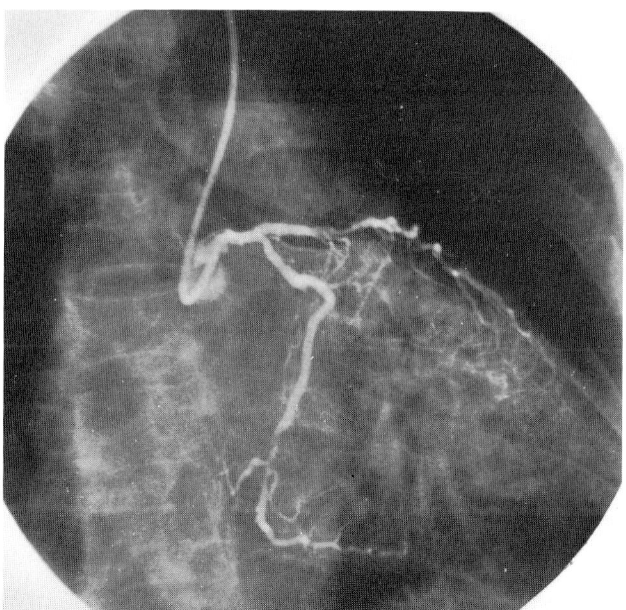

D

ADDITIONAL APPROACHES WITH THE MULTIPURPOSE CATHETER

When the patient has severe femoral or iliac disease precluding catheterization from the leg, the option has been to change to the Sones technique. It is possible, however, to use the percutaneous approach either from the brachial or the axillary artery. In our laboratory, we have performed approximately 200 brachial percutaneous coronary arteriograms from the right or left brachial artery. Patients selected for this technique are those with a large palpable brachial artery pulse and have been men in most cases. The incidence of loss of brachial pulse is quite low. The same precautions should be taken as for the Sones technique, namely checking the adequacy of the circulation of the arm and hand (see Chap. 6).

The Seldinger approach is accomplished in a similar manner as described for the leg and the guidewire inserted to the level of the shoulder. A no. 7 vascular dilator is inserted and removed and followed by a no. 7 multipurpose A2 catheter. The guidewire is passed all the way around the shoulder into the subclavian artery and into the ascending aorta. The subclavian vessel is frequently tortuous and therefore the guidewire is essential in making this maneuver so as to not cause damage to the subclavian artery. Manipulations of the catheter once it is in the ascending aorta are quite similar to those used in catheterizing the coronary arteries by the femoral approach (Fig. 8-18).

An alternate method of coronary arteriography has been described by Dr. Bernard Valeix and colleagues from Marseille, France.[7] They performed 105 transaxillary coronary arteriograms using both the left and right brachial arteries with a vascular sheath in place. The complication rate using this sheath in their hands has been quite low. They also have used the Judkins and Bourassa catheters from the left axillary approach in a manner similar to the femoral technique of coronary arteriography.

Both these approaches are alternatives to the Sones technique when the femoral approach is not possible due to lower extremity vascular disease. In our experience, the need to go to the arm is limited to under 1 percent of our cases.

REFERENCES

1 Schoonmaker FW, King SB III: Coronary arteriography by the single catheter percutaneous femoral technique: Experience with 6800 cases. Circulation, 50:735, 1974.
2 Seldinger SI: Catheter replacement of the needle in percutaneous arteriography: A new technique. Acta Radiol Scan, 39:368, 1953.
3 Ricketts HJ, Abrams HL: Percutaneous selective coronary cine arteriography. JAMA, 181:620, 1962.
4 Takaro T, Hultgren HN, Littman D, Wright EC: An analysis of deaths occurring in association with coronary arteriography. Am Heart J, 86:587, 1973.
5 Amplatz K, Formanck G, Stranger P, Wilson W: Mechanics of selective coronary artery catheterization via femoral approach. Radiology, 89:1040, 1967.
6 Judkins MP: Selective coronary arteriography. I. A percutaneous femoral technique. Radiology, 89:815, 1967.
7 Valeix B, Labrunie P, Levy S, Gerrard R: Selective coronary arteriography by percutaneous transaxillary approach: Value in peripheral arterial disease of the lower limbs (submitted for publication in "Archives des Maladies du Coeur et des Voisseaux.")

Chapter 9

New Radiographic Views for Imaging the Coronary Anatomy

John S. Douglas, Jr., M.D.
Spencer B. King III, M.D.

DEVELOPMENT OF SAGITTALLY ANGLED VIEWS

Since the performance of the first selective coronary arteriogram by Sones over 25 years ago,[1] angiographers have struggled with the problem of selecting angiographic views to clearly delineate coronary anatomy[2]. The tortuosity of the coronary arteries, multiple branch points, motion, vessel overlap, and the presence of eccentric atherosclerotic lesions provide a constant challenge. Basic rules in radiology applicable to all organ systems point out the need for at least two views of the region of interest with projections being roughly perpendicular to each other. When tubular structures such as arteries or bones are studied, the direction of the x-ray beam should be perpendicular to the long axis of the structure. However, during the first 15 years of coronary arteriography, visualization of coronary arteries was limited to views which were perpendicular to the long axis of the body rather than perpendicular to the arteries being examined. A conventional vertical x-ray beam was used, and the patient was simply rotated from side to side to obtain multiple views in the transverse plane (Fig. 9-1).

By 1972, over 20,000 coronary arteriograms had been done at the Cleveland Clinic alone, and other centers were reporting their large experiences with coronary arteriography using views limited to those in the transverse plane.[3–6] Not surprisingly, early reports of the interpretation of coronary arteriograms revealed a great interobserver and intraobserver variability. A study of cardiac anatomy quickly reveals that the orientation of the long axis of the heart is leftward and anterior and the course of the major epicardial coronary arteries from base to apex is also leftward and anterior. Although it may be

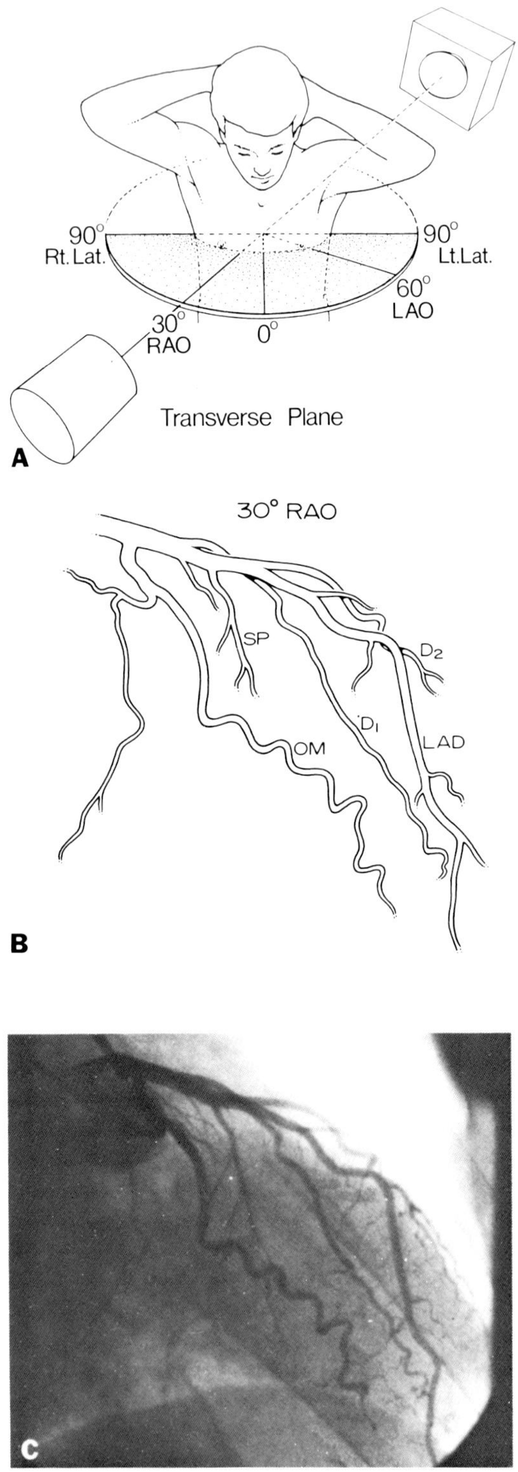

Figure 9-1 Diagrammatic representation of the standard right anterior oblique (RAO) view of the left coronary arteriogram. The x-ray source is beneath the patient, the x-ray beam travels in a posterior-to-anterior direction, and the image intensifier is overhead. Most of the left coronary artery is well-visualized in this projection, although there is considerable overlap of the mid–left anterior descending coronary artery and the diagonal branches. When the left main, circumflex, and diagonal branches have a leftward initial course, the long axis of these arterial segments is projected away from the image intensifier, preventing optimal visualization in this view. (*From King, Douglas, Morris,*[24] *with permission of the authors.*)

possible to solve some problems related to overlapping vessels by performing numerous views in the transverse plane (Figs. 9-2 and 9-3), one often is forced to make judgments about arterial segments seen "on end" or with considerable foreshortening. This is particularly true when the anterior descending, posterior descending, and obtuse marginal branches are visualized in left anterior oblique projections. This leads to misinterpretation. When eccentric stenoses are present, a decrease in opacity of an arterial segment may be the only clue to high-grade stenosis unless one views the artery from multiple projections perpendicular to the long axis of the artery. In addition, branch points of many coronary arteries are not well seen in any projection selected in the transverse plane.

In 1973, Bunnell[7] reported on the advantages of views of the left coronary artery obtained by angling the x-ray beam in the sagittal plane (Fig. 9-4), that is, the x-ray beam was angled along the long axis of the body. He reported that incorporating these sagittally angulated views materially improved angiographic assessment of the proximal left coronary artery in 33 of 72 (46 percent) unselected coronary arteriograms. Other angiographers quickly reported and continue to report their experiences with this new dimension.[8–23] Initially, standard large-film studies were performed.[7–9] However, by elevating the patient's upper trunk on pillows,[10] or on a polystyrene wedge,[16] investigators were able to utilize a conventional vertical x-ray beam to obtain cine coronary arteriograms with angulation of the x-ray beam in the sagittal plane. Subsequently, the radiological equipment industry, related to coronary arteriography, was revolutionized.

At the present time, there are a great variety of commercially available x-ray systems for coronary arteriography which are capable of directing the x-ray beam through a wide range of angles in sagittal and transverse planes. These modern systems have brighter images with better resolution. In addition, the availability of high-quality video tape and video disk systems permits immediate replay to determine adequacy of documentation of the anatomy. The burden has shifted more than ever to the angiographer to ensure that every coronary arterial segment is well-visualized by selection of proper views. One simply cannot assume that a fixed selection of left and right coronary views will be adequate.

TERMINOLOGY

The terms used in the literature to describe angle views in coronary arteriography (half axial, caudocranial, craniocaudal, lordotic, right posterior oblique, etc.) are confusing[7–9,12,23–25] (Table 9-1). This is related in part to the fact that radiologists and cardiologists use different nomenclatures. The radiologist defines x-ray beam orientation from the x-ray tube to the image intensifier (or film changer). This terminology results in the PA (posteroanterior) chest x-ray. In most coronary arteriography laboratories, the same x-ray beam orientation results in a "anterior or frontal" view. Similarly, when the under-the-table x-ray tube is moved toward the feet and the overhead image intensifier moved toward the head (30° cranial in Fig. 9-4 or Fig. 9-5*a*) the radiologist's term to describe this view is *caudocranial*, since the x-ray beam passes in a caudal to cranial direction. However, it is simpler to indicate angulation of the x-ray beam in the sagittal plane by referring only to the location of the image intensifier. If the image intensifier is moved toward the head 30° from vertical as in Fig. 9-5, this may be described as a 30° cranial view (rather than caudocranial), and if moved toward the feet 15° as in Fig. 9-6, this is a 15° caudal view.

This nomenclature has been adopted by the authors and others[21,23–25] and greatly simplifies terminology. The picture obtained is that which the viewer would have if his or her face were in the same position as the image intensifier. In the standard right anterior oblique (RAO) view, the viewer would be looking at the right anterior chest (Fig. 9-1), and in the left anterior oblique (LAO) cranial view, the coronaries would be viewed as if one were looking over the left shoulder of the patient (as in Fig. 9-5, 45° LAO, 30° cranial). The cranial

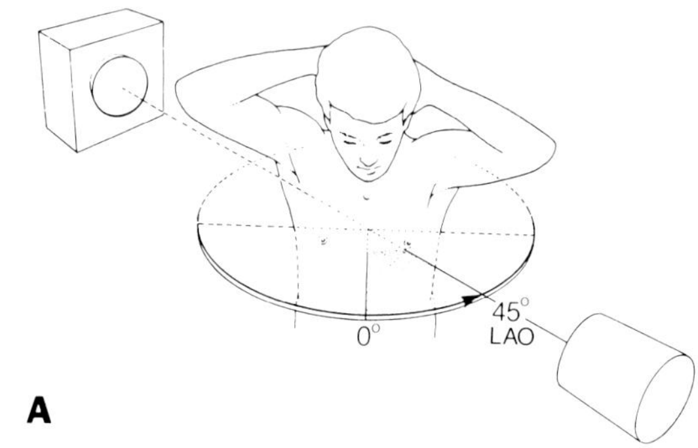

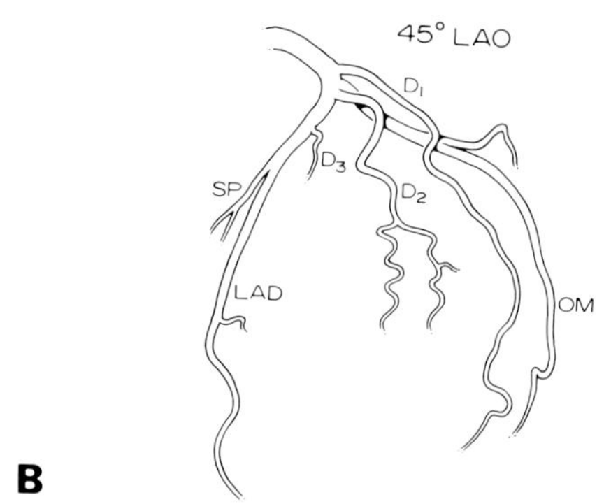

Figure 9-2 Diagrammatic representation of the left anterior oblique (LAO) left coronary arteriogram. The image intensifier is above the patient in the LAO position, and the x-ray beam travels in a posterior-to-anterior direction. The value of this view depends in large part on the orientation of the long axis of the heart. When the heart is relatively horizontal, the left anterior descending (LAD) coronary artery and diagonal branches are seen end on throughout much of their course. In this illustration, the heart is in an intermediate position, and there is moderate foreshortening of the LAD and diagonal branches in their proximal portions. The LAO projection is frequently inadequate to visualize the proximal LAD and its branches, the left main, which is directed toward the image tube and therefore foreshortened, and the proximal circumflex coronary artery, which may be obscured by overlapping vessels as in this illustration. The LAO projection is frequently used to visualize the proximal circumflex when there is not overlap, the distal LAD and its branches, the midcircumflex coronary artery in the atrioventricular groove, and the distal right coronary artery when it is filling via collaterals from the left coronary artery. (*From King, Douglas, Morris,*[24] *with permission of the authors.*)

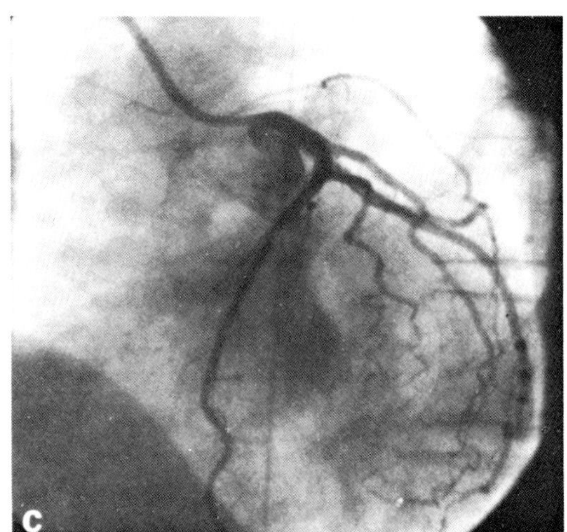

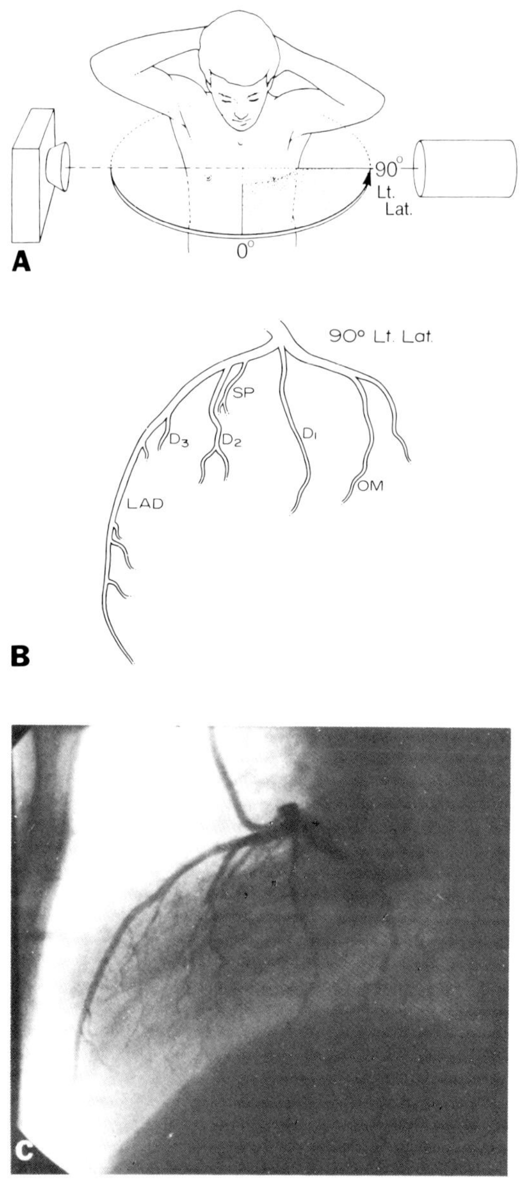

Figure 9-3 Diagrammatic illustration of the 90° left lateral coronary arteriogram of the left coronary. The image intensifier is on the patient's left and the x-ray beam has a right-to-left direction in the horizontal plane. The lateral view of the left coronary artery is most useful for analyzing the proximal and mid LAD by avoiding overlap with the diagonal branches, which commonly take an inferior course from the LAD in this projection. The most proximal portion of the diagonal branches may not be well-visualized since the long axis of these segments may be in the direction of the x-ray beam. The leftward-directed left main coronary artery segment and the proximal circumflex are foreshortened in this view (compare with Fig. 9-2). (*From King, Douglas, Morris,*[24] *with permission of the authors.*)

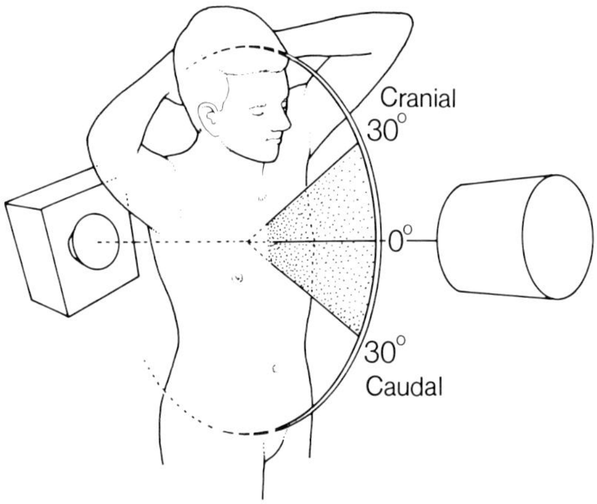

Figure 9-4 Illustration of angulation of the x-ray beam in the sagittal plane. The image intensifier is above the patient and the direction of the x-ray beam is posterior to anterior. (*From King, Douglas, Morris,*[24] *with permission of the authors.*)

RAO view allows one to peer at the coronary arteries from a position over the right shoulder (Fig. 9-7), while the caudal RAO and caudal LAO are views from the liver and spleen, respectively. The degree of rotation in the transverse plane is measured from the midline (i.e., a left lateral projection is a 90° left lateral) and angulation in the sagittal plane from the vertical as in Fig. 9-4. Using this simple terminology, all coronary arteriography views can be clearly described by the location of the image intensifier alone.

Table 9-1 Glossary of Terms

Old Term	New Term
Caudocranial	Cranial
Lordotic LAO	LAO cranial
Half-axial	LAO cranial
Prop-up view	Cranial
Lordotic right posterior oblique	LAO caudal
Craniocaudal	Caudal
"Liver" view	RAO caudal
"Spleen" view	LAO caudal
"Spider" view	LAO caudal
Lordotic RAO	RAO cranial

CHOICE OF VIEWS

To achieve optimal accuracy in evaluating a coronary arterial stenosis, it should be visualized perpendicular to the course of the arterial segment without overlap and circumferentially to detect maximal luminal reduction by an asymmetric lesion. In practice, this can be achieved best by the performance of several routine views of the coronary arteries and then special views to highlight segments of interest or segments not adequately visualized. The routine views in our laboratory are as follows: Left coronary artery: 10° RAO, 30° RAO, 45° to 60° LAO, 45° to 60° LAO/ 30° cranial, 45° RAO/15° cranial, 30° to 45° RAO with 15° caudal. Right coronary artery: 30° RAO, 45° to 60° LAO. LAO projections are selected to avoid superimposing the coronary arteries over the spine and in cranial LAO views, to display the coronary arteries between the spine and the right hemidiaphragm.

As indicated in Chap. 6 to 8 and 11, not all patients can tolerate a full coronary arteriogram, and procedures are tailored for the individual patient. In stable patients, the angiographer can choose the special views necessary to evaluate arterial segments in question by making mini-injections in various views, finally settling on the optimal view, which is filmed with a full 4-to 8-mL injection of contrast medium. The choice of special views will be influenced by orientation of the heart (horizontal versus vertical), by complexity of the arterial tree, and by location of disease: Our choice of views to evaluate problem areas in various arterial position is as follows.

Left Main Coronary

Visualization of the left main coronary artery is critical and problematic. Pathological studies commonly show a significant underestimation of disease by angiography. The single best view is a shallow RAO during which forceful contrast injection produces reflux into the aorta and visualization of the ostium. A second view is necessary, and the 45° LAO/30° cranial view is usually best

A

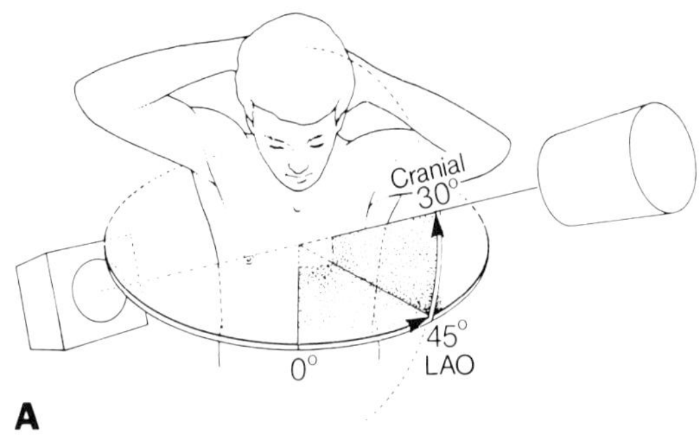

B

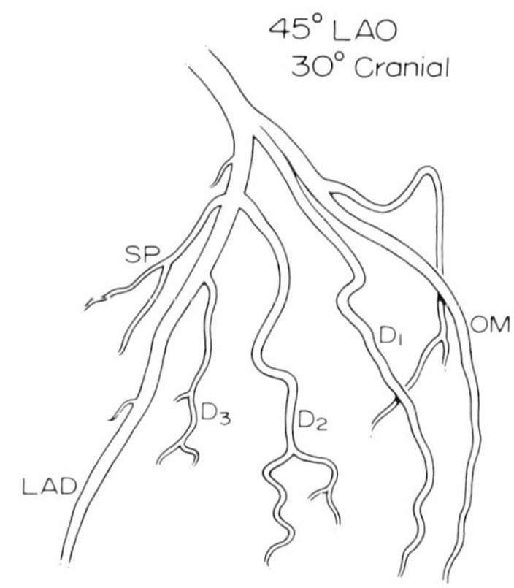

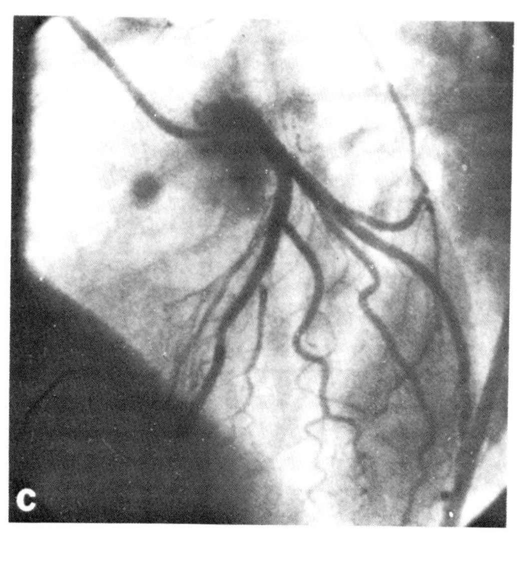

Figure 9-5 Diagrammatic illustration of the left coronary arteriogram in the 45° left anterior oblique (LAO) with 30° cranial angulation. The image intensifier is on the patient's left and the direction of the x-ray beam is posterior to anterior. This is the most valuable view of the left coronary artery in most patients. Foreshortening of the left main and proximal LAD and diagonal branches, which occurs in the LAO view, is usually overcome by cranial angulation of the intensifier. The proximal left coronary artery segments are usually visualized at an angle almost perpendicular to their long axis. The ostium of the left main coronary artery, the proximal portion of the LAD, and the origin of the diagonal branches are usually well-visualized without overlap (compare with Fig. 9-2). Some overlap may occur with branches of the proximal circumflex coronary artery, and this may be overcome by using a 60° LAO with 30° cranial angulation. The value of the LAO cranial view is considerably less when the proximal left coronary artery has a cephalad direction, in which case caudal angulation of the image intensifier is frequently helpful. (*From King, Douglas, Morris,*[24] *with permission of the authors.*)

C

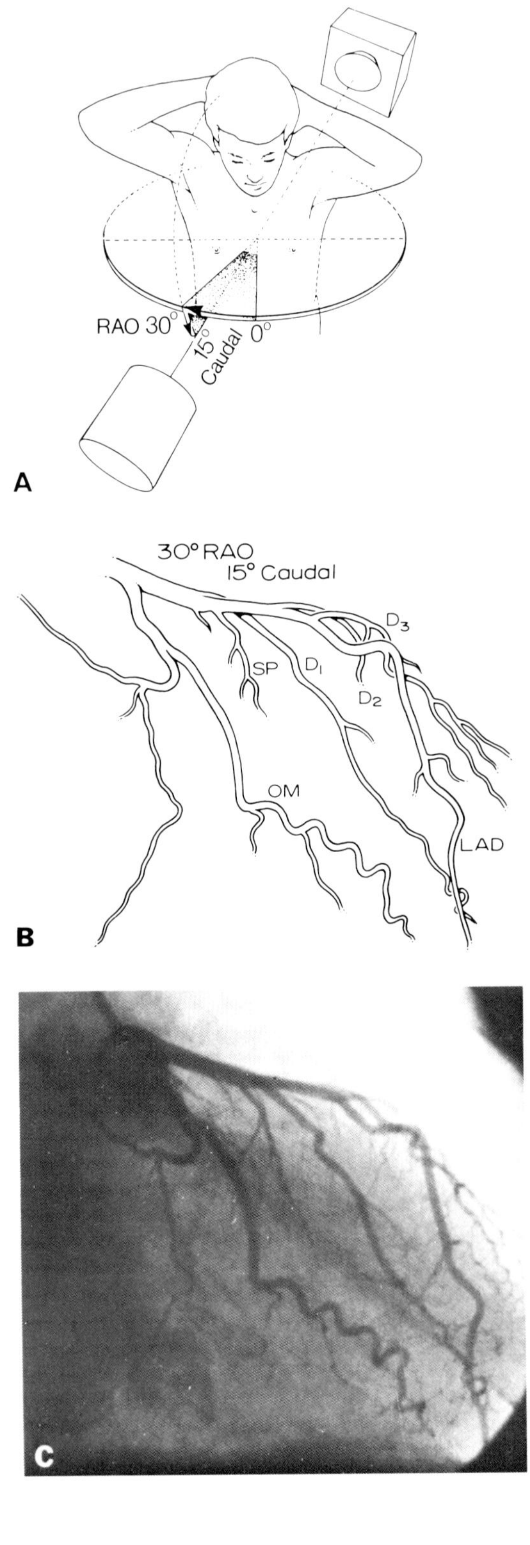

Figure 9-6 Diagrammatic illustration of the left coronary arteriogram in the 30° right anterior oblique (RAO) with 15° caudal angulation of the image intensifier. The image intensifier is positioned over the patient's liver and the direction of the x-ray beam is posterior to anterior. This view is helpful to unravel overlapping diagonal branches, to better visualize the proximal portion of the circumflex coronary artery, whose long axis was parallel to the x-ray beam in the routine RAO view, and to better visualize the mid LAD, which overlaps diagonal branches in the standard RAO views. In this illustration, the mid LAD is well-visualized, as is a portion of the first diagonal, not well-visualized in the RAO view. There is slight unfolding of the proximal circumflex artery, as well. (*From King, Douglas, Morris,*[24] *with permission of the authors.*)

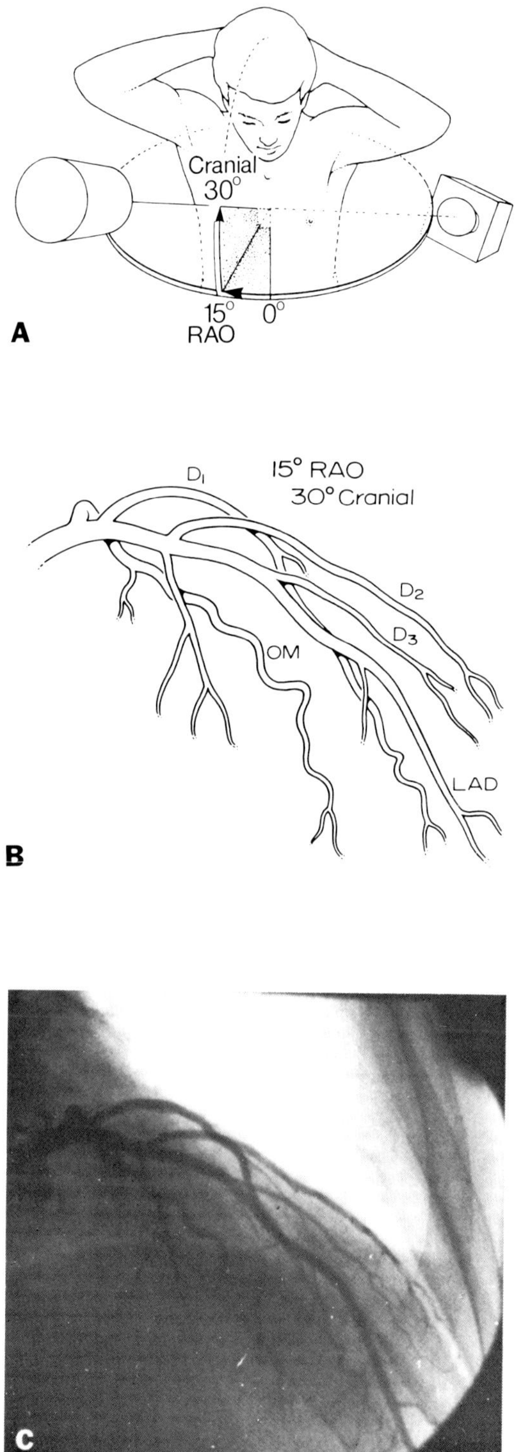

Figure 9-7 Diagrammatic illustration of the left coronary arteriogram in the 15° right anterior oblique view with 30° cranial angulation. This view is particularly helpful in analyzing the mid–left anterior descending coronary artery and the origin of diagonal arteries and septal perforating arteries. Overlap with diagonal branches is usually avoided. The origin of the circumflex artery may be well seen, as in this illustration. (*From King, Douglas, Morris,*[24] *with permission of the authors.*)

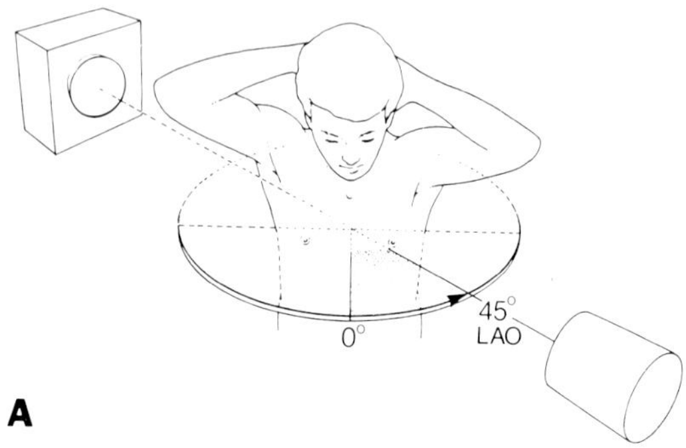

A

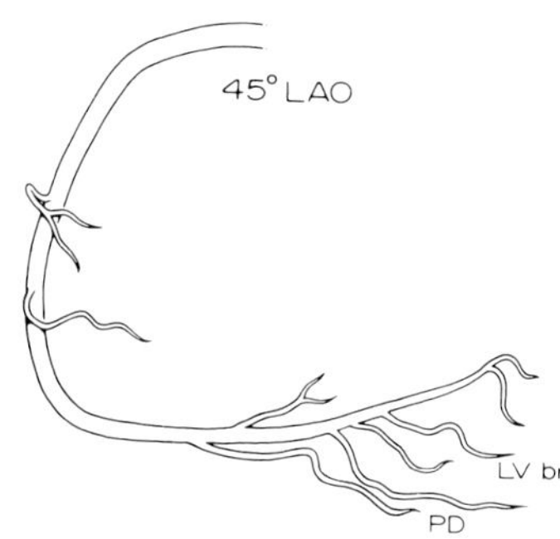

B

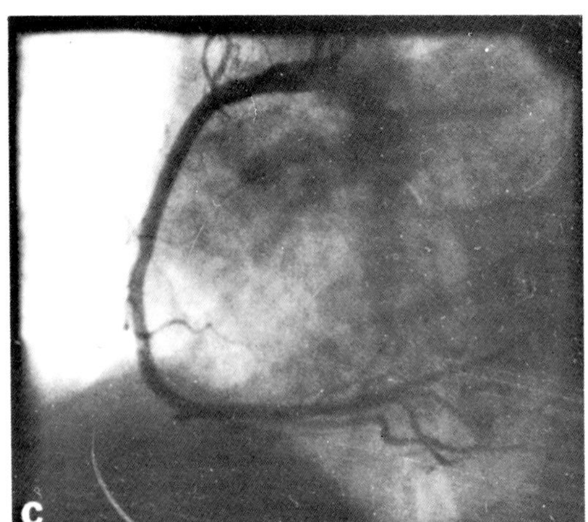

Figure 9-8 Diagrammatic illustration of the right coronary artery in the 45° left anterior oblique projection. The image intensifier is positioned on the patient's left and the x-ray beam travels in a posterior-to-anterior direction. This view is excellent for visualizing the proximal, mid, and distal right coronary artery in the atrioventricular groove since the direction fo the x-ray beam is perpendicular to these arterial segments. Ostial lesions of the right coronary artery are not well-visualized if the proximal right coronary artery takes an anterior direction from the aorta and therefore travels in a direction parallel to the x-ray beam. This can usually be overcome by turning to a more steep left anterior oblique projection. The posterior descending and left ventricular branches of the right coronary artery, which pass down the posterior aspect of the heart toward the apex, may be severely foreshortened since the long axis of these vessels is in the same direction as the x-ray beam. The proximal portion of the posterior descending branches can be visualized by cranial angulation of the overhead intensifier (see Fig. 9-9) or with a right anterior oblique view with cranial angulation. (*From King, Douglas, Morris,*[24] *with permission of the authors.*)

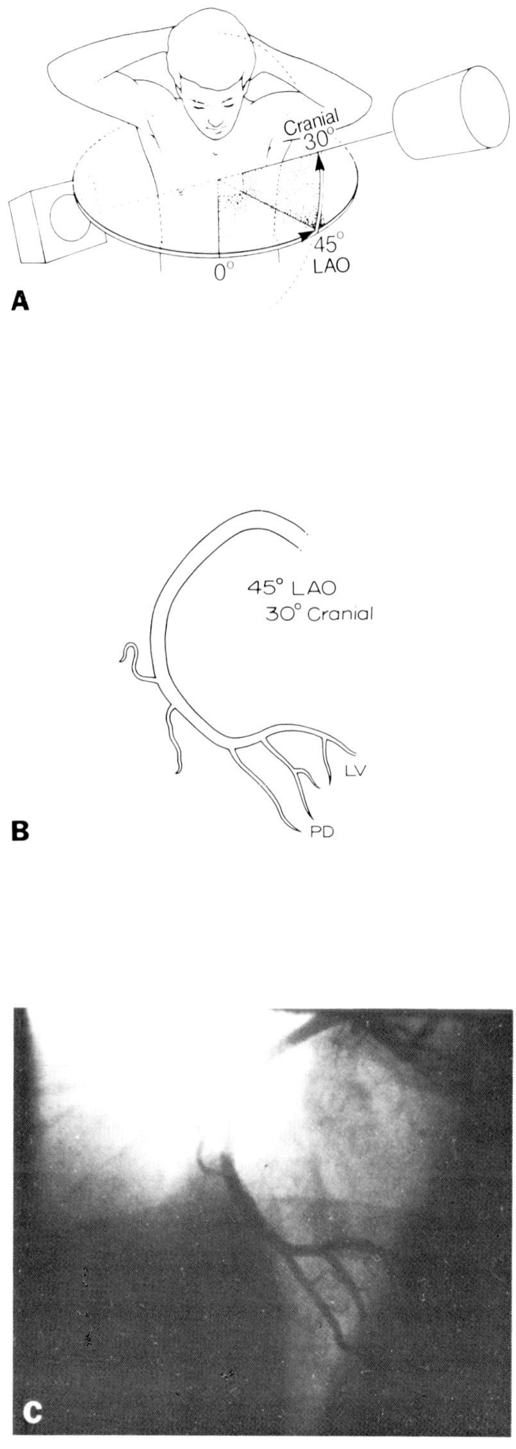

Figure 9-9 Diagrammatic illustration of the right coronary artery in a 45° left anterior oblique (LAO) view with 30° cranial angulation. Cranial angulation of the image intensifier overcomes the problem of foreshortening of the posterior descending and left ventricular branches observed in Fig. 9-8. Lesions in the posterior descending or left ventricular branches can be well-visualized. When the right coronary artery originates anteriorly from the aorta, the proximal portion of this vessel is frequently well seen in this projection. When the left anterior descending artery arises anomalously from the right sinus of Valsalva, this view is helpful since the standard LAO view produces considerable foreshortening of the anomalous artery. (*From* King, Douglas, Morris,[24] *with permission of the authors.*)

unless the left main has a cephalad orientation, and then 45° LAO/15° to 20° caudal ("spleen view") may be needed to visualize the left main and the origin of the left anterior descending (LAD) and circumflex.[22] When an eccentric distal left main stenosis is present, a frontal cranial 30° view (view from the patient's chin) may be the only one to show the stenosis. In the presence of very early bifurcation of the left main coronary artery, a 15° RAO/20° caudal view may elucidate the anatomy. Multiple injections may be needed at slightly different angles to evaluate difficult eccentric lesions.

Left Anterior Descending

The LAD gives rise to diagonal and septal branches which overlap the parent vessel in RAO and LAO views, respectively. We find the shallow RAO view with cranial angulation (Fig. 9-7) and the LAO cranial view (Fig. 9-5) to be excellent views to evaluate the proximal and mid LAD and the origin of diagonal and septal branches. Elliott reported the RAO cranial view improved assessment of the mid LAD in 80 percent of patients.[22] One must individualize, however, and select the degree of angulation that best visualizes the problem area. When the heart is horizontal and the proximal LAD has a cephalad direction, the LAO caudal view is better than the LAO cranial view.[11] When the mid LAD is tortuous and has eccentric stenoses, the cranial 30° view may visualize the anatomy best. To evaluate diagonal branches, one may need to perform multiple 30° RAO views with different amounts of caudal and cranial angulation to see the various overlapping segments (Figs. 9-1 and 9-6). By combining these RAO views with an LAO cranial view, one can usually evaluate diagonal arteries, including branch points.

Circumflex Coronary

There are several problem areas in evaluating the circumflex coronary artery. The origin of the circumflex is not well seen in the standard RAO views since this segment is seen on end. RAO caudal views (Fig. 9-6) may permit better visualization of the proximal circumflex coronary artery when it has an initial caudal direction, but the RAO cranial view is better when the circumflex is cranially directed (Fig. 9-7). The LAO cranial view is usually an excellent projection to visualize the proximal circumflex, takeoff of a ramus intermedius, or takeoff of obtuse marginal branches arising from the proximal portion of the circumflex artery. The mid-circumflex may not be well seen in RAO views if it is tortuous, and lesions may occur in segments seen end on. The 40° LAO view is commonly better than the LAO cranial to evaluate this segment. The mid and distal portions of obtuse marginal branches are usually well seen in RAO views. The best choice for a second view of these segments is usually an LAO cranial projection, since these segments are seen end on in standard LAO views.

Right Coronary Artery

The most difficult segments to visualize in the right coronary artery are the orifice when the takeoff from the aorta is quite anterior and the distal right coronary artery, takeoff from the posterior descending artery, or the origin of the left ventricular branch when the heart is in a horizontal position. In the former, a steep LAO or RAO cranial view may be helpful (Fig. 9-8). In the latter, LAO or RAO cranial views offer a means of avoiding viewing segments end on (Fig. 9-9).

REFERENCES

1 Sones F, Shirey EK: Cine coronary angiography. Mod Concepts Cardiovasc Dis, 31:735, 1962.
2 Sones FM: Indications and value of coronary arteriography. Circulation, 46:1155, 1972.
3 Amplatz K, Formanck G, Stranger P, Wilson W: Mechanics of selective coronary artery catheterization via femoral approach. Radiology, 89:1040, 1967.
4 Bourassa MG, Lesperance J, Campeau L: Selective coronary cine arteriography by the percutaneous femoral approach. Am J Roentgenol, 107:377, 1969.
5 Judkins MP: Selective coronary arteriography: A percutaneous transfemoral technic. Radiology, 89:815, 1967.

6 Ricketts HJ, Abrams HL: Percutaneous selective coronary cine arteriography. JAMA, 181:620, 1962.
7 Bunnell IL, Greene DG, Tandon RN, Arani DT: The half-axial projection: A new look at the proximal left coronary artery. Circulation, 48:1151, 1973.
8 Lesperance J, Saltiel J, Peticlerc R, Bourassa MG: Angulated views in the sagittal plane for improved accuracy of cine coronary angiography. Am J Roentgenol, 121:575, 1974.
9 Sos TA, Lee LG, Levin DG, Baltaxe HA: New lordotic projection for improved visualization of the left coronary artery and its branches. Am J Roentgenol Radium Ther Nucl Med, 121:575, 1974.
10 Eldh P, Silverman JF: Methods of studying the proximal left anterior descending coronary artery. Radiology, 113:738, 1974.
11 Arani DT, Bunnell IL, Greene DG: Lordotic right posterior oblique projection of the left coronary artery: A special view for special anatomy. Circulation, 52:504, 1975.
12 Aldridge HE, McLoughlin MJ, Taylor KW: Improved diagnosis in coronary cine arteriography with routine use of 110 oblique views and cranial and caudal angulations. Am J Cardiol, 36:486, 1975.
13 Eldh P: Axial views. Cathet Cardiovasc Diagn, 2:315, 1976 (editorial).
14 Aldridge HE: Better visualization of the asymptomatic lesion in coronary arteriography utilizing cranial and caudal angulated projections. Chest, 71:502, 1977.
15 Taylor KW, McLoughlin JH, Aldridge HE: Specification of angulated projections in coronary arteriography. Cathet Cardiovasc Diagn, 3:367, 1977.
16 Grollman JH, Barack BM, MacAlpin RN: A new wedge to facilitate obtaining half-axial views during coronary arteriography. Cathet Cardiovasc Diagn, 2:181, 1976.
17 Frederick PR, Fry WH, Russell JG, Marshall HW: Longitudinal angulation in coronary arteriography: Apparatus and evaluation. Cathet Cardiovasc Diagn, 3:305, 1977.
18 Sos T, Baltaxe H: Cranial and caudal angulation for coronary arteriography revisited. Circulation, 55:119, 1977.
19 Nath PH, Velasquez G, Castaneda-Zuniga WR, Zollikofer C, Formanek A, Amplatz K: An essential view in coronary arteriography. Circulation, 60:101, 1979.
20 Miller RA, Warkentin DL, Felix WG, Hashimian M, Leighton RF: Angulated views in coronary arteriography. Am J Roentgenol, 134:407, 1980.
21 Elliott LP, Bream PF, Soto B, Russell RO Jr, Rogers WJ, Mantle JA, Hood WP Jr: Significance of the caudal left-anterior-oblique view in analyzing the left main coronary artery. Radiology, 139:39, 1981.
22 Elliott LP, Green CE, Rogers WJ, Mantle JA, Papapietro SE, Hood WP Jr, Russell RO Jr: Advantage of the cranial–right anterior oblique view in diagnosing mid left anterior descending and distal right coronary artery disease. Am J Cardiol, 48:754, 1981.
23 Gomez A, Esposito V, Grollman J, O'Reilly R: Angled views in the evaluation of the right coronary artery. Cathet Cardiovasc Diagn, 8:71, 1982.
24 King SB III, Douglas JS Jr, Morris DC: New angiographic views for coronary arteriography, in Hurst JW (ed): *Update IV: The Heart*. McGraw-Hill, New York, 1981, p 193.
25 Grover M, Slutsky R, Higgins C, Atwood JE: Terminology and anatomy of angulated coronary arteriography. Clin Cardiol 7:37, 1984.

Chapter 10

Quantitative Evaluation of Left Ventricular Function

Douglas C. Morris, M.D.
John S. Douglas, Jr., M.D.
Spencer B. King III, M.D.

The purpose of left ventriculography during cardiac catheterization is to define the size and contour of the left ventricular chamber, to outline the shape and mobility of related valvular structures, and to assess ventricular function. Frequently, an accurate assessment of segmental ventricular function requires intervention techniques in an attempt to unmask reversible asynergy. Unless contraindicated by the patient's clinical status, left ventriculography should be a routine part of any left-sided heart catheterization. Furthermore, the recognized temporary depressive effect of previous intracoronary injection of contrast material upon ventricular function,[1,2] persuades many angiographers to perform left ventriculography as the initial angiocardiographic procedure.

TECHNIQUE

In adults, left ventriculography is optimally performed by injecting contrast material directly into the left ventricular chamber. An alternative, but less acceptable, technique is to perform ''levophase filming'' of the left ventricle during a pulmonary angiogram. In certain instances, injection of contrast material into the left atrium during a transseptal catheterization or into the ascending aorta in a patient with severe aortic regurgitation will allow adequate opacification of the left ventricle.

The preferred catheter position within the left ventricular chamber depends primarily on the contour of the distal portion of the catheter used. The catheter must sit free in the chamber with the tip removed from the ventricular wall. End-hole catheters must be positioned further removed from the wall than tip-occluded or pigtail catheters. Conversely, if the catheter is positioned too high in the chamber, recoil during the pressure injection may propel the catheter into the aorta. An NIH catheter, a multipurpose catheter, a Lehman ventriculography catheter, and an angulated pigtail catheter should all be positioned in the plane of the long axis of the ventricle. A nonangulated pigtail catheter is generally most stable when positioned in the inflow tract of the left ventricular chamber. The same position is preferred for a Sones catheter if it is being used for ventriculography. The proper position of the catheter should always be confirmed by a test injection of 5 to 10 mL of contrast material under fluoroscopic visualization.

The rate of the injection and the volume of contrast material to be used depend primarily upon the size and function of the left ventricle and the clinical state of the patient. To a lesser extent, these parameters depend on the catheter used. For example, the injection rate with an end-hole catheter should seldom exceed 10 to 12 mL/s. The catheter is less important than the ventricle in determining the injection rate and volume of contrast material because catheter selection should also be predicated upon ventricular size and function. A normal-size left ventricle can be adequately opacified with 32 to 45 mL of contrast material delivered over no more than 4 s while a dilated ventricle may require 60 mL. If the stroke volume is low to normal, an injection rate of 8 to 12 mL/s is adequate, while a large stroke volume may require 15 to 18 mL/s. If the patient has severe left ventricular failure or unstable angina pectoris, the total volume of contrast delivered should be reduced and preferably delivered following the administration of sublingual nitroglycerin or intravenous nitroglycerin or nitroprusside. An end-diastolic pressure over 20 mmHg or a pulmonary capillary wedge pressure over 25 mmHg in a patient with myocardial ischemia or impaired left ventricular contractility or valvular regurgitation also warrants the administration of nitroglycerin prior to ventriculography. Patients with severe aortic stenosis should, likewise, receive a significantly reduced contrast load.

PROJECTION

Biplane ventriculography is preferable to single plane ventriculography, particularly in patients with coronary artery disease. The 30° right anterior oblique (RAO) single plane projection, however, is certainly adequate in many circumstances and, if carefully reviewed, will provide almost as much information as biplane projections. The left ventricular segments which are best delineated on the left anterior oblique (LAO) projection are the septal and posterolateral segments. Evidence of asynergy of these segments, however, is usually also evident on the RAO projection. Septal asynergy is evident on the RAO projection as anterior or apical asynergy while posterolateral asynergy manifests as inferior or anteroapical asynergy. A comparative study of the efficacy of biplane versus single plane ventriculography in 50 patients with coronary artery disease revealed that 20 percent of the patients had asynergy visible only on the RAO projection but no patient has asynergy isolated to the LAO projections.[3] In addition, on the LAO projection the septal motion is often obscured by the overlying apical segments and frequently apical contraction or the lack of such is mistakenly attributed to the septum.

Recently, angled cineangiography has been demonstrated to be advantageous in left ventriculography. The cranial LAO view profiles best the lateral wall of the left ventricle and its outflow tract, composed of the ventricular septum and the anterior leaflet of the mitral valve. Since these are the areas of particular interest on the LAO view, the angled projection seems to be preferable to the routine LAO view in those systems with triaxial motion capability. The cranial LAO view is a relatively steep 60° to 70° LAO view with the image intensifier positioned over the left shoulder and the x-ray beam angled caudocranially 20° to 45°. The degree of angulation depends upon the position of the heart in the chest cavity. A rather vertical heart is best defined by 20° angulation, while a more horizontal heart is better defined with a higher degree of angulation.[4]

FILMING TECHNIQUE

Cineangiography, utilizing intensification and amplification fluoroscopy, is the preferred means of filming the ventriculogram. This technique provides the following advantages over serial angiocardiography: the ability to monitor the injection, better appreciation of dynamic events during the cardiac cycle, less x-ray exposure to the patient, and more cost and time efficiency. The cine filming is generally performed at rates of 30 or 60 frames per second. The only two real advantages of serial angiography (large-size x-ray films taken using cut film or roll film changers at a filming rate as fast as 12 frames per second but usually at 4 to 6 per second) are better definition of anatomic detail and a larger field size. A spot film fluorographic camera using roll film may be used as an adjunct to cineangiography. These 105-mm films taken at a rate of up to 12 frames per second allow direct visualization during the filming.

EVALUATION OF VENTRICULOGRAPHY

Global and segmental left ventricular function is frequently determined by visual estimation of ventricular wall motion on the cineangiogram. It has been demonstrated, however, that such a subjective evaluation is highly variable[5] and tends to overestimate wall motion in some segments (anterolateral) and underestimate it in other segments (inferior).[6] The reproducibility and accuracy of ventricular wall motion is greatly enhanced by utilization of quantitative techniques.

The Dodge area-length technique is the most widely utilized method for quantitating the left ventricular volume.[7] This technique is based upon the premise that an ellipsoid is the most representative geometric figure for the left ventricle. The volume of an ellipsoid is derived from the equation

$$V = \frac{4}{3}\pi abc$$

where a = one-half the length of the major axis
b,c = one-half the lengths of the minor axis and diameter, respectively

The length of the major axis (L_m) is measured directly in each plane as the longest measurable axis within the ventricular silhouette from the apex to the aortic valve. The longest measurable length (regardless of the plane in which it occurred) is used as the major axis. The length of the minor axes may be calculated in two different ways: first, by direct measurement either of the largest diameter (D) perpendicular to the major axis or of the diameter located at the midpoint of the major axis; second, and this is probably more accurate, by calculating the minor axis diameter by measuring the long axis and planimetering the area of the chamber and substituting both results into the equation $A = \pi L_m D/4$. The length of the major axis and diameter are then inserted into the equation

$$V = \frac{4}{3}\pi \times \frac{L_m}{2} \times \frac{D_{RAO}}{2} \times \frac{D_{LAO}}{2}$$

The angiographic estimates of ventricular volumes generally overestimate the true volume. This overestimation probably arises because of the inadequacy of the ellipsoid reference figure in characterizing the left ventricular chamber and the inability to account for the portion of the ventricular chamber occupied by the papillary muscles and trabeculae carneae. The angiographic assessment of end-systolic volume is perhaps even less accurate than the end-diastolic volume assessment. This results from the following: the eccentric shape of the end-systolic ventricle is less adequately represented by the ellipsoid model applied to ventricular volume measurements, and there is loss of a greater portion of the end-systolic volume in the form of blood within the trabeculae.

Several investigators have derived regression equations by comparing the measured volume of postmortem hearts with the calculated angiographic volume. Dodge and associates concluded that with anteroposterior and lateral biplane projections

$$V_{true} = 0.928\ V_{calculated} - 3.8\ cm^3$$

Subsequently, Wynne and associates found that using biplane oblique projections

$$V_{true} = 0.989\ V_{calculated} - 8.1\ cm^3$$

In single plane angiography, the two minor axes are assumed to be equal.[8] This assumption results in the following equation:

$$V = \frac{4}{3}\pi \frac{L_m}{2} \times \frac{D^2}{4}$$

Studies in which the minor semidiameters were compared have demonstrated that their equality is generally a reasonable assumption.[8] The regression equation for volumes derived from single plane films as developed by Sandler and Dodge[8] is

$$V_{true} = 0.951\ V_{calculated} - 3.0\ cm^3$$

A magnification factor must be incorporated into these calculations in order to correct for magnification of the image due to divergence of the x-ray beam and for the possibility of greater magnification at the periphery than in the center of the field (pin-cushion effect). A calibrated grid is filmed at the estimated level of the left ventricle to enable the physician to determine the magnification factor. It is worth emphasizing that a calibrated grid is preferable to other calibration devices because only the grid allows one to correct for the pin-cushion distortion. The calibration grid must be traced from its projected image, and the squares which are closest in position to the image of the left ventricle are planitered (Fig. 10-1).

Once the end-diastolic volume (EDV) and end-systolic volume (ESV) are calculated, the stroke volume (SV = EDV − ESV) and the ejection fraction (EF = SV/EDV) can then be determined. Left ventricular mass can also be computed from angiocardiograms. The left ventricular wall is measured at the junction of the middle and lower thirds of anterior segment. This total thickness is then added to each of the dimensions used to compute chamber volume. The resulting volume represents the volume of the chamber plus wall thickness. This volume less the chamber volume and the specific gravity of heart muscle

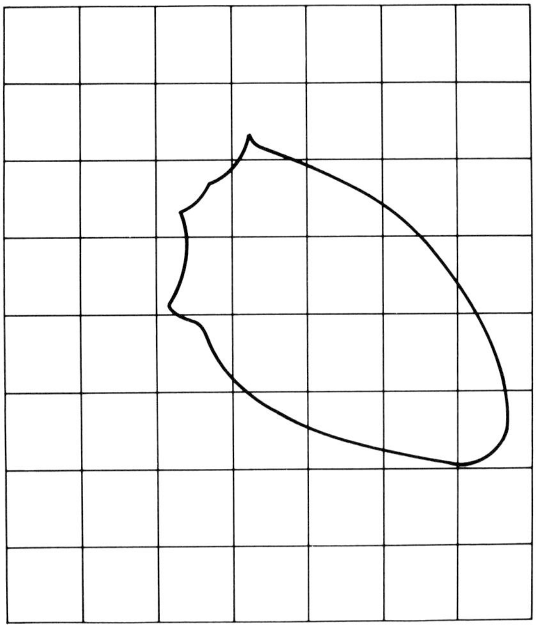

Figure 10-1 Diastolic outline of left ventricle superimposed on calibration grid. Squares which are closest in position to ventricular image should be planimetered.

(1.050) provides a value for left ventricular mass (Fig. 10-2).

A step-by-step approach to the calculation of ventricular volumes and function would be as follows:

Step 1: The outline of the left ventricle is traced in systole and diastole in each of the projections filmed as seen in Fig. 10-1, ignoring the papillary muscle and trabecular projections. (Repeatedly scan the entire cineventriculogram and select the best cardiac cycle in terms of opacity and rhythm; do not select a premature beat or a postextrasystolic beat.)

Step 2: Measure the major axis in the RAO or AP projection from the apex to the midpoint of the aortic valve and in the LAO projection from the apex to the junction of the aorta and mitral valve (Fig. 10-2).

Step 3: Calculate D_{RAO} and D_{LAO} from the equation $D = 4A/L_m$, where A = area, using the planimetered area and measured major axis for each projection.

Table 10-1 Normal Values for Left Ventricular Volumes in Adults

Volumes*	Wynne et al.[9]	Kennedy et al.[10]	Hammermeister et al.[11]
EDVI (mL/m^2)	72 ± 15	70 ± 20	78 ± 15
ESVI (mL/m^2)	20 ± 8	24 ± 10	
SVI (mL/m^2)	51 ± 10	45 ± 13	50 ± 13
EF	0.78 ± 0.08	0.67 ± 0.08	0.65 ± 0.07
Angiographic techniques	Biplane oblique projections	Biplane AP and lateral projections	Single plane RAO or AP projection

*EDVI = end-diastolic volume index, ESVI = end-systolic volume index, SVI = stroke volume index, EF = ejection fraction.

Step 4: Simplify formula for ventricular volume as follows:

$$V = \frac{4}{3}\frac{L_m}{2} \times \frac{D_{RAO}}{2} \times \frac{D_{LAO}}{2}$$

$$V = \frac{1}{6}L_m \times D_{RAO} \times D_{LAO}$$

$$V = 0.85\ L_m \times D_{RAO} \times D_{LAO}$$

Step 5: Insert L_m and calculated diameter (D) into this formula.

Step 6: Determine x-ray magnification factor (F) with the formula:

$$F = \frac{A_{true}}{A_{planimetered}}$$

Step 7: Determine the observed volume from the calculated volume with the formula:

$$V_{observed} = V_{calculated} \times F$$

Step 8: Correct the observed volumes using one of the linear regression equation formulas:

$$V_{true} = 0.928\ V_{calculated} - 3.8\ cm^3$$

(biplane AP and lateral)

or

$$V_{true} = 0.989\ V_{calculated} - 8.1\ cm^3$$

(biplane RAO and LAD)

or

$$V_{true} = 0.951\ V_{calculated} - 3.0\ cm^3$$

(single plane)

Step 9: Calculation of left ventricular mass would proceed as follows[12]:

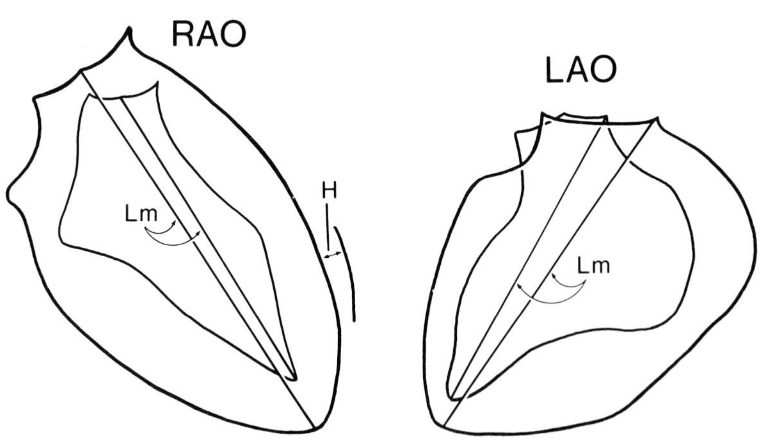

Figure 10-2 Right anterior oblique and left anterior oblique projections of left venticle depicting proper position of the major axis. H = wall thickness, L_m = length of the major axis.

(a) Measure wall thickness h (Fig. 10-2)
(b) Total EDV $= 0.85\ (L_m + h)\ (D_{RAO} + h)$
(c) Muscle volume = total EDV − EDV
(d) Muscle mass = muscle volume × 1.05

Since coronary atherosclerosis (the most common reason for performing left ventriculography) is a segmental disease, it is frequently important to make accurate regional evaluations of left ventricular function. Again, the substantial error rate associated with qualitative analysis requires that a quantitative regional analysis system be used. Quantitative left ventricular wall motion may be analyzed by the area, chord, or radial methods (Fig. 10-3). In each system, the major axis for the RAO view is a line from the apex to the midpoint of the aortic valve plane and in the LAO view a line from the aortic-mitral valve junction to the apex. Systolic

Figure 10-3 Quantitative evaluation of left ventricular function by the radial, chord, and area methods. In each method the major axis is drawn in both views. In the chord and area method lines are drawn on the right anterior oblique projection perpendicular to the major axis so as to divide it into thirds. In the left anterior oblique projection a single line is drawn perpendicular to the major axis as its midpoint. In the radial methods radii are drawn through the midpoint of the major axis at 45° intervals. L_m = length of the major axis.

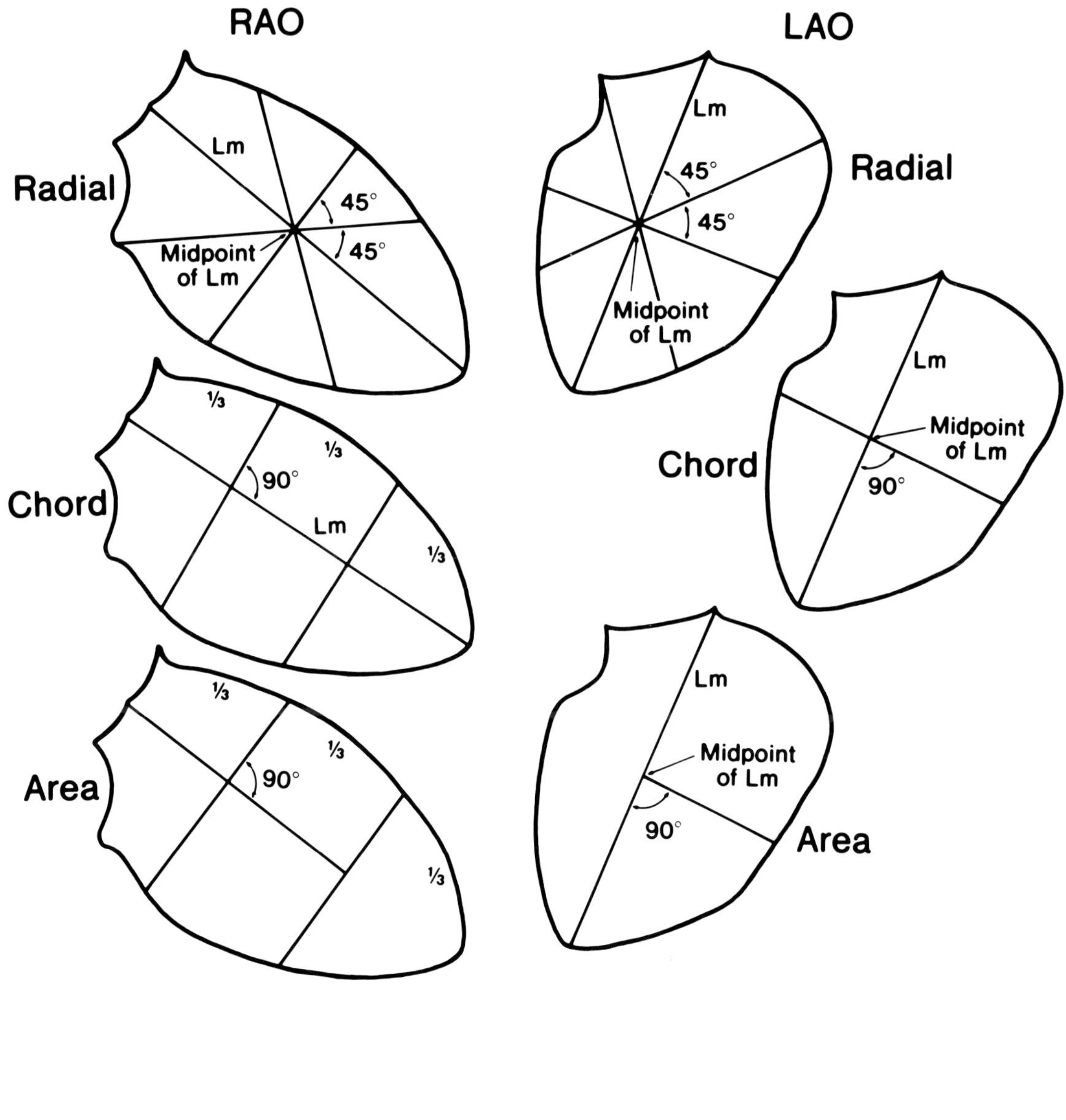

apical rotation and aortic motion is compensated for by overlapping the long axis of diastole and systole. In the chord and radial methods, regional function is reflected by the shortening of the chord or radius extending to any particular segment of the left ventricular wall. Clearly, the larger the number of measured radial or chord lines, the more adequately regional wall motion will be characterized. The area method, which is based on changes in the area of various left ventricular segments, proved to be the best of the three methods in both the detection of abnormal regional contraction patterns and the illustration of normal function.[3]

INTERVENTIONS IN LEFT VENTRICULOGRAPHY

In patients with coronary atherosclerotic heart disease, segments of the left ventricle displaying asynergy may represent compromised but viable muscle rather than infarcted muscle. It is important for the angiographer to unmask those segments with reversible asynergy. The two safest and most effective means of unmasking reversible asynergy are the sublingual administration of nitroglycerin[14–16] or postextrasystolic potentiation[16,17] (PESP). If nitroglycerin is used, it should be given as a 0.6-mg or 0.4-mg sublingual dose and the ventriculogram repeated 2 to 6 minutes later. The patient should demonstrate a reduction of both systolic and end-diastolic pressures in response to the nitroglycerin for the results to be reliable. Postextrasystolic potentiation is accomplished by producing an extrasystolic beat and evaluating ventricular function during the subsequent normal beat. The timing of the extrasystolic beat does not seem important.[16] A comparative study of the two methods indicated that they were equally efficacious in denoting compromised but viable myocardium.[16] It should be noted that dyskinetic segments do not improve with interventions; consequently, hypokinetic or akinetic segments do warrant evaluation by intervention, but dyskinetic segments do not.

Two other approaches to evaluating the contractile response to myocardial ischemia are the augmentation of contractility by the administration of an inotropic catecholamine[18] and the inducement of temporary ischemia through atrial pacing.[19] A failure of segmental contraction to improve during a 5- to 15-minute intravenous infusion of 1 to 4 μg/min 1-epinephrine indicates nonviable myocardium. Unlike the other two methods of demonstrating the contractile reserve (nitroglycerin or PESP), this intervention may cause angina (i.e., myocardial ischemia). The other method, atrial pacing at rates of 100 to 150 for 2 minutes, is predicated upon the production of myocardial ischemia. The ischemia will produce new or increased asynergy. The applicability of this last technique is limited to those patients in whom the clinical significance of a particular angiographic coronary artery obstruction is in dispute. With a few exceptions, thallium-201 scintigraphy will more accurately clarify these questions.

STRUCTURAL CONFIGURATION OF THE LEFT VENTRICULAR CHAMBER

Left ventriculography not only defines left ventricular function but also outlines the structural arrangements of the chamber. The angiographer must have a thorough knowledge of the configuration of the left ventricle and its valves in the various angiographic projections and the relationship between the left ventricular anatomy and the coronary arterial anatomy.

The American Heart Association has established the nomenclature for identifying the left ventricular segments in the RAO and LAO projections (Figs. 10-4 and 10-5).[20] The anterobasal segment is perfused by the proximal left anterior descending artery (LAD) and its first septal branch. Motion in this segment reflects motion in the upper septum. The anterolateral segment is generally perfused by the diagonal branches of the left anterior descending artery while the apical segment is supplied by the parent vessel (LAD) itself. The posterobasal segment is supplied by the posterior descending branch regardless of its origin (right coronary or circumflex). The diaphragmatic segment may be

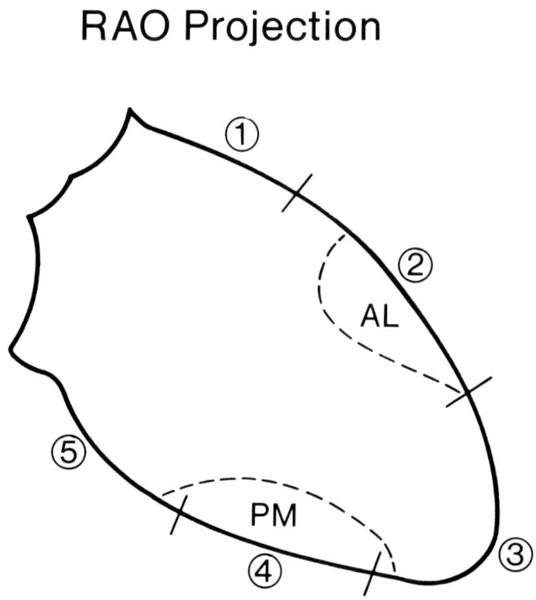

Figure 10-4 Nomenclature for identifying the left ventricular segments in the right anterior oblique projection as set forth by the American Heart Association in Circulation, 51:5–40, 1975. 1 = Anterobasal, 2 = Anterolateral, 3 = Apical, 4 = Diaphragmatic, 5 = Posterobasal, AL = Anterolateral, PM = Posteriomedial.

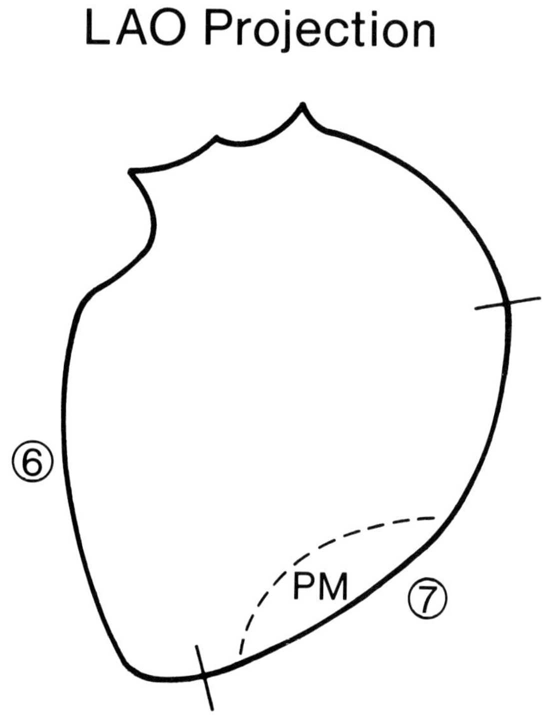

Figure 10-5 Nomenclature for identifying the left ventricular segments in the left anterior oblique projection as set forth by the American Heart Association in Circulation, 51:5–40, 1975. 6 = Septal, 7 = Posterolateral.

supplied by the same artery, but is frequently perfused by an obtuse marginal branch of the circumflex artery. The posterolateral segment outlined in the LAO projection is supplied by branches of the circumflex artery. While the anterior aspect of the ventricle in the LAO projection is identified as the septum, septal motion is often obscured by the overlying apical segments.

The anterolateral segment is generally indented by the anterolateral papillary muscle. The posteromedial papillary muscle is represented by indentation of the diaphragmatic segment on the RAO projection and either indentation of the posterolateral segment or by an oval "filling defect" near the posterolateral edge on the LAO projection. The posterobasal segment on the RAO projection terminates at the mitral annulus. The mitral annulus is generally in profile on the RAO projection and extends from the inferior left ventricular wall to the aortic valve. The normal mitral valve shows minimal systolic bulging beyond the mitral annulus. Conversely, patients with mitral valve prolapse manifest a distinct bulge into the left atrium during systole. The posterior leaflet is a triscalloped structure with a large middle scallop and two smaller commissural scallops. The scallop which is most likely to prolapse either as a single scallop prolapse or more often a multiple scallop prolapse is the middle scallop. Prolapse of this scallop produces a central bulge posterior to the mitral annulus. Prolapse of the posteromedial commissural scallop produces an oval or beak-shaped bulge at the inferior edge of the mitral annulus. The prolapsed anterolateral commissural scallop produces a bulge in the superior portion of the annulus (Fig. 10-6). Contrast in the aortic root often obscures this bulge.[21] Prolapse of the anterior leaflet of the mitral valve

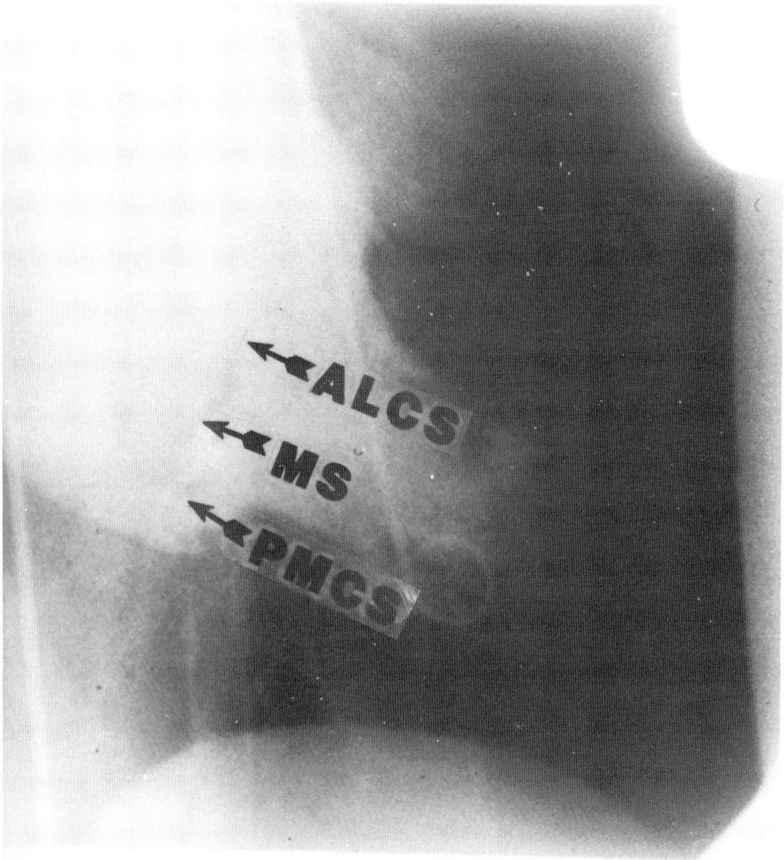

Figure 10-6 Left ventricle in systole demonstrating prolapse of three scallops of posterior mitral valve leaflet. ALCS = anterolateral commissural scallop, MS = middle scallop, PMCS = posteromedial commissural scallop.

often overlaps prolapse of the middle scallop on the RAO projection. Anterior mitral valve leaflet prolapse is better defined in the LAO projection,[22] particularly a cranial LAO view or in a straight lateral view.

The normal left ventricular outflow tract is a tubular space extending between the aortic valve and the left ventricular chamber. It is bounded anteriorly and medially by the interventricular septum. The anterior leaflet of the mitral valve forms the posterior wall of the outflow tract except for a small contribution by the posterior leaflet to the inferior aspect of the outflow tract.

The muscular portion of the interventricular septum forms the anterior wall of the left ventricular chamber. It actually extends around the left ventricle to form a portion of the inferior wall in the RAO projection.

In idiopathic hypertrophic subaortic stenosis the outflow tract is markedly narrowed by the hypertrophic septum. During diastole the narrowed outflow tract is portrayed on the LAO view as an inverted cone bordered by the septum anteriorly and the open anterior mitral leaflet posteriorly. On the RAO view, the hypertrophied septum produces a bulge into the left ventricular cavity in the region of the anterobasal segment. The large septal mass also is characteristically visualized as a bulge into the left ventricular cavity inferiorly. During systole in the LAO projection the septum bulges into the outflow tract and the anterior leaflet of mitral valve creates a curved, shelflike deformity extending toward the septum. The abutment of the anterior mitral valve leaflet against the septum is portrayed on the RAO view as an irregular linear radiolucency.[23]

The diastolic contour of the left ventricle can be

altered from its normal spherical shape to a more oval configuration by any condition which increases the diastolic volume. Mitral regurgitation, aortic regurgitation, and a dilated cardiomyopathy are the most common causes of an increased diastolic volume. The other common cause of an alteration of the diastolic contour of the left ventricle is an aneurysm. An aneurysm is defined as a localized bulge in the diastolic contour with paradoxical systolic expansion of this bulge. The vast majority of left ventricular aneurysms involve the anteroseptal segment,[24] but frequently adjacent segments are also involved.[25] Attempts at quantitating ventricular function have been reported to be of value in evaluating the feasibility of surgical resection of the aneurysm. Those patients with an ejection fraction of greater than 45 percent for the contractile section of the ventricle had significantly better surgical results than those with poor function in the contractile segment.[26]

MEASUREMENTS OF LEFT VENTRICULAR PRESSURE

In addition to left ventricular angiography, left ventricular pressure recordings are made at rest and, in some instances, following interventions. Two left ventricular pressures are usually measured: peak systolic pressure and end-diastolic pressure. Left ventricular end-diastolic pressure (LVEDP) is measured at the point where the downslope of the a-wave of the left ventricular pressure tracing reaches the initial upslope that occurs with ventricular systole (Fig. 10-7). Alternatively, the LVEDP may be measured at the peak of the R wave of the electrocardiogram. The normal range of LVEDP is 3 to 12 mmHg.

Measurement of left ventricular pressure in the coronary angiography laboratory is usually performed using external pressure transducers mounted on the radiographic table at the level of the patient's heart. Changes in pressure at the catheter tip are transmitted to the transducer by movements of the saline column in the catheter, manifold, and high-pressure tubing linking the manifold and transducer (Fig. 10-8). Movement of the fluid column alters the position of a diaphragm in the pressure transducer producing a proportional change in resistance in a Wheatstone bridge circuit which is converted to an electrical potential that represents the change in pressure. The fact that the fluid column must move limits the frequency response of fluid-filled systems. This results in an "overshoot" of the early systolic peak pressure tracing and an "undershoot" (lower than the true value) in early diastole (see Fig. 10-7). It is important to recognize the limitations of these low-resonance frequency systems. If measurement of "contractility indexes" (such as left ventricular) dp/dt or V_{max} are desired, catheter-tipped micromanometers are usually required. This is also true if precise timing of intracardiac pressure with simultaneous echo- or phonocardiography is desired since there is an approximately 40-ms delay in pressure recording in the fluid-filled catheter external transducer system. However, the external pressure transducer system is well-suited for most clinical applications. Important practical points in obtaining reliable pressure recordings include: (1) ascertaining proper zero adjustment of the system, (2) checking the calibration of the system by applying known pressures to the transducer using a mercury manometer, (3) minimizing the length of connecting tubing and use of stopcocks between the catheter tip and transducer, (4) ensuring adequate flushing of the catheter with saline solution prior to pressure recordings to remove contrast medium.

UTILITY OF LEFT VENTRICULAR PRESSURE MEASUREMENTS

In the resting state, a combination of elevated left ventricular end-diastolic volume and evidence of reduced cardiac performance point to the presence of impaired myocardial contractility. However, an elevation of LVEDP does not necessarily mean that left ventricular end-diastolic volume is elevated. Elevation of LVEDP may be due to a decrease in the diastolic compliance of the left ventricle caused by myocardial ischemia, hypertrophy, fibrosis, pericardial disease, and other factors.

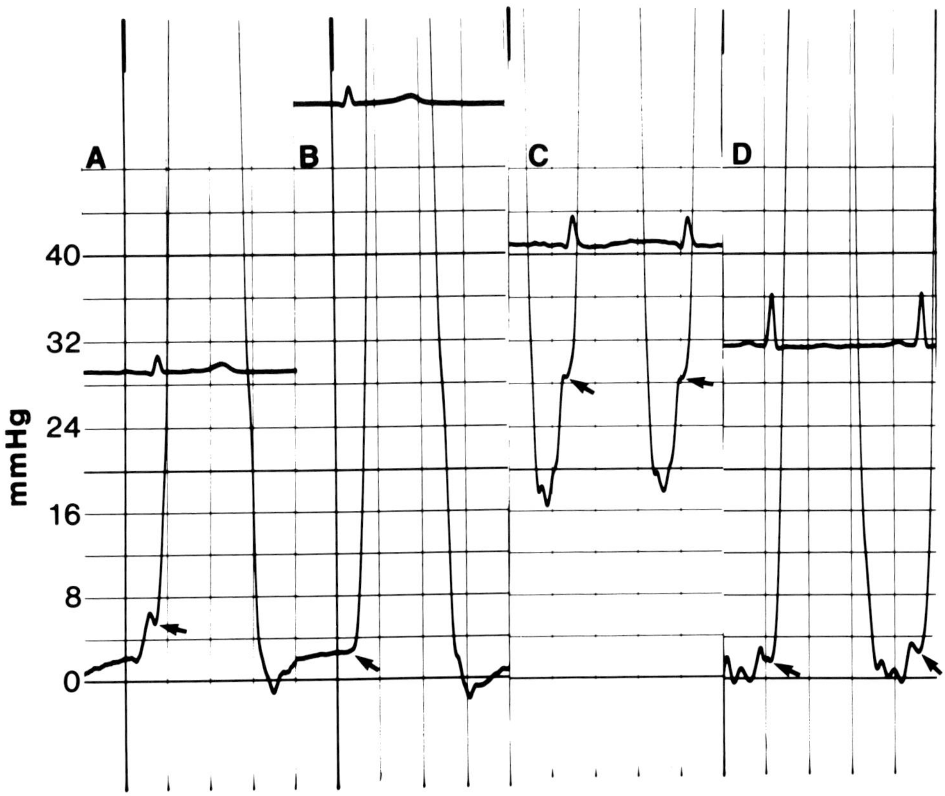

Figure 10-7 Left ventricle end-diastolic pressure. Arrows indicate point of measurement. (*a*) Normal left ventricular pressure tracing. The mass and inertia of the fluid-filled catheter pressure measurement system results in "undershoot" of the pressure tracing in early diastole. (*b*) Patient in junctional rhythm. (*c*) Elevated end-diastolic pressure in patient with acute myocardial ischemia. (*d*) Patient with reduced intravascular volume and a left ventricular end-diastolic pressure of 3 mmHg.

Measurement of the LVEDP provides information that may be useful during the performance of coronary arteriography and subsequently, as inferences are made regarding left ventricular performance. During the performance of coronary arteriography an unusually low LVEDP (less than 5 mm; see Fig. 10-7) suggests hypovolemia and may be a clue to a need for volume replacement or expansion in patients who are hypotensive due to simple dehydration, loss of blood into the retroperitoneal space, allergic reactions to contrast media, or excessive vasodilatation due to nitrates or calcium antagonists. That is, systemic arterial hypotension with a low LVEDP should suggest certain etiologic possibilities and therapeutic strategies. The contour of the aortic and left ventricular pressure tracings may be the first clue to impending vascular collapse due to an anaphylactoid reaction. The aortic pressure tracing in this situation may show an early systolic spike with subsequent abrupt collapse of the pressure tracing after this spike due to a dilated arterial vascular bed and poor left ventricular filling resulting in a small stroke volume. During coronary arteriography, changes in LVEDP are commonly due to myocardial ischemia. When marked increases in LVEDP occur in a patient with coronary artery disease, it is usually, but not invariably, associated with angina pectoris, and the effectiveness of acute therapy can be monitored by following the left ventricular end-diastolic pressure. Not

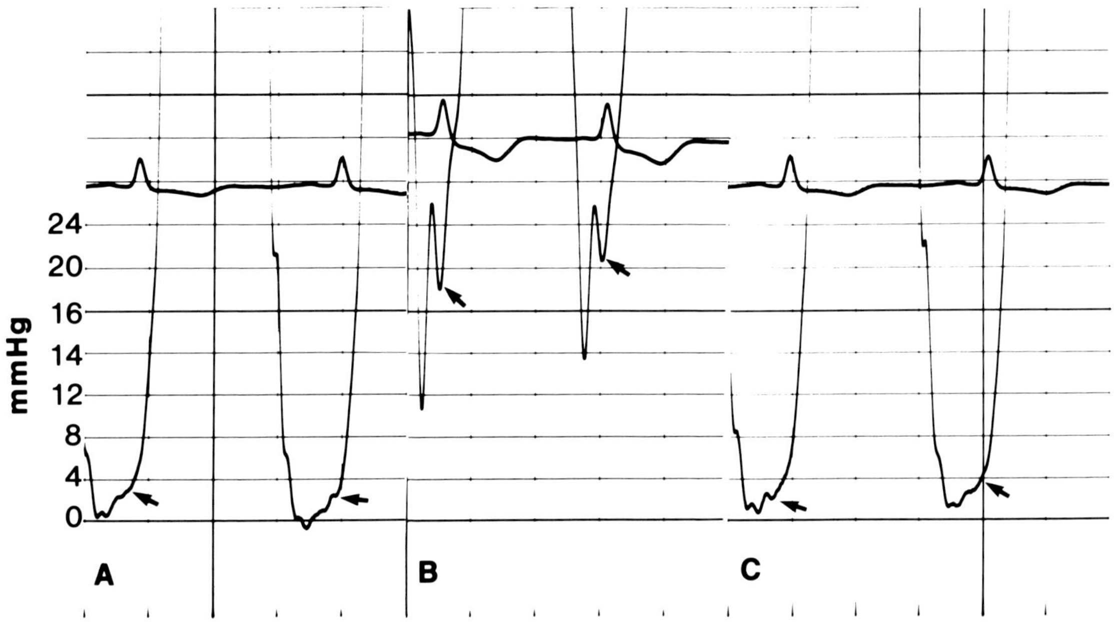

Figure 10-8 Left ventricular pressure tracings obtained in a 54-year-old male during coronary arteriography. Prior to coronary injections (*a*) left ventricular end-diastolic pressure was normal and the electrocardiogram showed slight ST-segment depression. Immediately following left coronary injection (*b*) the patient developed typical ischemic pain, tachycardia, marked ST-segment depression, and elevated left ventricular end-diastolic pressure. Following treatment with sublingual nitroglycerin and propranolol 1 mg intravenously, the chest discomfort abated, and the left ventricular end-diastolic pressure and electrocardiographic changes returned to baseline. (*c*).

infrequently, patients with severe coronary disease may have a resting LVEDP of 12 mmHg which increases to 40 mmHg following coronary or left ventricular injections. After administration of nitroglycerin and oxygen, angina pectoris, if present, abates and LVEDP returns to 12 mmHg. When a markedly increased LVEDP (greater than 20 mmHg) is recorded in a patient prior to left ventriculography, consideration is given to administration of nitroglycerin on the presumption that ischemia may be present leading to a falsely low estimation of left ventricular function by left ventricular angiography. In patients with high LVEDP associated with suspected severe left ventricular dysfunction (as estimated by symptomatic status, physical examination, chest x-ray, and/or electrocardiogram), attempts are made to minimize injections of contrast medium. In this situation, biplane left ventriculography is helpful in minimizing contrast medium load.

On a clinical level, the assessment of left ventricular function is increased by a knowledge of LVEDP. Normal ejection fraction and LVEDP provide more accurate indicators of normal contractility than either measure alone. The mildest disturbance of left ventricular performance in ischemic heart disease is a focal contraction abnormality with normal LVEDP, left ventricular end-diastolic volume, and ejection fraction. More severe is a reduced ejection fraction and an elevated LVEDP in the presence of normal end-diastolic volume. When abnormal wall motion involves more than approximately 15 percent of the endocardial surface of the left ventricle, the left ventricular end-diastolic volume rises and cardiac output decreases when abnormal contraction involves more than 20 to 25 percent of the endocardial surface. In the presence of frank left ventricular aneurysm, left ventricular function may be difficult to judge. We have been impressed that a near-normal LVEDP is a good predictor of ability to tolerate aneurysm resection in patients with large left ventricular aneurysms.

REFERENCES

1 Guzman SV, West JW: Cardiac effects of intracoronary arterial injections of various roentgenographic contrast media. Am Heart J, 58:597–607, 1959.

2 Friesinger GC, Schaffer J, Criley JM, Gaertner RA, Ross RS: Hemodynamic consequences of the injection of radiopaque material. Circulation, 31:730–40, 1965.

3 Cohn PF, Gorlin R, Adams DF, Chahine RA, Vokonas PS, Herman MV: Comparison of biplane and single plane ventriculograms in patients with coronary artery disease. Am J Cardiol, 33:1–6, 1974.

4 Elliott LP, Green CE, Rogers WJ, Hood WP, Mantle JA, Papapietro SE: Advantages of the caudocranial left anterior oblique left ventriculogram in adult heart disease. Am J Cardiol, 49:369–380, 1982.

5 Chaitman BR, DeMots H, Bristow JD, Rosch J, Rohimtoola SH: Objective and subjective analysis of left ventricular angiograms. Circulation, 52:420–425, 1975.

6 Leighton RF, Wilt SM, Lewis RP: Detection of hypokinesis by a quantitative analysis of left ventricular cineangiograms. Circulation, 50:121–127, 1974.

7 Dodge HT, Sandler H, Ballew DW, Lord JD Jr: The use of biplane angiocardiography for the measurement of left ventricular volume in man. Am Heart J, 60:762–776, 1960.

8 Sandler H, Dodge HT: The use of single plane angiocardiograms for the calculation of left ventricular volume in man. Am Heart J, 75:325–334, 1968.

9 Wynne J, Green LH, Mann T, Levin D, Grossman W: Estimation of left ventricular volumes in man from biplane cineangiograms filmed in oblique projections. Am J Cardiol, 41:726–732, 1978.

10 Kennedy JW, Baxley WA, Figley MM, Dodge HT, Blackman JR: Quantitative angiocardiography: I. The normal left ventricle in man. Circulation, 34:272–278, 1966.

11 Hammermeister KE, Brooks RC, Warbasse JR: The rate of change of left ventricular volume in man: I. Validation and peak systolic ejection rate in health and disease. Circulation, 49:729–738, 1974.

12 Rackley CE, Dodge HT, Coble YD, Hay RE: A method for determining left ventricular mass in man. Circulation, 29:666–671, 1964.

13 Gelberg HJ, Brundage BH, Glantz S, Parmley WW: Quantitative left ventricular wall motion analysis: A comparison of area, chord and radial methods. Circulation, 59:991–1000, 1979.

14 Helfant RH, Pise R, Meister SG, Feldman MS, Trout RG, Banks VS: Nitroglycerin to unmask reversible asynergy: Correlation with post coronary bypass ventriculography. Circulation, 50:108–113, 1974.

15 McAnulty JH, Hottenhauer MT, Rosch J, Kloster FE, Rahimtoola SH: Improvement in left ventricular wall motion following nitroglycerin. Circulation, 51:140–145, 1975.

16 Klausner SC, Ratchin RA, Tyberg JV, Lappin HA, Chatterjee K, Parmley WW: The similarity of changes in segmental contraction patterns induced by post extrasystolic potentiation and nitroglycerin. Circulation, 54:615–623, 1976.

17 Dyke SH, Cohn PF, Gorlin R, Sonnenblick EH: Detection of residual myocardial function in coronary artery disease using post-extrasystolic potentiation. Circulation, 50:694–699, 1974.

18 Horn HR, Teichholz LE, Cohn PF, Herman MV, Gorlin R: Augmentation of left ventricular contraction pattern in coronary artery disease by an inotropic catecholamine: The epinephrine ventriculogram. Circulation, 49:1063–1071, 1974.

19 Pasternac A, Gorlin R, Sonnenblick EH, Hoft JI, Kemp HG: Abnormalities of ventricular motion induced by atrial pacing in coronary artery disease. Circulation, 45:1195–1205, 1972.

20 Austen WG, Edwards JE, Frye RL, Gensini GG, Gott VL, Griffith LSC, McGoon DC, Murphy ML, Roe BB: AHA Committee Report: A reporting system on patients evaluated for coronary artery disease. Circulation, 51:5–40, 1975.

21 Ranganothan N, Silver MD, Robinson TI, Kostuk WJ, Felderhof CH, Pott NL, Wilson JK, Wyle ED: Angiographic-morphologic correlation in patients with severe mitral regurgitation due to prolapse of the posterior mitral valve leaflet. Circulation, 48:514–518, 1973.

22 Ranganothan N, Silver MD, Wigle ED: Mitral valve prolapse. Circulation, 49:1268–1269, 1974.

23 Simon AL, Ross J Jr, Gault JH: Angiographic anatomy of the left ventricle and mitral valve in idiopathic hypertrophic subaortic stenosis. Circulation, 36:852–867, 1967.

24 Burton NA, Stinson EB, Oyer PE, Shumway NE: Left ventricular aneurysm: Preoperative risk factors

and long-term postoperative results. J Thorac Cardiovasc Surg, 77:65–73, 1979.

25 Grondin P, Kretz JG, Bical O, Donzeau-Gouge P, Petitclerc R, Campeau L: Natural history of saccular aneurysms of the left ventricle. J Thorac Cardiovasc Surg, 77:57–64, 1979.

26 Watson LE, Dickhaus DW, Martin RH: Left ventricular aneurysm: I. Preoperative hemodynamics, chamber volume, and results of aneurysmectomy. Circulation, 52:868–873, 1975.

Chapter 11

Management of Complications

John S. Douglas, Jr., M.D.
Spencer B. King III, M.D.

Coronary arteriography is an invasive procedure with certain inherent risks. Complication rates depend on a host of factors, including the skill of the angiographer, the clinical stability of the patient, and the seriousness of underlying disease processes. Several large, multihospital surveys have been conducted to assess the risk of coronary arteriography. Adams et al. undertook a nationwide survey of complications of coronary arteriography from 1970 to 1971 and reported the results from 173 responding hospitals analyzing 46,904 coronary arteriographic procedures.[1] The total mortality rate was 0.45 percent; major complications (death, acute myocardial infarction or cerebral embolus) occurred in 1.3 percent; and a total of 5.1 percent of patients had at least one complication. Nonfatal complications included myocardial infarction (0.61 percent), ventricular fibrillation (1.3 percent), arterial thrombosis (1.4 percent), hemorrhage from the arterial entry site (0.12 percent), pseudoaneurysm at the arterial entry site (0.06 percent), cerebral emboli (0.23 percent), reaction to contrast medium (0.14 percent), and other complications (0.21 percent).

In this survey, the occurrence rate of all complications listed except pseudoaneurysm was higher with the femoral percutaneous technique than with the brachial approach. This increased complication rate of the femoral percutaneous method was attributed by Judkins and Gander[2] to the competence of the angiographer (complication rates were higher in low-volume laboratories) and to thromboembolism which occurred as a result of poor technique, long procedures, and catheter exchanges over guidewires. The inherent thrombogenicity of all catheters and guidewires and the injury at the entry site may be contributing factors to the formation of a doughnut or Cheeriolike thrombus at the entry site produced as thrombus elements are stripped from a catheter on removal and carried on the tip of succeeding catheters into the ascending aorta, where embolization to the brain or myocardium may occur (Fig. 11-1).[2,3] Judkins and Gander recommended single dose total body heparinization on the basis of studies showing that heparin reduced thromboembolic complications when multiple catheter changes were performed.[4,5]

Abrams and Adams[6] repeated the nationwide survey of complications of coronary arteriography in 1973 to 1974 analyzing data from 89,079 coronary arteriograms from 176 institutions, finding a striking drop in mortality rate with the femoral approach from 0.78 to 0.16 percent. Death rate and major complications were similar for femoral and brachial approaches, and there was no difference in results with and without heparin (except that a higher death rate occurred when heparin was omitted in the brachial approach). Davis reported 7553 consecutive patients in the Coronary Artery Surgery Study (CASS) study from 13 institutions studied in 1975 to 1976 and noted similar complication rates with femoral and brachial approaches except in centers with less than 80 percent brachial procedures, and in those centers, a higher risk occurred with brachial procedures.[7] As in the Abrams and Adams study, risk in femoral procedures was not altered by heparin. It was observed that the presence of left main coronary disease increased the

Figure 11-1 Mechanism of clot embolization with catheter exchanges. Clot may form at the puncture site as a result of the injury of entry. This clot and platelet aggregates adherent to the catheter surface are stripped from the catheter at the entrance site during removal of the first catheter. The second catheter carries the thrombus material to the ascending aorta, where embolization may occur. (*From Judkins MP, Gander MP: Prevention of complications of coronary arteriography, Circulation, 49:599, 1974, with permission of the authors and publisher.*)

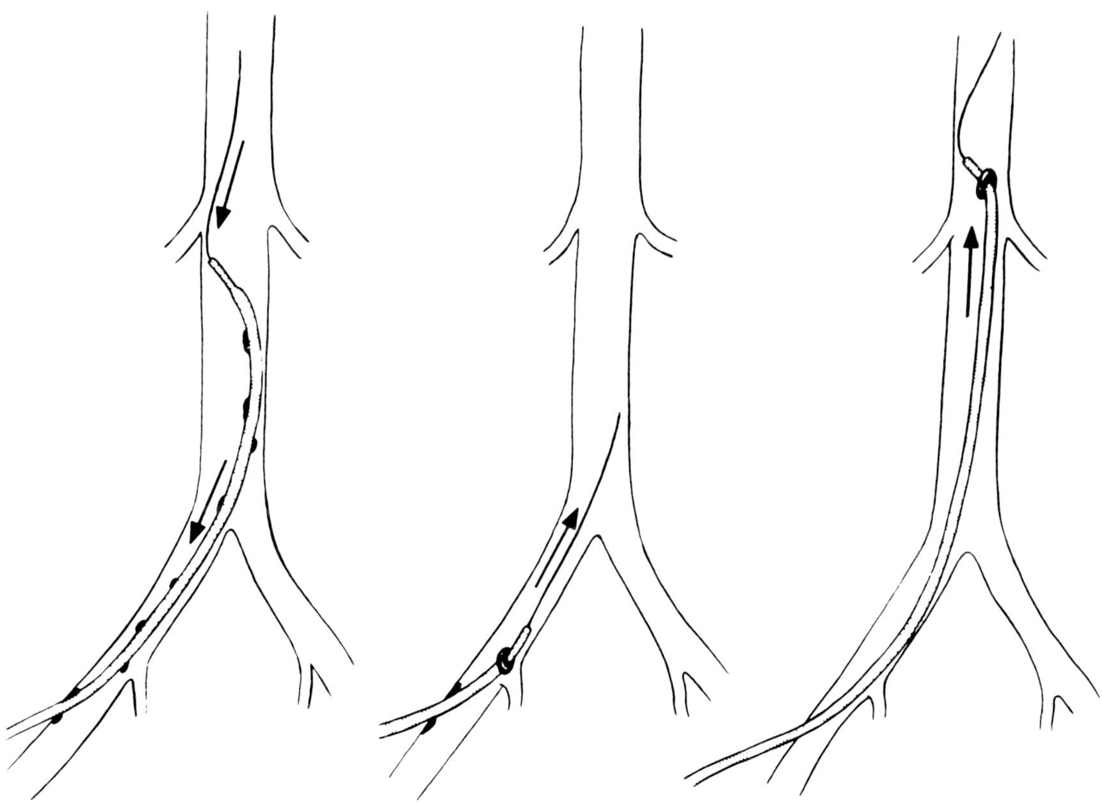

risk of death by 6.8 times (total mortality rate 0.2 percent, left main mortality rate 0.76 percent, non–left main mortality rate 0.12 percent). All patients dying in the report of Davis had severe coronary artery disease.

In the most recent report from the CASS study[8] complications encountered in almost 20,000 coronary arteriograms were outlined (Table 11-1). The complications reported in this CASS study were quite similar to those reported by the Society for Cardiac Angiography in a prospective study of 53,581 cardiac catheterization procedures done in 66 laboratories in 1978 to 1979.[9] In the Society for Cardiac Angiography study which included noncoronary procedures, mortality was 0.14 percent; 1.8 percent of patients had at least one significant complication which included vascular complications (0.57 percent), myocardial infarction (0.07 percent), cerebral vascular accident (0.07 percent), and arrhythmias (0.56 percent). The mortality rate was 0 in over 11,000 patients with minimal or no coronary artery disease. In both the CASS study and in the Society for Cardiac Angiography study, the mortality rate was higher for patients over age 60 to 65 (0.19 and 0.25 percent, respectively). The similarity of the results in these two large studies suggests that they closely reflect the true incidence of complications associated with cardiac catheterization and coronary arteriography as they are performed today.

It has become increasingly clear that the risk of coronary arteriography in a good catheterization laboratory is primarily determined by the severity of coronary anatomy and factors such as left ventricular dysfunction, advanced age, and instability of clinical course. Complications rates in a given laboratory, therefore, will be strongly influenced by the mix of patients studied. If a large proportion of patients studied have left main artery disease or cardiogenic shock, or if patients with evolving infarction are studied, a higher complication rate will occur than that expected if mostly stable patients are studied. Published figures suggest that most laboratories can achieve a mortality rate of less than 0.1 percent and a myocardial infarction rate of approximately the same order if mostly stable patients are studied. Mortality rates, however, will be higher in those laboratories studying high-risk patients.

A complication of coronary arteriography that is not dealt with in these reports is the incomplete or

Table 11-1 Complications of Coronary Arteriography in 19,309 CASS Patients[8]

Complication	Number of patients	Percent
Death	14	0.07
Nonfatal infarction	66	0.34
Definite	53	0.27
Probable	13	0.07
Vascular complication	162	0.83
Arterial thrombosis	101	0.52
Dissection or rupture	35	0.18
Hematoma	21	0.11
Pseudoaneurysm	3	0.02
Thrombophlebitis	2	0.01
Arterial embolism	13	0.07
(To central nervous system)	(6)	(0.03)
Neurological complication	26	0.13
Transient	19	0.09
Permanent	7	0.03
Ventricular fibrillation (without infarction)	74	0.38
One or more complications per patient	323	1.67

nondiagnostic study. In this situation, the patient must undergo the risk of a second procedure or be treated with incomplete information. Fortunately, the currently available video tape and video disk recorders provide immediate replay of high-quality images that greatly enhance the ability of the angiographer to carefully evaluate the adequacy of a study. If there is uncertainty about a particular arterial segment, additional views can be taken to clarify the problem area.

The optimal approach to complications of coronary arteriography is to avoid them by excellent preparation of the patient to enable them to tolerate the stress encountered, by tailoring procedures for each patient, and by prompt therapeutic interventions when required. The following is a description of our management of complications encountered during and following coronary arteriography.

MANAGEMENT OF COMPLICATIONS OCCURRING DURING OR AS A RESULT OF CORONARY ARTERIOGRAPHY

Ischemic Pain

Development of ischemic pain during coronary arteriography is common when patients with severe coronary arterial disease are studied. *Preparation of the patient is critical*. Key elements in preparing severely symptomatic patients for coronary arteriography are beta-adrenergic blockade and maximal therapy with nitrates and calcium channel–blocking agents to achieve stability of symptoms prior to the study if possible (using intravenous nitroglycerin if necessary). Consequences of inadequate beta-adrenergic blockade include tachycardia, hypertension, and prolonged ischemic pain, which lengthens the arteriographic procedure and increases risk. It is important to carefully plan each procedure in severely symptomatic patients and those anticipated to have severe obstructive disease. Provision on the operating room schedule for the most severely symptomatic patients should be ensured prior to the study. In these fragile patients, coronary injections are usually done first (or following a small-volume left ventricular injection), and the number of intracoronary injections is minimized consistent with clear identification of all important anatomy.

The first coronary injection in our laboratory is of the left coronary in a shallow right anterior oblique view, which allows visualization of the left main and also all left coronary branches. One or two left coronary injections may be sufficient in some high-risk patients. Prompt *treatment* of ischemic pain with sublingual nitroglycerin is usually effective alone in adequately prepared patients. If pain is not relieved in a few minutes following nitroglycerin, attention is directed to the determinants of myocardial oxygen consumption. Measurement of heart rate, systemic blood pressure, and left ventricular end-diastolic pressure (LVEDP) are made and utilized as a basis for therapy. If systemic blood pressure is adequate or elevated, we administer additional nitroglycerin, elevate the patient's upper trunk on a foam rubber wedge, and give oxygen. Increments of propranolol (1 mg intravenously) are administered at 2-minute intervals to achieve a heart rate of approximately 60 beats per minute. Hypertension is effectively controlled with nifedipine 5 to 10 mg sublingually repeated to a total dose of 20 to 40 mg over 10 to 20 minutes.

Monitoring of ischemic symptoms, LVEDP, and electrocardiographic evidence of ischemia will allow one to assess effectiveness of treatment. Institution of intravenous nitroglycerin and use of small increments of intravenous narcotics (morphine 2 to 4 mg) may be required in difficult patients. The basis for refractory ischemic pain may be the stress of the procedure, which tips a previously delicately balanced supply-demand relationship, or thromboembolism, air embolism, or coronary arterial damage by the catheter may be responsible. Reinjection of the coronary arteries may be necessary if pain cannot be controlled or if ST-segment shifts (elevation) suggest a major coronary artery occlusion has occurred. In the rare case of spontaneously occurring coronary spasm which is unresponsive to sublingual nitrates intracoronary nitroglycerin 100 to 200 μg is administered if coronary occlusion is documented, and consideration is given to thrombolytic therapy if thrombus is evident or to emergency bypass surgery. The intraaortic balloon pump is inserted percutaneously if pain is uncontrolled by medical means, and emergency surgical consultation is sought if bypassable disease is present.

In occasional patients, emergency balloon angioplasty may correct severely symptomatic single vessel disease, with a happy outcome for all concerned. If the patient with severe obstructive coronary disease can be stabilized adequately, attention must be directed to optimizing therapy during the waiting period prior to surgery. This includes rehydration to overcome the osmotic diuresis, coronary care unit monitoring, and intravenous nitroglycerin. Heparin anticoagulation is frequently used in patients with near total occlusion of major coronary arteries with and without visible intracoronary thrombi. In our experience, the development of acute myocardial infarction during coronary arteriography is exceedingly rare. A more common sequence of events is the development of pain and evidence of myocardial infarction in 8 to 24 hours following coronary arteriography due to progression of a high-grade stenosis to total occlusion.

Acute Congestive Heart Failure

The development of pulmonary edema during coronary arteriography is a rare complication in adequately prepared patients. In general, all signs of congestive heart failure should be absent before coronary arteriography is attempted, but this goal is not possible in all patients. It is well known that the adverse effects of contrast media on cardiac physiology include depression of generated myocardial force.[10–12] Heart failure during coronary arteriography is usually due to a combination of factors: prior infarction, acute increase in intravascular volume, negative inotropic effects of contrast media, regional myocardial ischemia, and/or mitral regurgitation due to papillary muscle dysfunction. Treatment is directed at reducing left ventricular wall stress by reducing left ventricular volume (elevating the patient's upper trunk on a foam rubber wedge, morphine, nitrates, diuretics, and control of hypertension) and maximizing oxygen delivery (oxygen administration, nitrates to improve collateral flow). In severe congestive heart failure, afterload reduction with nitroprusside or intraaortic balloon pumping may be required.

"Anaphylactoid Reactions" to Contrast Medium

As the term implies, anaphylactoid reactions to contrast medium lack elements of classical anaphylaxis. Contrary to true anaphylaxis, these reactions to contrast medium occur without participation of IgE antibody or antigen[13–15] except in a few rare instances.[16] This nonimmunologic basis explains the occurrence of anaphylactoid reactions on first exposure to contrast medium and the similar severity of subsequent reactions. The clinical features, however, are identical to true anaphylaxis and occur as a result of degranulation of circulating basophils and tissue mast cells with liberation of histamine and other toxic vasoactive mediators[17,18] The precise mechanism that leads to degranulation of these cells is unknown. A direct effect of contrast medium or complement activation (producing C5a, C3a, and C4a anaphylatoxins) or other mechanisms may be responsible.

The clinical manifestations of anaphylactoid reactions to contrast media (Table 11-2) are determined by the amount and location of histamine

Table 11-2 Anaphylactoid Reactions to Contrast Medium

Cutaneous and mucosal
Urticaria
Pruritis
Flushing
Angioedema
Laryngeal edema
Cardiovascular
Vasodilatation
Hypotension (shock)
Arrhythmia
Smooth muscle
Bronchospasm
Gastrointestinal spasm
Uterine contraction

release and the interaction of H_1 and H_2 membrane receptors. Consequences of H_1- and H_2-receptor stimulation include pruritis, vasodilatation, increased vascular permeability, reduction in threshold for ventricular fibrillation, and gastric hyperacidity. Release of histamine in the skin produces flushing and urticaria; in the lung, bronchoconstriction and mucus production; in the vascular system, hypotension and arrhythmia. Urticaria is reported to occur in 1 to 2 percent of patients initially exposed to contrast medium,[19] but may be present in milder degrees in up to 10 percent of patients.[20] Although pruritis may be intense, urticaria is transient, well-tolerated, and does not imply a more severe reaction on subsequent exposure to contrast medium. Intense flushing occurs in less than 1 percent of patients.[19] Angioedematous swelling of subcutaneous tissue (most commonly lips and eyelids) occurs in 0.03 percent of patients.[19] Fortunately, life-threatening laryngeal edema is quite rare, occurring in 7 of 32,000 patients in Witten's experience[19] and less often in our experience. Unfortunately, similar reactions are common on reexposure to contrast medium, unless prophylaxis is provided. Bronchospasm is reported in 0.03 percent, shock in 0.05 percent, and death due to anaphylactoid reactions in approximately 1 in 50,000 patients.[13,19]

Recognition and Prophylaxis of High-risk Patients

Administration of antihistamines and corticosteroids prior to contrast medium has been carried out with the hope of avoiding undesirable symptoms and serious reactions. In general, prophylaxis of all patients has not been recommended because of the clinical impression that only minor reactions were prevented by antihistamine premedication. Patients are characterized as to risk of anaphylactoid reactions based on previous contrast media exposures. Low-risk patients are those with no prior contrast medium exposure and with no allergic history.

Although anaphylactoid reactions to contrast medium are nonimmunologic in most cases, patients with "allergic histories" have roughly twice the risk of mild anaphylactoid reactions but no increase in severe reactions.[19] Patients with mild previous reactions to contrast media or allergic histories appear to have slightly increased risk on exposure to contrast medium, and patients with prior serious reactions to contrast medium are at high risk. Attempts to identify high-risk patients by pretesting with small amounts of contrast medium have proved unreliable and have been abandoned by most investigators.[19] Some advocate the use of intravenous pretesting in patients with prior contrast medium sensitivity, but the usefulness of this technique is limited by the observation that up to 20 percent of negative reactors may experience anaphylactoid reactions on full exposure to the agent.[21] In the future, in vitro testing of blood for complement activation, basophil degranulation, histamine production, or other markers may offer means for clinical identification of patients at risk for serious anaphylactoid reactions to contrast medium.[18,22,23] For the present, the clinical angiographer must rely on historical aspects for estimation of this risk.

Recent studies have shown the value of antihistamines (H_1 agents alone or combined with H_2 agents) in reducing the incidence of minor anaphylactoid reactions in low-risk patients.[20,21] It has not been our practice, however, to administer antihistamines routinely in low-risk patients. Of most concern, of course, are those patients who have had prior reactions to contrast medium but require another contrast study. Risk of anaphylactoid reactions on reexposure to contrast media is 15 to 35 percent in these patients.[19,21,24]

Most studies report results of pretreatment of high-risk patients with corticosteroids with or without type H_1 antihistamines, and with this pretreatment, the occurrence of minor anaphylactoid reactions is reduced to 5 to 10 percent and of severe reactions to less than 1 percent.[21,24,25] In a report of 318 procedures in patients with prior reactions to contrast media, pretreatment (prednisone 50 mg orally every 6 hours for three doses ending 1 hour before the procedure, and diphenhydramine 50 mg intramuscularly 1 hour before the procedure) was highly effective; 20 (6.2 percent) had minor reactions, 3 (0.9 percent) generalized urticaria, and in only 3 (0.9 percent) serious anaphylactoid reactions occurred.[24] In 84 patients whose prior anaphylactoid reactions were serious (hypotension, laryngeal edema, marked wheezing, or syncope) only 5 (6 percent) had repeat reactions, none serious. Similar favorable results have been reported using pretreatment with high-dose steroids alone.[25] Although pretreatment with steroids and type H_1 antihistamines is highly effective, severe reactions and death have been reported in high-risk patients pretreated with these agents (see Fig. 11-2).[26,27] It has been suggested that the use of nonionic contrast medium[28] and the addition of H_2 antihistamines to the pretreatment regimen[20,27] be considered in high-risk patients. Both suggestions need further study.

Because complete reassurance cannot be given to high-risk patients, we believe the following are minimal requirements which should be met before the contrast study is carried out: (1) The procedure requiring contrast medium must be essential. (2) The patient must be fully informed of the potential risks of a reaction equal to or of greater severity than that previously experienced. (3) Prophylaxis with H_1 antihistamines and corticosteroids should be provided (for example, prednisone 40 mg orally the night before and repeated several hours prior to the study and diphenhydramine 50 mg intravenously 5 minutes prior to contrast administration). H_2 Antihistamines may be considered as well. (4)

Figure 11-2 A 60-year-old male with a history of cardiac arrest during a previous renal arteriogram required coronary arteriography because of disabling chest pain. The patient was pretreated with diphenhydramine 50 mg intravenously and hydrocortisone 100 mg intravenously 30 minutes prior to administration of contrast medium. (*a*) Baseline arterial pressure tracing with blood pressure 142/80 mmHg. Following intracoronary injection of 8 to 10 mL of Renografin 76, blood pressure dropped to 85/50 mmHg, and the arterial pressure tracing developed a narrow spikelike contour (*b*) and the patient developed marked generalized erythema. Blood pressure subsequently dropped to 55/35 mm Hg(*c*), and following administration of intravenous epinephrine and volume expansion, blood pressure stabilized at 110/75 mmHg (*d*) and a limited coronary arteriogram was completed. The coronary arteriogram was normal.

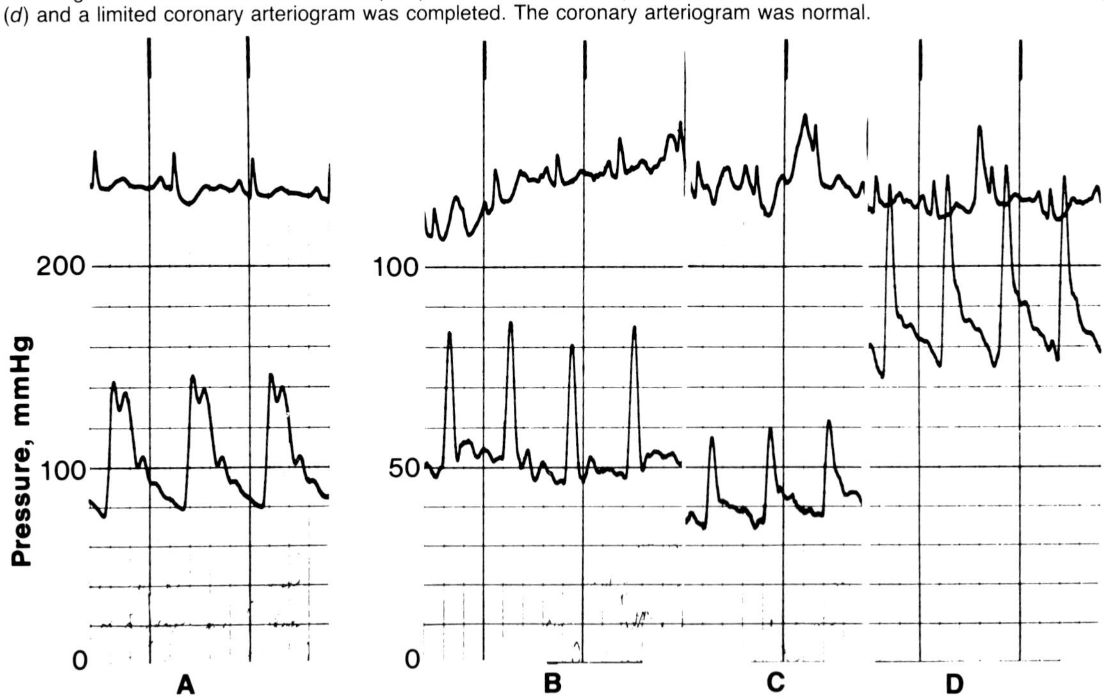

The ability to ensure an airway and treat all manifestations of anaphylaxis must be ensured.

Treatment of Anaphylactoid Reactions

Minor Reactions The vast majority of anaphylactoid reactions to contrast media are mild and self-limiting (urticaria, erythema, itching, angioedema). Antihistamines act by binding histamine receptor sites and are of limited value in treating acute reactions. Antihistamines do not hasten resolution of urticaria and angioedema already present, but do reduce itching and block further histamine binding. We administer diphenhydramine hydrochloride 25 to 50 mg intravenously when these mild reactions occur during coronary arteriography and recommend that pretreatment with antihistamines and/or corticosteroids be considered when subsequent studies requiring contrast medium. Corticosteroids and/or small doses of subcutaneous epinephrine (0.2 to 0.3 mg) may be administered for acute reactions in which the seriousness of the evolving reaction is difficult to ascertain and there is concern that more than a minor reaction may be present.

Major Reactions Treatment of more severe reactions (bronchospasm, laryngeal edema, hypotension, vascular collapse) must be prompt and specific. Commonly, diffuse erythema and urticaria provide early clues to the etiology of the evolving reaction. A very valuable early sign of impending shock and cardiovascular collapse is the spikelike arterial contour in Fig. 11-2. The mainstay of therapy of severe anaphylactoid reactions is epinephrine (increments of 0.2 to 0.4 mg intravenously at 2-to 5-minute intervals). Profound hypotension is the rule in serious reactions in our experience. Peripheral and splanchnic vasodilatation and increased capillary permeability lead to low effective circulating blood volume, and massive volume replacement may be required. Corticosteroids (hydrocortisone 200 to 500 mg intravenously) and antihistamines (diphenhydramine 50 mg intravenously) are administered, but only after epinephrine and volume expansion are begun.

Promptness of the institution of therapy may determine the outcome in patients with severe multivessel or left main coronary disease. We have had experience with one patient whose clinical findings strongly suggested left main coronary disease who experienced cardiovascular collapse immediately after a normal left ventriculogram. This patient remained in shock despite maximal medical measures, and immediate multivessel ''blind'' coronary bypass surgery was lifesaving. Bronchospasm is treated with aminophylline (20 mg/min to a total dose of 500 mg). Endotracheal intubation or tracheostomy have not been needed for laryngeal edema in our experience; however, anesthesiology support is immediately requested to assist in airway maintenance when laryngeal edema occurs. Pathological studies by James and Austen in fatal cases of anaphylaxis showed upper airway edema and obstruction were predominant abnormalities.[29] Oxygen administration and arterial blood gas monitoring are carried out until respiratory function normalizes. It has been suggested that antihistamines of the H_2 type be utilized in acute anaphylactoid reactions when response to therapy is not immediate, and this seems reasonable. H_2-receptor blockers appear to be indicated when contrast angiography must be carried out in patients who have experienced anaphylactoid reactions in spite of pretreatment with steroids and H_1 antihistamines.

Arrhythmia

Bradyarrhythmia Injection of contrast medium into the coronary arteries, especially into the branches supplying the inferior left ventricular wall, commonly produces marked bradycardia and hypotension. This is a clinical example of the Bezold-Jarisch reflex in which myocardial receptors in the inferior left ventricular myocardium send impulses via the vagus nerve to vasomotor centers which inhibit sympathetic discharge and activate parasympathetic efferents with resultant bradycardia and peripheral vasodilatation.[30–31a] This reflex is blocked by atropine,[32,32a] and most, but not all, coronary angiographers administer atropine 0.4 to 0.6 mg intravenously prior to coronary injections to avoid the transient bradycardia and hypotension that would otherwise occur. Marked bradycardia may also occur after coronary injections due to sinus arrest in patients with sick sinus syndrome. Most often this is also the result of the Bezold-Jarisch reflex and occurs when the artery supplying the inferior wall is injected, independent of the origin of the sinus node artery. Transient complete heart block will occur in some patients with right bundle branch block when a catheter crossing the aortic valve stimulates the conduction system in the upper interventricular septum.

The treatment of severe persisting bradycardia during coronary arteriography includes atropine up to 1 to 2 mg and transvenous pacing; intravenous infusion of isoproterenol is only rarely needed to support a patient until pacing can be accomplished. Indications for prophylactic pacemaker insertion during coronary arteriography in our laboratory include sick sinus syndrome, complete or transient atrioventricular (AV) block, trifascicular conduction system disease, suspected Stokes-Adams attacks, evolving inferior infarction, and probable right coronary artery spasm in patients undergoing ergonovine testing. Cardiac pacing prevents bradycardia but not the cholinergic-mediated hypotension that occurs during coronary arteriography, whereas atropine prevents both.

Tachyarrhythmia Ventricular fibrillation is the most common serious arrhythmia during coronary arteriography, occurring in 0.3 to 0.5 percent of patients. Treatment is prompt DC cardioversion using 300 watt-seconds. Vigorous coughing has been shown to maintain forward blood flow transiently and is helpful if a delay in cardioversion occurs. External cardiac massage is usually unnecessary. Following defibrillation, the coronary arteriogram can usually be completed. Ventricular fibrillation is most often the result of overzealous injection of contrast medium (excessive volume injected over too long a period of time or too soon after previous injections). Ventricular fibrillation is more likely to occur in patients with active ischemia or evolving infarction but also occurs in patients with normal coronary arteriograms. Ventricular fibrillation may be induced by pacing stimuli falling in the vulnerable period. Contrast medium reduces the threshold for ventricular fibrillation by prolonging depolarization and repolarization permitting a reentry mechanism.[33–35] Nonionic contrast agents are less likely to cause ventricular fibrillation and may become the agents of choice in higher-risk patients undergoing coronary thrombolysis, percutaneous coronary angioplasty, or even coronary arteriography, although the cost of these agents may be substantially greater than currently used ionic agents.

Ventricular tachycardia or multiform ventricular premature beats occurring in a patient undergoing coronary arteriography are usually suppressed effectively with intravenous injections of lidocaine 50 to 75 mg. Supraventricular tachyarrhythmias occur quite rarely during coronary arteriography. Paroxysmal atrial tachycardia commonly can be reverted to sinus rhythm by simply stimulating a premature ventricular beat, which blocks the reentry circuit. Control of supraventricular tachycardia can usually be achieved with intravenous verapamil 5 to 10 mg, small doses of propranolol, or by digitalization. Atrial flutter can frequently be converted to atrial fibrillation or sinus rhythm by rapid atrial pacing.

Cardiogenic Shock

Cardiogenic shock is a rare but frequently fatal complication of coronary arteriography. The cardiac pathology in patients with this complication is most often left main and triple vessel coronary obstruction in our experience. The common denominator is global left ventricular ischemia produced by a vicious cycle of contrast medium–induced hypotension,[30–32,36] decreased coronary perfusion, progressive and massive left ventricular ischemia, ischemic paralysis of the left ventricle, and progressive hypotension. Cardiogenic shock is recognized by the presence of a low cardiac output state accompanied by increased left ventricular filling pressure. In the presence of critical left main coronary artery disease, cardiogenic shock is usually fatal unless immediate therapeutic measures, including coronary bypass surgery, are available. Treatment of cardiogenic shock occurring during coronary arteriography includes the use of catecholamines[37,38] and intraaortic balloon support.[39] Vasodilators are not usually indicated in treatment of cardiogenic shock in the coronary arteriography laboratory because of the threat of reducing coronary perfusion. The first order of therapy is to establish adequate arterial pressure. Norepinephrine has been shown to be transiently effective in increasing arterial blood pressure and cardiac output in severe cardiogenic shock,[39a] but other sympathomimetic amines or intraaortic balloon pumping may be needed. Intraaortic balloon pumping reduces ischemia by augmenting diastolic aortic pressure, reducing left ventricular afterload during systole, increasing coronary artery perfusion, and reducing myocardial oxygen consumption. Emergency coronary bypass surgery can be lifesaving. If surgery must be carried out without complete angiographic data, it should be assumed that triple vessel coronary disease is present and bypass to all three coronary arteries should be performed as suggested by Roberts et al.[40]

It must be kept in mind that in addition to global left ventricular ischemia and evolving infarction, the differential diagnosis of cardiogenic shock includes pericardial tamponade. We have not seen pericardial tamponade as a complication of coronary arteriography, but have had three patients with pericardial tamponade occurring as a complication of percutaneous coronary angioplasty. In each case, it appeared to result from perforation of the right ventricle with a pacing catheter in a patient who was heparinized. In two patients, only needle aspiration of the pericardium was required to restore normal hemodynamics.

Arterial Entry Site Complications

Femoral Complications at the femoral puncture site are minimized by meticulous attention to catheter removal and arterial compression as described in Chap. 8. *Hematoma formation*, the most frequent puncture site complication, may occur due to leaking around the catheter during coronary arteriography, leaking during compression of the femoral artery, or as a result of late bleeding. Surgical evacuation of the hematoma is not required, even for large hematomas, unless there is undue tension on adjacent structures or in the case of a truly huge hematoma. Surgical evacuation and arterial repair are required when the hematoma is pulsatile and expanding indicating communication of the hematoma with the femoral artery and the presence of a *false aneurysm*. In our experience, false aneurysms occur disproportionately in elderly women and in the presence of predisposing factors such as warfarin anticoagulation or aortic regurgitation. Bleeding from a femoral puncture site may occur into the retroperitoneal space with no external evidence of blood loss. In this case, symptoms of lower abdominal or flank discomfort may occur, or there may be no symptoms other than those related to a reduced circulating blood volume.

Retroperitoneal bleeding should be considered in patients experiencing significant hypotension within 12 hours following coronary arteriography. A reduction in hemoglobin may be the only firm clue to the diagnosis. Bleeding from a puncture site into the retroperitoneal space is self-limiting unless the patient is anticoagulated, in which case transfusion may be required. This complication is commonly not recognized, and therefore, its frequency is grossly underestimated. When the ipsilateral femoral artery and vein are catheterized, there is the theoretical possibility of arteriovenous fistula formation when the catheters are removed. Fortunately, this complication is exceedingly rare, having occurred in only two or three patients in our experience.

Occlusion of the femoral artery may occur due to thrombosis or local arterial injury. This complication, which occurs in less than 0.1 percent of patients, is confined almost exclusively to women with small femoral arteries which are completely blocked by the catheter during the procedure and in the rare patient in whom the superficial femoral artery rather than the common femoral is catheterized. In an effort to minimize this complication, we use heparin when very small femoral arteries are suspected. If previously palpable distal pulses are absent following catheter removal, we obtain immediate consultation with our vascular surgery colleagues. Intraarterial injection of 25 mg tolazoline may relieve femoral artery spasm if present. In the presence of significant distal vascular disease or if distal embolization has occurred (popliteal pulse is present but no pedal pulses), an arteriogram may be needed. Surgical exploration and passage of a Fogarty catheter is almost uniformly successful in restoring circulation in our experience.

Brachial Complications at the brachial artery entry site include infection, median nerve injury, brachial artery spasm, and brachial artery occlusion. Segmental occlusion of the brachial artery occurs in 2 to 3 percent of patients (see Chap. 6). Fortunately, when occlusion of the brachial artery occurs at the antecubital fossa in the absence of proximal occlusion, collateral circulation around the elbow will prevent major disability or tissue loss in almost all cases where adequate repair cannot be achieved. Fortunately, median nerve injury and false aneurysms at the brachial arteriotomy site are rare complications. When false aneurysms do occur, surgical repair is usually recommended.

Contrast Nephropathy

Nephrotoxicity is a well-recognized complication of radiographic procedures using intravascular contrast medium. Recent studies suggest that the incidence of acute renal failure (increased serum creatinine greater than 2 mg/dL) following arteriography procedures is approximately 0.5 percent.[42] Typically, the patient with contrast-induced renal failure develops oliguria within the initial 24 hours after exposure to the contrast agent. Oliguria persists for 2 to 4 days. Serum creatinine levels peak within 7 days and return to baseline in 80 to 90 percent of cases. Dialysis is rarely required in patients whose baseline renal function is normal. Irreversible renal failure has occurred in patients with diabetes or renal insufficiency, and the presence of these problems greatly increases the risk of contract nephropathy (Table 11-3). In patients with nondiabetic

Table 11-3 Incidence of Contrast Nephropathy* by Risk Factor

Risk factor	Incidence (%)
Normal renal function	0–0.6
Nondiabetic renal insufficiency	
Serum creatinine 1.5–4.5 mg/dL	0–60
Serum creatinine > 4.5 mg/dL	30–86
Diabetic nephropathy	
Serum creatinine < 1.5 mg/dL	0–0.6
Serum creatinine 1.5–2 mg/dL	16
Serum creatinine 2–4.5 mg/dL	50–92
Serum creatinine > 4.5 mg/dL	76–93
After renal transplant	36–65
Multiple myeloma	1–2

*Contrast nephropathy defined as a rise in serum creatinine > 1 mg/dL.
SOURCE: Adapted from Massry et al.[43]

renal insufficiency, the incidence of nephrotoxicity correlates directly with the level of renal impairment. There is increased filtration of contrast medium per functioning nephron with renal insufficiency. Of 28 well-hydrated patients with mean creatinine 3.8 mg/dL, 61 percent developed evidence of nephrotoxicity (serum creatinine level increased more than 1 mg/dL), while 86 percent of 22 patients with creatinine clearance less than 15 mL/min developed nephrotoxicity, which was reversible in most.[43] Although diabetics with normal renal function do not have significantly increased risk of contrast nephropathy, those with renal insufficiency are at substantial risk. In diabetics with serum creatinine levels 2 to 4.5 mg/dL, 50 to 90 percent experienced contrast nephropathy, but when the serum creatinine level exceeded 5 mg/dL, over 90 percent of patients experienced nephrotoxicity, and one-half required maintenance dialysis following the episode of contrast nephropathy.[43] The risk of contrast nephropathy in multiple myeloma has been overemphasized in the past. The incidence of this complication in myeloma patients is only slightly greater than in the population at large. Other significant risk factors for contrast nephropathy include advanced age, renal transplantation, dehydration, a previous episode of contrast nephropathy, and multiple contrast studies within 24 to 48 hours.

Important in the prevention of contrast nephropathy is the avoidance of the use of these agents in high-risk patients unless the potential benefits outweigh the risk. When use of contrast agents cannot be avoided, the risk of nephrotoxicity can be minimized by volume expansion and diuresis with furosemide or mannitol.[43] Whether the protective effect of these agents is due to an increased renal tubular flow preventing tubular obstruction or increased renal blood flow is unclear.

REFERENCES

1 Adams DF, Fraser DB, Abrams HL: The complications of coronary arteriography. Circulation, 48:609, 1973.

2 Judkins MP, Gander MP: Prevention of complications of coronary arteriography. Circulation, 49:599, 1974.

3 Takaro T, Hultgren HN, Littman D, Wright EC: An analysis of deaths occurring in association with coronary arteriography. Am Heart J, 86:587, 1973.

4 Eyer KM: Complications of transfemoral coronary arteriography and their prevention using heparin. Am Heart J, 86:428, 1973.

5 Walker WJ, Mundall SL, Broderick HG, et al: Systemic heparinization for femoral percutaneous coronary arteriography. N Engl J Med, 288:826, 1973.

6 Abrams HL, Adams DF: The complications of coronary arteriography. Circulation, 52(suppl II):II-27, 1975.

7 Davis K, Kennedy JW, Kemp HG, Judkins MP, Gosselin AJ, Kilip T: Complications of coronary arteriography from the collaborative study of coronary artery surgery (CASS). Circulation, 59:1105, 1979.

8 Gersh BJ, Kronmal RA, Frye RL, et al: Coronary arteriography and coronary bypass surgery: Morbidity and mortality in patients ages 65 years or older. A report from the coronary artery surgery study. Circulation, 67:483, 1983.

9 Kennedy JW: Symposium on catheterization complications: Complications associated with cardiac catheterization and angiography. Cathet Cardiovasc Diagn, 8:5, 1982.

10 Gusman SV, West JW: Cardiac effects of intracoronary arterial injections of various roentgenographic contrast media. Am Heart J, 58:597, 1959.

11 Tragardh B, Lynch PR, Vinciguerra T: Cardiac function during coronary arteriography with calcium-enriched diatrizoate and metrizamide. Invest Radiol, 11:569, 1976.

12 Popio KA, Ross AM, Oravec JM, Ingram JT: Identification and description of separate mechanisms for two components of Renografin cardiotoxicity. Circulation, 58:520, 1978.

13 Patterson R, Anderson J: Allergic reactions to drugs and biologic agents. JAMA, 248:2637, 1982.

14 Kolb WP, Lang JH, Lasser EC: Nonimmunological complement activation in normal serum induced by radiographic contrast media. J Immunol, 121:1232, 1978.

14a Westaby S, Pridie RB, Dawson P, et al: Angiography and complement activation: Evidence for generation for C3a anaphylatoxin by intravascular contrast media. Circulation, 68(suppl III):III-64, 1983.

15 Lieberman P, Siegle RL, Taylor WW: Anaphylactoid reactions to iodinated contrast material. J Allergy Clin Immunol, 62:174, 1978.

16 Brasch RC: Accumulated evidence for allergy to radiographic contrast media: Clinical studies and a new model of fatal anaphylaxis in immature animals. Am J Roentgenol, 139:1030, 1982.

17 Rockoff SD, Brasch R, Kuhn C, et al: Contrast media as histamine liberators:1. Mast cell histamine release in vitro by sodium salts of contrast media. Invest Radiol, 6:503, 1970.

18 Rice MC, Lieberman P, Siegle RL, Mason J: In vitro histamine release induced by radiocontrast media and various chemical analogues in reactor and control subjects. J Allergy Clin Immunol, 72:180, 1983.

19 Witten DM: Reactions to urographic contrast media. JAMA, 231:974, 1975.

20 King JF, Manley JC: The effectiveness of cimetidine and hydroxyzine prophylaxis for prevention of contrast media reactions in patients undergoing coronary arteriography. Circulation, 66(suppl II):II-324, 1982.

21 Yocum MW, Heller AM, Abels RI: Efficacy of intravenous pretesting and antihistamine prophylaxis in radiocontrast media–sensitive patients. J Allergy Clin Immunol, 62:309, 1978.

22 Siegle RL, Lieberman P, Rice MC: In vitro complement consumption by contrast materials and analogues: Reactors vs. nonreactors. Invest Radiol, 18:387, 1983.

23 Stratta P, Camussi G, Porcellini G, et al: The usefulness of the basophil degranulation test in the study of hypersensitivity reactions to iodinated contrast media. Minerva Med, 72:1703, 1981.

24 Greenberger PA, Patterson R, Simon R, et al: Pretreatment of high-risk patients requiring radiographic contrast media studies. J Allergy Clin Immunol, 67:185, 1981.

25 Zweiman B, Mishkin MM, Hildreth EA: An approach to the performance of contrast studies in contrast material–reactive persons. Ann Intern Med, 83:159, 1975.

26 Madowitz JS, Schweiger MJ: Severe anaphylactoid reaction to radiographic contrast media. JAMA, 241:2813, 1979.

27 Myers G, Bloom F: Cimetidine (Tagamet) combined with steroids and H_1 antihistamines for the prevention of serious radiographic contrast material reactions. Cathet Cardiovasc Diagn, 7:65 1981.

28 Rapoport S, Bookstein JJ, Higgins CB, et al: Experience with metrizamide in patients with previous severe anaphylactoid reactions to ionic contrast agents. Radiology, 143:321, 1982.

29 James LP Jr, Austen KF: Fatal systemic anaphylaxis in man. N Engl J Med, 270:597, 1964.

30 Perez-Gomez F, Garcia-Aguado A: Origin of ventricular reflexes caused by coronary arteriography. Br Heart J, 39:967, 1977.

31 Abboud FM, Heistad DD, Mark AL, Schmid PG: Reflex control of the peripheral circulation. Prog Cardiovasc Dis, 18:371, 1976.

31a Mark AL: The Bezold-Jarisch reflex revisited: Clinical implications of inhibitory reflexes originating in the heart. J Am Coll Cardiol, 1:90, 1983.

32 Zelis R, Caudill CC, Baggett K, Mason D: Reflex vasodilation induced by coronary arteriography in human subjects. Circulation, 53:490, 1976.

32a Eckberg DL, White CW, Kioschos JM, Abboud FM: Mechanisms mediating bradycardia during coronary arteriography. J Clin Invest, 54:1445, 1974.

33 Wolff GL, Mulry CS, Laski PA, Kilzer K: Changes in ventricular fibrillation threshold induced by contrast agents during acute coronary artery occlusion. Invest Radiol, 18:145, 1983.

34 Murdock DK, Euler DE, Scanlon PJ, Gunnar RM: Mechanisms responsible for ventricular fibrillation during coronary arteriography. Circulation, 68(suppl III):III-147, 1983.

35 Franz MR, Gottlieb SO, Brinker JA: Renografin-76 but not Iopamidol produces marked local prolongation of canine monophasic action potential duration. Circulation, 68(suppl III):III-350, 1983.

36 Chahine RA, Raizner AE: The mechanism of hypotension following angiography. Invest Radiol, 11:472, 1976.

37 Rackley CE, Russell RO Jr, Mantle JA, Moraski RE: Cardiogenic shock: Recognition and management. Cardiovasc Clin, 7:251, 1975.

38 Gunnar RM, Loeb HS: Shock in acute myocardial infarction: Evolution of physiologic therapy. J Am Coll Cardiol, 1:154, 1983.

39 Dunkman WB, Leinbach RC, Buckley MJ, Mundth ED, Kantrowitz AR, Austin WG, Sanders CA: Clinical and hemodynamic results in intraaortic balloon pumping in surgery for cardiogenic shock. Circulation, 46:465, 1972.

39a Gunnar RM, Cruz A, Boswell J, Co BS, Pietras RJ, Tobin JR Jr: Myocardial infarction with shock: Hemodynamic studies and results of therapy. Circulation, 33:753, 1966.

40 Cabin HS, Roberts WC: Fatal cardiac arrest during cardiac catheterization for angina pectoris: Analysis of 10 necropsy patients. Am J Cardiol, 48:1, 1981.

41 Warnes CA, Kishel JC, Roberts WC: Fatal cardiac arrest during cardiac catheterization for angina pectoris: A marker of quadruple vessel disease. Chest, 84:631, 1983.

42 Byrd R, Sherman RL, Radiocontrast-induced acute renal failure: A clinical and pathophysiologic review. Medicine, 58:270, 1979.

43 Abraham P, Harkonen S, Kjellstrand C: Contrast nephropathy, in SG Massry, RJ Glassock (eds): *Textbook in Nephrology*. Williams & Wilkins, Baltimore, 1983, p 6.206.

Chapter 12

Interpretation of Coronary Arteriograms and Left Ventriculograms

Spencer B. King III, M.D.
John S. Douglas, Jr., M.D.

Interpretation of coronary arteriograms and left ventriculograms is usually accomplished by evaluation of 35-mm cine film. While other methods are occasionally practiced, cineangiograms are the final common language used by most arteriographers in describing the coronary circulation and left ventricular function. In order for adequate interpretation, the final image that is viewed must be of good quality. A superb film interpreted by a novice is of more value than an inadequate film interpreted by an expert. This final image for interpretation is determined by the entire sequence of events that go into producing the picture. Techniques for filling the coronary arteries with contrast medium are described elsewhere in this book and are of course essential for adequate film interpretation.

OBTAINING ADEQUATE IMAGES FOR INTERPRETATION

Assuming that adequate injections are performed, the elements responsible for the quality of the picture include the x-ray generator and tube, the image intensifier, the television chain, the cine camera, processing equipment, and the projector itself. The television fluoroscopy is an important aspect of this sequence even though it is not directly related to the production of film. If one is not able to visualize in real time the pictures that are being taken, then there is little chance that adequate films will be obtained. All manufacturers now have generators and x-ray tubes capable of delivering adequate energy to produce x-rays to penetrate even the obese patient with an effective focal spot size of 1 mm or less. Image tubes have become much more sensitive, allowing a lower dose rate and therefore less scatter radiation, which improves image quality. The lens system and cine cameras have changed little in recent years. They are of very high quality and are seldom a problem in the overall film result. Processing equipment is a critical step in the entire chain of producing adequate images. The most powerful generators with high-quality image intensifiers can all go for naught if the film is processed using outdated or improperly mixed chemicals. The principles of cineradiography and videofluorography are discussed in depth in Chap. 14.

The projector used to view the film can make up for a lot of shortcomings. The commonly used Tagarno-type projectors are well-suited to rapid viewing of film but do not have the light intensity to handle films with any degree of base fog or inherent background density. Ordinarily, fairly high-contrast clear-base film works best with those type projectors. If the film has a wide gray scale with fine gradations between densities, then projectors with more light intensity, such as the Vanguard or Cepro projectors, are superior. Frequently a film which is almost uninterpretable using a low-intensity light projector can be interpreted quite readily using a projector with a high-intensity beam.

The ability to angle the patient or the x-ray beam in multiple views including sagittal angles permits the operator to take pictures that eliminate foreshortening and overlap of coronary arteries. If these types of views are obtained, then the interpretation of the coronary arteriogram becomes much easier and, more importantly, more accurate. A discussion of the particular advantages of these views is found in Chap. 9.

Finally, the experience of the angiographer counts for a great deal in interpretation of cine films. Angiographers who are fully committed to cardiac catheterization laboratory activity and who are engaged on a daily basis with surgical and pathological correlations of their angiographic findings will obviously benefit and become the most reliable interpreters of coronary arteriograms. Daily interaction with surgical colleagues also improves the diagnostic accuracy of coronary arteriography. The correlations to be found in the operating room are valuable lessons that should not be passed up by the angiographer. An ongoing evaluation of postmortem material and its relationship to the degree of coronary stenosis is also valuable.

IDENTIFICATION OF VESSELS

Although coronary arteriograms are viewed in many ways, it is important in evaluating a film to systematically go through every arterial segment, first of all to identify that it is indeed present, and then to ensure that every part of each artery is seen without overlap or foreshortening so that the presence or absence of disease can be identified. A brief scanning of the film will not suffice since often on more careful review areas of obstruction are identified that were not originally seen.

Since the coronary anatomy is quite variable, the cardinal rule to be remembered is that the myocardium is served in all its segments by terminal branches of coronary arteries. It is therefore crucial that each coronary segment be accounted for, so that the supply of the entire myocardium is seen, regardless of the variability of the anatomy or the origin of the arteries. One should be intimately familiar with the coronary artery anatomy and its special relationships as described in Chap. 2.

Certain views are usually most suitable for identifying certain arteries, but these must be modified in accordance with the variations in coronary anatomy for each individual patient. The main left coronary is of course of critical importance and underestimation of stenosis must be carefully avoided. The best views are the frontal or shallow right anterior oblique (RAO) or left anterior oblique (LAO) as well as a severe cranial view in the frontal projection, as will be indicated under "Pitfalls" (Fig. 12-1). The proximal left anterior descending (LAD) is usually well seen in the RAO, LAO cranial, and the lateral views (Fig. 12-2). There may be overlap so that the lesion is obscured in one or more views. Since this area is critical, stenoses should be carefully looked for in all views required to free the

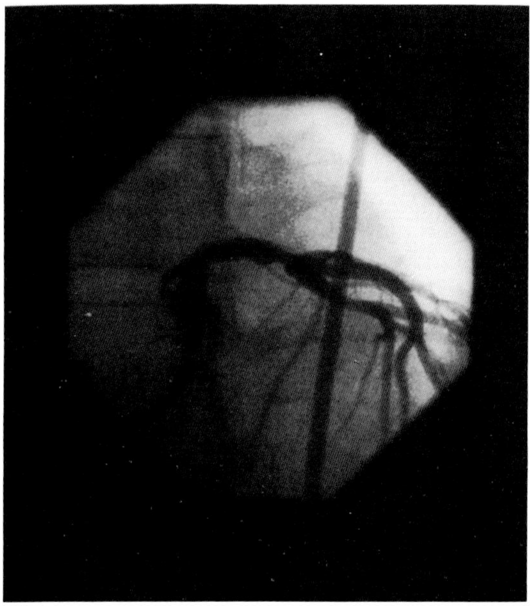

A

Figure 12-1 (*a*) Frontal view of left main coronary artery segment showing significant stenosis of the distal part just prior to the bifurcation. (*b*) LAO cranial view of left main artery showing severe stenosis.

artery from overlying structures (Figs. 12-1, 12-3, and 12-5). The diagonal branches of the LAD are frequently overlapped with the LAD when viewed in the standard RAO views. These vessels will almost always be identified in the LAO view with cranial angulation. This has proved to be the most valuable view for the diagonal origins (Fig. 12-3). Prior to the ability to do cranial angulation, lateral views were frequently obtained in an attempt to identify the diagonal branches, but this view produces overlap of the origin of the vessels with the LAD in most cases. The RAO view with cranial angulation will frequently give good visualization of the diagonal branches and LAD as well (Fig. 12-4).

The septal perforators are overlapped and frequently obscured by the LAD when viewed in the LAO view. Since the septal perforators arise at almost right angles from the LAD in most cases and dive deep into the muscular septum, the RAO view will usually show the septal perforators quite well (Fig. 12-5). In this view, there is sometimes overlap with diagonal branches, and when that is the case, viewing the septals in the left lateral view

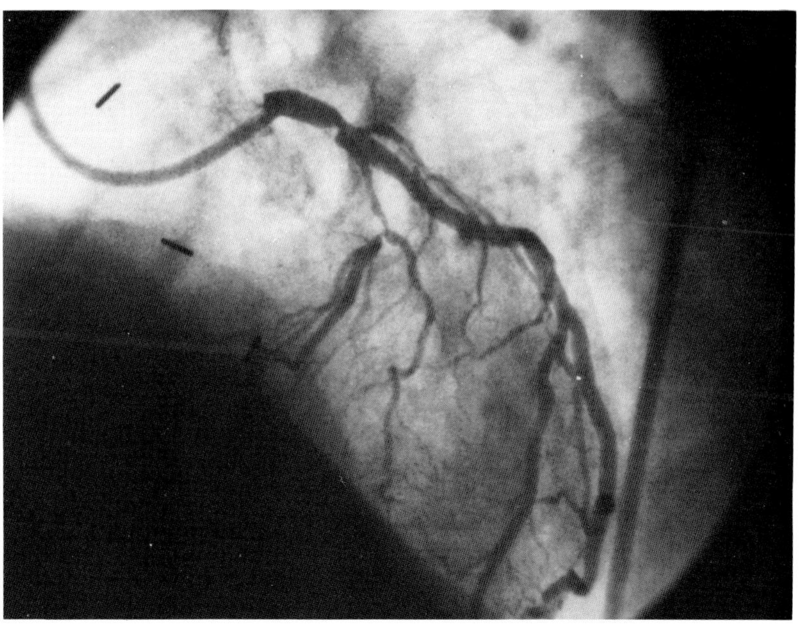

B

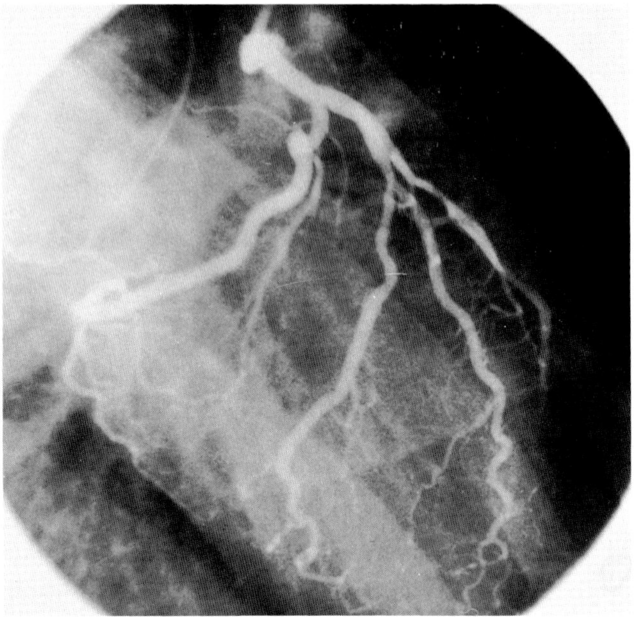

A

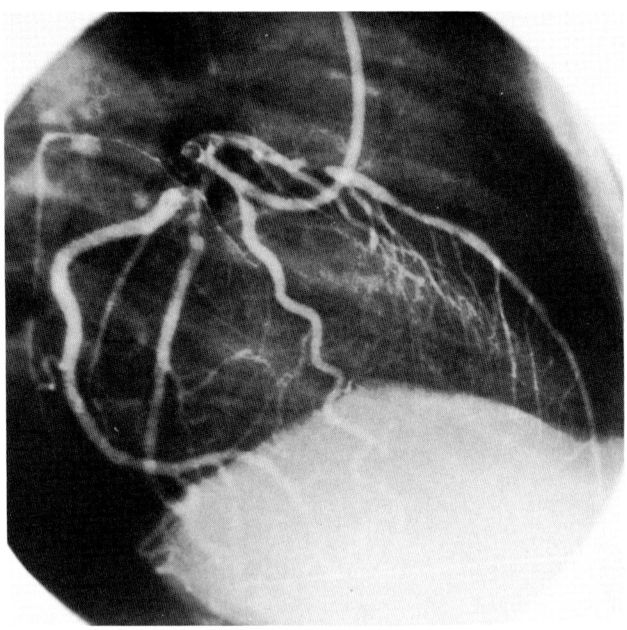

B

Figure 12-2 (*a*) RAO view of left coronary artery showing decreased flow in the LAD, but the lesion is not seen. (*b*) The lateral view shows a subtotal occlusion of the proximal LAD.

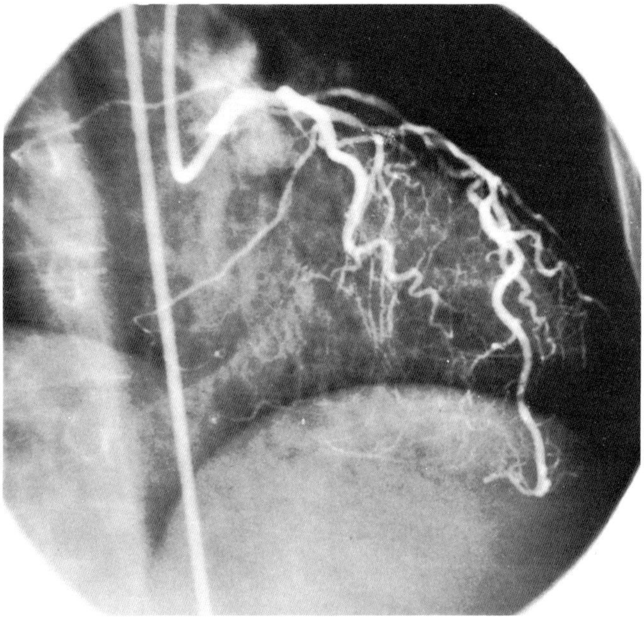

A

Figure 12-3 (*a*) RAO of left coronary artery showing overlap of proximal diagonal branches. (*b*) LAO cranial view showing the diagonal stenosis clearly. (*c*) LAO cranial view of left coronary artery showing diagonal origins.

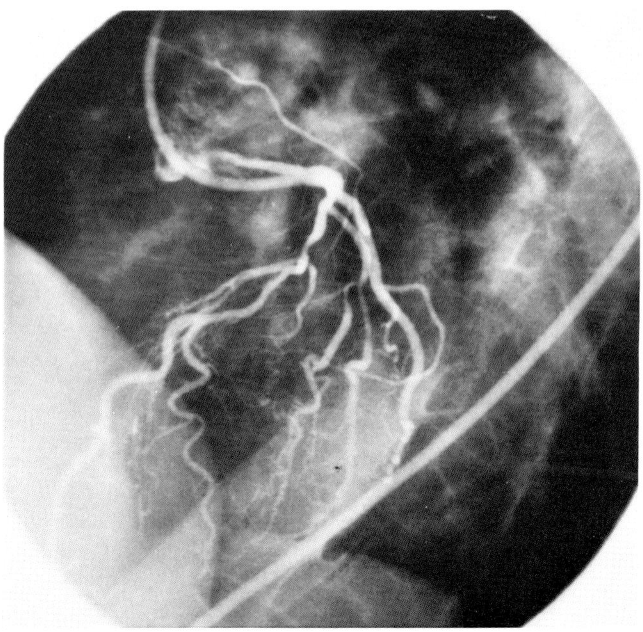

B

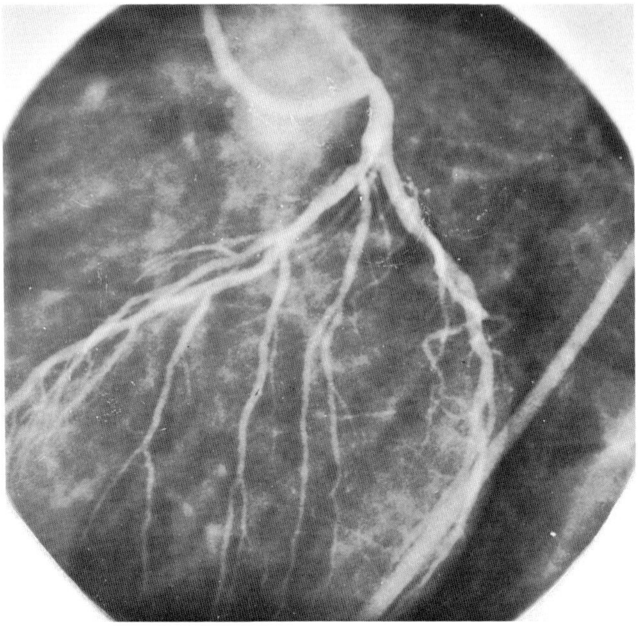

C *(Figure 12-3, continued)*

will be helpful. Septal perforators differ from epicardial vessels in that they are straighter and move in a different plane when compared to their epicardial counterparts. Sometimes a large branch arises from the LAD and travels just below the anterior descending artery almost parallel to it and then divides into the septal perforating branches. When this is the case, this artery may become confused with the LAD, especially if there is total occlusion of the LAD itself. That could be a serious error if bypass to this large septal perforating vessel was contemplated and when the surgeon tried to identify the vessel, could not find it because of its deep intramyocardial position.

The proximal circumflex travels posteriorly and may be obscured by the left main or LAD in the RAO views. The LAO or lateral view will best show the proximal circumflex (Fig. 12-6*a*). The circumflex marginal branches are usually best seen and delineated in the RAO views since they overlap the circumflex in the atrioventricular (AV) groove and each other in the LAO projections. Addition of caudal angulation will best separate the marginal branches in the RAO (Fig. 12-6*b*). This caudal angulation will widen the angle between the circumflex and the LAD, thereby separating the diagonal branches from the marginal branches. When the circumflex artery gives rise to the posterior descending branch, it should be viewed both in an LAO cranial projection to observe the portion of the vessel in the left ventricular groove which is proximal to the crux and in the RAO view so that the posterior descending artery can be seen on its side demonstrating the posterior septal perforators (Fig. 12-7).

The right coronary artery is examined in at least two views. The LAO view gives the best assessment of the conduit portion of the right coronary artery as it travels in the atrioventricular groove (Fig. 12-8*a*). Often, however, the posterior descending artery is obscured in this view. From its origin and throughout its course, it is traveling toward the viewer: therefore assessment of a lesion here is difficult. RAO views of the right coronary artery give a good evaluation of the mid-conduit portion and the best assessment of the posterior

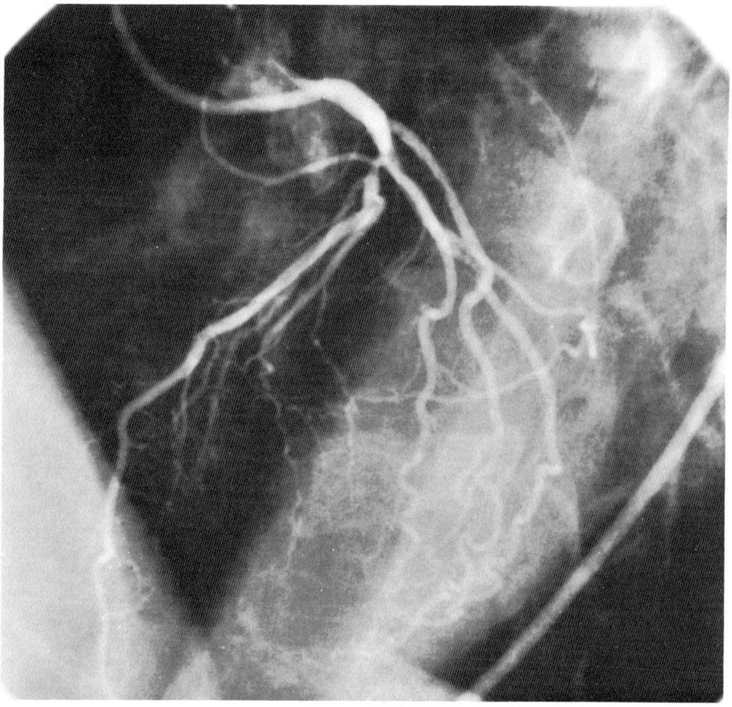

A

Figure 12-4 (*a*) LAO cranial view of left coronary artery showing proximal LAD stenosis, but the overlap of the diagonal branch is obscured by the proximal circumflex artery. (*b*) RAO cranial view of the left coronary artery showing the proximal LAD stenosis and also a high-grade lesion in the diagonal branch.

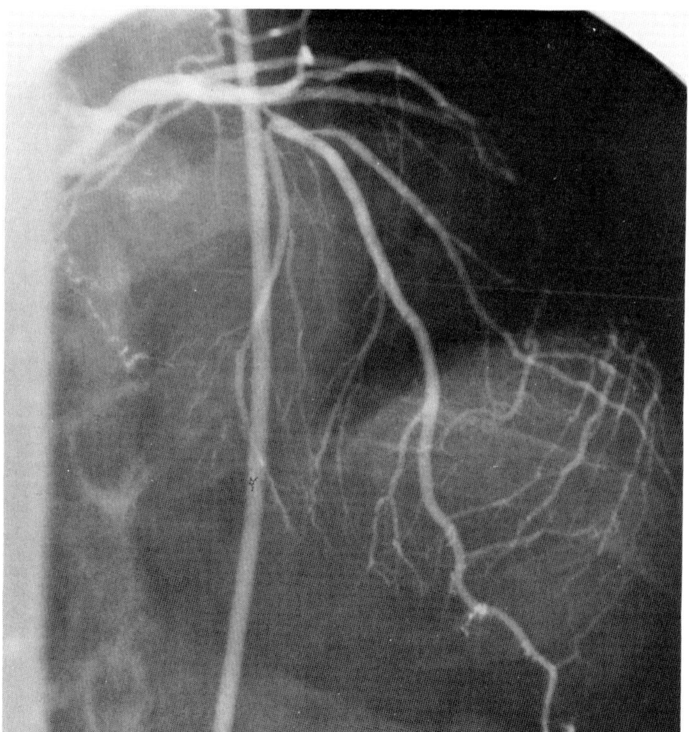

B

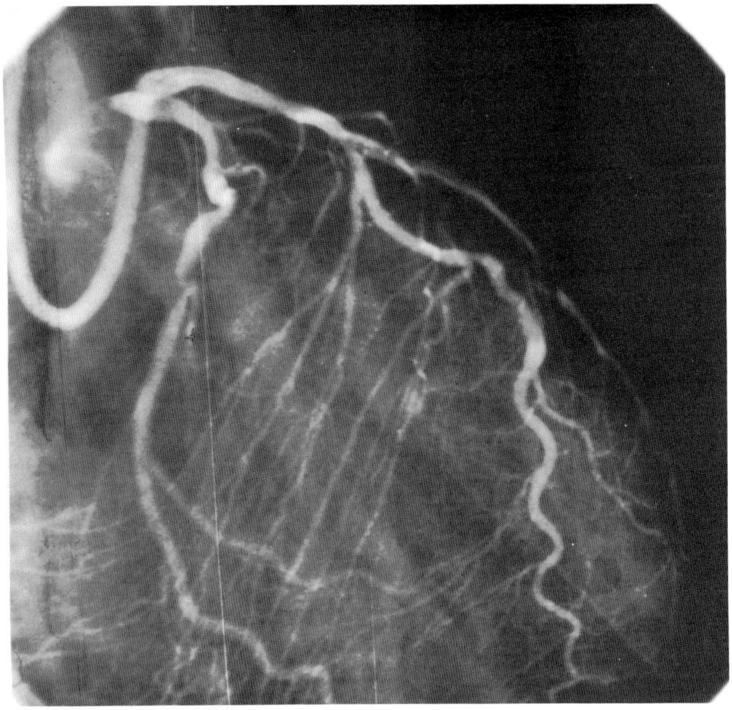

Figure 12-5 RAO view of left coronary artery showing septal perforating branches penetrating the interventricular septum. The septal perforators in this case are unusually large because of occlusion in the right coronary artery and secondary hypertrophy of the septal vessels to supply collaterals to the posterior circulation.

descending branch and its posteroseptal perforating arteries (Fig. 12-8*b*). If there is a large left ventricular branch distal to the posterior descending artery, this also can be evaluated in the RAO views. Addition of cranial angulation in the LAO view will give a good view of the bifurcation of the right coronary artery into its left ventricular branches and the posterior descending artery (Fig. 12-9). Often this view is essential in order to see this bifurcation, which is a frequent site of coronary atherosclerosis.

When the right coronary artery is nondominant, that is, when the posterior descending branch arises from the circumflex, the right coronary artery commonly bifurcates early, within 2 to 3 cm of its origin, into an equal-sized conus branch and a branch traveling in the right atrioventricular groove which stops prior to the crux of the heart. Differentiation between a totally occluded right coronary artery (RCA) and a nondominant right coronary artery is important and is facilitated by the knowledge of this early bifurcation and by the evaluation of the diameter of the proximal right. In a nondominant right coronary artery, the proximal segment is very small, whereas a totally occluded right coronary artery should have a large proximal segment prior to giving rise to right ventricular or conus branches. The conus artery may arise separately from the nondominant RCA (Fig. 12-10). The right coronary artery may be extremely tortuous, and therefore slight alterations in cranial or caudal angles may be necessary in order to avoid kinking and overlap.

When vessels are totally occluded, they are usually identified by a stub of a vessel or by the distal segment of the vessel filling via collateral vessels. This is not always the case, and therefore all segments of the myocardial surface should be inspected and if a zone void of vessels is detected, there should be a high index of suspicion that a vessel previously located in that area has been totally occluded. Usually if a coronary artery be-

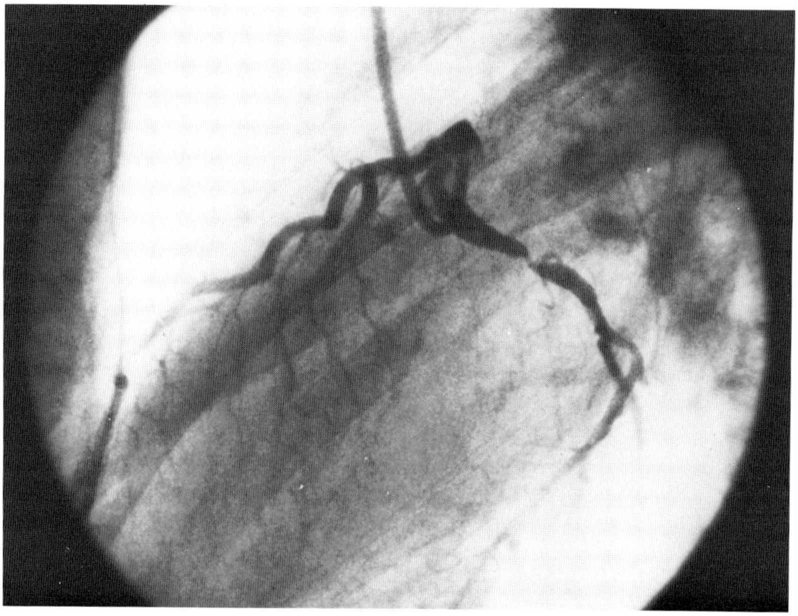

A

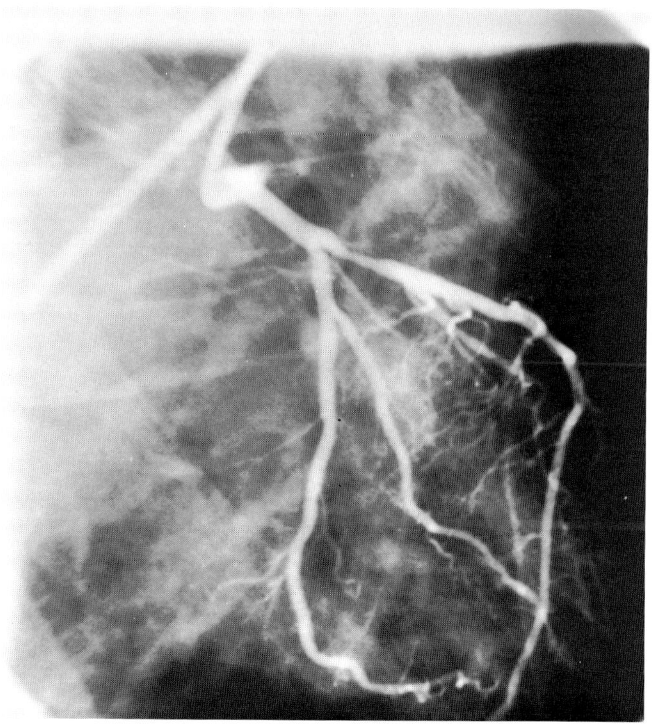

B

Figure 12-6 (*a*) Lateral view of left coronary artery (LCA) showing proximal circumflex lesion. (*b*) RAO caudal view of LCA showing the circumflex marginal arteries clearly separated from the LAD and the diagonal.

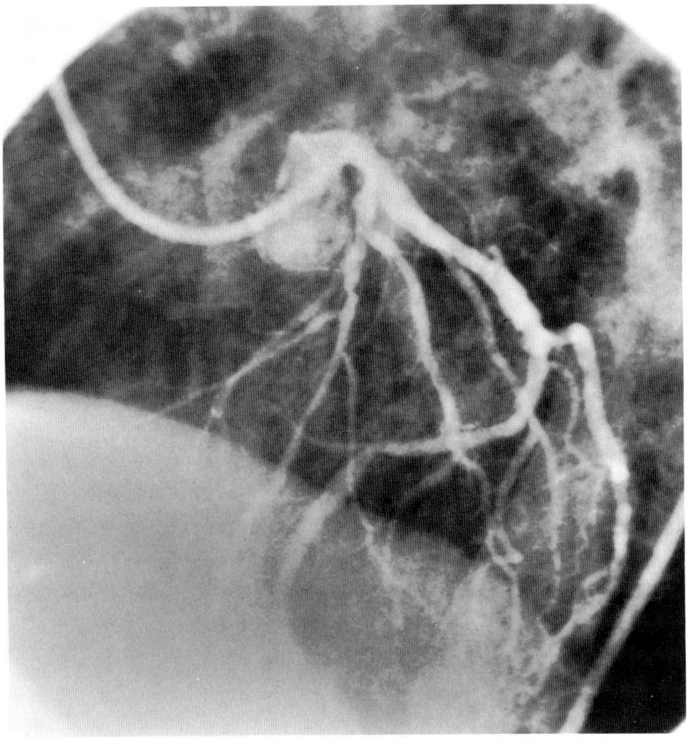

A

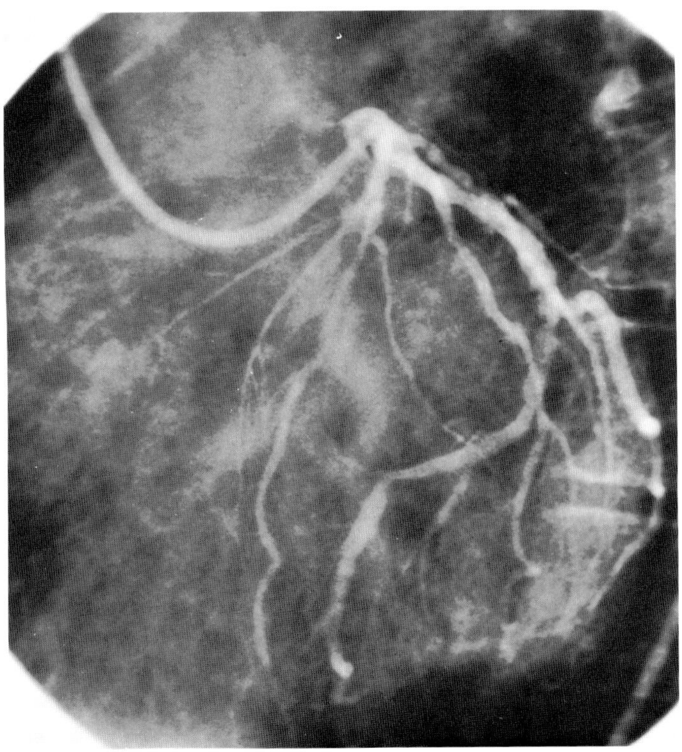

B

Figure 12-7 (*a*) LAO view of dominant left coronary artery. Posterior descending artery obscured by diaphragm. (*b*) LAO cranial view of dominant left coronary artery. Notice how the cranial view and deep inspiration brings the posterior descending artery into clear view.

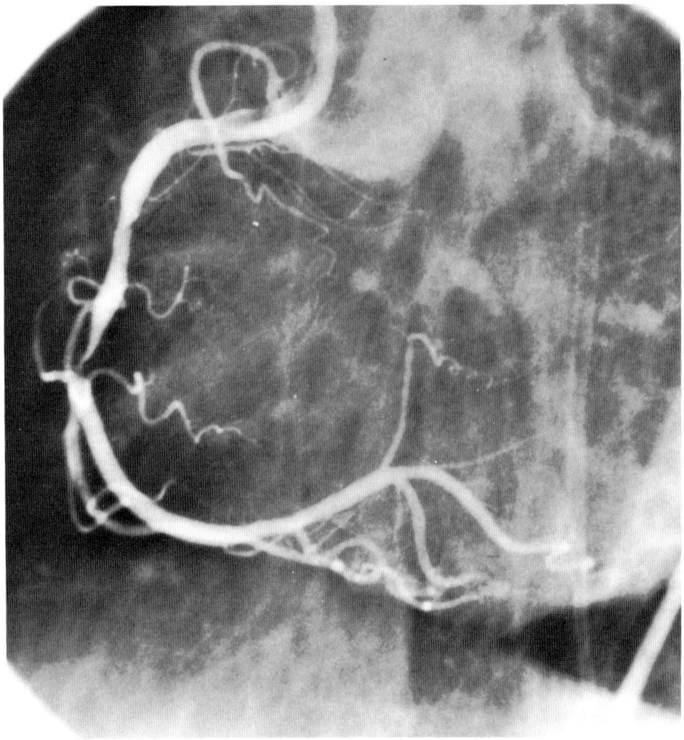

A

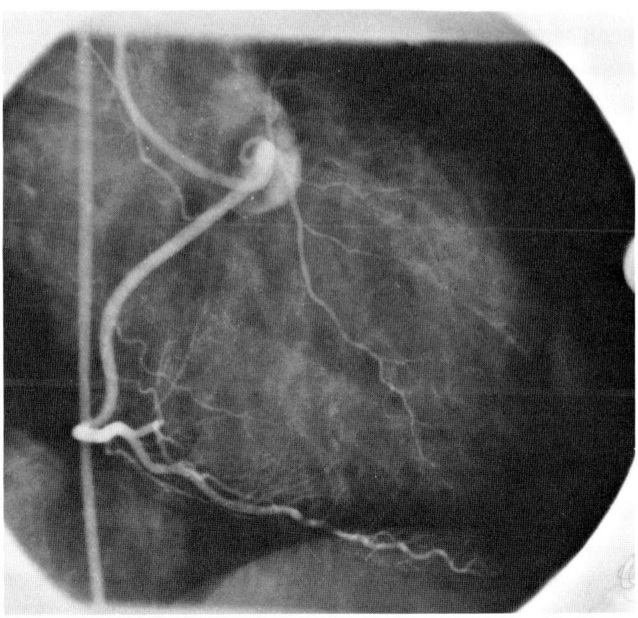

B

Figure 12-8 (*a*) LAO of right coronary artery (RCA) showing severe mid-RCA stenosis. (*From King SB III, Douglas JS Jr: Coronary arteriography and left ventriculography, in Hurst JW (ed)*: The Heart (4th ed). *McGraw-Hill, New York, 1978, p 409, fig 29D-12.*) (*b*) RAO of RCA showing the posterior descending artery on side.

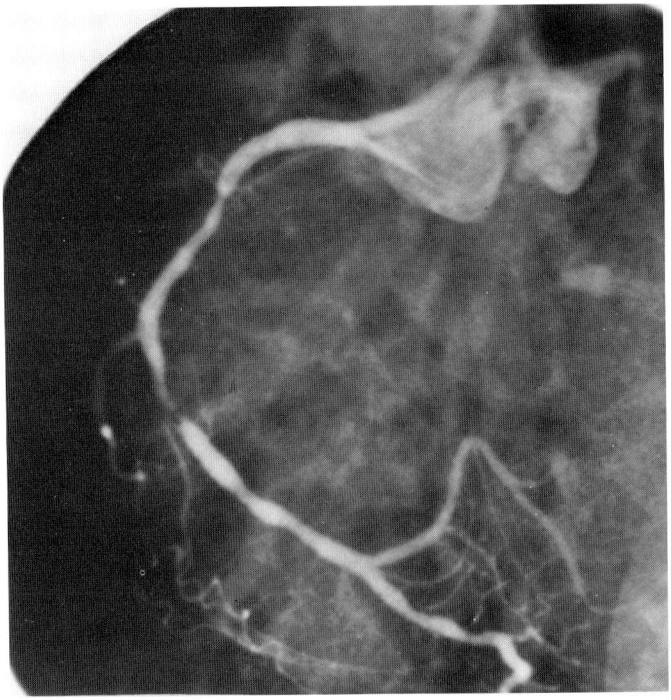

Figure 12-9 LAO cranial view of right coronary artery (RCA) showing mid-RCA lesion and severe diffuse disease. Notice the excellent view of the bifurcation of the RCA into the posterior descending and left ventricular branch.

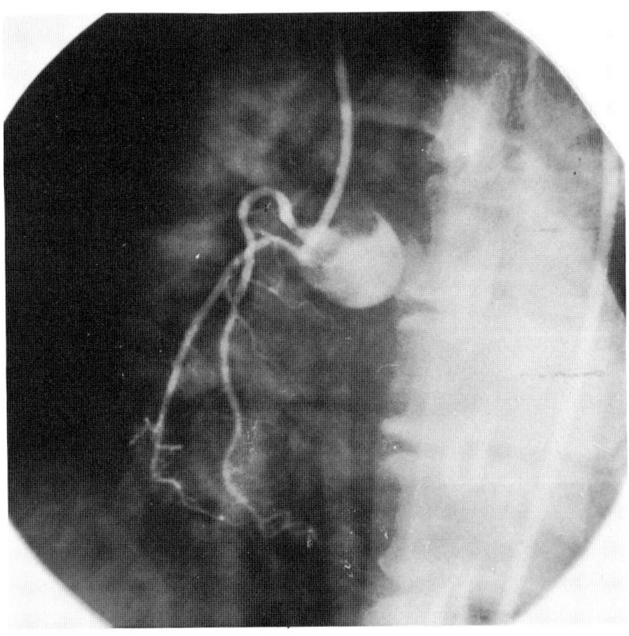

A

Figure 12-10 (*a*) LAO view of nondominant right coronary artery (RCA) showing separate right ventricular branch. (*b*) LAO of the dominant left coronary artery. (*From King SB III, Douglas JS Jr: Coronary arteriography and left ventriculography, in Hurst JW* (*ed*): The Heart (4th ed). *McGraw-Hill, New York, 1978, p. 409, fig 29D-10.*) (*c*) LAO of occluded RCA.

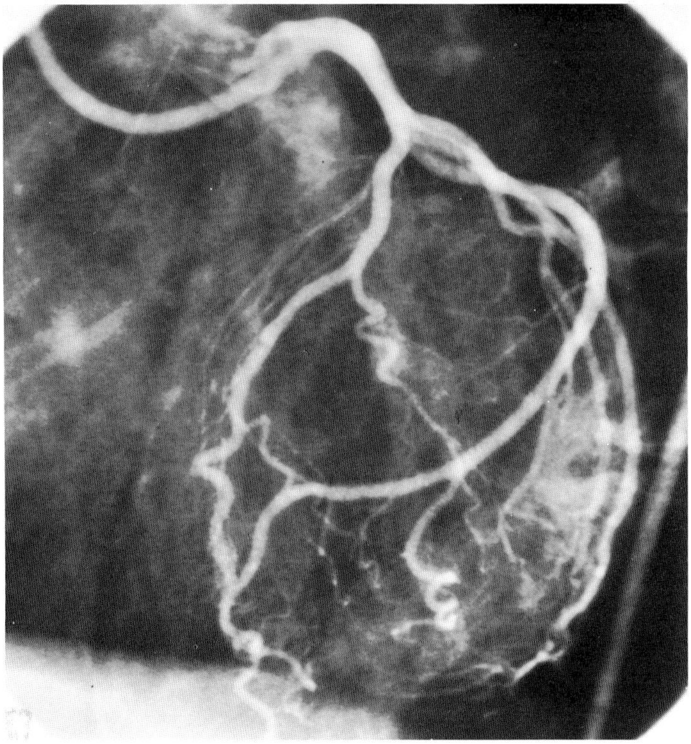

B

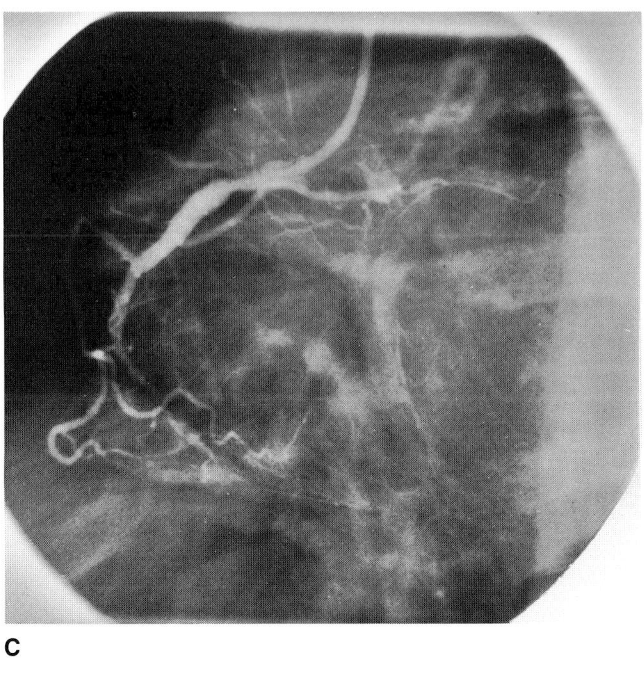

C

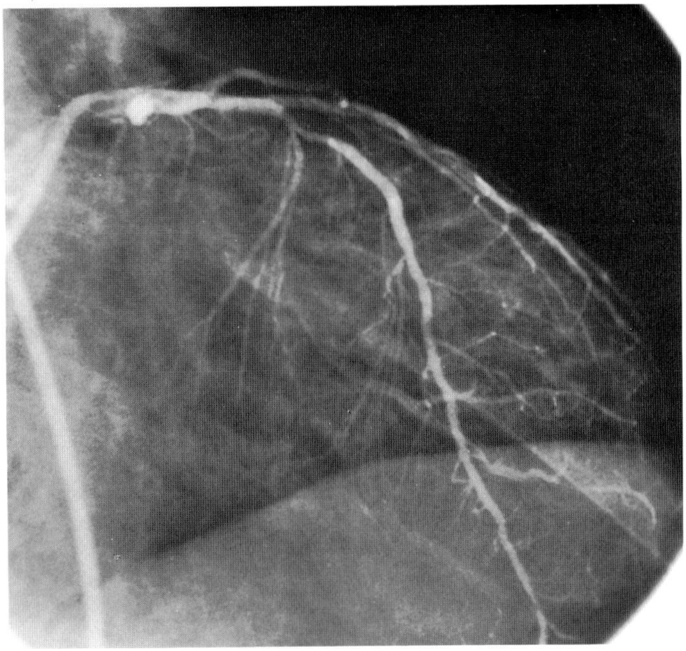

A

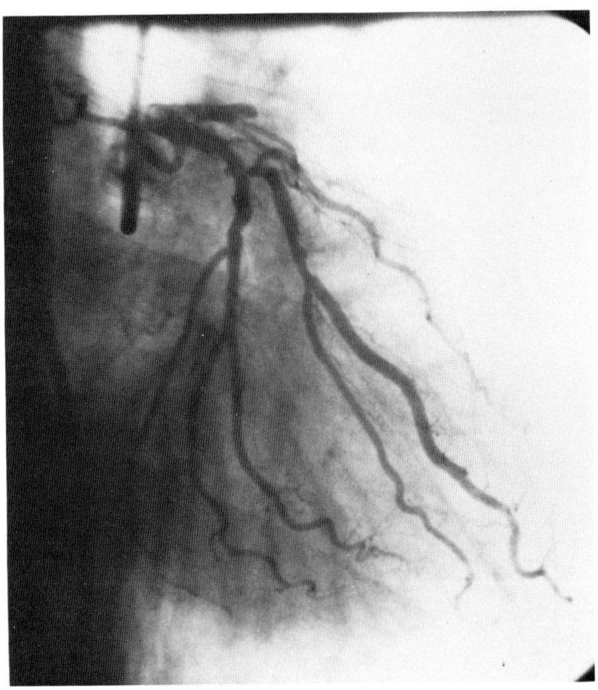

B

Figure 12-11 (*a*) RAO view of left coronary artery (LCA). Note the late filling of the circumflex marginal artery. (*b*) RAO of LCA with acutely occluded left anterior descending (LAD). Note acute cutoff. (*c*) RAO of LCA. Chronically occluded LAD.

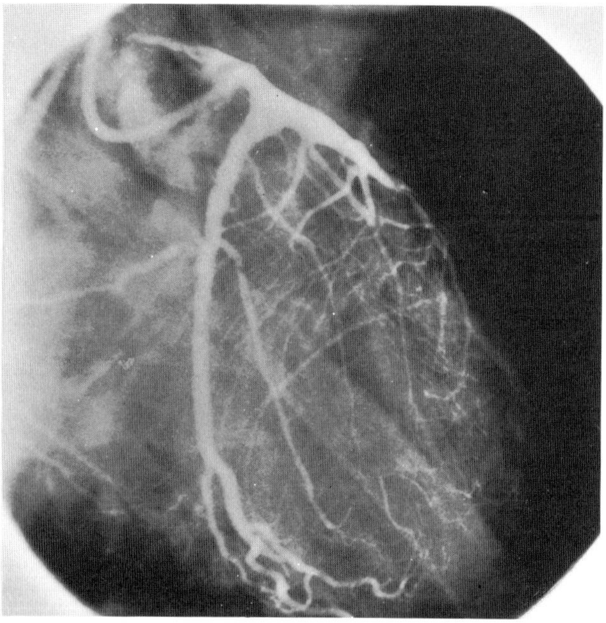

c

comes totally occluded, infarction occurs or collateral vessels develop and maintain viability of the segment affected. Acute total occlusion may leave a stump or cul-de-sac with an abrupt cutoff or even concave end, indicating thrombus (Fig. 12-11*b*). With passage of time, the artery will thrombose off to the last side branch, forming a smooth tapering with termination into that branch (Fig. 12-11*c*).

Late filling indicates collateral perfusion distal to a total occlusion. If a late-filling vessel is observed, then the stub of the occluded artery should be identified (Fig. 12-11*a*). Sometimes the vessels filling via collateral circulation are difficult to identify, particularly when they occur in the posterior circulation. In order to distinguish whether a collaterally filled vessel is part of the circumflex or the right coronary artery, one should remember that as coronary arteries branch, they form an acute angle pointing toward the origin of the artery. In other words, the point of the acute angle points against the direction of flow. Using this rule, one can easily identify in the LAO view whether the "V" formed by the branches of the totally occluded vessel point leftward, which would indicate that it rose originally from the circumflex, or rightward, which would indicate that it arose from the right coronary artery (Fig. 12-12).

A comparative evaluation of each lesion should be made in all views taken. The angiographer who is reviewing a cine film should be able to identify the point of stenosis or obstruction in a vessel in views in which that stenosis is not optimally seen by knowing the anatomy in all views. Sometimes logical deduction is necessary in reading a coronary arteriogram. In other words, if in viewing a left coronary artery in the RAO view one sees an artery with a high-grade obstruction running parallel to the marginal branches but in the careful assessment of this vessel it is determined to be moving discordantly with those vessels, then it cannot be on the same surface, namely the lateral wall. Further evaluation may prove that this vessel lies on another surface, such as the anterior interventricular sulcus, the right ventricular free surface, or in the interventricular septum. Observation of the artery in the LAO view may be necessary to determine on which of these the artery is located. This motion

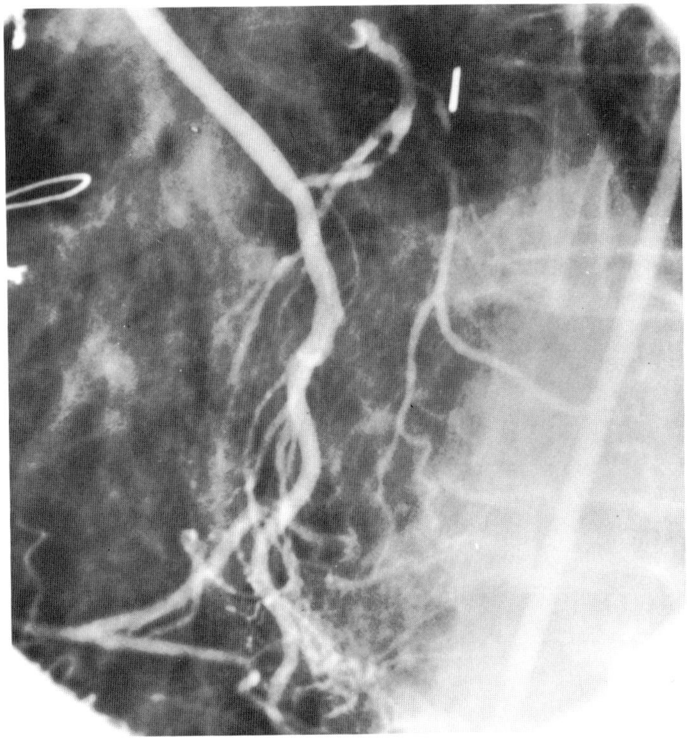

Figure 12-12 LAO view of graft to LAD showing collateral filling to the posterior artery. The "V" formed by the bifurcation of the vessel proves that this is the distal right coronary artery and not the circumflex.

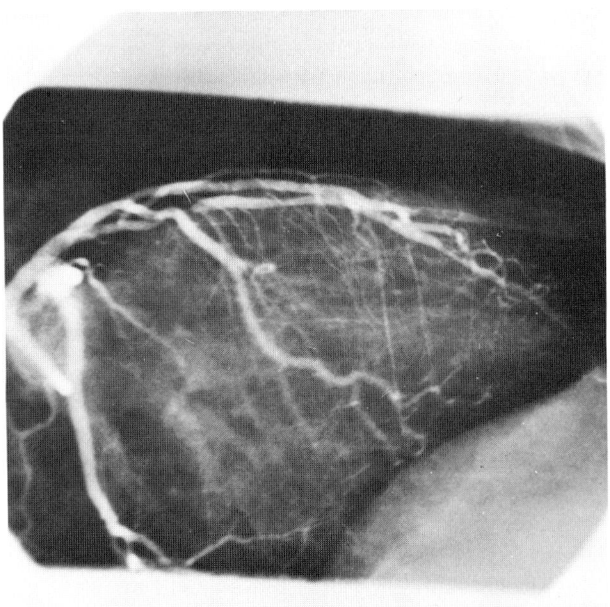

A

Figure 12-13 (*a*) RAO view of left coronary artery (LCA) with overlap of LAD and marginal arteries. (*b*) RAO of LCA with branches separated. (*c*) Note the concordant motion of the lateral marginal arteries (downward-pointing arrows) and the opposite motion of the LAD (upward-pointing arrow).

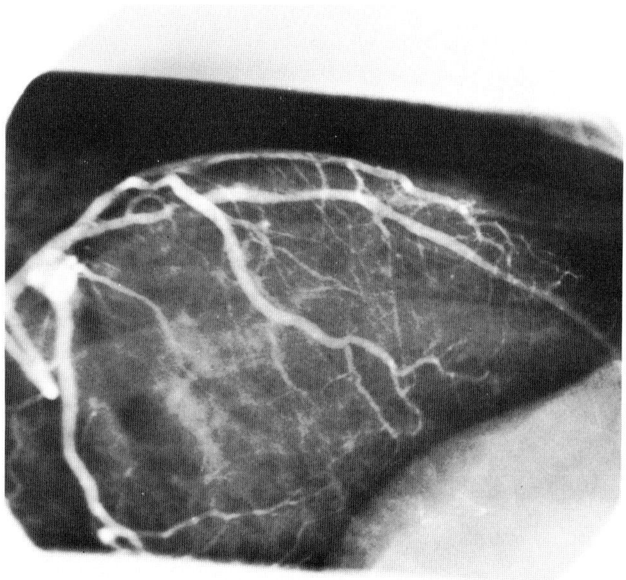

B

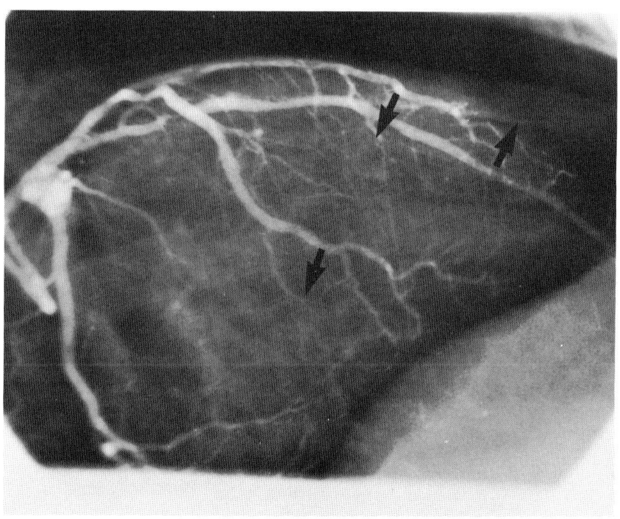

C

of coronary arteries can be used very effectively to identify arteries which lie adjacent to each other and to separate them from arteries which are obviously moving in a different plane (Fig. 12-13). In the RAO view, the diagonal branches are on the tangent of the heart, the marginal branches are on the lateral wall, and the LAD in the anterior septal sulcus. Motion of these vessels clearly indicates that the LAD and marginal branches are not on the same surface due to discordant motion. Vessels which move together are in the same plane and on the same surface. Septal perforators are seen moving on a different surface when compared to the LAD and marginals. A pseudo-three-dimensional perspective can be obtained when observing these vessels in motion.

Another rule is that vessels on the same surface never cross each other. If a distal left ventricular (LV) branch of the right coronary artery rises high on the lateral wall, then no marginal branch will be present in that same area, since to do so it would have to cross the terminal right coronary branches.

A strong advantage of cineangiography over cut film is the presence of many exposures throughout the cardiac cycle. It is tempting when looking at a single exposure to make assessments about the lesion; however, one should view the angiographic lesion throughout the cardiac cycle in order to best evaluate the true degree of stenosis. Sometimes buckling of an artery will totally obscure the lesion during a portion of the cycle and only reveal the stenosis at another time. On the other hand an overlying vessel may move into place during a portion of the cycle, causing a normal vessel to appear to have a lesion because of heavy opacification on either side of a less-opacified portion of the vessel. This same effect can be obtained by kinking of a vessel, which may give the appearance of a lesion when none is present.

ASSESSING STENOSIS

In making a decision regarding the degree of stenosis, one should look at the lesion in all views in which the lesion can be seen, and assessment should be made when the lesion can be seen without overlap from other vessels and when as little motion as possible is occurring. If motion is present, then there may be blurring of the margins of the lesion and the adjacent artery, making direct assessment of the degree of stenosis difficult. Usually the end-diastolic frames are best suited for elimination of motion. In any case, lesions should be examined in the frames in which the borders of the lesion are best seen so that they may be measured accurately.

The percent stenosis of a vessel has been expressed in two ways, and methods of measuring have varied widely. The stenosis may be expressed as a percent reduction in the diameter of the artery or, by assuming a certain geometry of the stenosis, as a percent reduction in cross-sectional area.[1,2] It is very important to communicate which method is being used when describing a stenosis (Fig. 12-14). (See Chap. 4 for a discussion of the pathophysiology of coronary obstruction.) Regardless of whether the percent diameter or the percent cross-sectional area method is used, it is important to evaluate every view in which the lesion is adequately seen. Since stenoses are not always concentric, a lesion may appear more severe in one view than in another. This, in fact, reflects the true state of affairs and should be taken into account when reporting the degree of stenosis. If the arterial segment that is narrowed is measured in two or three different views and compared to the best evaluation of a normal segment nearby, then an average-diameter stenosis can be determined. That average-diameter reduction can be expressed itself or converted to an average cross-sectional area reduction (see Chap. 4).

When the disease is not discreet, it is often difficult to decide what to designate as the normal segment. Adjacent segments of the artery without intervening side branches should be selected for comparison to the lesion. Often that is difficult,

Figure 12-14 Diameter versus cross-sectional chart. (*From King, Douglas, Morris*[2], *p 200, fig 9.*)

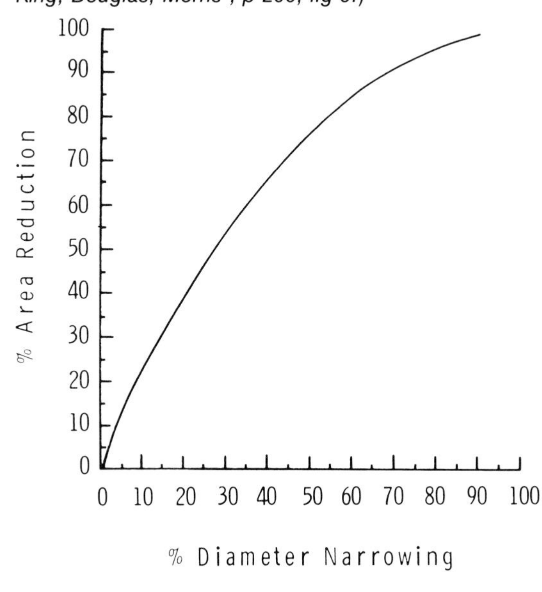

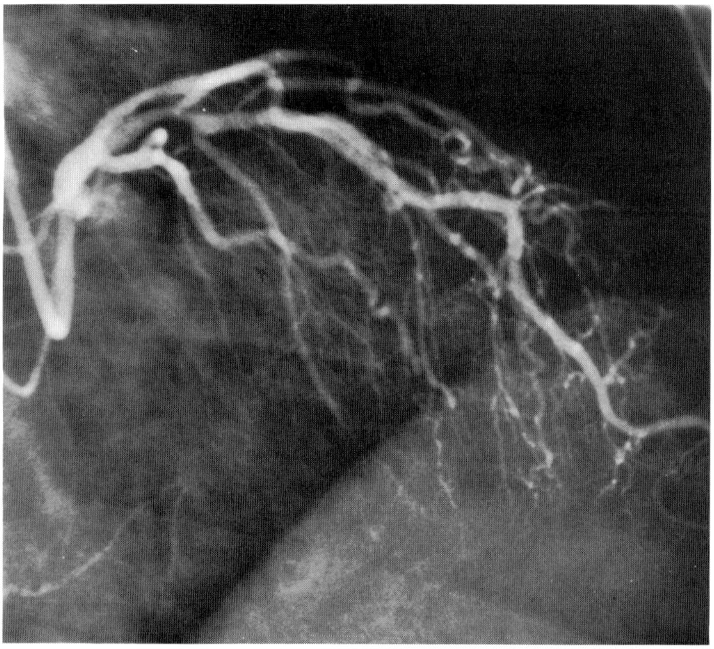

A

Figure 12-15 (*a*) RAO cranial view of left coronary artery. The proximal LAD stenosis extends to and involves the diagonal. The normal diameter of the proximal LAD must be estimated because overlap with the intermediate branch precludes measurement of the segment directly. The distal LAD cannot be used for comparison because of the intervening diagonal branch. (*b*) RAO view of left coronary artery. The entire length proximal to the severe stenosis is involved. Note the small diameter of the proximal .AD compared to the distal LAD.

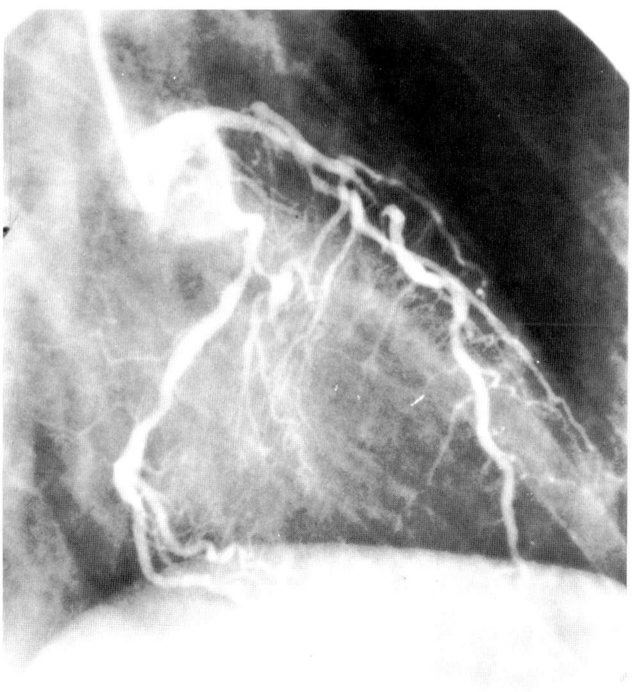

B

when more distal segments are the only normal zones. The normal reduction of the arterial lumen after the takeoff of a large side branch must be taken into account when estimating the normal diameter of the stenosed segment (Fig. 12-15).

Long lesions which taper gradually give the visual impression that they are less severe than a very abrupt short lesion. This is another reason that direct measurement of the lesion is important (Fig. 12-16). When arteries are heavily calcified, additional clues can be obtained by viewing the calcified wall of the artery and comparing that to the lumen which remains. Sometimes this is quite surprising because the lumen diameter reduction seems insignificant compared to adjacent segments; however, the true diameter of the artery as revealed by the calcified wall is much larger, indicating diffuse disease throughout the entire vessel (Fig. 12-16). Remember that coronary arteriography reveals only the lumen of the vessel; therefore any assessment of the degree of stenosis depends on the assumption that the adjacent segment which is called normal in fact is normal. The left main segment of the coronary artery can be diffusely diseased and uniformly reduced in diameter but appear to be normal or to have only mild narrowing. In evaluating the left main segment, one should look at the distal distribution of the anterior descending and circumflex vessels to see whether the left main segment is the expected size or not. If a circumflex marginal branch is larger than the left main, then something is wrong in that there is obviously disease and reduction in lumen in a uniform fashion of the left main. Attention to this concept will prevent underestimation of left main stenosis. A lesion of the ostium of the left main, and to a lesser extent the right coronary, can be missed due to the deep insertion of the angiographic catheter. If there is no backflow of contrast medium into the aorta from such injections, the left main orifice cannot be evaluated (Fig. 12-17).

Some clues to ostial disease are failure of contrast medium to reflux into the aorta despite apparently vigorous injections fully opacifying the artery and failure of contrast material to clear from the artery until the catheter is removed.

MORPHOLOGY OF CORONARY LESIONS

There has been little emphasis placed on the morphology of lesions in the coronary arteries; rather the obstruction has been expressed as a percent stenosis and left at that. As better resolution of lesions is obtained, we can now differentiate in some cases between smooth intimal surfaces and irregular or ulcerated ones and also identify filling defects. The prognosis of a lesion for progression to occlusion is likely to be related to its morphology.[3–6] Attention to this morphology has been heightened because of the use of coronary angioplasty. A postmortem radiographic study of excised hearts demonstrated the ability to predict complicated stenoses characterized by plaque rupture, plaque hemorrhage, superimposed partly occluding thrombus, or recanalized thrombus by the angiographic morphology.[7] Although in vivo angiograms cannot give the degree of detail provided by these postmortem radiographic techniques, it is still possible to identify complicated stenoses in some patients (Figs. 12-18 and 12-19).

ASSESSING THE VALUE OF A CORONARY ARTERIAL SEGMENT

The size of a coronary artery is determined by the flow which is required of it. In a general sense, the largest coronary arteries serve the largest amount of myocardium and therefore pose the most important problem should they become diseased.

Directly related and of equal importance is the distribution of the coronary artery over the myocardial surface. In reading a coronary arteriogram, one should judge the percentage of myocardium served by each of the major coronary arteries and its branches. Obstructions of the anterior descending artery vary widely in importance. Lesions occurring before takeoff of the diagonal and septal perforating branches may affect a large segment of myocardium, approaching 50 percent, whereas ste-

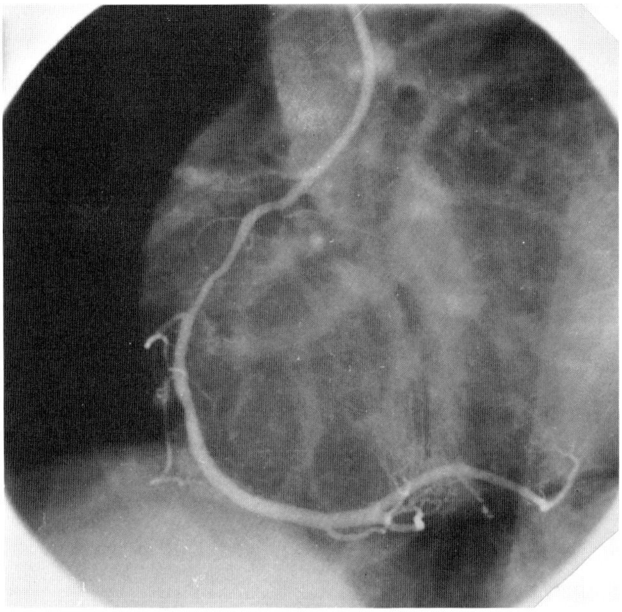

A

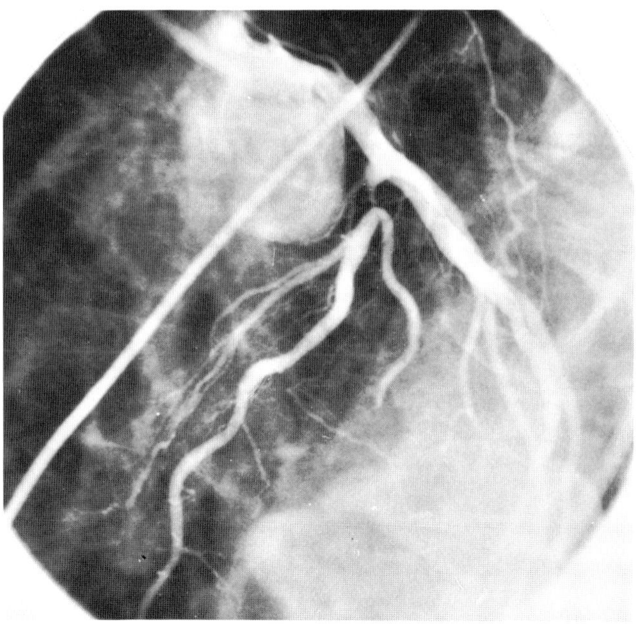

B

Figure 12-16 (*a*) LAO view of right coronary artery showing long diffuse-diseased segment. (*b*) LAO cranial of left coronary artery showing discreet proximal LAD stenosis.

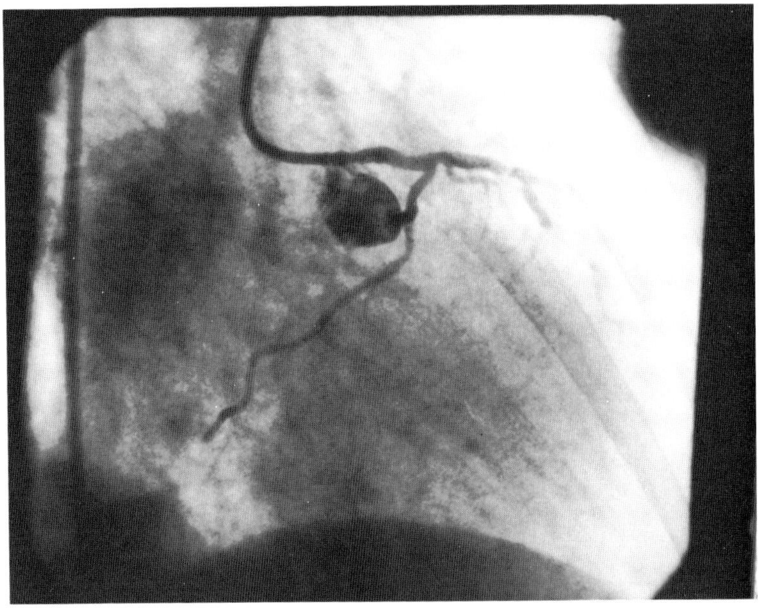

Figure 12-17 Left main orifice stenosis. Note the size of the catheter and the distal arterial segments compared to the left main coronary.

nosis after a large diagonal branch and septal perforator may affect less than 25 or 30 percent. These same comparisons can be made for all arterial segments and are crucial in evaluating the value of a coronary arterial obstruction. (Refer to Chap. 2 for the distribution of the coronary anatomy.)

Some common distribution patterns of the major coronary arteries will now be discussed.

The Anterior Descending Coronary

The anterior descending coronary artery commonly serves the entire septum by way of the septal perforating vessels with the exception of the high posterior one-third, and by the diagonal branches serves most of the anterior wall. The LAD may distribute to the apex and around it, extending partially up the inferior wall of the left ventricle. Smaller LADs may stop short of the apex and be rather sparse as far as the distribution of their diagonal branches are concerned.

The Circumflex

The circumflex artery may send marginal branches over the entire lateral surface of the heart, continuing posteriorly to supply the inferior surface and posterior interventricular groove. On the other hand, the circumflex may give rise to only one or two marginal branches which serve the anterolateral portion of the heart, or the circumflex branches may be quite rudimentary. A lesion of one marginal branch of the circumflex is less important if there are two or three other branches of similar size than if the circumflex terminates in one large marginal branch which has a lesion.

The Right Coronary Artery

The right coronary artery varies in its distribution. It may be a small, nondominant vessel which gives branches only to the right ventricle; an average-sized right coronary artery, which supplies the posterior descending branch and a small left ventricular branch; or a very dominant right coronary artery, which supplies the inferior surface and then gives off several left ventricular branches which take the place of the posterior marginal branches of the circumflex to supply the majority of the posterior and lateral wall of the left ventricle. A system of segmenting the left ventricle so that no avascular zones are missed, such as that suggested by Paulin, may be helpful.[8] Obstructions in each of these arterial segments should be weighed in light of the amount of myocardium in jeopardy.

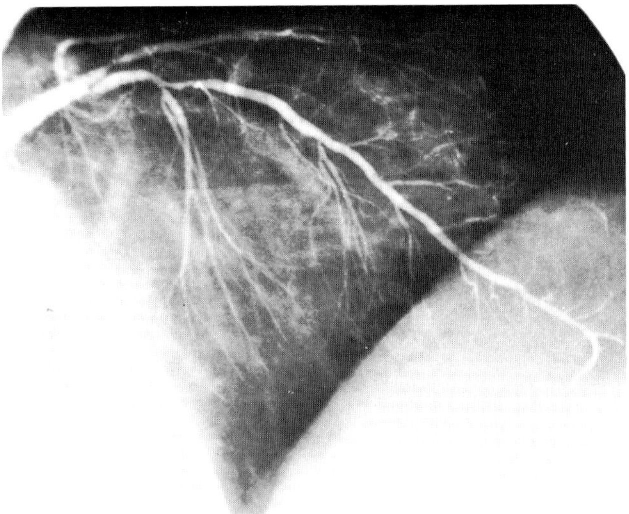

A

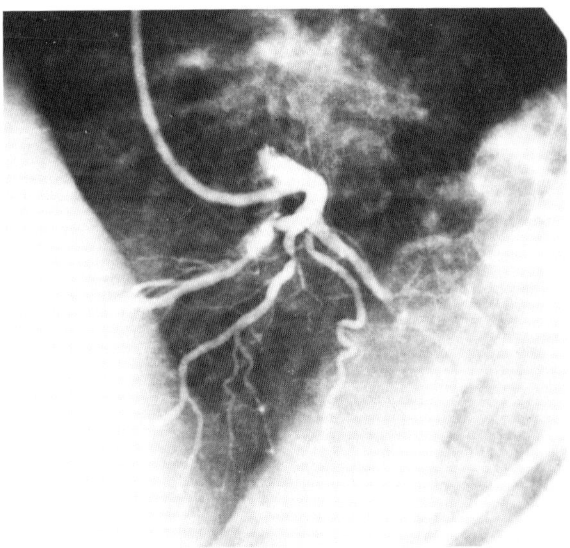

B

Figure 12-18 (*a*) RAO view of left coronary artery showing proximal LAD and diagonal stenoses, both of which have smooth borders. (*b*) LAO cranial view showing the diagonal stenosis.

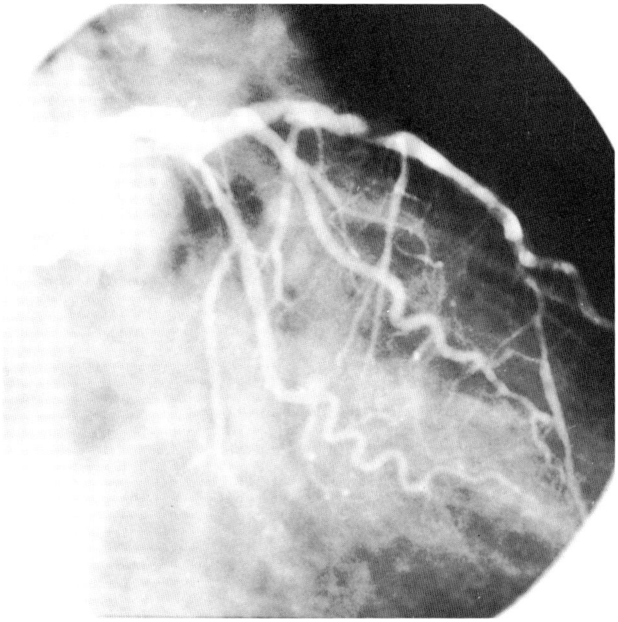

A

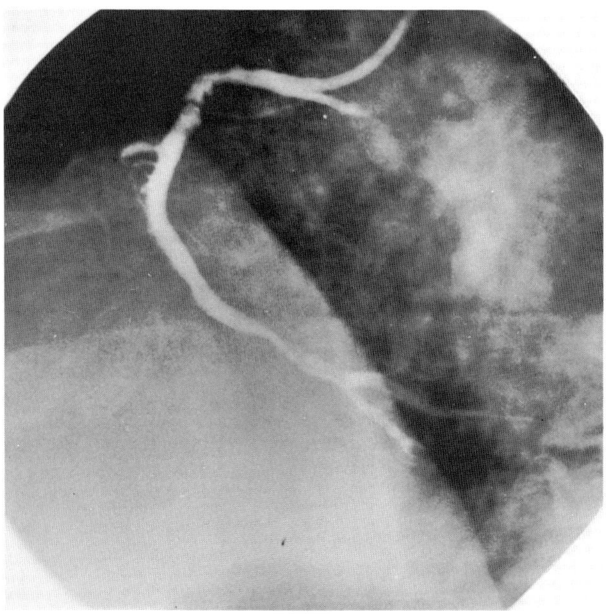

B

Figure 12-19 (*a*) RAO view of left coronary artery. The LAD has a very eccentric and complex obstruction. (*b*) Proximal right coronary artery has a membranelike transverse lesion with plaque ulceration.

Adequacy of Collaterals

When vessels become severely occluded so that there is a significant pressure drop distally, the stimulus for collateral development exists. Totally occluded arteries almost always have collateral vessels filling the distal vessel except in the case of acute occlusion, when collaterals have not had time to develop, or of complete avascular scar, when there is no need for blood flow.

Measurement of distal coronary occlusion pressure at coronary angioplasty has taught several lessons regarding the functional adequacy of collateral vessels. When a coronary artery which has no collaterals is suddenly obstructed, the distal pressure is very low, in the 15 to 25 mmHg range. On the other hand, if the distal occlusion pressure is above 30 to 40 mmHg, then collateral vessels are uniformly demonstrable. Collateral vessels are responsive to the hemodynamic forces applied; therefore they will be seen to apparently disappear suddenly when the obstructed artery is reopened and will reappear when the obstruction is reapplied.

The angiographic demonstration of collaterals depends on (1) an adequate injection of the artery supplying the collaterals (a wedged injection into an artery, however, may force collateral flow in a direction it would not take under normal conditions); (2) a lumen size of the collaterals large enough to be resolved with the angiographic technique used (many times the distal occluded coronary artery is visualized without actual visualization of the small collateral vessels); and (3) filming long enough for the contrast medium to concentrate in the occluded segment. Common collateral connections are illustrated in Chap. 3.

The important aspects of collateral filling of a vessel are that (1) it always means severe hemodynamic obstruction has occurred, resulting in reduced distal pressure; (2) collaterals can almost never accommodate increased flow to the degree the native unobstructed coronary can; (3) collateral filling of vessels signifies their presence but may not accurately define the true size of the distal artery since the lower perfusion pressure applied does not fully distend the walls. This third point is very important in surgical selection since a collaterally filled vessel appearing less than 1 mm in diameter may actually be 1.5 or 2 mm when filled to normal pressures by a vein bypass graft (Fig. 12-20).

Collateral vessels are obviously necessary to protect the myocardium from infarction when an artery becomes totally occluded. There has been some confusion on this point when patients with collaterals are compared to patients without collaterals for ventricular contractility.[10] Collaterals indicate more severe obstruction; therefore, it is not surprising that the patients with collaterals have worse left ventricular function. However, when total occlusion is considered, presence of collaterals and the extent of distal filling correlates with preservation of regional wall motion.[11] If wall motion is demonstrated distal to a total occlusion, then collateral filling must be present.

PITFALLS IN INTERPRETATION

Short or Absent Left Main Artery

The left main coronary artery may present difficulties in interpretation because it is very short or in fact may be totally absent. The very short left main arteries give rise almost immediately to the anterior descending and circumflex branches, so stenosis in the main artery is extremely difficult to assess. In evaluating any left main, one should search for views taken in the frontal or near-frontal projection. The left main can often be seen well also in the shallow right oblique or shallow left oblique view and again in a left anterior oblique with cranial angulation. If the left main artery is short and the angiographic catheter selectively enters the anterior descending or circumflex vessel, then the vessel not entered will not be opacified at all. This could lead to the impression that the other vessel is totally occluded or was congenitally absent. Evaluation of angiograms often gives a hint of the presence of the other vessel by backflush from the injection, or the left ventriculogram may be reviewed to see if the missing vessel is identified in that injection (Fig. 12-21).

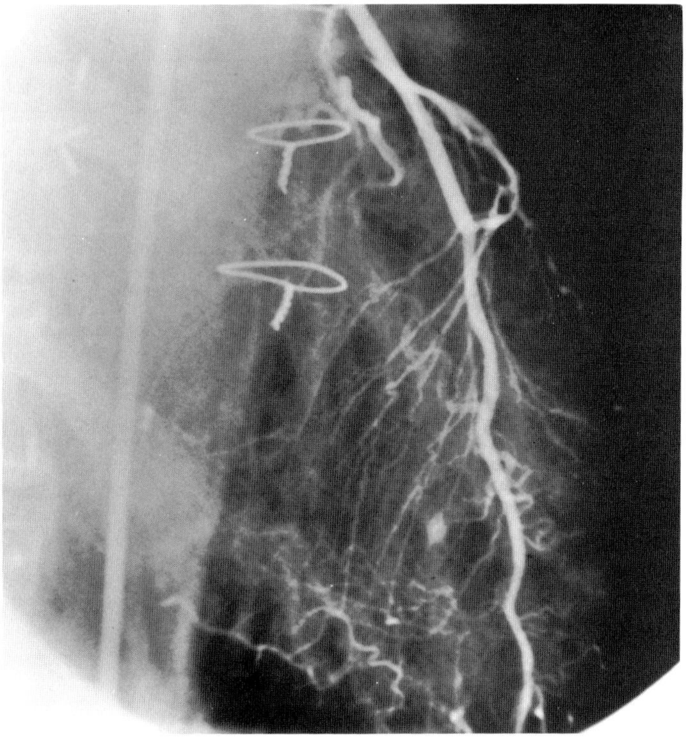

A

Figure 12-20 (*a*) Collateral vessels from LAD filling the distal right coronary artery through the septum. (*b*) Collateral from proximal circumflex filling into atrioventricular node artery and distal portion of right coronary artery. Note marked tortuosity of the collaterals. (*c*) Old, well-developed collateral from proximal right coronary artery coursing over right ventricular epicardium to fill left anterior descending.

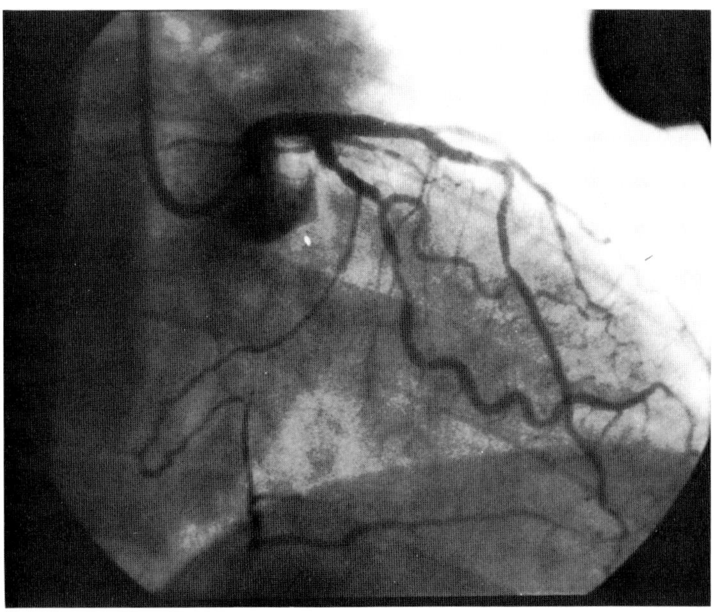

B

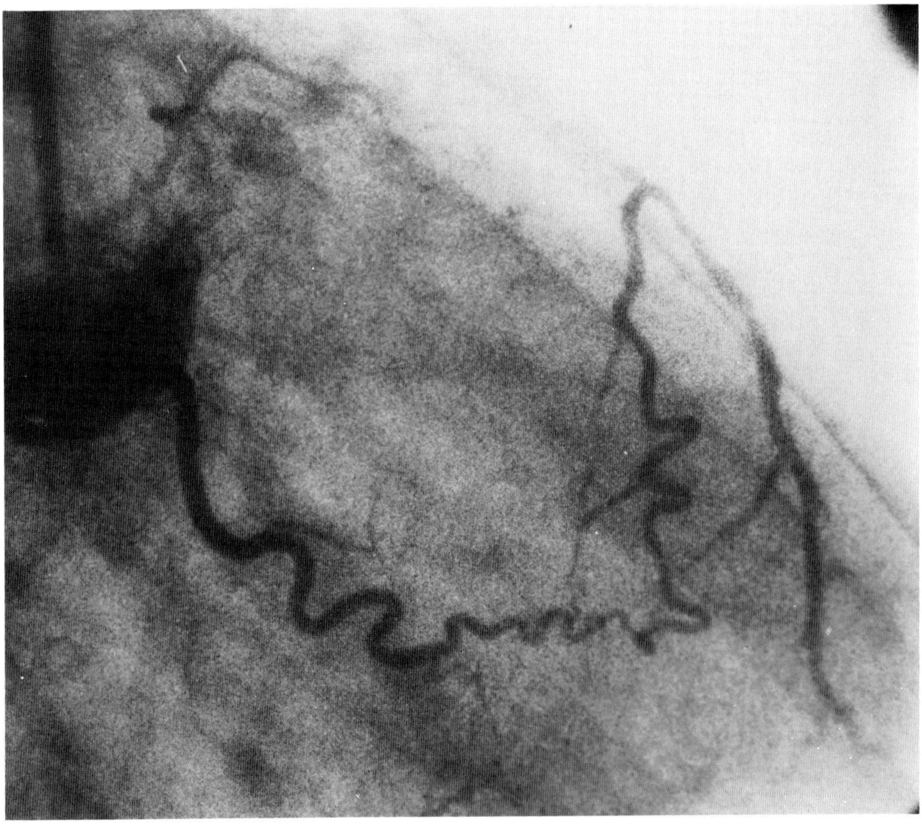

C

Total Occlusion

If a total occlusion of an artery occurs so that there is no stub left, there will be no clue in evaluating the coronary artery that an occlusion is present. The identification of the distal vessel will be possible only through filling by collaterals, as is usually the case, or by identification of a segment of the myocardium that is devoid of coronary arteries (Fig. 12-22).

Orifice Lesions

Orifice lesions of the left or right coronary arteries have been frequently missed for two reasons. One is that the catheter may be advanced distal to the lesion and adequate back flushing of contrast medium does not occur; therefore the lesion is missed. This most commonly occurs with the Judkins or Sones techniques and is unlikely with the multipurpose technique since the distal tip of the catheter is larger and does not enter the left main artery very far. The other reason for missing the orifice lesion is the fact that the orifice is obscured by contrast medium spilled into the aortic cusps. This, in fact, is more common with the multipurpose technique. When reviewing films, views should be looked for which place the coronary orifice on tangent, thereby eliminating the possibility of obscuring the orifice with the contrast material–filled aortic cusp.

Myocardial Bridging

The coronary segment should be viewed throughout the cardiac cycle, and any fixed obstruction should be present throughout. If long areas of nar-

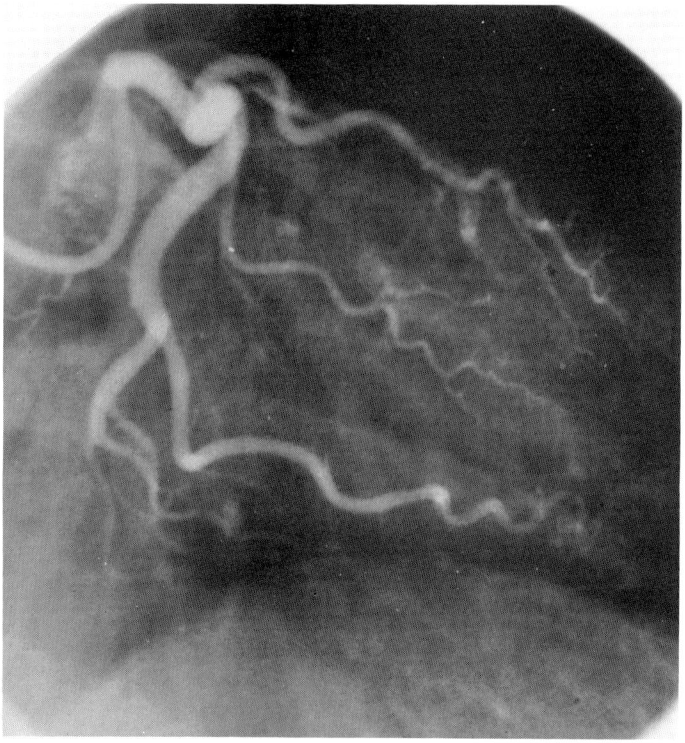

A

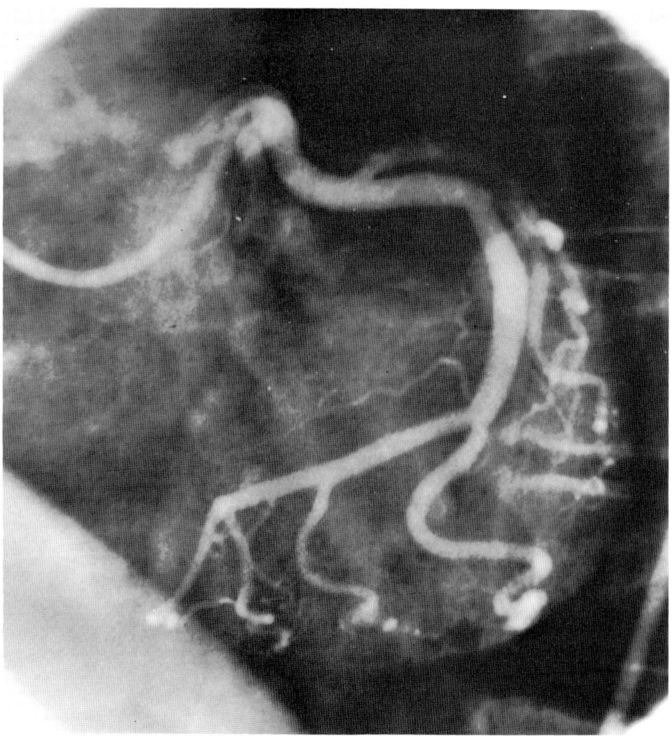

B

Figure 12-21 (*a*) RAO view of left coronary artery (LCA) injection showing nonfilling of the LAD. (*b*) LAO view of LCA confirming that LAD is not filling. (*c*) LAO view of selective LAD injection with only slight filling in the circumflex. (*From King SB III, Douglas JS Jr: Coronary arteriography and left ventriculography, in Hurst JW* (*ed*): The Heart (4th ed). *McGraw-Hill, New York, 1978, p 403, fig 29D-2.*)

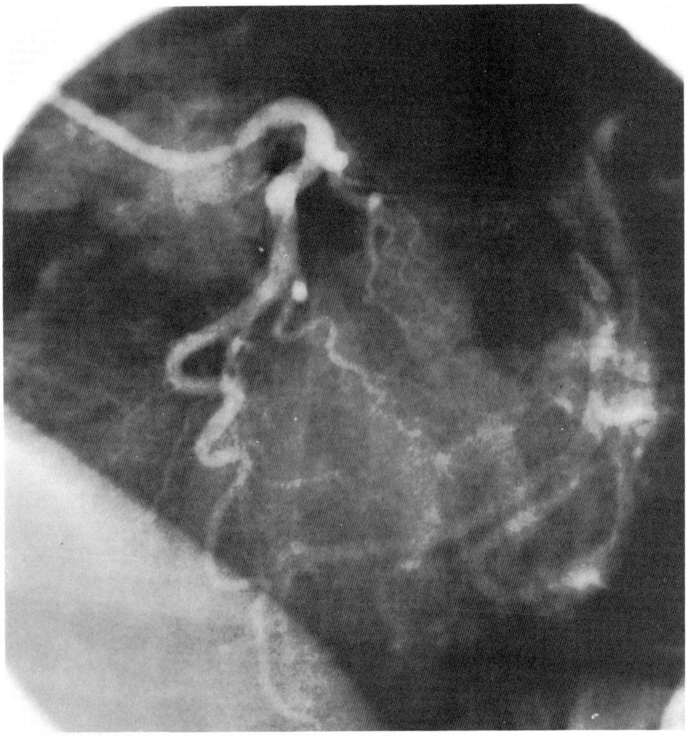

C (*Figure 12-21, continued*)

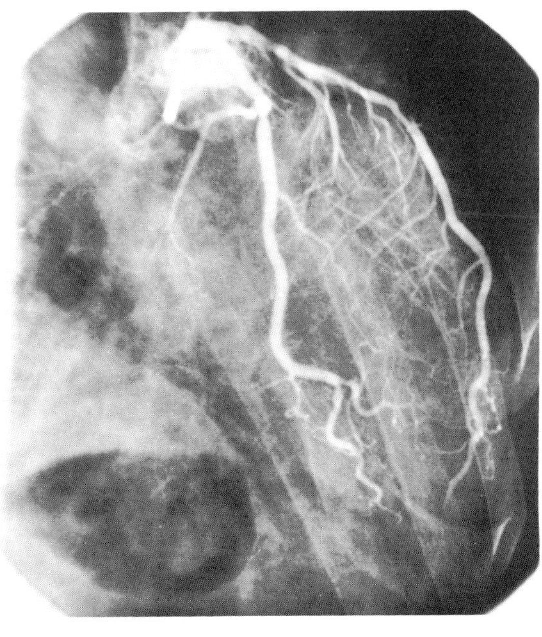

A

Figure 12-22 (*a*) RAO of left coronary artery (LCA) showing proximal left anterior descending artery and circumflex disease. Diagonal occlusion not suspected. (*b*) LAO cranial view of LCA shows a vacant area in the normal distribution of the diagonal branches. (*c*) Late filling in lateral view demonstrates opacification of one diagonal branch confirming the total occlusion.

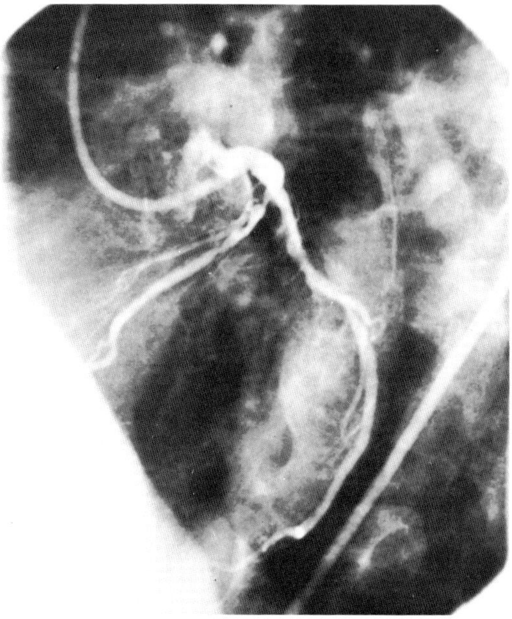

B

(Figure 12-22, continued)

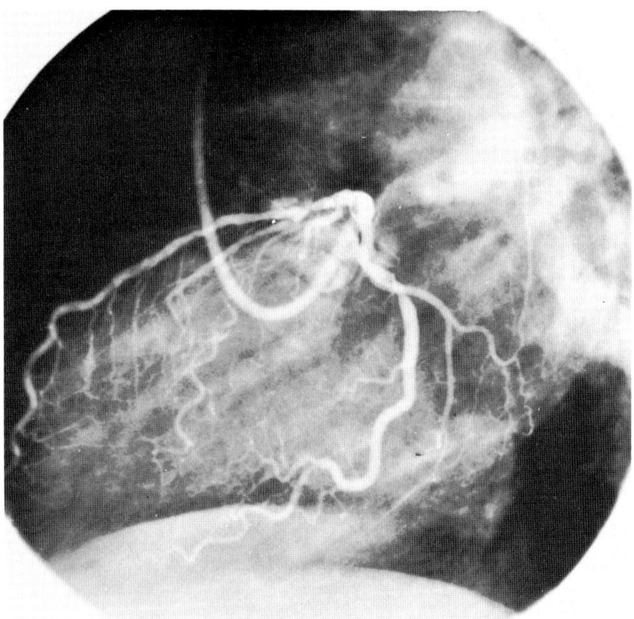

C

rowing appear in systole, this is most likely due to compression of the artery by overlying muscular bridges of myocardium. It has been suggested that this systolic compression may be a cause of myocardial ischemia.[12,13] This seems unlikely in most cases since the bulk of coronary flow is in diastole, when the artery is widely patent. Bridging occurs most commonly in the anterior descending artery but also has been seen in the diagonal and marginal branches as well as in the septal perforators (Fig. 12-23).

Coronary Artery Aneurysms and Ectatic Enlargment

Coronary aneurysms may be congenital as well as the result of medial destruction by atherosclerosis or vasculitis or other processes. Aneurysmal dilatation has been reported in 1.5 percent of patients studied

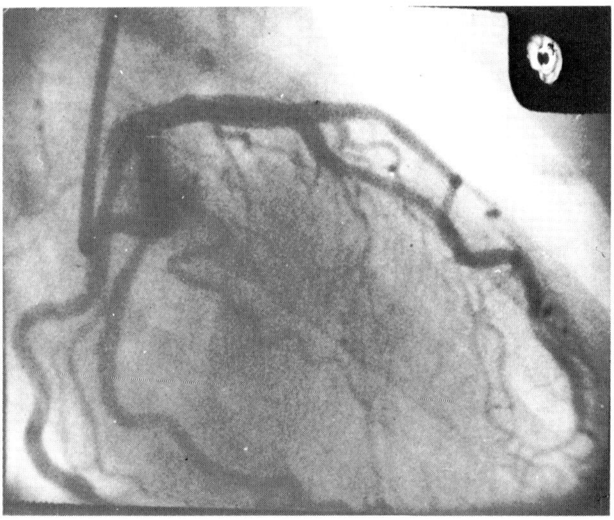

A

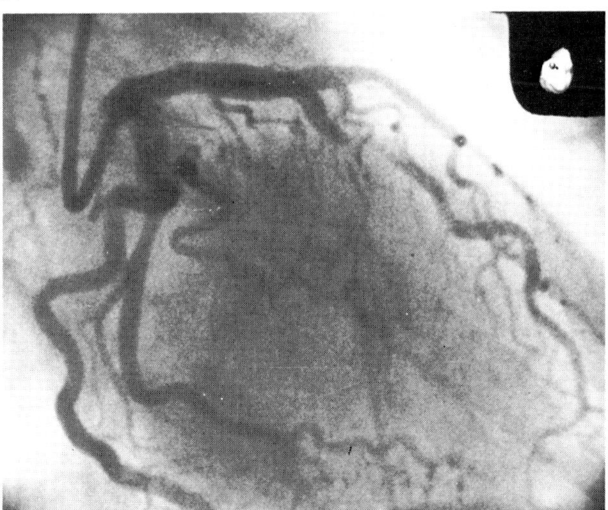

B

Figure 12-23 (*a*) RAO view of left coronary. Appearance in diastole of LAD showing no narrowing. (*b*) Systolic appearance showing obliteration of lumen by overlying muscular bridge. (*From Franch RH, King SB III, Douglas JS Jr: Techniques of cardiac catheterization including coronary arteriography, in Hurst JW (ed)*: The Heart (5th ed) *McGraw-Hill, New York, 1982, p 1875, fig 98–41.*)

at autopsy or coronary arteriography.[14] Aneurysms may or may not be associated with stenosis. Multiple views will be necessary to exclude overlap of dilated segments obscuring tight stenosis (Fig. 12-24).

Foreshortening and Overlap

When coronary arteries are viewed end on, there is marked foreshortening, so that the vessel cannot be properly evaluated. When this occurs, areas of increased density can, when compared to areas where the density is less, produce the confusing appearance of a lesion.

Overlapping vessels can obscure a lesion or cause normal vessels to appear diseased. The movement of the coronary arteries seen on cineangiography is advantageous in eliminating overlap since vessels sometimes separate for only two to three frames throughout the cardiac cycle. These brief periods of separation should be examined and lesions evaluated. Lesions should also be searched for in every view in order to minimize overlap problems (Fig. 12-25).

Coronary Spasm

Since coronary artery spasm is a transient event, it may or may not be discovered at the time of coronary arteriography. Methods of provoking and relieving spasm are discussed in Chaps. 4 and 8.

Transient catheter-induced spasm may be unrelated to any clinical problem but may produce confusion in interpreting angiographic films. Coronary spasm induced by the catheter is most commonly located at the tip of the catheter in the right coronary artery. A smooth lesion in that area in the absence of disease elsewhere in the coronary arteries should raise the question of spasm. If adequate injections following nitroglycerin have not been used, then spasm may not have been ruled out. One should evaluate each angiographic view of the coronary artery in question in order to assess

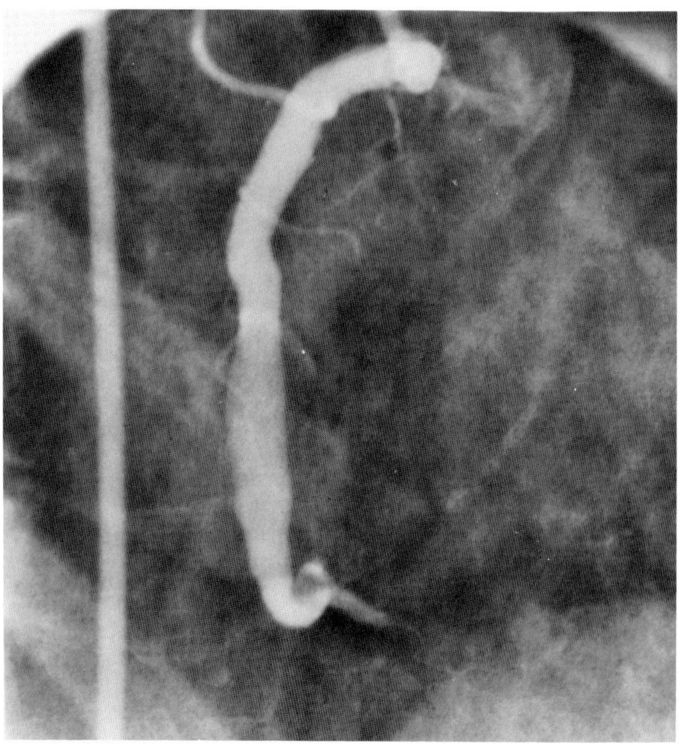

A

Figure 12-24 (*a*) Diffuse ectatic enlargement of right coronary artery without obstruction. (*b*) Multiple coronary aneurysms with severe distal stenoses (RAO). (*c*) Same artery (LAO).

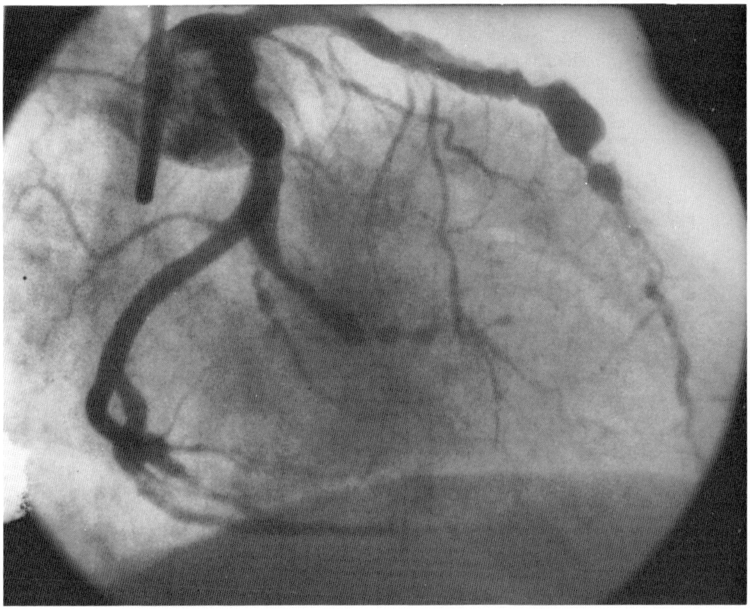

B

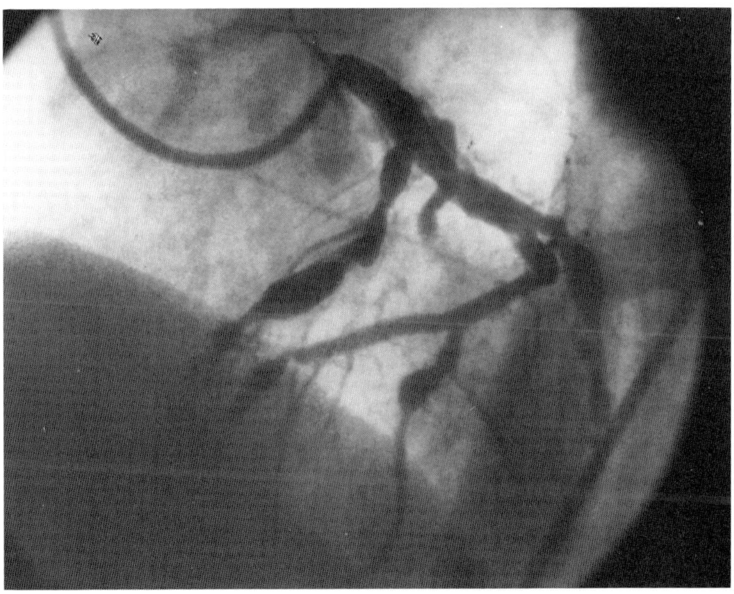

C

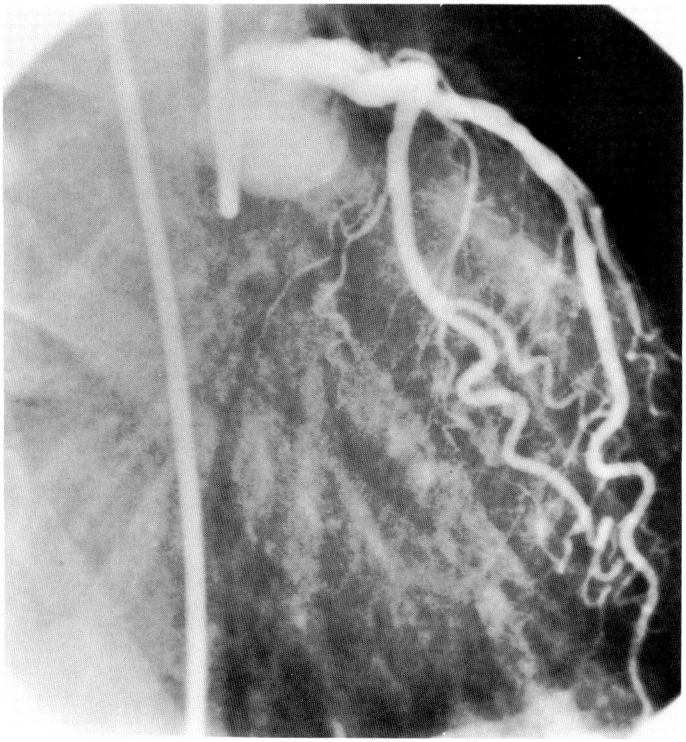

A

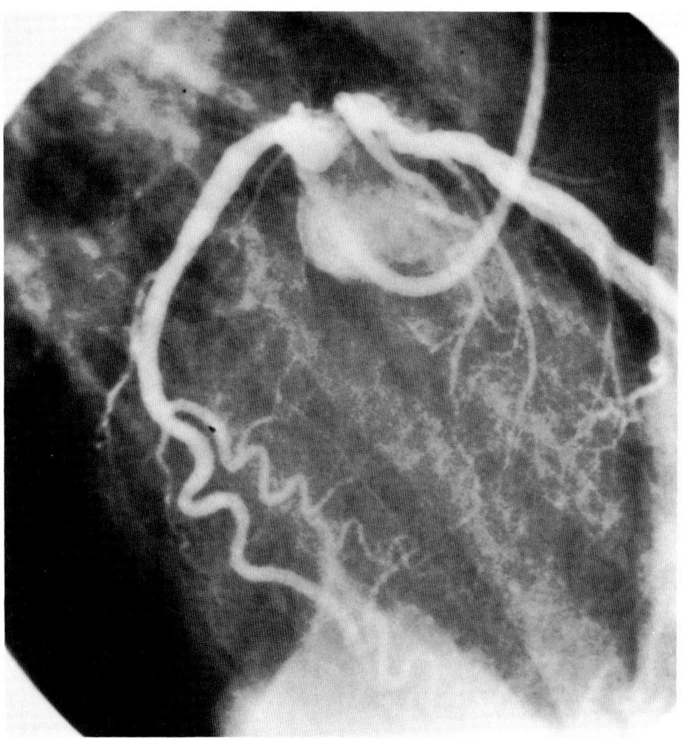

B

Figure 12-25 Overlap of proximal LAD lesion prevents proper assessment in (*a*) RAO, (*b*) lateral view, and (*c*) LAO. (*d*) LAO cranial view shows the lesion clearly. (*From King SB III, Douglas JS Jr: Coronary Arteriography and left ventriculography, in Hurst JW* (*ed*): The Heart (4th ed). *McGraw-Hill, New York, 1978, p 408, fig 29D-9.*)

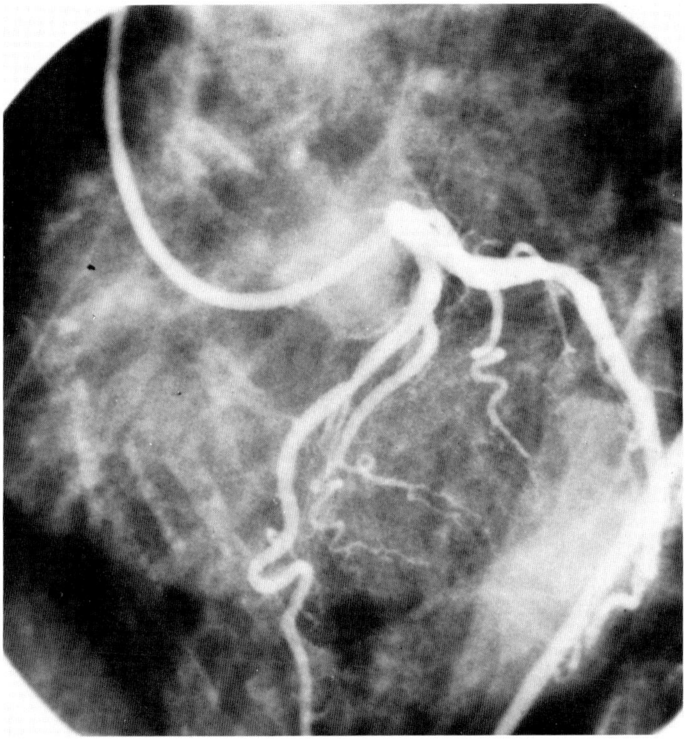

C

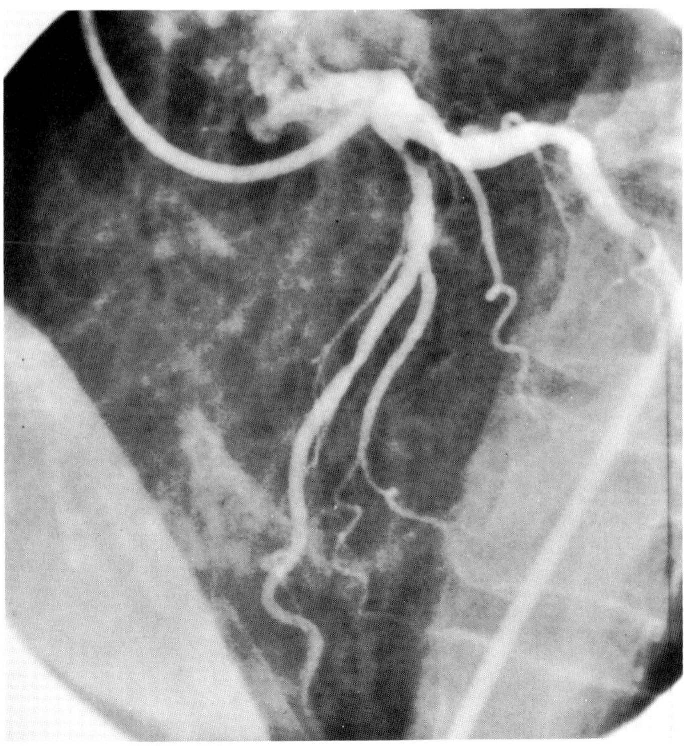

D

whether there is a change in lumen size from one injection to another. Contrast medium is a vasodilator in itself and may partially reduce or relieve spasm on successive angiographic views. Spasm occurring remote from the catheter has the characteristic appearance of a very smooth lesion which is indistinguishable from some fixed concentric coronary plaques. Sometimes it is impossible on reviewing film to eliminate coronary spasm if this has not been done at the time of the catheterization. In such cases, repeat angiography may be necessary to answer the question (Fig. 12-26).

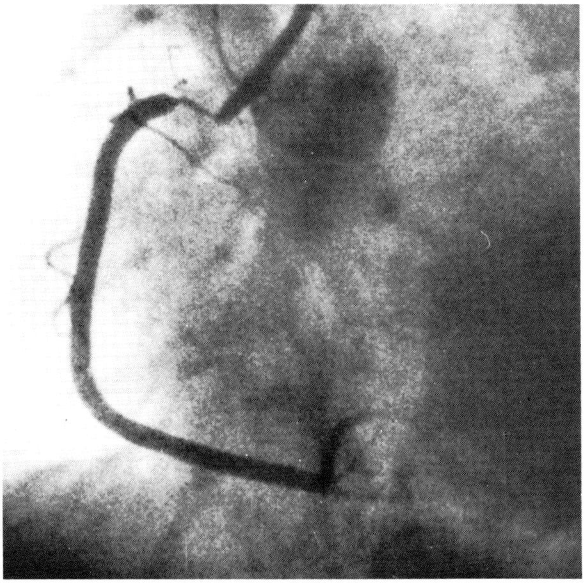

A

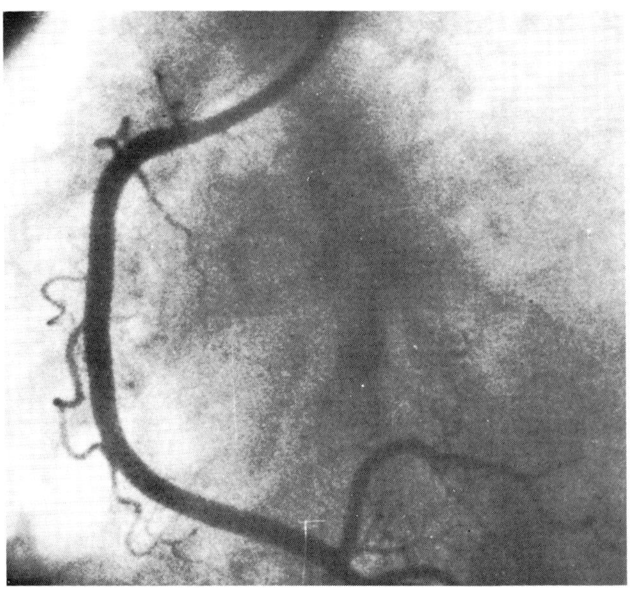

B

Figure 12-26 (*a*) Proximal spasm of right coronary artery. (*b*) Spasm relieved following sublingual nitroglycerin. (*From Franch RH, King SB III, Douglas JS Jr: Techniques of cardiac catheterization including coronary arteriography, in Hurst JW (ed)*: The Heart (5th ed), *McGraw-Hill, New York, 1982, p 1876, fig 98–42*)

EVALUATING CORONARY BYPASS GRAFT STUDIES

Coronary bypasses are constructed from saphenous veins or from internal mammary artery direct anastomoses. The angiographic appearance should be smooth, with the graft equal or slightly larger than the recipient artery (Fig. 12-27). If the large thigh veins are used, then there will be a greater discrepancy between the vein size and the artery size. Obstructive lesions can appear in (1) the aortic anastomosis, (2) the body of the graft, (3) the distal graft-artery anastomosis, or (4) in the native artery distal to the graft. Since there is a section of aorta removed at the proximal anastomosis, stenosis of this area is rare. If graft occlusion occurs anywhere in the graft, however, the vessel will clot off back to this aortic anastomosis. Injection into that area will show only a dimple indicating the site of the previous bypass. When the aortic connection is viewed on tangent, midgraft stenoses are of two types. Intimal fibrosis secondary to vein damage at surgery can develop relatively early postoperatively and present as a smooth concentric constriction or several constrictions.[15–17] Later typical atherosclerotic change can develop in the veins.[15,18] Distal anastomotic stenosis occurs early following coronary artery bypass graft surgery. These lesions may form from the suture line as a thrombotic or proliferative event.[18–20,21] In evaluating the hemodynamic significance of vein graft stenosis, the narrowed area should be compared to the size of the native artery or arteries being served rather than to the adjacent vein segment.

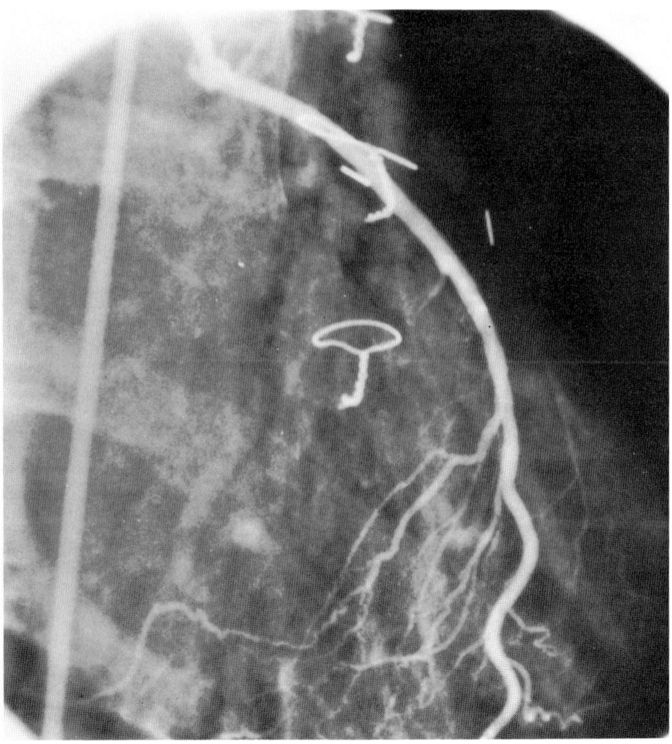

A

Figure 12-27 (*a*) Saphenous vein graft to LAD. Note smooth appearance and the fact that the vein has assumed the same size as the distal LAD. (*b*) Internal mammary graft to LAD. (*c*) Total occlusion of vein graft site. (*d*) Vein graft stenosis 5 years postoperative. Note the irregular appearance and filling defects in the proximal graft. (*e*) Smooth concentric vein graft stenosis.

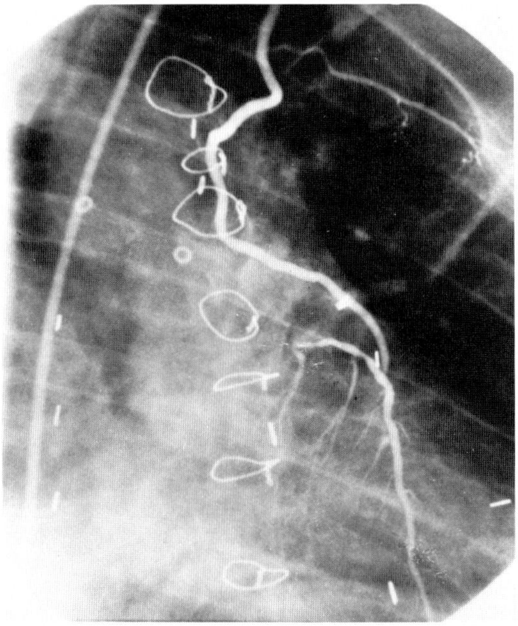

B

(Figure 12-27, continued)

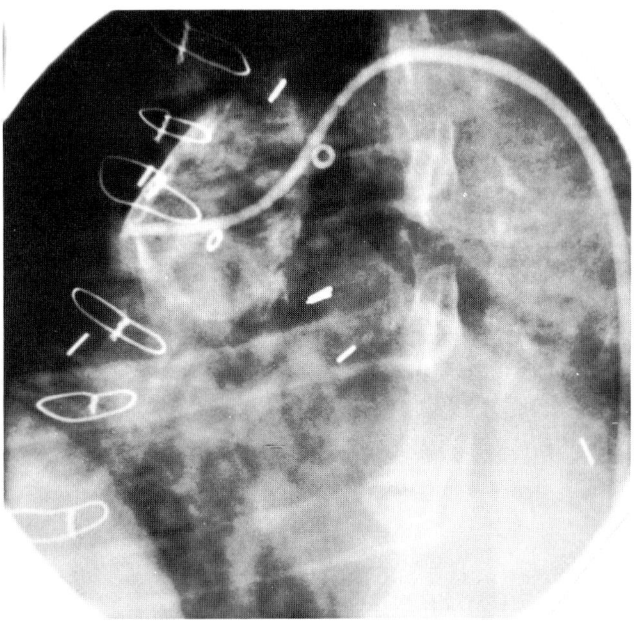

C

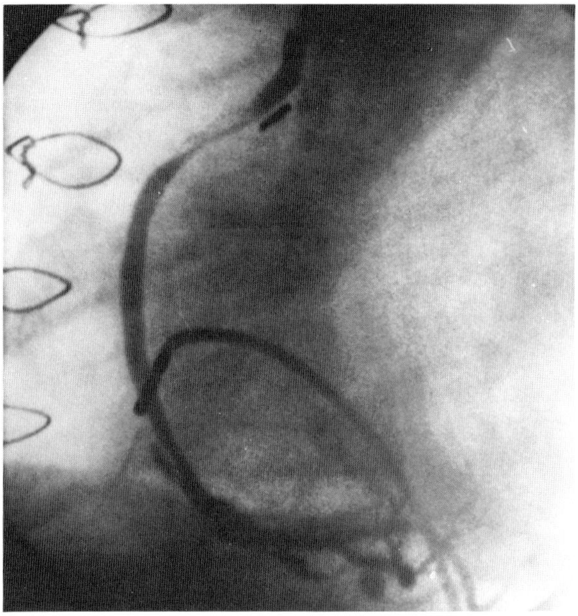

D

(Figure 12-27, continued)

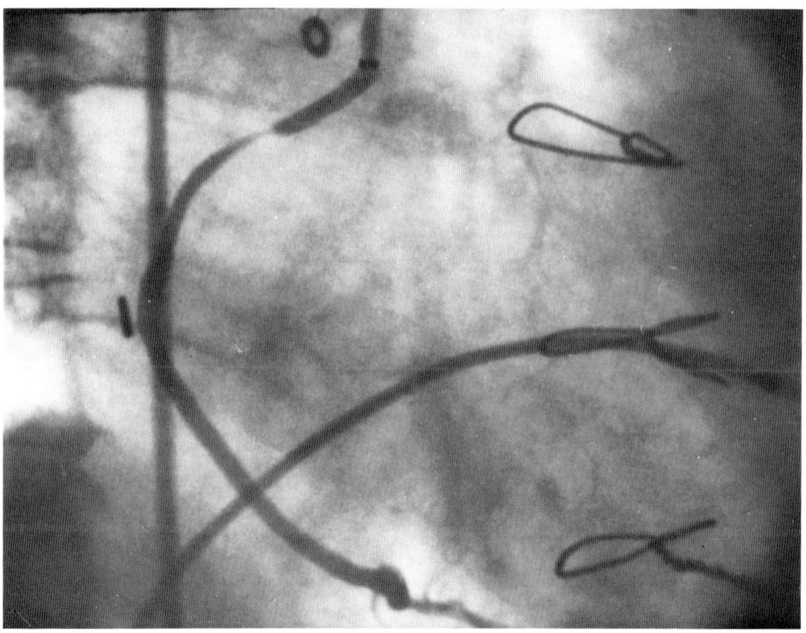

E

EVALUATION OF LEFT VENTRICULAR FUNCTION

The performance of the left ventricle may be altered by medications administered prior to the study, by ischemia during the study, and by contrast media, particularly if coronary arteriography precedes left ventriculography. Injection of contrast medium directly into the ventricle has little effect on the ventricular contractility or volume measurements during the first three or four cycles following injection. Therefore the left ventricular systolic function reflected by the angiogram should give an accurate representation of the motion of the left ventricle.

Assessment of the regional left ventricular wall motion is made by visual inspection of the cineventriculogram. The normal pattern of left ventricular contraction is a uniform and almost concentric inward movement of all areas of the endocardial surface during systole. Harrison[22] introduced the term "asynergy," which has been used to indicate a disturbance of the normal contraction pattern. The Ad Hoc Committee for Grading of Coronary Artery Disease of the American Heart Association has recommended that five RAO segments and two LAO segments be defined and characterized as to wall motion (Fig. 12-28). Herman et al.[23] classified ventricular asynergy according to the severity of the contractile abnormality, and a similar classification of left ventricular wall motion is recommended by the Ad Hoc Committee.[24] These designations are *normal* (normal wall motion of indicated ventricular segment), *reduced* (velocity or amplitude of indicated wall segments are/is reduced), *none* (absence of appropriate wall motion of indicated ventricular segment), *dyskinetic* (paradoxical wall motion of indicated segment), *aneurysmal* (aneurysmal bulging with sharply defined margins of indicated ventricular segment), or *undefined wall motion*. Many angiographers use the term *akinesis* when no wall motion is present and *hypokinesis* when wall motion is reduced.

It has been shown that contractile abnormalities not observed under basal conditions may be elicited by stress in the form of exercise, atrial pacing, handgrip, or a negative inotropic agent such as propranolol. It is also clear that localized contractile abnormalities may be due to chronically ischemic but viable myocardium. Inotropic agents, postextrasystolic potentiation, and nitrates have been used to identify those segments with potentially reversible contraction abnormalities, and a significant correlation has been observed between pharmacological responsiveness and improvement in contraction of a segment following coronary bypass surgery.[25–27] In evaluating the effect of interventions on regional left ventricular wall motion, objective methods are necessary. There is no current uniformity as to the method of superimposing end-diastolic and end-systolic silhouettes. Recommended methods include the use of the aortic valve plane, the longitudinal axis, and the use of external and internal reference points[23,28] (see Chap. 10).

QUANTITATIVE VENTRICULOGRAPHY

The ability of the left ventricle to function as a pump is best analyzed by left ventricular volume determinations. By assuming the left ventricular chamber to be ellipsoid in shape and using the area length method of Dodge[29] it is possible to calculate left ventricular volumes, and regression equations can be utilized to correct the consistent overestimation. Although the majority of volume studies have been performed using biplane filming, good correlations have been reported between single and biplane volume studies in patients with valvular heart disease.[30] It is clear, however, that single and biplane volumes may differ significantly in patients with coronary artery disease and regional contraction abnormalities. In particular, the single plane RAO view frequently underestimates overall left ventricular contraction because it selectively visualizes the anterior and inferior free walls of the left ventricle. These are the most commonly involved segments in coronary artery disease; however, the septum and lateral walls remain unvisualized. Vogel et al.[31] found that single plane RAO ventriculography underestimated ejection

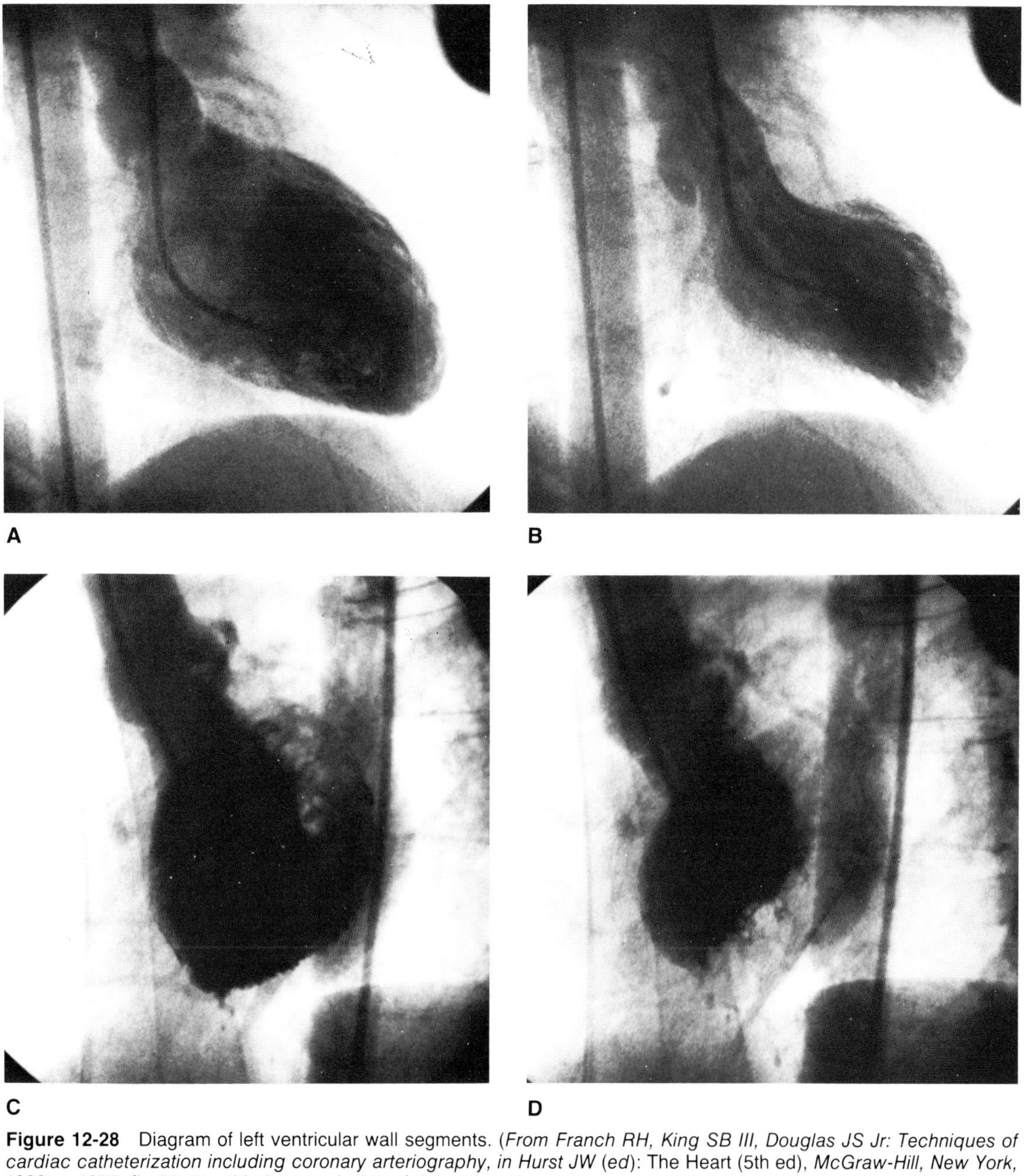

Figure 12-28 Diagram of left ventricular wall segments. (*From Franch RH, King SB III, Douglas JS Jr: Techniques of cardiac catheterization including coronary arteriography, in Hurst JW (ed)*: The Heart (5th ed), *McGraw-Hill, New York, 1982, p 1877, fig 98-43, with the permission of the authors.*)

Name ____________ Cath. Date ____________ Normal LCA ______

ID # ____________ Hosp. ____________ Normal RCA ______

Dominant Cor. R ___ L ___ Balanced ___

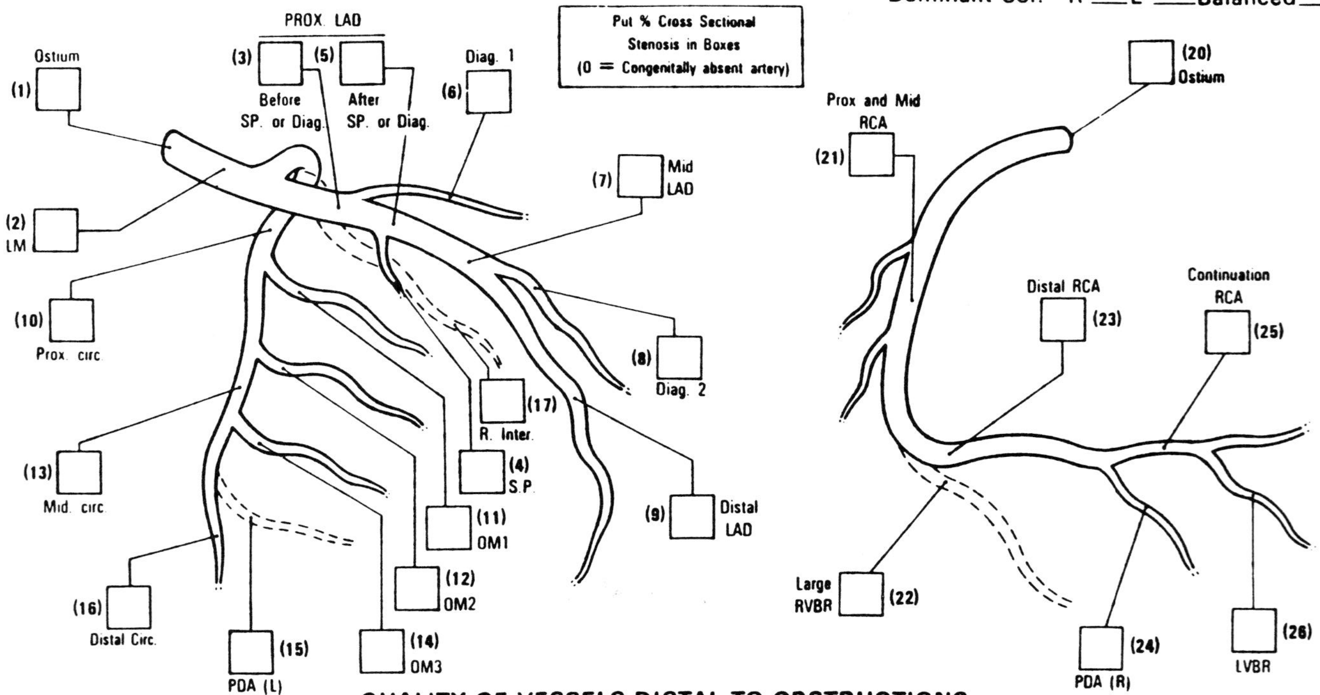

QUALITY OF VESSELS DISTAL TO OBSTRUCTIONS

Disease Code			DISEASE CODE	SIZE mm.	SUITABLE FOR BYPASS		DISEASE CODE	SIZE mm.	SUITABLE FOR BYPASS	Suitable For Bypass
Normal	2	LAD	___	___	___	OM 3	___	___	___	Yes = Y
Lumen Irreg.	3	DIAG 1	___	___	___	PDA (L)	___	___	___	No = N
Not Visualized	4	DIAG 2	___	___	___	PDA (R)	___	___	___	Uncertain = U
Severe Diffuse Disease	5	OM 1	___	___	___	RCA	___	___	___	
Distal Stenosis	___%	OM 2	___	___	___	LVBR	___	___	___	

Figure 12-29 Arterial segments form for recording coronary artery obstructions.

fraction in 70 percent of the patients with coronary artery disease. A more detailed discussion of left ventriculography is found in Chap. 10.

RECORDING AND REPORTING RESULTS OF CORONARY ARTERIOGRAMS

Many methods of reporting coronary arteriographic findings have emerged. Every laboratory has its own catheterization report format. In a laboratory with a large volume, we find a structured recording and report method works best. It forces each angiographer to consider each arterial segment and record its condition. Figure 12-29 is the recording form we use. All these arterial segments do not exist in every patient, and some patients have more segments than are indicated; however, this format describes the coronary distribution without being overburdensome.

REFERENCES

1 Austin WG, Edwards JE, Frye RL, Gensini GG, Gott VL, Griffith LSC, McGoon DC, Murphy ML, Roe BB: A reporting system on patients evaluated for coronary artery disease: Report of the Ad Hoc Committee for Grading of Coronary Artery Disease, Council on Cardiovascular Surgery, American Heart Association. Circulation, 51(suppl 4):30, 1975.

2 King SB III, Douglas JS Jr, Morris D: New angiographic views for coronary arteriography, in Hurst JW (ed): *Update IV: The Heart*. McGraw-Hill, New York, 1982, pp 198–201.

3 Friedman M: The coronary canalized thrombus: Provenance, structure, function, and relationship to death due to coronary artery disease. Br Exp Pathol, 48:556, 1967.

4 Roberts WC: Coronary arteries and fatal acute myocardial infarction. Circulation, 45:215, 1972.

5 Ridolfi, RL, Hutchins, GM: Relationship between coronary artery lesions and myocardial infarcts: Ulceration of atherosclerotic plaques precipitating coronary thrombosis. Am Heart J, 93:468, 1977.

6 Horie T, Sekiguchi M, Hirosawa K: Relation between myocardial infarction and preinfarction angina: A histopathologic study of coronary arteries in two sudden death cases employing serial section. Am Heart J, 95:81, 1978.

7 Levin DC, Fallon JT: Significance of the angiographic morphology of localized coronary stenoses: Histopathologic correlations. Circulation, 66:316–320, 1982.

8 Paulin S: Normal coronary anatomy, in Abrams HL (ed): *Coronary Arteriography, A Practical Approach*. Little, Brown, Boston, 1983, p 165.

9 Paulin S: Intra-arterial coronary anastomoses in relation to arterial obstruction demonstrated in coronary arteriography. Invest Radiol, 2:147, 1967.

10 Helfant RH, Kemp HG, Gorlin R: Coronary atherosclerosis, coronary collaterals and their relations to cardiac function. Ann Intern Med, 73:189, 1970.

11 Levin DC, Sos TA, Lee JG, Baltaxe HA: Coronary collateral circulation in distal coronary runoff: Key factors in preserving myocardial contractility in patients with coronary artery disease. AJR, 119:474, 1973.

12 Noble J, Bourassa MG, Petitclerc R, Dyrda I: Myocardial bridging and milking effect of the left anterior descending coronary artery: Normal variant or obstruction. Am J Cardiol, 37:993, 1976.

13 Farukui AMA, Maloy WC, Felner JM, Schlant RC, Logan WD, Symbas P: Symptomatic myocardial bridging of coronary artery. Am J Cardiol, 41:1305, 1978.

14 Glickel SZ, Maggs PR, Ellis FH Jr: Coronary artery aneurysm. Ann Thorac Surg, 25:372, 1978.

15 Smith SH, Geer JC: Morphology of saphenous vein coronary artery bypass grafts: 7–116 Months after surgery. Arch Pathol Lab Med, 117:13–18, 1983.

16 Spray TL, Roberts WC: Changes in saphenous veins used as aortocoronary bypass grafts. Am Heart J, 94:500–516, 1977.

17 Vlodaver Z, Edwards JE: Pathologic changes in aortic coronary arterial saphenous vein grafts. Circulation, 44:719–728, 1971.

18 Lie JT, Lawrie GW, Morris GC Jr: Aorto coronary bypass saphenous vein graft atherosclerosis: Anatomic study of 99 vein grafts from normal and hyperlipoproteinemic patients up to 75 months postoperatively. Am J Cardiol, 40:906–914, 1977.

19 Bulkley BH: Advances in cardiac pathology in Hurst JW (ed): *Update I: The Heart*. McGraw-Hill, New York, 1979, pp 83–114.

20 Moore GW, Hutchins GM: Coronary artery bypass grafts in 109 autopsied patients: Statistical analysis of graft and anastomosis patency in regional myocardial injury. JAMA, 246:1785–1789, 1981.

21 Douglas JS Jr, Gruentzig AR, King SB III, Hollman

J, Ischinger T: Percutaneous transluminal coronary angioplasty in patients with prior coronary bypass surgery. J Am Coll Cardiol, 2(4): October 1983, p 745–754.

22 Harrison TR: Some unanswered questions concerning enlargement and failure of the heart. Am Heart J, 69:100, 1965.

23 Herman MV, Heinle RA, Klein MD, Gorlin R.: Localized disorders in myocardial contraction. N Engl J Med, 277:222, 1967.

24 Austin WG, Edwards JE, Frye RL, et al: A reporting system on patients evaluated for coronary artery disease: Report of the Ad Hoc Committee for Grading of Coronary Artery Disease, Council on Cardiovascular Surgery, American Heart Association. Circulation, 51(suppl 4):30, 1975.

25 Helfant RH, Pine R, Meister SG, Feldman MS, Trout RG, Banka VS: Nitroglycerin to unmask reversible asynergy: Correlation with post coronary bypass ventriculography. Circulation, 50:108, 1974.

26 Horn HR, Teicholz LE, Cohn PF, Herman MV, Gorlin, R: Augmentation of left ventricular contraction pattern in coronary artery disease by inotropic catecholamine: The epinephrine ventriculogram. Circulation, 49:1063, 1974.

27 Dyke SH, Cohn PF, Gorlin R, Sonnenblick EH: Detection of residual myocardial function in coronary artery disease using post extrasystolic potentiation. Circulation, 50:694, 1974.

28 Chaitman BR, Bristow JD, Rahimtoola SH: Left ventricular wall motion assessed by using fixed external reference systems. Circulation, 48:1043, 1973.

29 Dodge T, Sandler H, Ballew DW, Lord JH: The use of biplane angiocardiography for the measurement of left ventricular volume in man. Am Heart J, 60:762, 1960.

30 Greene DG, Carlisle R, Grant C, Bunnell IL: Estimation of left ventricular volume by one-plane cineangiography. Circulation, 35:61, 1967.

31 Vogel JHK, Cornish D, McFadden RB: Underestimations of ejection fraction with single plane angiography in coronary artery disease: Role of biplane angiography. Chest, 64:217, 1973.

Chapter 13

Prevalence and Distribution of Disease in Patients Catheterized for Suspected Coronary Disease

James Campbell, M.D.
Spencer B. King III, M.D.
John S. Douglas, Jr., M.D.
James M. Bradford, Ph.D.

Coronary arteriography is performed on various indications. A good deal of information which may help in predicting the prevalence of disease in the patients studied is available prior to catheterization. This chapter will analyze the results of over 10,000 coronary arteriograms performed over a 5-year period at Emory University Hospital Cardiac Catheterization Laboratory. We will look at the prevalence and distribution of disease and the effect of sex, age, risk factors, duration of symptoms, chest pain symptomatology, and the history of prior myocardial infarction on this prevalence and distribution.

Prior to catheterization, all patients were seen by an attending cardiologist and fellow, and a questionnaire and physical examination were completed. On the questionnaire basic information is recorded about age, sex, race, the chest pain history, duration of symptoms, presence of risk factors, history of prior cardiac events, and cardiac medications (Fig. 13-1). The data from these forms was then transferred to the computer of the Cardiac Data Bank, and it is this information which provides the data for the study.

EXCLUSIONS

Between January 1, 1978, and December 31, 1982, there were 15,523 patients catheterized at Emory University Cardiac Catheterization Laboratory. All patients with congenital heart disease, valvular heart disease, and cardiomyopathy including idiopathic hypertrophic subaortic stenosis (IHSS) and congestive or restrictive cardiomyopathies have been eliminated from consideration. Also all second catheterizations, all repeat catheterizations at the time of percutaneous transluminal coronary angioplasty (PTCA) and all follow-up post-PTCA and

OK for Computer Entry ______
Completed By ________
(*) Codes on Back

Cardiovascular Laboratory
Patient Information Form
SUBJECTIVE DATA

PATIENT'S NAME, PHYSICIAN'S NAME, HOSPITAL #

DATE	PREVIOUS CATH DATE	HOSPITAL*	POST SURGERY CATH? Yes ___ No ___
__ __/__ __/__ __ Y Y M M D D	__ __/__ __/__ __ Y Y M M D D		POST PTCA CATH? Yes ___ No ___

AGE: ____ **SEX:** (circle) M F **RACE:** (circle) White Black Other ________

CARDIAC DIAGNOSES: (*) Fill in Appropriate Data
(1) ________ (3) ________
(2) ________ (4) ________

CHEST PAIN SUBSETS: (*) (check)
__ A. Stable Angina (*)
__ B. Stable Disabling Angina
__ C. Recent Onset (≤ 60 days)
__ D. Recent Onset + Rest Pain
__ E. Progressive without Rest Pain
__ F. Progressive with Rest Pain (Not Disabling)
__ G. Progressive with Rest Pain (Disabling)
__ H. Prolonged (> 20 min.) without Previous Pains (≤ 30 days)
__ I. Prolonged with Previous Pain or Objective Evidence (≤ 30 days)
__ J. Chest Discomfort Not Characteristic of Myocardial Ischemia
__ K. No Chest Discomfort
__ L. Asymptomatic with Positive Exercise Tolerance Test

DURATION OF ISCHEMIC SYMPTOMS ____ mths.
RECENT CHANGE ____ wks.

GALLOP RHYTHM (✓) ___ S_3 ___ S_4 ____ None
ELEVATED VENOUS PULSATION (✓) ___ Yes ___ No ___ Unknown
TOTAL NO. MI's ____
MOST RECENT MI __ __/__ __/__ __ Y Y M M D D
CAROTID BRUIT: Yes No R ___ ___ L ___ ___

MURMUR: Yes ___ No ___ Grade: 1 2 3 4 5
A. SYSTOLIC: Apex ___ Base ___ LLSB ___ 2nd LICS ___
Holosystolic ___ Late Systolic ___ Spindle Shaped ___
Other ________
B. DIASTOLIC:
Diastolic Blow: Faint ___ Moderate ___ Loud ___
Apical Diastolic Rumble: Faint ___ Moderate ___ Loud ___
Other ________

LOCATION OF MI'S
___ A. Anterior ___ E. Posterior
___ B. Septal ___ F. Subendocardial
___ C. Lateral ___ U. Unknown
___ D. Inferior

HISTORY OF CHF: (✓)
___ Yes
___ No
___ Unknown

CANADIAN (*) HEART CLASS:
___ (CHF)
___ (Angina)

RISK FACTORS	YES	NO	DURATION
HBP	___	___	__ __ . __ YRS.
Diabetes:	___	___	__ __ . __ YRS.
(if yes, insulin therapy?)	___	___	__ __ . __ YRS.
Hyperlipidemia:	___	___	__ __ . __ YRS.
Menopause Occurred?	___	___	__ __ . __ YRS. AGO
Oral Contraception Ever?	___	___	__ __ . __ YRS.

(if stopped, date stopped: __ __/__ __) Y Y M M
No. of Family Members < 55 with Coronary Event: ____

SMOKING HISTORY
___ Never Smoked
___ Former Smoker
Date Stopped __ __/__ __ Y Y M M
___ Smoking Now
__ . __ Pks/Day when Smoking
__ __ . __ No. of Years Smoking

THERAPY 0 = NONE
Nifedipine (Mg/day) ____
Nitroglycerin (Tabs/wk) ____
Propranolol (mg/day) ____
Lopressor (Mg/day) ____
Corgard (Mg/day) ____

	Yes	No	Unknown
Digitalis	___	___	___
Long Acting Nitro	___	___	___
Diuretics	___	___	___

Figure 13-1 Questionnaire for inputting clinical patient information prior to catheterization.

postsurgical catheterizations were eliminated. This gave a total of 10,489 patients who were catheterized for the first time for evaluation of coronary artery disease. Of these, 7732, or 74 percent, were males. The mean age for males was 54.6 years, and the age distribution for the male population showed a bell-shaped curve with 29 percent under the age of 50, 43 percent in their 50s, and 28 percent greater than 60 years of age. There were 2757 females catheterized, and they were significantly older than the males, mean 57.1 years, with 22 percent being under the age of 50, 39 percent in their 50s, and 39 percent greater than 60 years of age. According to race, 9737 patients (93 percent) were white, 259 (2.5 percent) were black, and 428 (4.0 percent) were of other races.

CHEST PAIN SUBSETS

Following the precatheterization interview, all patients were classified into 1 of 12 symptom subsets. These subsets can be grouped into four general categories: unstable angina, stable angina, no chest pain or nonischemic chest pain, and a fourth and smaller group of patients who were asymptomatic but had a positive electrocardiographic response on exercise testing. Most of the patients (53 percent) belong to the broad unstable angina category. This category was defined as recent onset of chest pain (less than 60 days) with or without rest pain, progression of symptomatology within the last 60 days, again with or without rest pain, or a prolonged episode of chest pain (greater than 20 minutes) within the last 30 days prior to catheterization. A slightly higher percentage of the males belonged to this category than females (55 percent of the males, 48 percent of the females). The next largest group represented those patients with no chest discomfort or nonischemic chest pain. This group made up 26 percent (2710 people) of the series. A higher percentage of the females belonged to this group than males (36 percent of the females, 23 percent of the males). Stable angina was represented by 19 percent (2002) of the total population (20 percent of the males, 15 percent of the females). The classification asymptomatic with a positive exercise test was represented by an interesting but small group of 184 patients, or 1.7 percent of the total. Of these, 173 were males.

RISK FACTORS AND OTHER PREDICTORS OF CORONARY DISEASE

Five generally accepted risk factors for coronary artery disease were evaluated: smoking, diabetes, hypertension, hyperlipidemia, and a positive family history for coronary artery disease.

The criteria for these risk factors is entirely historical:

Smoking—Those patients currently smoking or who have smoked greater than 20 pack-years. (1 pack-year equals 1 pack per day for a year.)

Diabetes—Those patients who responded positively to the question, "Do you have diabetes?"

Hypertension—Those patients who have been diagnosed as having hypertension.

Hyperlipidemia—Those patients who responded positively to the question, "Have you ever been told you have elevated cholesterol or blood fats?"

Positive family history—Those patients who have had an immediate family member with a coronary event, i.e., angina, myocardial infarction, sudden cardiac death, coronary bypass surgery, or catheterization-proven coronary disease prior to age 55 years.

The most frequently encountered risk factor in our population was smoking (53 percent). There was a significant difference between the male and female populations with this risk factor (males 60 percent, females 35 percent). Hypertension was the next most frequently encountered risk factor, occurring in 40 percent of the population. Females were more likely to have hypertension (48 percent) than males (37 percent). Of all patients 34 percent gave a positive family history for coronary disease. The proportions of the males and the females were roughly equal (32 percent of the males, 36 percent of the females). A history of diabetes was given by 11 percent of the patients. Again the percentages of males and females were roughly equal (10 percent of the males, 14 percent of the females). The figure for history of hyperlipidemia obviously underestimates the extent of true hyperlipidemia, but 11 percent of the patients gave such a history. The male and female populations were equal in this history of hyperlipidemia (12 percent of the males, 11 percent of the females). Fourteen percent of the patients gave no history of any of the known risk factors.

Forty-four percent of the patients gave a history of having had a prior myocardial infarction (males

49 percent, females 30 percent), while 31 percent had Q waves on their precatheterization ECG. In 10 percent of the patients there was a history of congestive heart failure (males 9 percent, females 12.4 percent).

INTERPRETATION OF THE CORONARY ARTERIOGRAMS

All coronary arteriograms were interpreted by the cardiac fellow and attending cardiologist performing the procedure, and the amount of narrowing was assessed in terms of cross-sectional narrowing. The amount of coronary occlusion was then further divided into four subgroups based on the extent of cross-sectional narrowing: no coronary artery disease, mild coronary artery obstruction, representing patients whose most significant coronary narrowing was felt to be 1 to 49 percent cross-sectional narrowing, moderate coronary artery obstruction, representing patients whose most significant lesion was between 50 and 74 percent cross-sectional narrowing, and significant coronary artery obstruction, made up of patients whose most significant lesion was greater than 75 percent cross-sectional narrowing. It is to be remembered that a 75 percent cross-sectional obstruction is equal to a 50 percent diameter narrowing as assessed from the two-dimensional cineangiogram.

PREVALENCE OF CORONARY DISEASE IN THE TOTAL SERIES

Of this total series of persons catheterized for evaluation of coronary artery disease, 22 percent were found to have no coronary artery obstruction, while 5 percent had mild disease, and 4 percent had moderate disease. There were 7182 patients who had significant coronary artery obstruction (68 percent). As one can see by referring to Table 13-1, the majority of the patients with significant coronary disease were males, which was not only due to the greater number of males in this study but also the increased percentage of males with significant disease compared to females (males, 77 percent, females, 46 percent). It can also be noted from Table 13-1 that the percentage of males with significant disease within each group is always greater than the percentage of females, and the incidence of significant disease increases with increasing age for both sexes.

Single vessel disease was defined as a significant lesion in major divisions of the left anterior descending, (LAD), circumflex, or right coronary ar-

Table 13-1 Prevalence of Disease in Total Group

Age	N	No disease	Mild disease	Moderate disease	Significant disease
Male					
<50 yr	2266	617 (27%)┐	108 (5%)	79 (4%)	1462 (65%)┐
50–60 yr	3294	384 (12%)┤ *	153 (5%)	143 (4%)	2614 (79%)┤ *
>60 yr	2174	162 (8%)┘ *	77 (4%)	87 (4%)	1846 (85%)┘ *
Total	7732	1163 (15%)	338 (4%)	309 (4%)	5922 (77%)
Female					
<50 yr	603	375 (62%)┐	39 (7%)	21 (4%)	168 (28%)┐
50–60 yr	1063	459 (43%)┤ *	75 (7%)	50 (5%)	479 (45%)┤ *
>60 yr	1091	310 (28%)┘ *	96 (9%)	72 (7%)	613 (56%)┘ *
Total	2757	1144 (42%)	210 (8%)	143 (5%)	1260 (46%)

* = $p < 0.001$

tery (RCA), while double vessel disease represented significant disease in two of these three territories. Any significant lesion in the left main with or without other coronary obstruction was considered left main disease. Figure 13-2 outlines the coronary circulation. The territory of the LAD considered in this survey was defined as the proximal-to-mid LAD, positions 3, 5, and 7 on the schematic. Because of the variability of the circumflex coronary artery, the common circumflex and all three marginals were considered part of this distribution, positions 10 to 15. The right coronary artery was defined as the proximal right coronary artery through its long conduit portion down to and including the posterior descending artery, positions 18, 19, 21, and 22. The fifth category was described as *distal vessels* and included the septal perforator, position 4, both first and second diagonals, positions 6 and 8, distal LAD, position 9, distal circumflex, position 16, and posterior descending if it arose from the circumflex artery, position 17. Also included were a large right ventricular branch of the right coronary artery if present, position 20, and the distal right coronary circulation, including a left ventricular branch of the right coronary distal to the posterior descending

Figure 13-2 Diagram of the coronary circulation with the segments which were used for this study identified.

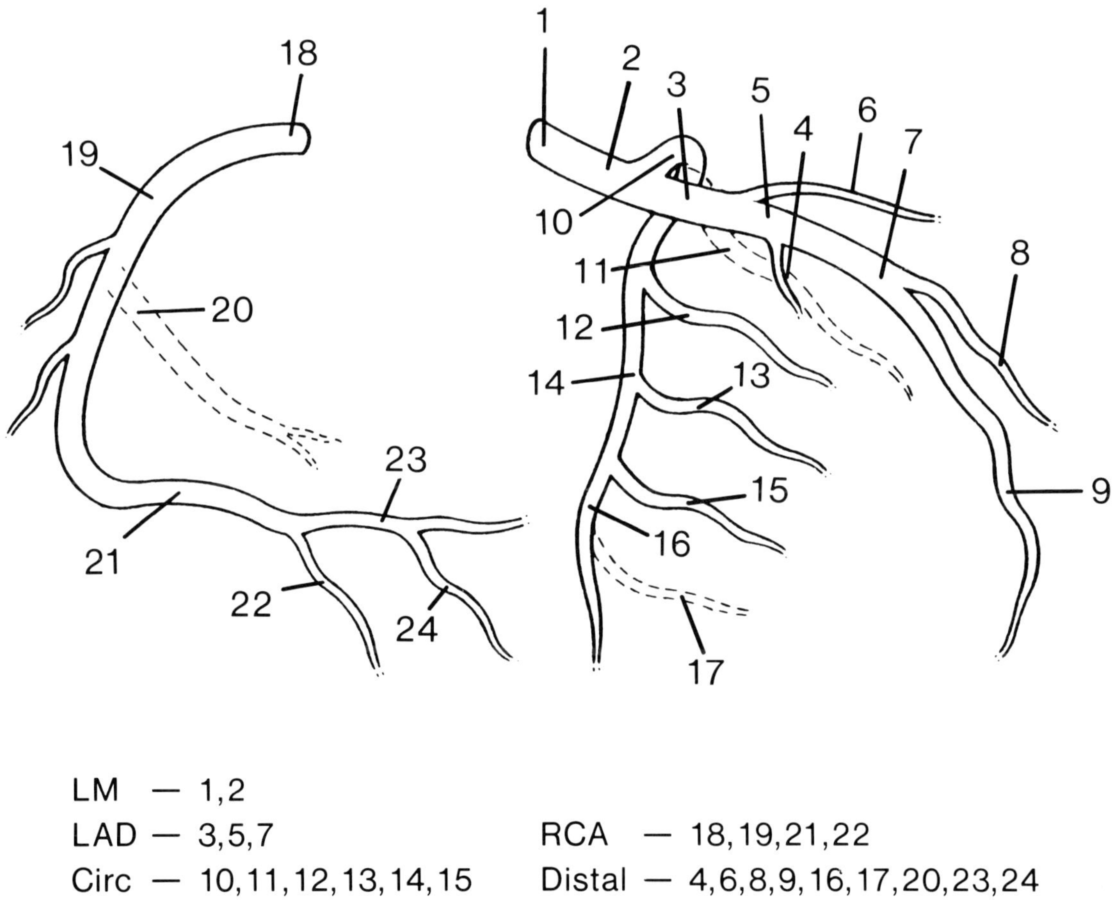

branch, positions 23 and 24. For a patient to be grouped in the distal vessel category, there had to be significant disease only in these distal vessels without significant obstructions in any of the territories of either the left main, LAD, circumflex, or RCA.

DISTRIBUTION OF CORONARY DISEASE IN PATIENTS WITH SIGNIFICANT OBSTRUCTION

Table 13-2 outlines the distribution of disease in those patients with significant coronary artery obstruction. Of the males with significant coronary artery obstruction, 32 percent had single vessel disease while another 32 percent had double vessel disease. Triple vessel disease represented 28 percent, while left main disease was found in only 7 percent. In the male population with significant coronary disease, only 2 percent had significant disease confined to the smaller and more distal vessels. In the male group under the age of 50 with significant disease, 41 percent had single vessel disease, but this percentage dropped to only 25 percent of the group older than 60 years. Triple vessel and left main disease became increasingly common with age. Disease limited to the smaller and more distal vessels was equally uncommon throughout the three age groups.

In the female group with significant coronary disease, 40 percent had single vessel disease while 30 percent had double vessel disease. Triple vessel disease occurred in 22 percent, while 5 percent had left main disease. Again the percentage with disease limited to the smaller and more distal vessels is quite small (40 patients or 3 percent of the total female group with significant disease and equal in the three age groups). As with the male group, the females showed more single vessel disease in the younger age groups, and this decreased with increasing age while double and triple vessel disease became more prevalent. However, even in the older than 60-year-old group, 35 percent of the females had single vessel disease. The percentage of left main disease did not increase in the female population with age, and the percentage of smaller vessel or distal disease remained small throughout all three age groups.

PREVALENCE AND DISTRIBUTION RELATED TO SYMPTOMATIC SUBSETS

Each patient's history of chest pain was elicited prior to catheterization, and the patient was placed into one of the four groups: stable angina, unstable angina, no pain or nonischemic pain, or asymptomatic with a positive exercise test. Table 13-3

Table 13-2 Distribution of Significant Disease

Age	N	Single vessel disease	Double vessel disease	Triple vessel disease	Left main disease	Distal
Male						
<50 yr	1462	592 (41%)	448 (31%)	312 (21%)	60 (4%)	50 (3%)
50–60 yr	2614	855 (33%)	825 (32%)	740 (28%)	136 (5%)	58 (2%)
>60 yr	1846	452 (25%)	590 (32%)	584 (32%)	186 (10%)	34 (2%)
Total	5922	1899 (32%)	1863 (32%)	1636 (28%)	382 (7%)	142 (2%)
Female						
<50 yr	168	87 (52%)	44 (26%)	22 (13%)	6 (4%)	9 (5%)
50–60 yr	479	201 (42%)	145 (30%)	97 (20%)	19 (4%)	17 (4%)
>60 yr	613	216 (35%)	184 (30%)	161 (26%)	38 (6%)	14 (2%)
Total	1260	504 (40%)	373 (30%)	280 (22%)	63 (5%)	40 (3%)

* = $p < 0.001$.
△ = $p < 0.05$.

Table 13-3 Prevalence by Chest Pain Subsets

Subset	N	No disease	Mild disease	Moderate disease	Significant disease
Male					
Stable angina	1586	138 (9%)	51 (3%)	68 (4%)	1329 (84%)
Unstable angina	4243	456 (11%)	140 (3%)	150 (4%)	3497 (82%)
Other pain	1726	520 (30%)*	134 (8%)*	80 (5%)△	992 (58%)*
Asymptomatic with positive exercise test	173	49 (28%)	13 (8%)	11 (7%)	100 (58%)
Female					
Stable angina	416	136 (33%)	40 (10%)	17 (4%)	223 (54%)
Unstable angina	1345	386 (29%)	96 (7%)	84 (6%)	779 (58%)
Other pain	984	616 (63%)*	72 (7%)	42 (4%)	254 (26%)*
Asymptomatic with positive exercise test	11	6 (55%)	2 (18%)	0 (0%)	3 (27%)

* = $p < 0.001$
△ = $p < 0.05$

outlines the extent of disease in both males and females according to their precatheterization chest pain subset. The stable and unstable male groups had a higher percentage of significant disease than the total male group, and their incidence of no coronary disease was about 10 percent. There was no difference in the extent of disease as defined between the stable and unstable angina groups, but as expected these groups had more coronary disease than the remaining two groups. In the no pain or nonischemic pain group and the asymptomatic with positive exercise test group, only 58 percent of the males catheterized had significant coronary obstructive disease, while almost one-third had no coronary artery disease.

Within the female population, those thought to have stable and unstable angina had a much lower incidence of coronary disease than the men. There was only a slight increase in significant coronary disease in the unstable group as compared to the stable angina group, 58 versus 54 percent. Of the females who had no pain or nonischemic pain symptoms prior to catheterization, only 26 percent had significant coronary obstruction, and 63 percent had no coronary artery disease. Only 11 females were thought to be asymptomatic with positive exercise test, and of this group, 3, or 27 percent, had significant coronary disease.

The distribution of disease in those male patients who had significant coronary artery obstruction was not different between the stable and unstable angina and no pain or nonischemic pain groups (Table 13-4). There was a slight decrease in the amount of triple vessel disease in the asymptomatic with positive exercise test group.

The distribution of significant disease in the female population does show some differences when broken down into various symptom groups. Of those females thought to have unstable angina prior to catheterization, the percentage of single vessel disease (37 percent) was significantly less than it was in the no pain or nonischemic pain group (47 percent), while the percentage of triple vessel disease was increased (25 versus 16 percent). The extent of left main disease was similar in all three groups, as was the amount of disease limited to smaller and more distal vessels.

DURATION OF SYMPTOMS

The distribution of disease in all patients with significant coronary obstruction is also outlined in Table 13-5 based on the duration of symptoms. The percentage of single vessel disease is greatest in those with no history of chest pain or duration of pain under 3 months and decreases with longer

Table 13-4 Distribution by Chest Pain Subsets

Subset	N	Single vessel disease	Double vessel disease	Triple vessel disease	Left main disease	Distal
Male						
Stable angina	1324	405 (31%)	407 (31%)	396 (30%)	85 (6%)	36 (3%)
Unstable angina	3497	1124 (32%)	1117 (32%)	954 (28%)	226 (7%)	76 (2%)
Other pain	992	335 (34%)	302 (30%)	264 (27%)	66 (7%)	25 (3%)
Asymptomatic with positive exercise test	100	33 (33%)	36 (36%)	21 (21%)	5 (5%)	5 (5%)
Female						
Stable angina	223	94 (42%)	66 (30%)	46 (21%)	11 (5%)	6 (3%)
Unstable angina	779	289 (37%)	235 (30%)	193 (25%)	40 (5%)	22 (3%)
Other pain	254	120 (47%)	71 (28%)	40 (16%)	11 (4%)	12 (5%)
Asymptomatic with positive exercise test	3	0 (0%)	1 (33%)	1 (33%)	1 (33%)	0 (0%)

△ = $p < 0.05$

duration of angina to the point that the patients who have a greater than 2-year history of angina have only a 23 percent chance of having single vessel disease at catheterization. Conversely the amount of triple vessel disease increases with increasing duration of angina. The percentage of left main disease was small throughout but showed a steady increase as the duration of symptoms increased.

PREVALENCE AND DISTRIBUTION OF CORONARY DISEASE RELATED TO RISK FACTORS

Smoking

Of the five stated risk factors, smoking was the most prevalent in the men, with 60 percent of the male population fitting into this subgroup. Among males, smoking had an effect on the percentage of patients with significant coronary disease for each of the three age groups. Significant disease occurred in 69 percent of smokers versus 52 percent of nonsmokers in the under 50-year-old age group, 81 versus 72 percent in the 50- to 59-year-old age group, and for the greater than 60-year-old age group, the percentages were 86 percent against 82 percent. Table 13-6 outlines the effect of smoking on the total group. Among males with significant coronary artery obstruction, there is a significant difference in the percentage of single vessel disease (35 versus 31 percent) and in triple vessel disease (25 versus 30 percent) between the smoking and nonsmoking groups.

The percentage of females with a smoking history was much less than the males, only 35 percent.

Table 13-5 Distribution by Duration of Symptoms

Symptoms	N	Single vessel disease	Double vessel disease	Triple vessel disease	Left main disease	Distal
None	477	208 (44%)	142 (30%)	97 (20%)	12 (3%)	18 (4%)
<3 mo	1465	667 (46%)	429 (29%)	267 (18%)	59 (4%)	32 (3%)
3–6 mo	899	324 (36%)	285 (32%)	214 (24%)	52 (6%)	24 (3%)
7–24 mo	1215	397 (33%)	381 (31%)	339 (28%)	67 (6%)	31 (3%)
>24 mo	2057	465 (23%)	655 (32%)	724 (35%)	173 (8%)	40 (2%)

* = $p < 0.001$
△ = $p < 0.05$

Table 13-6 Smoking

Prevalence in total group

Sex	Smoking	N	No disease	Mild disease	Moderate disease	Significant disease
Males	Yes	4266	549 (13%)	194 (5%)	183 (4%)	3340 (78%)
	No	2824	585 (21%) *	137 (5%)	115 (4%)	1987 (70%) *
Females	Yes	917	267 (29%)	97 (11%)	53 (6%)	500 (55%)
	No	1699	857 (50%) *	113 (7%) *	87 (5%)	642 (38%) *

Distribution of significant disease

Sex	Smoking	N	Single vessel disease	Double vessel disease	Triple vessel disease	Left main disease	Distal
Males	Yes	3340	1167 (35%)	1070 (32%)	839 (25%)	190 (6%)	74 (2%)
	No	1987	613 (31%) △	589 (30%)	593 (30%) *	131 (7%)	61 (3%)
Females	Yes	500	229 (46%)	146 (29%)	93 (19%)	16 (3%)	16 (3%)
	No	642	232 (36%) *	189 (29%)	159 (25%) △	38 (6%) △	23 (4%)

* = $p < 0.001$
△ = $p < 0.05$

The relationship of smoking to the extent of disease in females, however, was more marked than among the males. In the female population under age 50, significant disease was present in 40 percent of those who had a positive smoking history and only 16 percent in the nonsmoking group. In the 50-year-old age group, the percentages were 57 and 33 percent, and in the group older than 60, the percentages were 66 and 51 percent. In the females with significant disease, there was also more single vessel disease among the smokers than the nonsmokers (46 versus 36 percent), and there was a higher percentage of triple vessel disease in the nonsmoking group (25 versus 19 percent). Rather than protecting against the development of triple vessel disease, smoking may accentuate some of the nonatherogenic components of coronary disease as proposed by Cobbs, i.e., spasm or thrombosis. This leads to earlier symptomatology, hence earlier catheterization in those patients with less extensive disease.

History of Hypertension

A history of hypertension was elicited in 37 percent of the males catheterized at Emory (Table 13-7). The effect of this history was not evident on the occurrence rate of significant disease in any of the three age groups. Among males with hypertension and significant disease, there was a mild alteration in the distribution of the disease, with decreased single vessel disease and more triple vessel and left main disease when compared to the nonhypertensive group.

Of the females 48 percent had a history of hypertension. This history was associated with an increased prevalence of coronary disease which was most pronounced in the 50-years-and-older age groups. In the females under the age of 50, significant coronary disease occurred in 29 percent with and 25 percent without a history of high blood pressure, while for the group in their 50s, 50 percent with high blood pressure history and 37 percent without had coronary disease. In those over 60 years, 60 percent with and 49 percent without hypertension had coronary disease. Among patients who had coronary disease, there was less single vessel disease in the group with the history of hypertension (37 versus 45 percent) and consequently more multivessel involvement when compared to the nonhypertensive group.

Table 13-7 Hypertension

Prevalence in total group

Sex	Hypertension	N	No disease	Mild disease	Moderate disease	Significant disease
Males	Yes	2651	364 (14%)	115 (4%)	143 (5%)	2029 (77%)
	No	4598	788 (17%)	222 (5%)	157 (3%)	3431 (75%)
Females	Yes	1270	455 (36%)	108 (9%)	69 (5%)	638 (50%)*
	No	1380	682 (49%)	102 (7%)	71 (5%)	525 (38%)*

Distribution of significant disease

Sex	Hypertension	N	Single vessel disease	Double vessel disease	Triple vessel disease	Left main	Distal
Males	Yes	2029	602 (30%)△	658 (32%)	577 (28%)△	139 (7%)△	53 (3%)
	No	3431	1209 (35%)△	1058 (31%)	892 (26%)△	187 (6%)△	85 (3%)
Females	Yes	638	238 (37%)*	199 (31%)	144 (23%)	32 (5%)	25 (4%)
	No	525	236 (45%)*	138 (26%)	115 (22%)	21 (4%)	15 (3%)

* = $p < 0.001$
△ = $p < 0.05$

History of Diabetes

Diabetes in the male population catheterized was associated with a greater likelihood of coronary disease in all age groups. In men under age 50, 67 percent with and 62 percent without a history of diabetes had significant coronary disease. For those in their 50s, 84 percent with and 77 percent without diabetes had significant disease and for the group over age 60, 91 and 83 percent, respectively. The values for the total group are given in Table 13-8. In males with a history of diabetes there was also an effect on the distribution of disease, with less single vessel disease (22 versus 35 percent) and more triple vessel disease (36 versus 26 percent) compared to the nondiabetic population.

In females, a similar association was noted between diabetes and the prevalence and distribution of coronary disease. The percentages of females with a history of diabetes who had significant disease were 49 percent in the group under the age of 50, 71 percent in the group in their 50s, and 75 percent in the group older than 60. This is in contrast to the 24, 39, and 51 percent, respectively, for the similar age groups in the nondiabetic patients. Diabetic women over age 50 had the same prevalence of disease as the total male population. Among the diabetic women with disease, there was less single vessel disease than among nondiabetic women (24 versus 45 percent), more triple vessel disease (37 versus 18 percent), and more left main disease (7 versus 4 percent).

History of Hyperlipidemia

Hyperlipidemia is a difficult diagnosis to document by history alone. Bearing this in mind, for the male group, this history was associated with a significant increase in disease in the population we catheterized. This was most marked in the under 50-year-old group. In this group, the percent having significant coronary disease was 77 while in the group without a history of hyperlipidemia, the percent was only 60. For the 50- to 60-year-old group, the percent was 88, while in the 60-plus group it was 90 compared to 76 and 83 percent, respectively, for the same age groups in the nonhyperlipidemic male population. See Table 13-9 for the results in the group as a whole. As far as distribution, there was a mild but significant decrease in single vessel disease with a concomitant increase in triple vessel

Table 13-8 Diabetes

Prevalence in total group

Sex	Diabetes	N	No disease	Mild disease	Moderate disease	Significant disease
Males	Yes	750	81 (11%)	27 (4%)	22 (3%)	620 (83%)
	No	6445	1077 (17%) *	307 (5%)	275 (4%)	4786 (74%) *
Females	Yes	368	79 (22%)	21 (6%)	16 (4%)	252 (69%)
	No	2270	1052 (46%) *	187 (8%)	122 (5%)	909 (40%) *

Distribution of significant disease

Sex	Diabetes	N	Single vessel disease	Double vessel disease	Triple vessel disease	Left main	Distal
Males	Yes	620	133 (22%)	213 (34%)	223 (36%)	38 (6%)	13 (2%)
	No	4786	1664 (35%) *	1477 (31%)	1231 (26%) *	288 (6%)	126 (3%)
Females	Yes	252	60 (24%)	77 (31%)	92 (37%)	17 (7%)	6 (2%)
	No	909	413 (45%) *	259 (29%)	167 (18%) *	36 (4%)	34 (4%)

* = $p < 0.001$

disease in the population with a history of hyperlipidemia.

The effect of a positive history for hyperlipidemia had a more impressive effect on the percentage of females with significant disease. Of women with a history of hyperlipidemia 61 percent as opposed to 41 percent without this history had significant coronary artery disease. The distribution of coronary disease was similar in women to the findings in the male population. There was less single vessel disease in those with a history of hyperlipidemia (34 versus 43 percent) and a recip-

Table 13-9 Hyperlipidemia

Prevalence in total group

Sex	Hyperlipidemia	N	No disease	Mild disease	Moderate disease	Significant disease
Males	Yes	809	73 (9%)	29 (4%)	26 (3%)	681 (84%)
	No	6102	1057 (17%) *	295 (5%)	261 (4%)	4489 (74%) *
Females	Yes	271	71 (26%)	20 (7%)	14 (5%)	166 (61%)
	No	2256	1033 (46%) *	181 (8%)	125 (6%)	917 (41%) *

Distribution of significant disease

Sex	Hyperlipidemia	N	Single vessel disease	Double vessel disease	Triple vessel disease	Left main	Distal
Males	Yes	681	191 (28%)	221 (33%)	214 (31%)	40 (6%)	15 (2%)
	No	4489	1545 (34%) △	1392 (31%)	1158 (26%) △	274 (6%)	120 (3%)
Females	Yes	166	57 (34%)	45 (27%)	51 (31%)	9 (5%)	4 (2%)
	No	917	393 (43%) △	263 (29%)	187 (20%) △	40 (4%)	34 (4%)

* = $p < 0.001$
△ = $p < 0.05$

rocal increase in triple vessel disease (31 versus 20 percent).

Positive Family History

As one can see from Table 13-10, there was a surprisingly weak association between a positive family history for coronary disease and the finding of significant coronary disease among the males. In this case, 77 percent with a positive family history versus 74 percent without had significant coronary disease. A positive history had no effect on the distribution of disease in those males with significant disease. In the female population, the findings were slightly more impressive: 48 percent with the family history versus 41 percent without a family history had coronary disease. There was no effect on the distribution of disease.

History of No Risk Factors

It is also interesting to look at a small group of patients who listed none of the five risk factors (Table 13-11). There were 968 males who fell into this category, and of that number, 64 percent had significant disease compared to 78 percent for those males with at least one risk factor. The absence of risk factors was associated with a greater likelihood of single vessel disease (37 versus 32 percent) and a decrease in double vessel disease (26 versus 32 percent) when compared to the group with one risk factor.

There was an impressive negative association between the absence of risk factors and coronary disease in the females. Of the 468 females who were catheterized in this designation, only 110, or 24 percent, had significant coronary artery obstruction, compared to 50 percent of the female population with at least one risk factor. The distribution of disease is virtually identical between the females with no risk factors and the female population with at least one risk factor. Women under the age of 60 with none of the five stated risk factors had a chance of significant coronary disease of only 12 percent.

HISTORY OF PRIOR MYOCARDIAL INFARCTION

A history of prior myocardial infarction was a very positive predictor of significant coronary disease, as one would expect. Of the males with this history

Table 13-10 Positive Family History

Prevalence in total group

Sex	History	N	No disease	Mild disease	Moderate disease	Significant disease
Males	Yes	2235	325 (15%) △	102 (5%)	92 (4%)	1716 (77%) △
	No	4666	789 (17%)	225 (5%)	190 (4%)	3462 (74%)
Females	Yes	909	354 (39%) *	73 (8%)	46 (5%)	436 (48%) *
	No	1613	739 (46%)	129 (8%)	86 (5%)	659 (41%)

Distribution of significant disease

Sex	History	N	Single vessel disease	Double vessel disease	Triple vessel disease	Left main	Distal
Males	Yes	1716	569 (33%)	518 (30%)	489 (29%)	100 (6%)	40 (2%)
	No	3462	1157 (33%)	1093 (32%)	913 (26%)	207 (6%)	92 (3%)
Females	Yes	436	163 (37%)	130 (30%)	109 (25%)	20 (5%)	14 (3%)
	No	659	281 (43%)	190 (29%)	133 (20%)	29 (4%)	26 (4%)

* = $p < 0.001$
△ = $p < 0.05$

Table 13-11 No Risk Factors

Prevalence in total group

Sex	Risk factors	N	No disease	Mild disease	Moderate disease	Significant disease
	At least one	5264	718 (14%)	229 (4%)	225 (4%)	4092 (78%)┐
Males	risk factor					*
	No risk factors	968	251 (26%)	60 (6%)	34 (4%)	623 (64%)┘
	At least one	1926	723 (38%)	140 (7%)	102 (5%)	961 (50%)┐
Females	risk factor					*
	No risk factors	468	298 (64%)	37 (8%)	23 (5%)	110 (24%)┘

Distribution of significant disease

Sex	Risk factors	N	Single vessel disease	Double vessel disease	Triple vessel disease	Left main	Distal
	At least one	4092	1310 (32%)┐	1313 (32%)┐	1124 (27%)	250 (6%)	95 (2%)
Males	risk factor		△	△			
	No risk factors	623	230 (37%)┘	164 (26%)┘	165 (27%)	41 (7%)	23 (4%)
	At least one	961	379 (39%)	288 (30%)	215 (22%)	47 (5%)	32 (3%)
Females	risk factor						
	No risk factors	110	43 (39%)	34 (31%)	22 (20%)	6 (6%)	5 (5%)

* = $p < 0.001$
△ = $p < 0.05$

93 percent had significant coronary disease as contrasted with 59 percent of males who gave no history of a prior myocardial infarction. If males gave a history of a prior myocardial infarction, only 4 percent had no coronary disease. Of the females with a history of infarction 74 percent had significant coronary disease; 31 percent who did not give this history had significant coronary artery obstruction. The history of infarction was not associated with a difference in the distribution of disease in the males who had coronary artery obstruction but in the female population was associated with less single vessel disease and more double and triple vessel disease.

Q WAVES

Q waves on a precatheterization ECG had a very similar predictive value for coronary disease. Of the males with Q waves 94 percent had significant disease while only 65 percent without Q waves had disease. The effect on distribution of coronary disease was not significant. The prevalence of coronary disease in the female population was significantly higher in the women with Q waves as opposed to those without Q waves (78 versus 36 percent). Again there was a difference in the distribution of disease, with less single vessel disease and more triple vessel disease in females with precatheterization Q waves.

DISTRIBUTION OF DISEASE

Since June 1 of 1981, all coronary artery obstructions have been documented on a schema as demonstrated in Fig. 13-2 outlining the 24 discrete positions in the coronary artery tree. Since that date, there have been 1948 males found to have significant coronary artery obstruction, and the distribution of their coronary artery narrowing is graphed in Fig. 13-3. The Y axis represents the number of discrete obstructions found at that position while the X axis outlines the 24 vessel positions grouped according to their artery distribution. Numbered positions with asterisks represent those vessels in that artery distribution that we define as left main, left anterior descending (LAD), circumflex, or right coronary artery (RCA) distribution. All nonasterisk vessels represent the more distal vessel group.

Position 19, or the conduit portion of the RCA, is the most frequently encountered single site of significant coronary artery obstruction in this group of male patients. There were 958 significant coronary artery obstructions here; almost half of the 1948 males who had significant coronary artery obstruction had it at this position. Also of interest is the fact that 535, or 56 percent, of those significant obstructions were total obstructions. The great number of obstructions at this position may be influenced by the length of vessel subtended by this position which includes everything from the ostia around to the posterior surface of the right ventricle.

The next more frequently involved sites were the proximal LAD before and after the first diagonal or septal perforator. There were 528 and 666 significant obstructions for a total of 1194 obstructions at these two positions. These two positions taken together are more frequently involved than the conduit portion of the RCA alone. Only 34 percent of the significant obstructions were total occlusions. The next most frequently involved site was the first diagonal with 531 obstructions. Only 10 percent were totally occluded. The most commonly involved sites of the circumflex system were the proximal circumflex, with 449 obstructions of which 34 percent were totally occluded, and the first marginal or anterior lateral obtuse marginal, where there were 480 obstructions of which 18 percent were totally obstructed.

As one goes more peripherally, the incidence of

Figure 13-3 Distribution of significant disease in the male patients grouped by arterial segments.

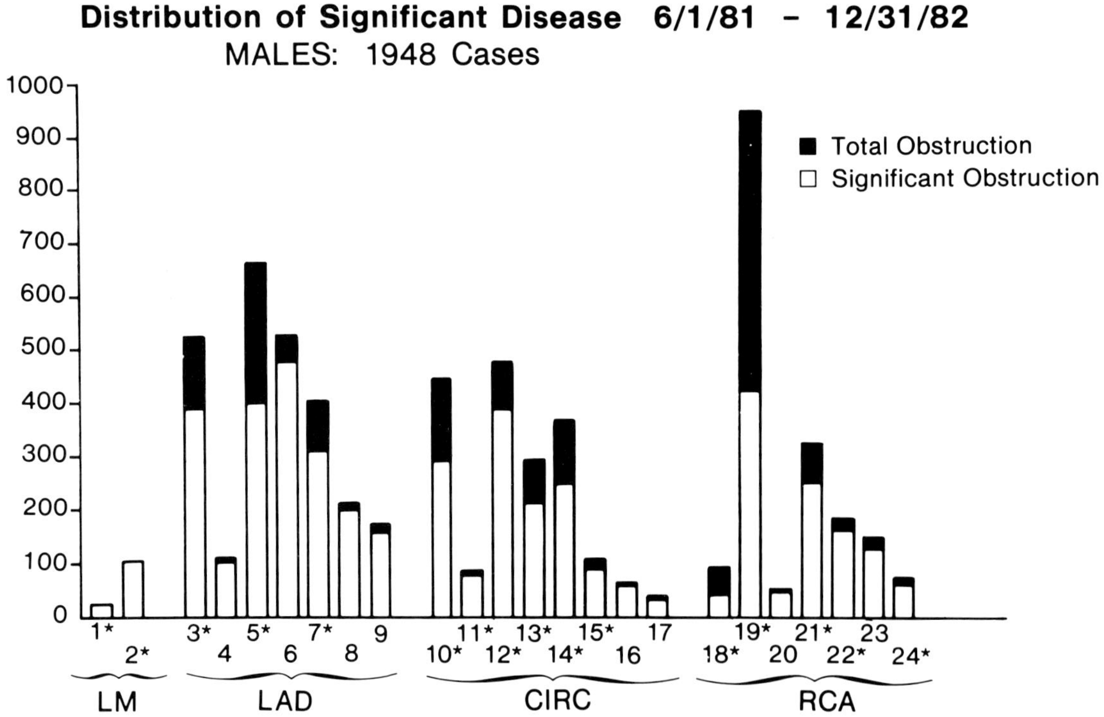

significant coronary artery obstruction decreases. Part of this can be explained by total proximal obstructions obscuring the distal vessels; however, even if nonvisualized vessels are removed from the calculations, this finding is still present, confirming the more proximal distribution of coronary disease.

Figure 13-4 outlines the distribution of disease in the female population. There were only 426 patients since June, 1981, with significant disease, and the distribution of disease looks remarkably similar to that found in the men. Position 19, or the conduit portion of the RCA, again was the most frequently encountered site of obstruction (201 or 39 percent were totally obstructed). The LAD before and after the first diagonal or septal perforator was the next most frequently encountered site again followed by the first diagonal (position 3 = 106, position 5 = 58, position 6 = 105). The distribution of disease in the left main and more distal vessels is basically similar in the male and the female populations.

Single Vessel Disease

In the total group, there were 1899 males with significant single vessel disease, of which 43 percent had left anterior descending disease, 38 percent RCA disease, and 20 percent circumflex disease. Distribution of single vessel disease in the female population was similar in 505 patients; 46 percent had LAD disease, 38 percent RCA disease, and only 15 percent circumflex disease.

Double Vessel Disease

Of the male patients with double vessel disease, 37 percent had LAD and RCA disease while another 37 percent had circumflex and RCA disease. The remaining 27 percent had LAD and circumflex disease. The female population showed a slight increase in the amount of LAD disease, with 41 percent having LAD and RCA disease while 32 percent had LAD and circumflex, and only 26 percent had circumflex and right disease.

Figure 13-4 Distribution of significant disease in the female patients grouped by arterial segments.

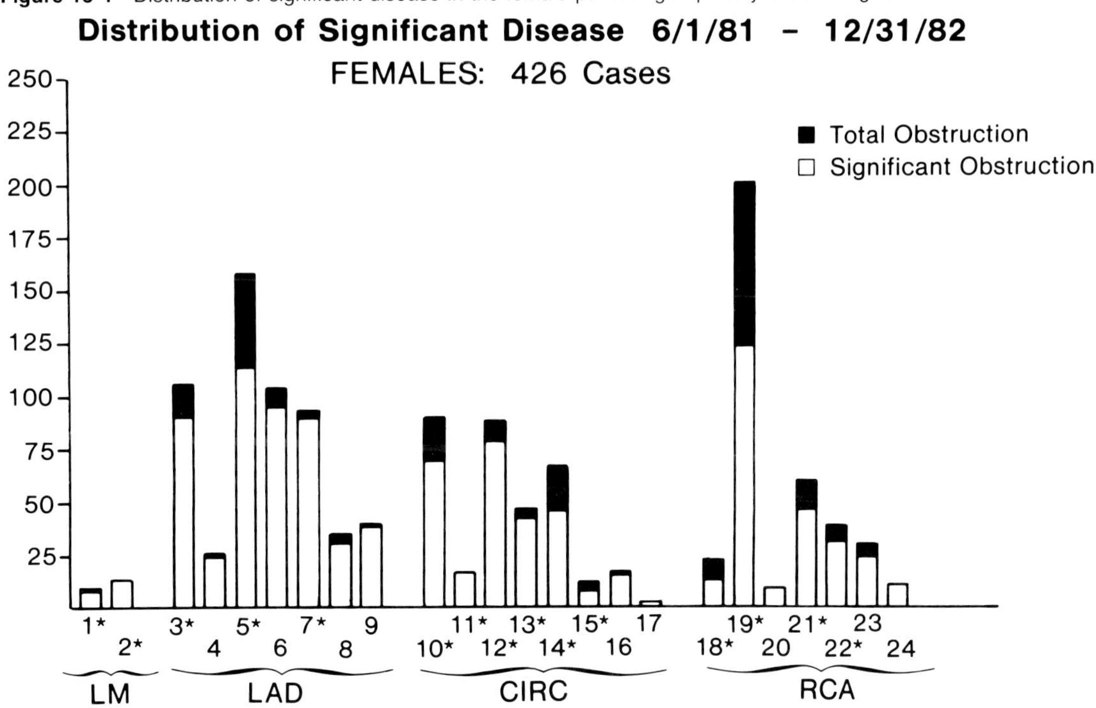

CONCLUSIONS

In reviewing this data collected in patients selected for coronary arteriography, it is obvious that the three variables most predictive for significant coronary artery disease are history of angina, age, and the male sex. In fact, of all the females catheterized for this study, only 46 percent had significant coronary artery obstruction. The percentage was even less if the female patient was felt to have either atypical chest pain, where only 26 percent had significant obstruction, or if the female patient had none of the five risk factors as defined; in that case only 24 percent had significant coronary artery obstruction. There was a significant increase in the incidence of coronary artery disease at each of the three age levels for both males and females.

Among the chest pain subsets, patients with stable and unstable angina have an equal prevalence of significant coronary artery obstruction. Patients thought to have "other pain" or who were asymptomatic with a positive exercise test had a much lower incidence of significant obstruction.

The effect of risk factors on the prevalence and distribution of disease was quite variable. The male and the female patients who smoked had a significant increase in the percent of significant coronary artery obstruction. The distribution of disease was modified in the smokers with an increased incidence of single vessel disease and a concomitant decreased incidence of triple vessel disease for both the male and the female populations. The reason for this is unclear but may be related to rapid progression of single lesions in smokers which produces symptoms before multivessel disease can occur. Patients with a history of diabetes and hyperlipidemia were found to have an increased incidence in both the prevalence of significant coronary artery disease and the occurrence of triple vessel disease in both the male and female populations. The presence of hypertension had no association with the prevalence of significant obstruction in the male population, while it was associated with an increase in the percent of significant disease in the female population. A positive family medical history was found to have a mild effect on the prevalence of significant disease in the male population, while the effect on the female population was more marked, but there was no effect on the distribution of coronary artery obstruction. Absence of risk factors was associated with a decrease in the prevalence of significant disease for both the male and the female populations. In the male population, there was a mild increase in single vessel disease and decrease in double vessel disease, while the absence of risk factors had no effect on distribution of disease in the female population.

When one looks at the distribution of significant coronary artery obstruction within the coronary arterial tree, one notes that the conduit portion of the RCA is the most commonly affected site of significant obstruction for both the male and the female populations. The second and third most frequently encountered sites of significant obstruction are the LAD before and after the first diagonal or septal perforator. For both the male and female populations significant disease at these two positions added together is found more frequently than in the conduit portion of the RCA alone. It appears that the distribution of disease within the coronary artery tree is basically similar for both the male and the female populations with some mild differences in the more distal vessels. When single vessel disease was found, it occurred in the LAD in 43 percent of the males and 46 percent of the females and in the RCA in 38 percent of both sexes.

Single vessel disease is more common in the female population than in the male population throughout all three age groups. The percentage of single vessel disease decreases with advancing age and duration of chest pain symptomatology. In the males with double vessel disease, the combination of LAD and RCA and of circumflex and RCA are of equal frequency, while the LAD and circumflex combination is the third most common. In the female population, the most commonly found pair in double vessel disease is LAD and RCA, followed by LAD and circumflex, and finally by circumflex and RCA obstructions.

Chapter 14

The Cardiac Catheterization Laboratory: Radiographic Equipment and Radiation Protection

Perry Sprawls, Jr., Ph.D.
Russell E. Aiken, M.S.
Spencer B. King III, M.D.

PLACEMENT OF CARDIAC CATHETERIZATION LABORATORIES

Only a few years ago, a cardiovascular laboratory was considered an investigational arm of very specialized hospitals and referral centers. Today, many hospitals consider a cardiovascular laboratory to be an essential element of a full-service hospital. Considering the aspects of cost efficiency in delivery of health care, the current reality probably lies somewhere between.

Certainly all hospitals with cardiovascular surgical programs must have a cardiovascular laboratory to support that surgical unit. Should cardiovascular laboratories be established in hospitals without cardiovascular surgery services? Experience has taught that free-standing laboratories can be developed and operated safely independent of cardiovascular surgical facilities. The Inter Society Commission for Heart Disease Resources,[1] although still expressing the opinion that the optimal arrangement is for laboratories to be located in hospitals with cardiovascular surgery, recognizes the feasibility in some cases of establishing laboratories in institutions without cardiac surgical programs. When this is the case, there must be close liaison between the laboratory and a surgical center. Cases must be selected so as to minimize the risk to the patient. High-risk patients and those undergoing procedures which may have surgical complications should be referred directly to a surgical center for catheterization in their laboratory.

The argument for having a catheterization laboratory in a general hospital without a surgical program is obvious. The availability of the laboratory in-house influences the selection of diagnostic studies in patients with suspected cardiac disease. In hospitals remote from cardiac catheterization facilities, practice is commonly toward investigating all noncardiac causes and utilizing all noninvasive procedures prior to selecting cardiac catheterization. This is often not cost-effective and may not be in the best interest of patient safety.

The argument against establishing a cardiovascular laboratory relates to the duplication and cost inefficiency if the caseload will be inadequate to maintain near capacity operation. Adequate caseloads are necessary to maintain the skills of the diagnostic team, to ensure patient safety, and to provide for cost efficiency so that the unit cost of procedures can be maintained at a reasonable level. If the volume in the catheterization laboratory falls below 300 cases per year, there is a sharp increase in the per case cost to the hospital related to amortization of equipment and salary reimbursement.

Providing quality cardiovascular services does not require that a cardiovascular laboratory be physically located in every hospital. There is ample opportunity to share facilities between hospitals which are located in reasonable geographic proximity. This is especially true when there are common hospital staffs as is usually the case in towns of moderate size. In urban areas, interhospital referral is readily available, and it is reasonable that some hospitals develop more sophisticated cardiac services than others. Patient care, however, is affected when there are areas that are totally unserved by cardiac catheterization facilities. Referral patterns vary, but often a situation exists in which a moderate-sized city is remote from an urban area, and therefore if no catheterization facilities exist, patients often undergo extensive evaluation before consideration of catheterization. As mentioned, this is not always in the best interest of patient safety or cost effectiveness. Such modest-sized cities may never have an adequate volume to justify a surgical center; however, if the laboratory director and physician users of the laboratory are well-trained, maintain adequate volume, cultivate a close working relationship with the surgical center, and exercise proper case selection, a high-quality freestanding laboratory can be operated.

In urban areas, it is perfectly reasonable for some hospitals to maintain cardiac catheterization laboratories which have close liaison with a surgical center but to have no cardiac surgery in their own hospitals. This provides for high-level cardiac diagnostic facilities with laboratories operating at near occupancy. At the same time, these hospitals are freed from the problem of operating a low-volume surgical center, allowing these cases to be concentrated into surgical referral centers which can operate at a high volume and maintain the complex, multidisciplined approach to cardiac surgical patients.

There will always be small towns and rural areas which cannot support cardiac catheterization facilities. It should, however, be the responsibility of physicians in those areas to become acquainted with the availability and proper indications for utilization of cardiac catheterization facilities so that effective referral relationship can be established.

STAFFING OF THE CARDIOVASCULAR LABORATORY

Laboratory Director

Although hospitals will have many different arrangements for the operation of the cardiac laboratory, it is essential that one individual be named the director and that he or she should have the overall responsibility for the direction of the laboratory, planning the annual budget and playing a major part in recommendations concerning the selection of equipment, supplies, and personnel within the laboratory. The training of the laboratory director should include cardiology, cardiovascular radiology, and radiation safety. Most laboratory directors will be cardiologists, and this is certainly the most appropriate avenue from which to enter this particular position. The cardiologist should be board-certified and complete an extensive training program in cardiology which includes at least 1 year working in a cardiac catheterization laboratory under supervision and performing a large number of cases. In addition, the director should have experience and training in the aspects of cardiovascular radiology applicable to the laboratory and should have become knowledgeable about the needs for radiation safety for the personnel in the lab. If possible, the director should also have experience working in a laboratory following the normal training.

If the director is a cardiovascular radiologist, he or she should be board-certified in radiology with subspecialty training in cardiac radiology but should also be thoroughly trained in all aspects of clinical cardiology which relate to patients seen in the cardiovascular laboratory. Although a program of this type is not standardized, it would seem reasonable that the radiologist should have a training period of 1 year or its equivalent in the basic disciplines of clinical cardiology in order to direct a cardiovascular laboratory.

If the laboratory is designed specifically for pediatric cases, then it should be directed by a pediatric cardiologist board-certified both in pediatrics and in pediatric cardiology. Regardless of who the laboratory director is, he or she should have a close working relationship with the departments of cardiology, radiology, cardiovascular surgery, and, if pediatric patients are addressed, pediatric cardiology within the hospital.

Physicians

Physicians performing coronary arteriography should be cardiologists who have completed a thorough training program with extensive experience in cardiac catheterization. Some training programs have a duration of 2 years, while others insist on a third year of catheterization training. In our institution, we require 12 full months of work in the cardiac catheterization laboratory in addition to the 2-year clinical cardiology program. The physician should be certified by the training center as competent to perform all procedures independently. It is not adequate to know just the technical aspects of cardiac catheterization and coronary arteriography. The physician performing the procedures is thought of as a consultant to the noninvasive cardiologist, the general internist, general practitioners, and surgeons who refer the patients. This physician must integrate the catheterization findings with the history and other noninvasive investigations in order to make proper recommendations to the referring physicians and the surgeons. This responsibility requires a high volume of cases, both during the training period and in practice, in order to maintain the technical skills needed as well as the broad experience required to make proper recommendations.

Support Personnel

There are four support functions within the laboratory which must be adequately staffed. The necessary skills will be supplied by

1 A nurse capable of assisting the physician in all aspects of care of the cardiovascular patient to include routine care as well as care in case of cardiovascular emergencies.

2 A scrub nurse, needed for assistance at the x-ray table to provide the operating physician with all the equipment and supplies needed to carry out the examination as well as to assist in the exchanging of catheters, etc.

3 A radiological technologist. The technologist should be completely trained in x-ray principles, especially as they relate to cardiovascular procedures and cineangiography and fluoroscopy. The technologist should also have complete knowledge of use of power injectors and proper use of x-ray generators, cine pulse systems, image intensifiers, and film processing equipment.

4 A monitoring and recording technician. One individual is responsible for monitoring the electrocardiogram and the pressures during catheterization and keeping the physician apprised of changes. This individual should be thoroughly trained in recognition of arrhythmias and appropriate interpretation of wave forms as well as in operation of all physiological recording equipment.

Every case of coronary arteriography does not require all of these people to be present. In our laboratories, we find that three assistants are required for each catheterization procedure. One person is scrubbed and assists the physician at the table. One is not scrubbed and circulates in the room providing patient care and procuring any supplies that are needed during the procedure, and one person performs the duties of recording technician and radiological technologist by selecting proper cineangiographic programs, field sizes, etc., as required.

Staffing for our laboratory, however, requires four assistants per room because of all day operations and the need for replacement personnel so that all three of these jobs may always be staffed. Cross-training of the individuals in the laboratory is helpful in maintaining the morale and competence in each job described. Cross-training also means that each individual in the laboratory will be competent to start up the laboratory and assist in operations on an emergency 24-hour basis when needed.

All members of the catheterization team should be fully trained in cardiopulmonary resuscitation and the use of the defibrillators. Additional personnel who process film, prepare catheter trays, and maintain equipment are of course essential to the efficient operation of a busy laboratory.

RADIOLOGICAL IMAGING

Radiological images are used to visualize the internal structure and function of the human body. The images are produced when a portion of the x-ray beam passes through the body and casts an invisible image on the input screen of the image intensifier tube. The intensifier tube converts the x-ray image into a light image which is either viewed through a closed-circuit videosystem during fluoroscopy or recorded on film as part of a cineradiographic procedure. The objective in cardiac imaging is to produce an image of adequate quality to provide all the information needed for diagnosis and interventional procedures. All radiological imaging systems do not produce the same degree of visibility or image quality. There are three primary factors which affect radiological image quality as it relates to cardiac anatomy and function. These factors are (1) contrast, (2) blur (unsharpness), and (3) image noise. These three factors are in turn affected by the design and condition of the imaging system and the manner in which it is operated.

The objective of this section is to review the components and operation of a typical radiological imaging system for cardiac applications and to give special attention to the factors which influence overall image quality and visibility.

Contrast

Image contrast is the variation in the shades of gray (image brightness) which correlates with anatomic structure. An object, such as a coronary artery, must produce a certain level of image contrast relative to its background in order to be visible. The level of contrast in an image is determined by the following factors:

X-ray Penetration No small anatomic object, such as a vessel filled with contrast medium, is completely radiopaque. The radiation which penetrates such an object reduces its contrast and perhaps its visibility within the image. The amount of x-ray penetration and contrast loss depends on the object size, the concentration of contrast medium, and the penetrating characteristics of the x-ray beam. The amount by which iodine contrast medium attenuates the x-ray beam and produces contrast is significantly affected by the energy of the individual x-ray photons as shown in Fig. 14-1. Maximum image contrast is produced with photon energies of approximately 35 keV. As the x-ray photon energies increase above this value, penetration increases and contrast is reduced. The penetrating ability of the x-ray beam can be controlled to some extent through the kilovoltage (kV). Image contrast can be enhanced by maintaining low kV values.

Scatter Radiation When the x-ray beam interacts with the patient's body, it produces a significant amount of scatter radiation, some of which exposes the image receptor. This unwanted exposure reduces the contrast content of the image.

Exposure Level In cardiac imaging, the contrast and visibility of vessels is sometimes seriously

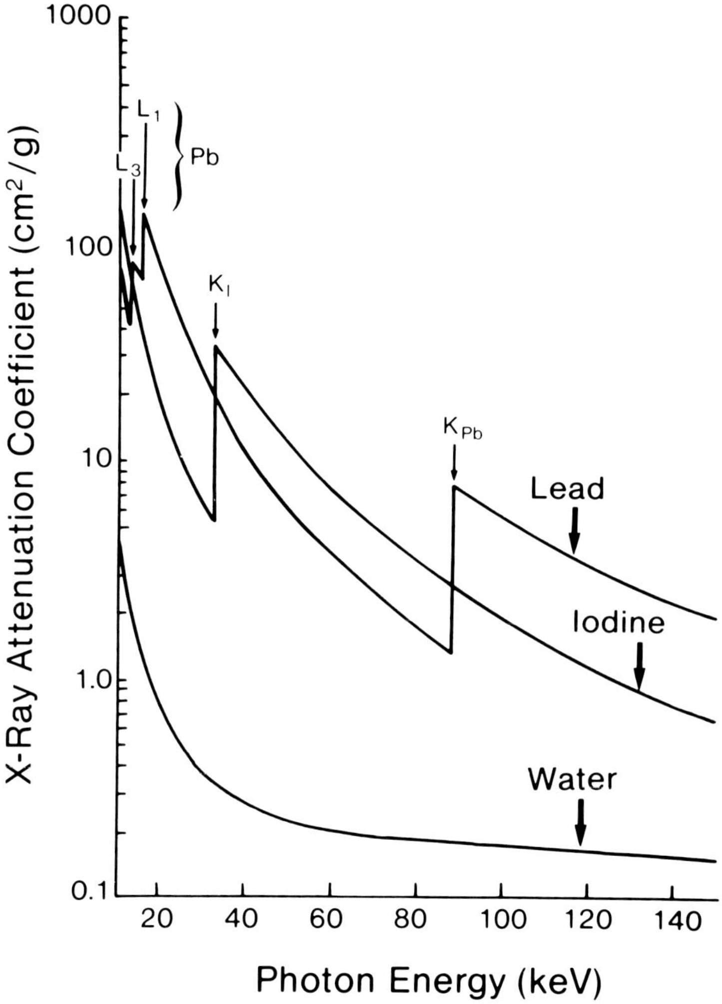

Figure 14-1 These curves describe x-ray attenuation as a function of x-ray photon energy in electronvolts for water, iodine (I), and lead (Pb). The higher the attenuation, the greater the image contrast. Notice iodine has greater attenuation than lead from 30 keV to approximately 90 keV.

reduced when the immediate image area surrounding the vessel is either under- or overexposed. An underexposed area has a washed-out appearance with very little image contrast. Overexposed areas are often too dark to see through under normal viewing conditions. In cardiac imaging, this is an especially significant problem because the variation in body density from the mediastinum to the lung area produces a variation in image exposure over which the arterial images are superimposed.

Receptor Contrast Characteristics Several components which make up the image receptor system have characteristics which may limit image contrast. These components include the image intensifier tube, the film, and the video system.

Blur (Unsharpness)

All imaging systems introduce some blur or unsharpness into the final image. The overall effect of the blur is to reduce the contrast and visibility of small objects and to give other structures a general unsharp appearance. The amount of blur is generally the limiting factor to the visibility of detail within an image. In a radiological imaging system, there are three principal sources of image blur.

Motion Movement of the anatomy is an obvious cause of image blur but is not a major problem in cardiac imaging because of the short exposure times normally employed.

Focal Spot Size A much more significant factor is the size of the x-ray source (focal spot) in the x-ray tube. The formation of a sharp image requires a small focal spot. Unfortunately, there are practical limits on focal spot size in cardiac imaging.

Receptor Characteristics Several of the components within the receptor system add blur to the image. These include the image intensifier tube, the optical system, and the video chain.

Noise

The textured or mottled appearance of radiological images is a form of image noise. The presence of noise reduces the visibility of low-contrast objects. The most significant source of noise in cardiac images is the random distribution of the x-ray photons which form the image. Image noise from this source is known as *quantum noise* or *quantum mottle*. The amount of noise in an image is inversely related to the quantity of radiation (exposure) used to form the image. The sensitivity and operating level of the cardiac imaging system is adjusted to give a compromise between image noise and patient exposure.

RADIOLOGICAL IMAGING SYSTEMS

The typical imaging system for cinefluorography contains a number of major components as shown in Fig. 14-2. The selection of these components and their integration into a fully optimized system is a significant factor in obtaining high-quality images.

Figure 14-2 Diagram of complete imaging system for cinefluorography.

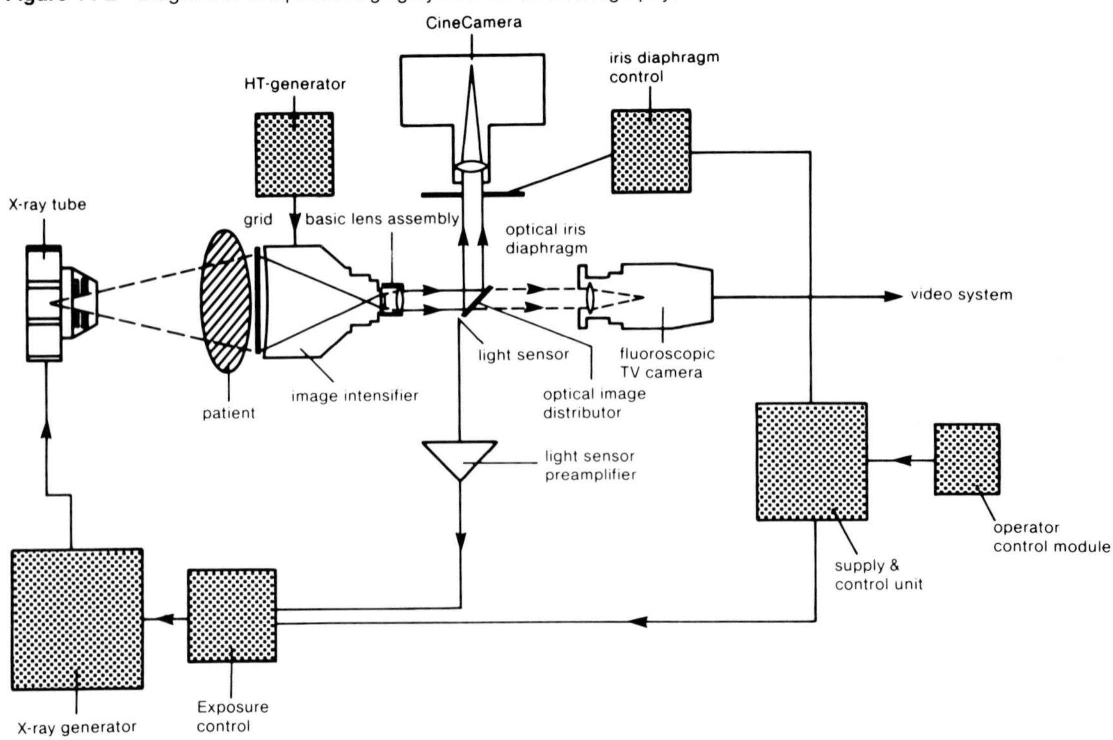

The characteristics of the various components which impact on image quality and system operation will now be considered.

X-ray Generators

X-ray generators are the ultimate power source for the production of roentgen rays. Modern systems for angiocardiography are equipped with 12 pulse or constant potential generators specifically designed for cine applications. Cine generators are pulsed by secondary switching vacuum tubes or the x-ray tube itself. There must be automatic exposure controls for cine recording and fluoroscopy. Light is measured from the image intensifier by a photo multiplier for control of cine recording. Fluoroscopic levels are controlled by the same photo multiplier or by the video signal from the television system.

X-ray Tube

The function of an x-ray tube is to convert electrical energy into a beam of x-ray energy. Unfortunately, they are rather inefficient as energy converters. Most of the input energy to the x-ray tubes is converted into heat. Less than 0.2 percent of this electrical energy is actually converted into image-producing x-ray photons.

The characteristic of an x-ray tube which has the greatest impact on image quality is the focal spot size. Small focal spots are needed to reduce image blurring. On the other hand, the focal spots must be large enough to accommodate the heat produced during the x-ray production process.

X-ray tubes contain rhenium molybdenum or rhenium tungsten anodes with graphite heat sinks. X-ray tube anodes are supported by a single or dual bearing structure capable of nearly 10,000 revolutions per minute (Fig. 14-3). Modern x-ray tubes

Figure 14-3 Drawing of all-metal x-ray tube insert without housing. The principle: rotating anode with dual bearing support (A) inside an all-metal insert (B) with ceramic inserts (C). D = filament.

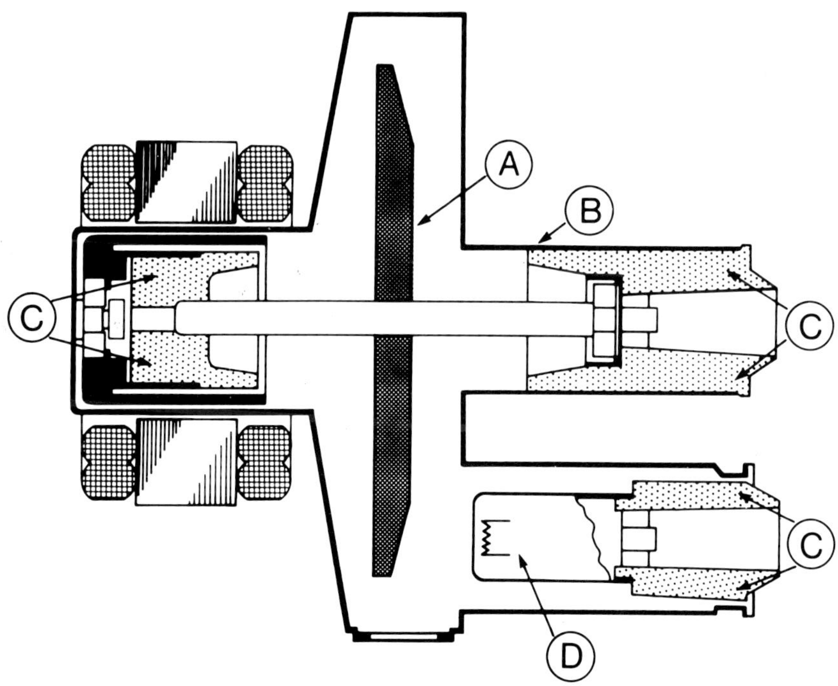

for coronary arteriography are constructed of all glass, glass-metal, or all metal composition. All metal construction has advantages over glass or glass-metal due to its possible higher vacuum, greater x-ray photon production efficiency, and less off focal radiation. Greater x-ray photon production efficiency is possible with all metal construction because of the higher vacuum within the insert, and the distance between the filament and rotating anode is reduced. The electron beam between filament and anode is more concentrated, giving greater x-ray photon yield. Focal spots range from 0.2 to 1.2 mm. Anode angles vary from 7° to 12°. The angles should be no greater than necessary to cover the largest image intensifier field. A small anode angle gives the best possible relationship between heat capacity and image quality.

The heat capacity of an x-ray tube target is determined by the melting point of the target material in the focal track, which is approximately 2500°C. As the focal spots or tracks become smaller, this temperature limit is reached at a lower energy input level. Focal spot sizes should be as small as possible for fluoroscopy and cine operation in order to produce sharp images and still have sufficient heat capacity to minimize times between cine runs. Fluoroscopic focal spots should be less than 0.6 mm and have a continuous heat dissipation rate of at least 750 watts. Cine focal spots should have the ability to operate at a minimum of 50 kilowatts with an anode loadability of at least 400,000 heat units. The instantaneous loading of the x-ray tube focal spot area is usually less for coronary arteriography than for other radiographic applications. However, with long fluoroscopic times and several cine runs, total anode capacity and tube housing capacity are major concerns. External oil cooling with some type of heat exchanger is preferable to only air cooling of the x-ray tube housing. Failures of coronary arteriography x-ray tubes are almost always caused by excessive temperatures of the anode causing a gas to form within the vacuum of the tube. If gassing has occurred, an x-ray tube replacement is usually necessary.

The size of the x-ray beam is determined by the collimator attached to the x-ray tube. Collimation of the x-ray beam should be automatic to the image field sizes of the image intensifiers. These collimators should have multiple leaves with some type of near focus shutters to reduce scatter radiation to a minimum. Semitransparent radiation filters which attenuate the lung field and are electrically operated

Figure 14-4 Principle of grid operation: A = x-ray photon source; B = grid; C = scatter radiation; D = primary radiation; and E = patient. Scatter radiation is reduced by grid in front of image intensifier.

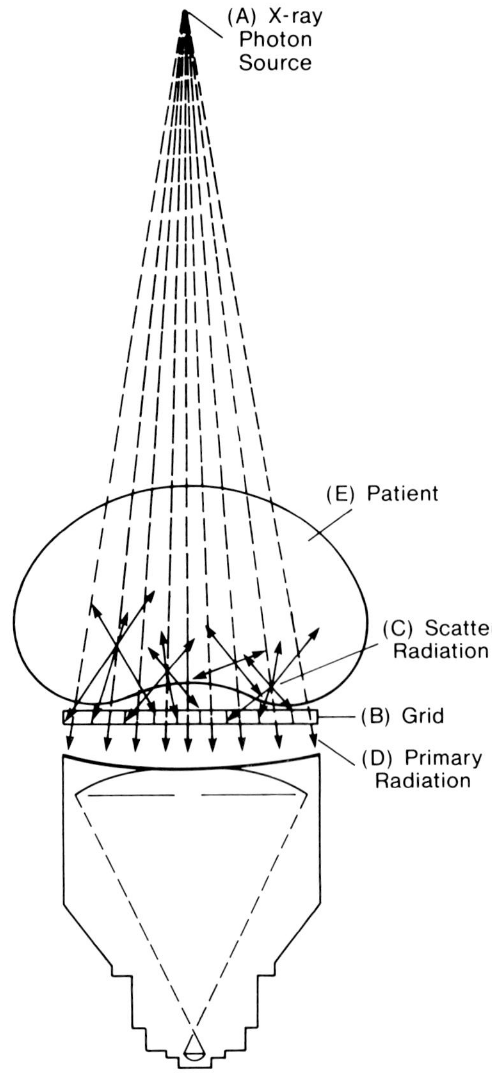

through 360° by the physician or laboratory technician can improve image quality. These filters correct the very annoying problem of lung field blooming which causes video overload of the television monitors and video recording devices.

Grid

X-ray grids are used in cinefluorography to reduce the scattered radiation reaching the image intensifier, as shown in Fig. 14-4. Scattered radiation will reduce contrast and visibility in the image. There is a trade off between a grid's ability to reduce scatter and the absorption of the primary x-ray beam. X-ray grids for cinefluorography must be designed for minimum primary x-ray photon absorption to prevent high KVP values which will reduce contrast. Carbon grids with ratios of 8:1 at 110 lines per inch fulfill the requirements of both low primary absorption and high scatter radiation attenuation.

Image Intensifier Tube

Image intensifiers are high-vacuum devices constructed of glass and metal (Fig. 14-5). These devices convert x-ray photons into the visible angiographic image and are therefore one of the most important components in the imaging chain.

As the image passes through the image intensifier tube, there is the possibility of some loss of contrast and some additional image blurring. The loss of contrast results from light scattering within the tube. Recent advances in tube design have minimized the contrast loss and significantly improved the quality of the images.

A major source of blur within the image intensifier tube is the finite thickness of the phosphor screens. A thin phosphor minimizes blur but can also have the disadvantage of low x-ray absorption and overall tube efficiency. Figure 14-6 compares the modulation transfer function (MTF) curve for three different phosphor thicknesses.

It is possible for the electron focus within the

Figure 14-5 Drawing of an image intensifier, where A = x-ray photon input window, B = cesium iodide surface where x-ray photons are converted to electrons, C = output window where angiographic image is formed.

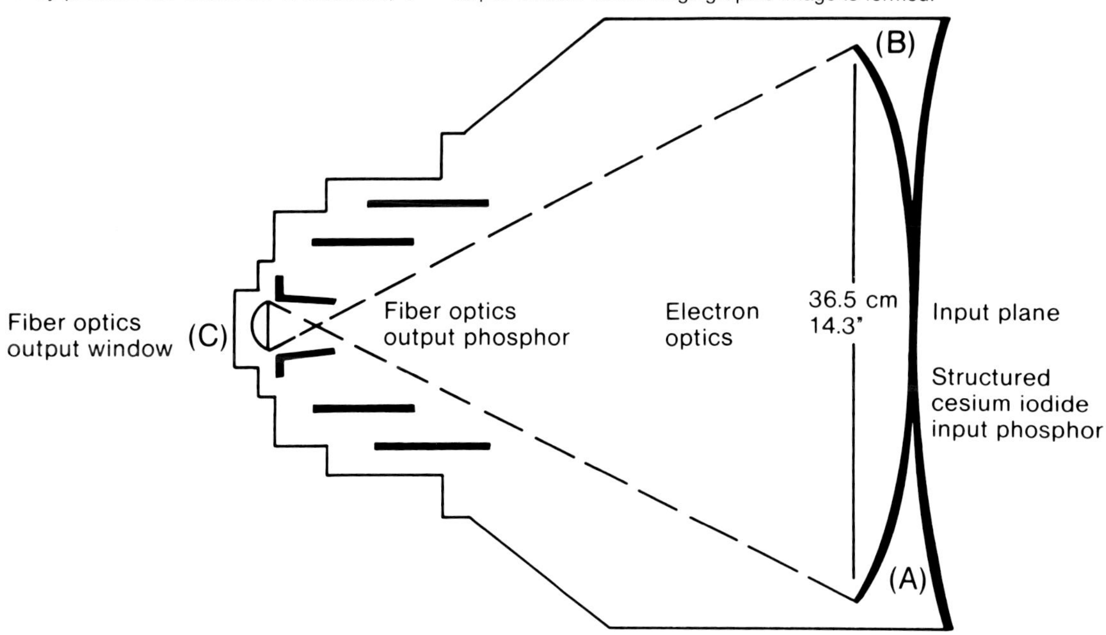

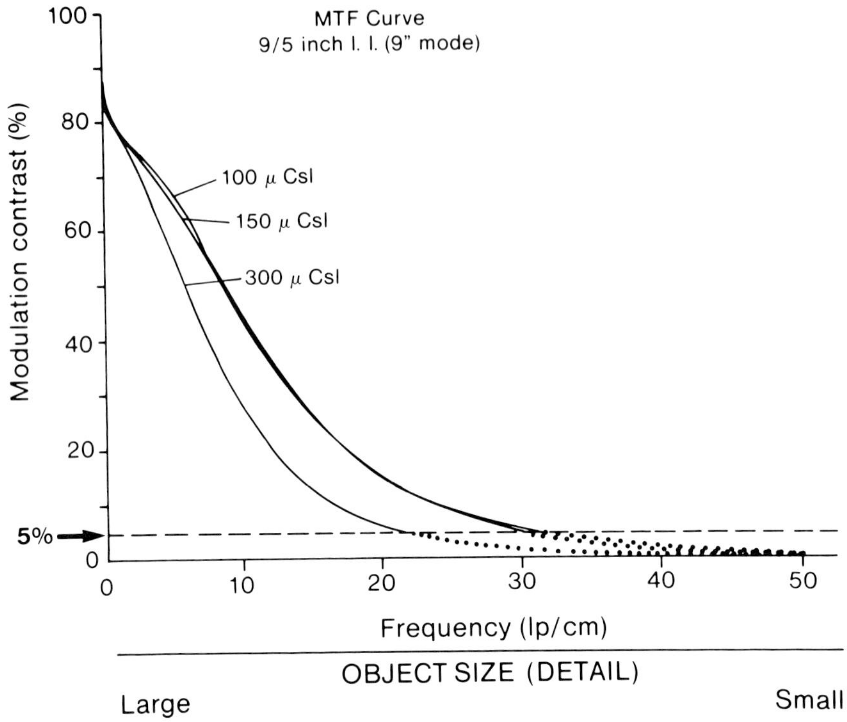

Figure 14-6 Modulation transfer function curves.

tube to become misadjusted and introduce additional image blur. Image intensifier input field sizes range from 4 to 14 inches. The efficiency of the image intensifier in converting x-ray photons to light images is critical for keeping the KVP as low as possible. The input window and input cesium iodide phosphor thickness should be designed for maximum efficiency with acceptable image sharpness.

Optical System

An optical system consisting of several lenses and an image distributor transfers the image from the output of the image intensifier to the appropriate cameras. These are typically a fluoroscopic television camera and a cine camera.

Magnification of the cine image is controlled by the focal length of the cine camera lens. Increased overframing is achieved by increasing the focal length. An 82-mm lens may give optimal framing of the image so that the lateral edges of the image intensifier image correspond to the lateral edges of the cine frame (maximum horizontal overframing). A 100-mm lens will produce more magnification but only 5½ × 7 inches of a 9-inch mode of the image intensifier would be seen on film. That degree of overframing is usually unnecessary with multiple mode intensifiers.

Video System

The very highest possible video image quality is required for modern coronary arteriography. Due to new interventional techniques, video systems require state-of-the-art technology. During the last few years, there has been increasing interest in high-resolution (low-blur) television systems. Recent advances in video signal processing techniques and the digitization of these signals have brought the picture quality near to that of traditional film systems.

Video images consist of a series of horizontal lines. The width of the individual lines is a major factor in image quality. Small objects within the image are blurred by the width of the line. Maximum visibility of detail is obtained by reducing line width. This can be achieved both by reducing the image size at the input to the image intensifier and increasing the number of lines in the image. The more conventional video systems use 525 lines to form an image, but systems are now available which use 1023 to 1049 lines for increased image detail.

The amount of noise (mottle) in a fluoroscopic image is determined primarily by the exposure level at the input to the image intensifier. In most systems, this can be adjusted to arrive at an appropriate compromise between image quality (noise) and patient exposure.

The bandwidth of the video system is a factor which affects both the blurring and the noise content of the images. Increasing bandwidth reduces blurring but also increases the visible noise. It should be adjusted for an appropriate compromise between these two factors.

Major components of video systems used in coronary arteriography are the television camera, camera control, video display monitors, and video recording equipment. Fluoroscopic television image quality (noise) is directly influenced by the fluoroscopic dose rates, television bandwidths, and the television scanning line rate. Multiple fluoroscopic dose rate selection should be part of the cinefluorographic equipment if interventional techniques are contemplated. A minimum of 50 μR/s measured at the image intensifier input up to several hundred μR/s for critical phases of interventional techniques is required. However, exceeding the Department of Health, Education, and Welfare fluoroscopic dose rate of 10 R/min at the tabletop will require that an audible signal from the x-ray generator be given or a continuous video recording be made during high-dose fluoroscopy.

Conventional 525-line television line rates are less suited for new interventional techniques due to objectionable television raster lines seen at close viewing distances (Fig. 14-7). If 525 systems are used, a method of optical or electrical magnification to a field size smaller than 4 inches is desirable. High-line 1049- or 1023-line television systems will eliminate seeing raster lines at close viewing distances. However, these television systems require special recording and display systems.

Camera tubes which are large-area, diode gun plumbicons have been developed especially for high-

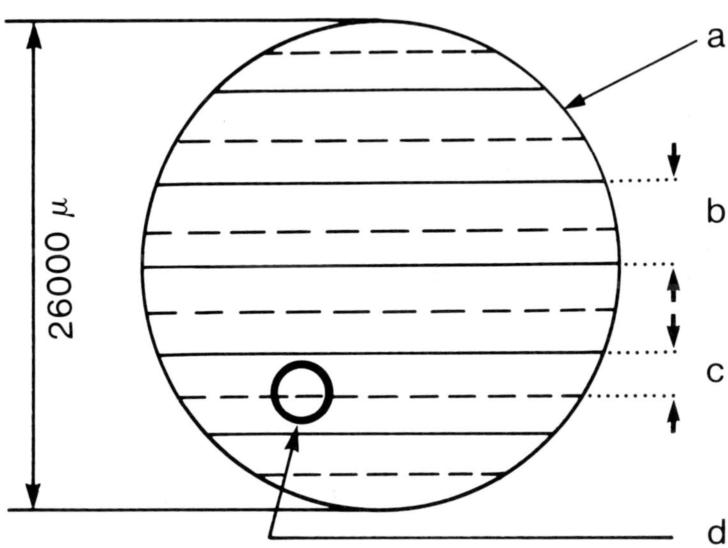

Figure 14-7 a = scanning area of a 2-inch camera tube, diameter = 26 mm, or 26,000 μ; b = distance between lines for 525 lines: 26,000/525 = 49.52 μ; c = distance between lines for 1049 lines: 26,000/1049 = 24.79 μ; d = diameter of scanning beam: approximately 16 μ.

resolution television systems. Lead oxide plumbicons have two important advantages in cardiac imaging: low lag and very fast signal buildup.

For standard angiographic labs, 525-line video recorders are satisfactory. For interventional procedures, however, video recording equipment should be designed to operate at high television line rates. These machines must operate at real time rates, store a large number of cases, and produce perfect stop frame or slow motion in either forward or reverse tape directions. Broadcast-type C-helical teleproduction videotape recorders fulfill these requirements. In addition to the videotape machine, a field or frame memory device is helpful for guiding information during interventional techniques.

Video display monitors are the final component in the video imaging system. Newly developed p-45 picture tube phosphors produce some very beneficial quantum noise integration. These phosphors also have an increased dynamic range of video levels. A minimum of 3 line pairs per millimeter resolution as seen on the display monitors on the maximum magnification mode of the image intensifier at 1:1 magnification is necessary for optimum television viewing for new interventional techniques.

Cine Film

The quality of the angiographic image transferred from the image intensifier to the cine film involves a number of variables. How the cine film variables affect cine film image quality is well-understood. Cine film is manufactured for specific film speeds and contrast gradients. Very fast cine film tends to be noisy. Modern image intensifiers generate adequate light levels so very fast cine films are not needed. Film speeds of 100 ASA and below are adequate for modern image intensifiers. Cine film contrast is determined by cine film type and processing variables. Characteristic curves are published by cine film manufacturers which describe average gradient, gamma, gross fog (defined below), and relative speed of films for cinefluorography.

Average gradient for cine film is the slope of line connecting 0.15 and 1.50 density values above base fog (Fig. 14-8). *Film gamma* is the slope of the straight-line portion of these characteristic curves. *Base fog* is the measured base density plus emulsion fog values. *Relative speed* is the speed measured at a density of 0.85 above gross fog. Cine film is manufactured for a range of contrast ranges from very high contrast to low-contrast films. Very high contrast films have a limited gray scale recording ability and thus some information could be lost in the angiographic image using very high contrast film. The characteristic curves given in Fig. 14-8 describe contrast ranges for five cine film types. Film CFH is the highest contrast film with the lowest or shortest gray scale. Film CFR is the lowest contrast with a longer gray scale. Also the processing variables of temperature, development time, and chemistry agitation are much more critical for the high-contrast films due to their limited latitude. Latitude of cine films is directly related to contrast ranges. In Fig. 14-8, film CFH would have a more limited latitude than film CFR.

Several film processors are capable of providing adequate conditions for processing. Examples are Jamieson, Combilabor, Houston Fearless, and Paco. If a large number of cases are to be processed daily, then processors which can handle these volumes should be chosen.

The commonly used Tagarno type of projectors are most convenient in rapid film handling and viewing. These projectors do not stop the film, and therefore some flicker is inevitable. Projectors which utilize still frame viewing give superior images but are more difficult to operate. The latter type of projectors usually have a greater light intensity which is an advantage when viewing low-contrast film or film with inherent base fog. Cine film viewing and analysis poses specific requirements for cine film projectors. These projectors must have variable frame rates with instantaneous forward and reverse film directions. Cine film projector focus should remain constant from single frame projection to maximum frame rates. The film transport mechanism should be designed to produce a flicker-free image. Op-

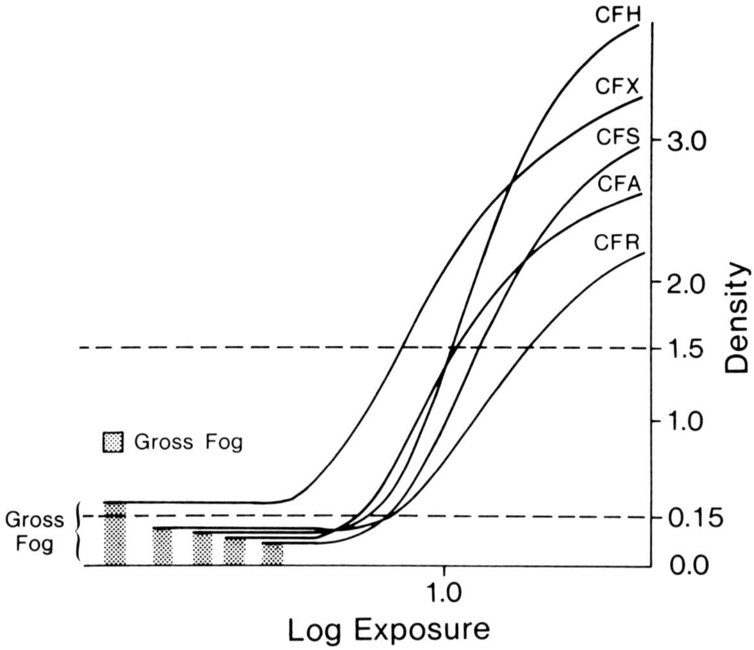

Figure 14-8 Characteristic curves for five different cine film types.

tical design and screen brightness without any degradation of the cine film sharpness.

RADIATION SAFETY

Introduction and Overview

The use of x-radiation carries with it some potential risk both to the patient and to the personnel conducting the procedure. A thorough understanding of the general characteristics of x-radiation, the potential biological effects, exposure levels and limits, and methods of personnel protection are helpful in minimizing this risk.

The objective of this section is to develop concepts and an understanding of x-radiation as it is used in cardiovascular procedures so that the professionals in the field can evaluate their particular environments and make decisions which will hopefully minimize the risk.

X-radiation is an invisible flow of energy which, when used appropriately, can make the hidden internal structures of the human body visible for diagnostic and therapeutic purposes. Because it is invisible, human nature might cause us to either ignore it or fear it to an extent not consistent with its real potential to produce biological damage.

Characteristics

X-radiation is created by electron interactions in the x-ray tube. Shutters or collimating devices shape the radiation into a well-defined beam as illustrated in Fig. 14-9.

The overall intensity (exposure rate) of the beam is determined by the technical factors, kilovoltage (kV) and milliamperage (mA), and the distance from the x-ray tube. The intensity is proportional to the mA value and increases even more rapidly with an increase in kV. In addition to increasing intensity, an increase in kV increases the penetrating ability of the beam. For a specific procedure, a pair of kV and mA values is selected which will produce adequate fluoroscopic image brightness or film exposure. The total radiation exposure

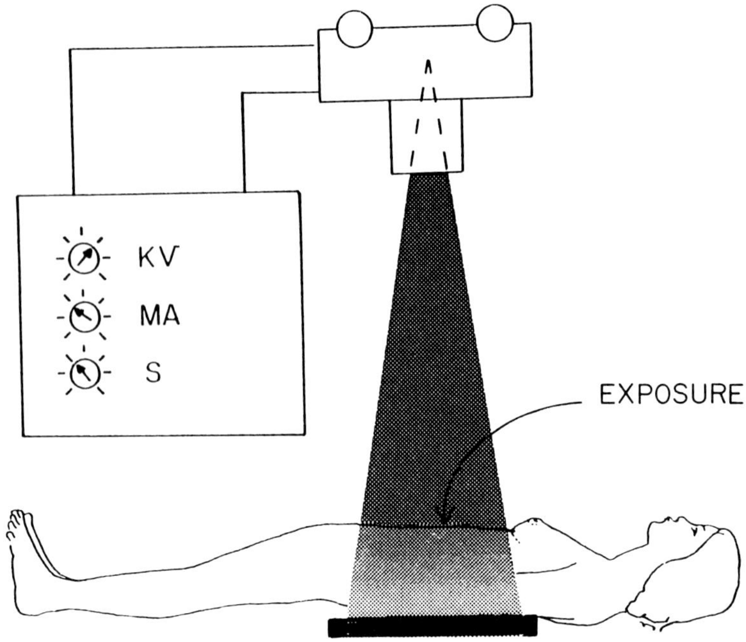

Figure 14-9 Collimated x-ray beam passing through body.

accumulated by a patient then depends on the duration.

Quantities and Units

Any consideration of radiation safety must take a quantitative approach. In most instances, the potential biological effects of radiation are related to the quantity of radiation energy absorbed by tissue. Also, most actions taken to reduce the potential hazard are only partially effective and must be evaluated in a quantitative manner.

In considering the quantity of radiation delivered to a human body, a clear distinction must be made between the total amount of radiation energy delivered to and absorbed by the body and the concentration of radiation to specific locations. The relationship between total radiation energy and concentration is determined by the amount of tissue exposed.

Although x-radiation is pure energy, it is generally not quantified in conventional energy units. The primary reason is that it is difficult to measure the precise energy content of an x-ray beam. On the other hand, it is quite easy to measure the amount of ionization produced by the radiation and use that as a quantifier. The radiation quantity, exposure, is proportional to the amount of ionization produced by radiation.

The quantification of x-radiation appears somewhat complex and confusing and requires an understanding of the difference between (1) total radiation and radiation concentration, (2) the different concentration quantities, i.e., exposure, absorbed dose, and dose equivalent, and (3) the use of conventional and contemporary SI units.

The concentration of x-radiation delivered to a specific point by an x-ray beam is properly referred to as *exposure*. The traditional unit of exposure is the roentgen (R) and the SI unit of exposure is the coulomb per kilogram (C/kg). In this section, all exposure values will be expressed in the units of roentgens or milliroentgens (mR). An exposure in roentgens can be converted to C/kg by multiplying by 2.58×10^{-4}.

Absorbed dose is the quantity of radiation energy deposited in a unit mass of tissue. The traditional unit for dose is the rad, and the SI unit is the gray, which is equivalent to 100 rad. When soft tissue is exposed to 1 roentgen, the absorbed dose will be very close to 1 rad. In bone, an exposure of 1 roentgen will generally produce an absorbed dose of 3 to 4 rad, depending on the characteristics of the radiation.

Another quantity, *dose equivalent*, is often used to express the biological impact of a specific exposure. The traditional unit for dose equivalent is the rem, and the SI unit is the sievert: 1 sievert is equivalent to 100 rem. For x-radiation, a dose of 1 rad will produce a dose equivalent of 1 rem.

The total radiation delivered to the body is essentially the product of the appropriate concentration quantity (exposure, dose, dose equivalent) and the amount of tissue receiving the radiation. The point which should be emphasized is that when assessing the radiation impact to a human body, we must not only know the concentration, i.e., exposure, but also the amount and location of the tissue receiving the radiation.

Interactions

An x-ray beam is essentially a shower of small individual units of radiation energy photons. As each photon encounters an object such as the human body, there is a possibility of three things happening:

1 Absorption. One possibility is that the photon will interact with and be absorbed by the body. In the absorption process, the energy of the photon is deposited in the body and contributes to the absorbed dose. As individual photons are absorbed from the beam, the intensity is reduced. During an x-ray procedure, at least 90 percent of the x-ray energy entering a body is absorbed.

2 Penetration. One of the significant characteristics of x-radiation is its ability to penetrate objects. In most instances, some of the photos are not absorbed and pass through or penetrate the object. The fraction of radiation which penetrates a specific object depends on characteristics of both the object and the x-ray beam. Certain materials are better x-ray absorbers and thus allow less penetration than other materials. Penetration generally decreases with increased material atomic number, density, and thickness. Lead, which has both a relatively high atomic number and density compared to most materials, is useful as a shielding material. Penetration through an object (material) decreases exponentially with increased object thickness. In theory, there is no object thickness which will completely eliminate penetration. The usual objective in radiation shielding is to use a thickness which reduces penetration to an acceptable level.

3 Scatter. The third possible fate of photons entering an object is that they will be deflected or scattered. This type of interaction is especially significant in relatively low atomic number materials such as soft tissue. The significance of this interaction is that the patient's body becomes a secondary source of radiation which exposes personnel and degrades image quality. In an x-ray procedure, only the portion of the patient's body which is within the primary x-ray beam becomes the radiation source which can expose personnel in the area.

Biological Effects and Risk

General Considerations When x-radiation is absorbed by the human body, a wide range of biological effects is possible. The specific effect is generally determined by the sensitivity of tissue or organ absorbing the radiation and the quantity of radiation energy actually absorbed. There are additional modifying factors such as the temporal distribution of the radiation exposure and the age of the person exposed.

In the cardiovascular laboratory, both the patient and the personnel conducting the examination are exposed to radiation. There is a difference, however. Typically, the patient is exposed to a relatively high level of radiation which is confined to a small portion of the body and is delivered in a short period of time. On the other hand, the personnel conducting the procedure are exposed to relatively low levels of radiation delivered to a larger area of the body and spread over a period of perhaps many years.

X-radiation has the potential for producing death, radiation sickness, cataracts, mutations, fetal malformations, cancer, and perhaps a general nonspecific reduction in life span. The relationship of specific biological effects to the radiation dose generally takes one of several specific forms. Some effects, such as death, radiation sickness, cataract formation, and the production of fetal malformations, appear to have threshold dose values. Exposures below the threshold value do not produce the effect. Above the threshold value, both the probability of occurrence and the severity of the effect generally increase with increased dose. The effects which appear to have thresholds, with the possible exception of fetal malformations, require exposure levels much greater than those experienced during a cardiovascular procedure. Other effects such as mutations and cancer induction might not have thresholds. For these effects, the primary variable is the probability of occurrence, which tends to increase with increasing radiation exposure. Numerous attempts have been made to develop a quantitative relationship between the risk of cancer induction and the amount of radiation.[2] However, at the present time there is no unified consensus as to the form of this relationship and the actual risk values. Many investigators tend to support a linear relationship between the risk of cancer and radiation dose. With this model, the actual risk is expressed in terms of the number of expected cancers induced by a dose of 1 rad/yr in a population of 1,000,000 persons. Specific values will be discussed later.[3]

The radiation exposure to the body of both the patient and staff personnel is distributed so that some parts of the body receive much greater exposures than other parts. Because of this distribution and the fact that some parts of the body are more sensitive than others, it is helpful to separate the body into three areas. These are (1) head and neck; (2) torso; and (3) limbs.

Head and Neck The major concern with radiation exposure to the head and neck is the possible induction of cataracts and thyroid cancer.

Cataracts Radiation-induced lens opacification has been observed in survivors of nuclear bomb explosions and patients undergoing radiation therapy. Cataract formation has occurred in humans after a single exposure of 200 R. When the exposure is fractionated over a period of months, it appears that the catarogenic threshold is in the range of 500 to 1000 R. It has been suggested that a cumulative lens dose of 1500 rad is below the threshold for the production of cataracts that would interfere with vision.

Thyroid Cancer The ability of radiation to produce thyroid neoplasms has been demonstrated in several populations. These include persons undergoing a variety of therapeutic radiation procedures, atomic bomb survivors at Hiroshima and Nagasaki, and persons exposed to nuclear fallout. The sensitivity of the thyroid to cancer induction is relatively high, but fortunately the induced malignancies are generally not lethal. There appears to be a latent period of at least 10 years, with the maximum incidence of cancer occurring about 20 years after exposure. Females appear to be more sensitive than males. The risk for radiation-induced cancers of the thyroid appears to be 20 to 150 carcinomas per 10^6 person-years per rad.

Torso Exposure to the torso has the potential of producing a variety of carcinomas, mutations, and fetal malformations (if the exposure occurs during pregnancy).

Cancer Cancer induction is perhaps the most serious effect resulting from radiation exposure during diagnostic x-ray examination. The cancers produced by radiation are not distinguishable from those produced by natural causes. While most human tissue is subject to cancer induction by radiation, there is a considerable variation in the sensitivity. In general, it appears that the probability of cancer occurrence increases with the radiation exposure. The elapsed time between the appearance of a carcinoma and the radiation exposure is generally quite long, 10 to more than 30 years. Within the torso, radiation-induced carcinomas can occur in the lungs and digestive organs. The female breast is especially sensitive to cancer induction. The risks (cancers per rad per 10^6 person-years) relative to torso exposure are as follows: (1) breast cancer, 30 to 200 cases; (2) lung cancer, 20 to 100 cases.

The ability of radiation to increase the incidence of leukemia has been demonstrated in several populations, including nuclear bomb survivors and patients undergoing radiotherapy. In general, the onset of leukemia appears within a few years after the radiation exposure and does not have the long latent characteristic of solid tumors. The risk is estimated to be 10 to 60 cases per rad per 10^6 person-years.

Mutations The ability of radiation to produce mutations has been demonstrated in experiments with small animals. The general effect is to increase the rate of naturally occurring mutations. While there is little direct evidence of the mutagenic effects in human beings, it is generally assumed that radiation can produce genetic change. The probability of a genetic change occurring increases with increased level of exposure, with a dose of 50 to 250 rad probably being sufficient to double the normal mutation rate in human beings.

Fetal Malformations Radiation-induced fetal malformations have been observed both in human populations receiving relatively high radiation exposures and in a variety of animal experiments. This does not appear to be a significant concern relative to cardiovascular examinations because of the low incidence of pregnancy among cardiovascular patients. Exposure limit guidelines for members of the staff who are pregnant will be given below.

Limbs The limbs are considered to be relatively insensitive in comparison to the head and trunk of the body.

Exposure Limits

From the biological point of view, the ideal situation is to protect the human body from all radiation exposure. Unfortunately, this is not possible for either the patient or the personnel performing x-ray procedures.

As we now consider permissible exposure limits, we must distinguish between the biological effects which appear to have exposure thresholds and those which can be induced by any level of exposure. Assuming that there is some risk of effects such as mutations and cancer associated with any level of exposure, decisions must be made as to what are acceptable exposure values. The general principle is that the benefit derived from the exposure should outweigh the risk. It is impossible to quantitate either the benefit or the risk for most specific exposure situations. Therefore, we must use professional judgment based on a general knowledge of both the risk (biological effects) and potential benefits from utilizing x-radiation.

Patients There are no established exposure limits for patients undergoing cardiovascular procedures. Even though the radiation exposure is relatively high in comparison to other x-ray procedures, the benefit of the procedure to the patient is also high in most cases.

Personnel For the personnel associated with an x-ray procedure, the radiation exposure becomes an occupational risk. The establishment of permissible exposure levels for occupationally exposed persons has received considerable attention since the introduction of x-radiation.

The National Council on Radiation Protection and Measurements (NCRP) is the organization whose dose limits are generally adopted by most agencies and institutions for guidance in radiation protection practices. The NCRP recommendations for the prospective maximum dose to occupationally exposed persons are as follows:[4]

Head and neck	5 rem/yr
Torso	5 rem/yr
Forearms	30 rem/yr
Hands	75 rem/yr
Fetus	0.5 rem in gestation period

These values do not necessarily represent safe radiation limits but dose levels (risk) which are acceptable for persons who use radiation in their professions and occupations.

Patient Exposure

A patient undergoing an x-ray cardiovascular examination is exposed to a relatively high intensity radiation delivered in a short period of time to a relatively small part of the body. The significance of this exposure is related to the total radiation energy imparted to the body and to the specific tissue which is exposed. The radiation energy deposited during an examination is determined by three primary parameters: (1) x-ray beam intensity, (2) exposed area, and (3) exposure time. A reduction in risk to the patient can, in principle, be affected by reducing any one of the parameters. However, there are limiting factors associated with each parameter.

X-ray Beam Intensity The intensity of the x-ray beam can be adjusted through two x-ray machine parameters, kV and mA. In most imaging systems, one or both of these factors is set by the automatic exposure control (AEC) circuit to compensate for variation in patient thickness and density. It is possible, however, to adjust both the sensitivity of the imaging system and the reference point for the AEC to operate over a wide range of x-ray beam intensities.

The limiting factor with respect to reducing x-ray beam intensity is the presence of noise (quantum mottle) within the image. Most imaging systems in use today could be adjusted to produce adequate film exposure or fluoroscopic image brightness with much lower intensities than are actually used. However, as the beam intensity is decreased, the random distribution of the individual x-ray photons begins to create the textured appearance within the image which is known as the image noise, or quantum mottle. The significance of image noise is that it reduces the visibility of small, low-contrast objects within the image. Since the amount of quantum noise present in an image is inversely related to the x-ray beam intensity, it places a definite limit on reducing patient exposure. The exposure level should be set to give an appropriate balance between image quality and patient (and personnel) exposure.

Typical image intensifier tube input exposure values are

Cine (6-inch mode)	20 μR per frame
Fluoroscopy (6-inch mode)	80 μR/s

The verification of the input exposure to the image intensifier tube and its adjustment to appropriate values is a significant factor in controlling patient radiation exposure.

The actual exposure to the patient's body is proportional to the exposure required by the image intensifier tube. The maximum exposure occurs at the entrance surface on the patient's body. As the x-ray beam passes through the body, it is absorbed and becomes less intense. When the beam exits the body, it is often reduced to close to 1 percent of the entrance exposure level.

Typical entrance exposure values for a patient are

Cine (6-inch mode)	12 mR per frame
Fluoroscopy (6-inch mode)	3 R/min

The specific entrance exposure values for individual patients will vary over a considerable range depending on the thickness and density of the body section being imaged and the penetrating ability of the x-ray beam. However, the values given above can be used in conjunction with the duration of a specific examination to provide an estimate of actual patient exposure.

Exposed Area The significant exposure to the patient's body is confined to the area traversed by the x-ray beam. In the cardiovascular examination, the tissue at risk is usually confined to a relatively small amount of bone marrow. The amount of tissue exposed is, in general, proportional to the size of the imaged area. However, with an image intensifier tube system reducing the field size by changing tube modes does not necessarily reduce the radiation impact to the patient.

The sensitivity of an image intensifier tube is proportional to the input image size. Therefore, switching to a smaller size decreases the tube sensitivity and requires a greater radiation intensity. The total radiation energy entering the patient's body is proportional to the product of the beam area and beam intensity. Since intensity changes to compensate for changing beam area, the product of these two factors does not change appreciably when changing field size.

Exposure Time For a given x-ray beam intensity and image area, the total radiation energy delivered to a patient's body becomes proportional to the duration of the exposure. This is the factor which must be monitored closely in order to prevent unnecessary patient exposure. Cine filming frequency of 30 frames per second is adequate for most diagnostic procedures; therefore higher frame rates should be avoided to minimize exposure.

Personnel Exposure

The exposure to persons conducting a cardiac procedure varies over a considerable range depending on the parameters of the examination. Factors which may vary from one examination to another and also within a single examination will now be considered.

Intensity and Penetrating Characteristics of Primary Beam When all other factors are constant, the intensity of scattered radiation is proportional to the intensity of the primary beam, which is, in turn, determined by the MA and KV values selected for the procedure. The intensity of the radiation is considerably greater during cineradiography than it is during fluoroscopy.

The penetrating ability of scattered radiation is directly related to the penetrating ability of the primary beam. Therefore, if the penetration is increased by increasing KV, the scattered radiation becomes more penetrating, and more of it escapes from the patient's body.

X-ray Beam Area (Field Size) If the x-ray beam intensity remains constant and the area is increased, the amount of scattered radiation produced will increase proportionately. This occurs in a fluoroscopic system which is equipped with shutters for altering the size of the beam. However, when the beam size is changed by switching the intensifier tube mode, the x-ray beam intensity also changes. Decreasing the intensifier tube field size also decreases the sensitivity of the tube. The x-ray tube intensity is then automatically increased in order to provide the same image brightness or film exposure. This results in relatively little variation in the amount of scattered radiation produced.

Distance As x-radiation moves away from its source, it is constantly spreading over a larger area and becomes less intense. When the radiation source is relatively small compared to the distance, the intensity of the radiation is reduced by a factor of 4 each time the distance is doubled (inverse-square law). Because of this, distance can be used as an effective means for reducing exposure.

X-ray Beam Orientation The intensity of scattered radiation is affected by the relationship of its direction to the orientation of the primary beam. Maximum intensity generally occurs in a direction toward the x-ray tube. Most of the scattered radiation is created in the first few centimeters of tissue within the primary beam. More of this scattered radiation escapes back toward the x-ray tube. For other scatter directions, the patient's body provides varying degrees of absorption (shielding) of the scattered radiation.

Since the intensity of scattered radiation is a function of both distance and direction, the distribution around the patient area becomes rather complex. The intensity (exposure rate) distribution is

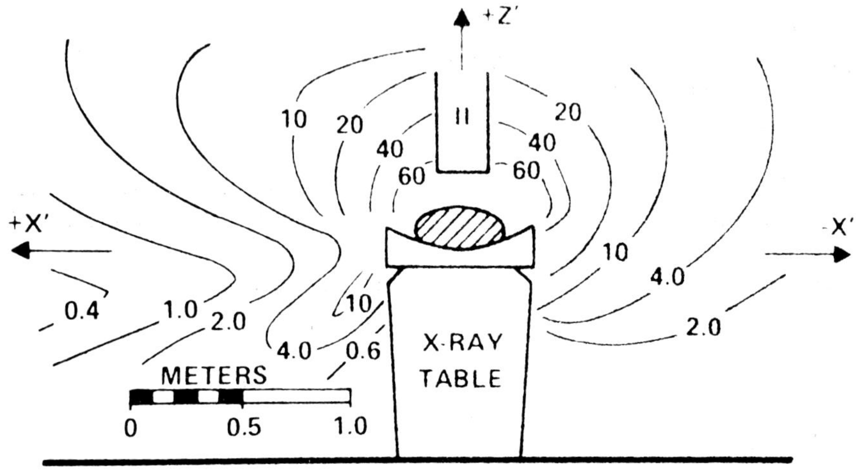

A

Figure 14-10 Scatter radiation pattern around the x-ray table. (*a*) Flat or cradle table. (*b*) U-arm in LAO view. (*c*) U-arm in RAO view. *(Part a from den Boer, Mohr,*[6] *with permission; parts* b *and* c *from Balter, Sones, Brancato,*[6] *with permission.)*

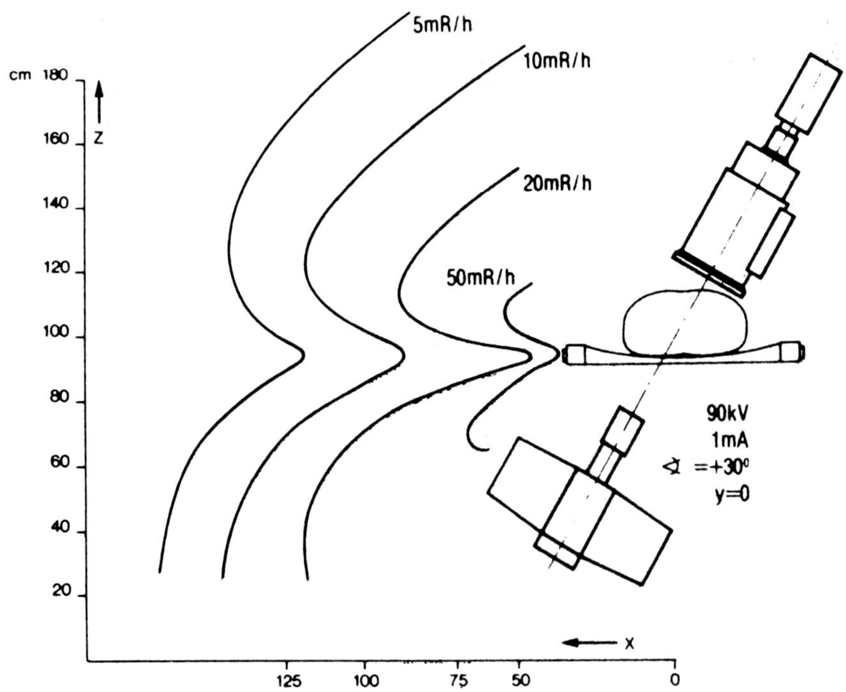

B

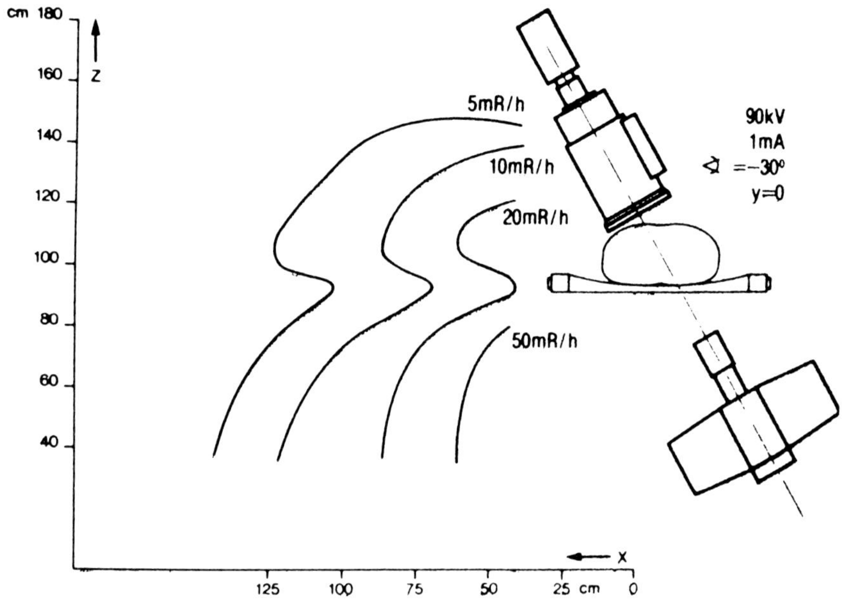

C

often mapped by means of isoexposure curves, as shown in Fig. 14-10.[5,6] Each line passes through the locations which receive the same radiation intensity.

Exposure Duration Perhaps the factor which causes the greatest variation in personnel exposure is time. Fluoroscopic time varies in proportion to the difficulty and complexity of the examination. The total duration of the cineradiography exposure is generally subject to less variation. The exposure to an individual is determined by how long the specific part of that person's body is located in a radiation field of given intensity (exposure rate). However, because of the complexity and the tremendous variation in these factors, it is difficult to give typical exposure values.

A number of investigators have measured the exposure to personnel conducting cardiovascular examinations. The results of several of these studies are summarized in Table 14-1 according to the different parts of the body. The values are the average and range of exposures for individual examinations.

It should be observed that there is a considerable range of exposure reported for a specific part of the body. This reflects the variations among cardiovascular examinations which have an effect on personnel exposure. It is beyond the scope of this chapter to attempt to develop a model or method for predicting the exposure to personnel conducting various examinations. However, it is obvious from the data shown above that without specific radiation protection, personnel can receive significant radiation exposure if they participate in cardiovascular examinations on a regular basis.

The levels of personnel exposure in a given facility can be determined only by a properly conducted radiation safety survey and the use of personnel monitoring devices such as film badges or thermoluminescent dosimeters.

Protection Radiation exposure to a specific body part can be reduced by using an appropriate shield. Lead is one of the most effective shielding materials and is generally incorporated into aprons, gloves, and into glass for transparent shields.

Table 14-1 Exposure to Radiation of Personnel Conducting Cardiovascular Examinations

Eye exposure		
	Exposure, mR	
Investigator	Average	Range
Balter[6]	6	5.6–6.7
Malsky[7]	13	10–26
Wold[8]	26	9.3–42
Rueter[9]	31	21–39
Thyroid exposure		
	Exposure, mR	
Investigator	**Average**	**Range**
Balter[6]	8.3	8.7–13.6
Malsky[7]	41	28–61
Wold[8]	28	19–46
Rueter[9]	27.6	25.8–33.8
Torso exposure		
	Exposure, mR	
Investigator	**Average**	**Range**
Balter[6]	5.8	4.6–7.6
Malsky[7]	560	320–800
Wold[8]	24	8.0–40
Hand and arm exposure		
	Exposure, mR	
Investigator	**Average**	**Range**
Balter[6]	6.5	4.6–10.1
Malsky[7]	143	119–177
Wold[8]	41	3.5–150
Rueter[9]	12.7	4–40

Eyes and Thyroid During procedures where the x-ray tube is superior to the patient's body, the head and neck of personnel close to the patient can receive relatively high exposures. A transparent lead glass shield can be used to reduce the exposure to an acceptable value.

Torso A conventional lead apron generally provides adequate shielding of the torso. It must be recognized, however, that the thickness of lead is not the same in all aprons. An apron with an equivalent thickness of 0.25 mm of lead can be expected to absorb 50 to 70 percent of the incident radiation. Using a heavier apron with an equivalent thickness of 0.5 mm of lead increases the absorption up to 70 to 90 percent.

Total Body Protection The importance of distance from the primary source of the scatter radiation cannot be emphasized enough. Personnel working around the patient should remain as far away as reasonable during fluoroscopy and espe-

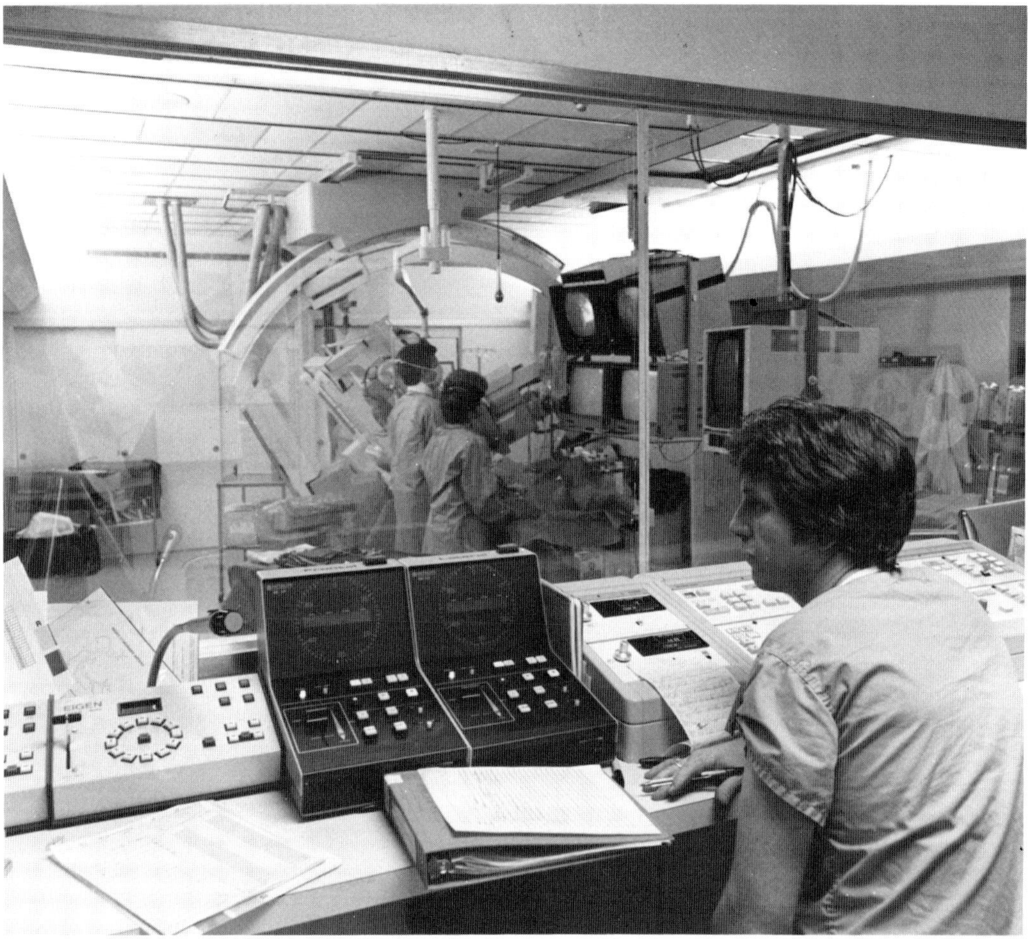

Figure 14-11 Separate control room for recording and x-ray technician and observers.

cially during cine filming. Floor-mounted leaded shields in the procedure room should be used for the circulating nurse. Monitoring technicians and x-ray technicians can perform their jobs in a separate control room with lead glass protection or behind a leaded shield (Fig. 14-11, picture of control room). Rotation of support personnel working in the lab can reduce the radiation exposure to any one individual.

At greatest risk of exposure is the physician operator. The usual protective measures of lead aprons should be supplemented by leaded glasses, thyroid shields, and leaded glass shields (Fig. 14-12). Working from the leg removes the operator from the scatter source somewhat more than working from the arm. Remember that the main source of scatter radiation is the point at which the primary x-ray beam enters the patient's body. Therefore, all left anterior oblique and left lateral views place the operator at increased exposure.

Habits of minimizing fluoroscopy time, reducing fluoroscopic dose, when possible, and proper use of shutters should become second nature to the angiographer.

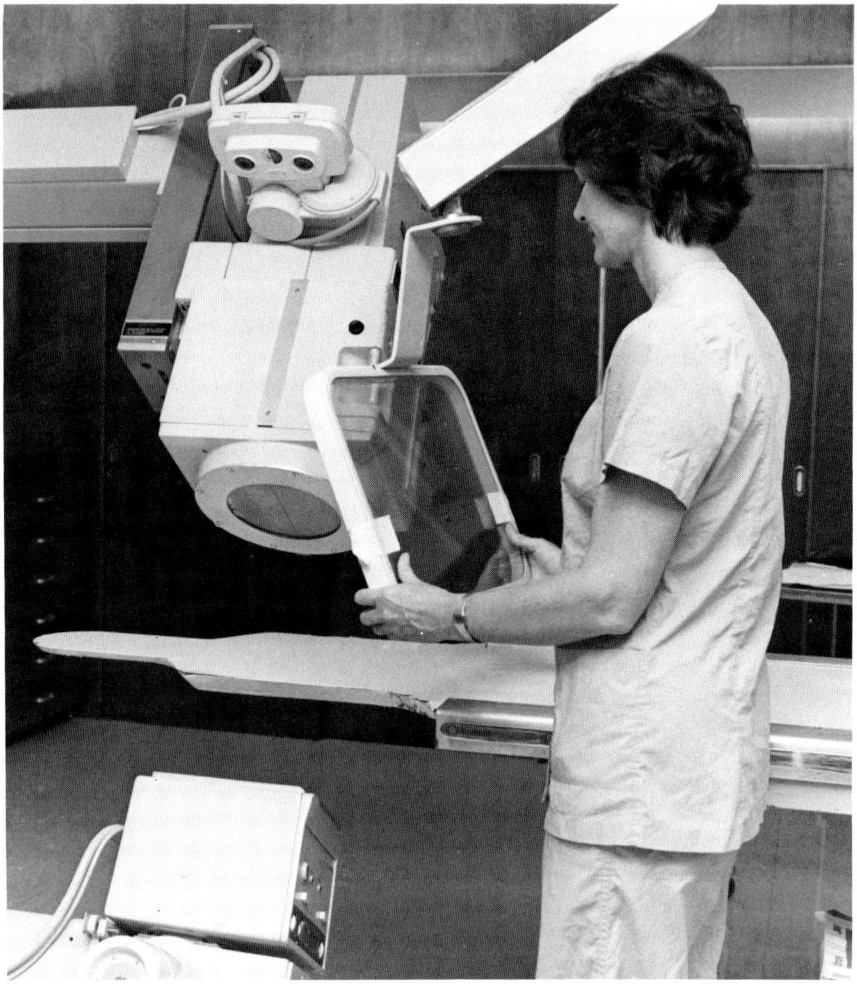

Figure 14-12 Leaded glass radiation shield.

REFERENCES

1 Friesinger GC, Adams DF, Bourassa MG, et al: Optimal resources for examination of the heart and lungs: Cardiac catheterization and radiologic facilities. Circulation, 68(4):893A–930A, October 1983.

2 The Effects on Populations of Exposure to Low Levels of Ionizing Radiation. National Academy of Sciences, Washington, 1980.

3 Pochin EE: Why Be Quantitative about Radiation Risk Estimates? National Council on Radiation Protection and Measurements, Washington, 1978.

4 Basic Radiation Protection Criteria. National Council on Radiation Protection and Measurements, Washington, 1971.

5 den Boer JA, Mohr H: Distribution of scattered radiation around the cardiodiagnost. Medicamundi, 21:121–126, 1976.

6 Balter S, Sones FM Jr, Brancato R: Radiation exposure to the operator performing cardiac angiography with U-arm systems. Circulation, 58:925–931, 1978.

7 Malsky SJ, Roswit B, Reid CB, Haft J: Radiation exposure to personnel during cardiac catheterization. Radiology, 100:671–674, 1971.

8 Wold GJ, Scheele RV, Agarwal SK: Evaluation of physician exposure during cardiac catheterization. Radiology, 99:188–190, 1971.

9 Rueter FG: Physician and patient exposure during cardiac catheterization. Circulation, 58:134–139, 1978.

Chapter 15

Selection for Surgery or PTCA

Spencer B. King III, M.D.
John S. Douglas, Jr., M.D.

The successful development of myocardial revascularization was the result of the understanding of the pathophysiology of myocardial ischemia combined with the technical developments which became available in the latter half of the twentieth century. The pathophysiology of atherosclerotic coronary heart disease was described by Alan Burns in 1809[1]:

> In health, when we excite the muscular system to more energetic action than usual, we increase the circulation in every part, so that to support this increased action, the heart and every other part has its power augmented. If, however, we call into vigorous action a limb, around which with a moderate degree of tightness we have applied a ligature, we find that then the member can only support its action for a short time; for now its supply of energy and expenditure do not balance each other; consequently, it soon from a deficiency of nervous influence and arterial blood fails and sinks into a state of quiescence. A heart, the coronary vessels of which are cartilaginous or ossified, is in nearly a similar condition; it can, like the limb, be girt with a moderately light ligature, discharge its functions so long as its action is moderate and equal. Increase, however, the action of the whole body, and along with the rest, that of the heart, and you will soon see exemplified the truth of what has been said; with this difference, that there is no interruption to the action of the cardial nerves, the heart will be able to hold out a little longer than the limb.

This dramatic insight into the origin of ischemic pain was not widely accepted until the twentieth century. Sir James MacKenzie described the relationship of the ischemic process to the observed obstructions in the coronary arteries[2]:

> That a muscle should evoke disagreeable symptoms when overfatigued is a principle applicable to all muscular structures of the body. In looking at the coronary arteries in certain typical cases of angina pectoris, one can reasonably infer one way in which the attacks are brought about. In some cases, the coronary arteries are so narrowed as scarce to permit the entrance of a pin. During life the stream of blood must have been greatly reduced, and if it were sufficient to supply the muscle during rest, it was demonstrably insufficient while the heart was in a state of activity. In this respect, there seems to be a distinct affinity between the origin of pain in these cases, and those cases of what is called intermittent claudication.

Prior to the development of cardiopulmonary bypass, many attempts were made to alleviate angina pectoris by surgical means. Thomas Jonnesco of France performed sympathectomy in 1916,[3] Claude Beck attached vascular pedicles to the inflamed surface of the heart in the 1930s,[4] internal mammary ligation was attempted as a means to increase coronary perfusion in the 1950s, and internal mammary artery implants into the myocardium were performed by Vineberg in the 1950s.[5] Each of these attempts was eventually discredited because the promised relief of angina pectoris was short-lived and was likely due to the placebo effect only. When the techniques of coronary arteriography and cardiopulmonary bypass became available, it was finally possible to apply the principles of Alan Burns to directly bypass the "cartilagenous or ossified coronary arteries." René Favaloro[6] and Dudley Johnson[7] performed direct coronary bypass surgery in 1967.

Coronary angioplasty grew out of the development of peripheral vascular angioplasty by Charles Dotter in 1964.[8] His technique involved insertion of multiple catheters of varying sizes to gradually increase the lumen of the artery. Zeitler in Germany improved the technique by developing the balloon catheters to enlarge the lumen, and these balloons were dramatically improved by Gruentzig, who also miniaturized the balloons for use in the coronary arteries. Percutaneous transluminal coronary angioplasty was first applied in September, 1977.

OBJECTIVES OF CORONARY ARTERY BYPASS GRAFT SURGERY AND PERCUTANEOUS TRANSLUMINAL CORONARY ANGIOPLASTY

Previous to development of coronary bypass surgery, most attempts at relieving ischemia were aimed at the demand side of the supply-demand formula. Although some effect on the blood flow to the myocardium has been demonstrated with medical therapy, the major impact of nitroglycerin, beta blockers, and calcium antagonists is on reducing the demand for blood by the myocardium by reducing myocardial work. If myocardial work can be reduced sufficiently to alleviate angina pectoris without producing unpleasant side effects while still allowing the patient to perform physical work at a level he or she deems adequate, then medical therapy is effective. If, however, angina pectoris is incompletely relieved or side effects or limitations in activity are unacceptable, then the objective of myocardial revascularization is to achieve those goals by improving the supply side of the equation.

The second objective of revascularization is to avoid the complications of infarction and extend longevity. It has now been demonstrated that coronary bypass surgery is effective in extending longevity in many subsets of patients with severe coronary obstructive disease.[9–19] Since percutaneous transluminal coronary angioplasty (PTCA) has largely been applied in patients with single vessel disease, a subset in which extension of longevity has been difficult to demonstrate by surgical intervention, and because the follow-up of patients undergoing PTCA is short, there has been no demonstrated statistical impact on survival by the technique as yet.

Evidence for Improved Myocardial Perfusion by Coronary Artery Bypass Surgery and Coronary Angioplasty

There has now been extensive documentation that coronary bypass surgery improves myocardial perfusion. Improved perfusion has been documented by xenon-flow studies with and without exercise,[20] postoperative exercise electrocardiographic stress testing,[21] atrial pacing studies with evaluation of myocardial lactate production,[22] electromagnetic flow probe measurements at surgery,[23] radionuclear blood pool imaging with exercise showing improvement in ejection fraction postoperatively,[24,25] digital angiographic studies pre- and postoperatively which show improved response to a hyperemic stimulus,[26] and the relationship of completeness of revascularization to symptomatic improvement.[25]

Although PTCA is a newer technique, extensive evaluations of the improvement in myocardial perfusion have been carried out. Improved perfusion has been demonstrated by exercise electrocardiographic stress testing,[27] thallium perfusion exercise stress testing,[28] radionuclear blood pool imaging with exercise,[29] and digital angiographic responses to hyperemic reperfusion.[30] Symptomatic improvement is demonstrable in PTCA patients right away since there is no masking of the improved symptomatic condition by the surgical procedure itself.

Angina relief has been documented in the vast majority of patients who have undergone either procedure. Although some improvement can be attributed to placebo effect, the magnitude of the improvement and the sustained benefit as well as the correlation between recurrent symptoms and obstructed bypass grafts or restenosed dilated segments indicates that increased myocardial perfusion is the principal reason for angina relief in revascularization procedures.

FACTORS INFLUENCING CONSIDERATION FOR CORONARY ARTERY BYPASS GRAFT SURGERY OR PTCA

Outcome of Medically Treated Patients

Before weighing the benefits of coronary bypass surgery or PTCA, one should consider the outcome of patients treated by medical means alone. Patients should always be considered from two points of view: (1) What is the current symptomatic status and how important is it to improve on any symptomatic relief that is achieved by medical therapy? (2) What are the chances of complications of coronary disease occurring, to include the possibility of early mortality?

Symptomatic Relief The possibilities for symptomatic improvement are usually determined by trial and error. Potent antianginal drugs are now available; however, the control of severe angina almost always includes a limitation in activity level. Sometimes this limitation is incompatible with a continued active and productive lifestyle when the alternative of myocardial revascularization exists. This is obviously a personal matter and would vary greatly between individuals. A retired person would have perhaps less incentive to seek myocardial revascularization if the anginal symptoms were well-controlled medically. A younger individual involved in active physical work or vigorous sports activities which were pleasurable might be reluctant to give up these activities in order to achieve freedom from angina pectoris. That individual might be much more willing to undergo myocardial revascularization to gain an improved symptomatic status which would allow these activities. Following coronary artery bypass graft surgery, greater than 90 percent of patients report they are free of symptoms or are significantly improved.[31]

Return to Work after Myocardial Revascularization The rehabilitative aspects of myocardial revascularization have been looked at by several investigators.[32–37] An evaluation of patients undergoing coronary bypass surgery at Emory University Hospital revealed that 66 percent of the patients either working at the time of coronary bypass surgery or who had discontinued work because of cardiac symptoms returned to work after surgery.[38] The variables that predicted patient's failure to return to work included residual chest pain, older age, not working prior to surgery, lower educational level, female sex, incomplete revascularization. Physicians' advice was cited as the most common reason for failure to return to work. Patients involved in professional activities had an 81 percent return to work rate while semiskilled workers had only a 34 percent return to work rate.

Since successful PTCA in properly selected patients almost always results in improvement in symptoms without a prolonged recovery period, there is little impact on the work status of the patient. The vast majority of patients anticipate returning directly to work following the procedure and do so. Patients undergoing emergency bypass surgery or elective surgery following failed PTCA are similar to patients operated on electively.

Prognosis of Medically Treated Patients

The second consideration, the prognosis of medically treated patients, has been extensively studied. Prognosis is closely tied to the extent of coronary disease and the left ventricular function. Evaluation of survival of medically treated patients was carried out prior to the availability of coronary bypass surgery. Significant variations exist between certain subgroups and between studies. A 4 percent annual mortality rate was found in patients developing angina pectoris in the Framingham study[39]; 13 percent annual mortality occurred over a 3-year period for patients with left main stenosis proved angiographically[9]; and a greater than 20 percent annual mortality rate existed in the subset of unstable angina patients who continued to have pain in the hospital setting.[40] Studies which relied entirely on symptomatic data without angiographic documentation tended to underestimate the risk of coronary disease because of the inclusion of patients with mild disease or no coronary disease at all. As has been mentioned earlier, a significant percentage of patients, especially women suspected of having coronary disease, are found to have no obstructions on angiography. The medical survival is dramatically influenced by the quality of the left ventricular function, the number of arteries affected and the location of these lesions, the presence of congestive heart failure or hypertension, and the patient's age.

Survival curves for medically treated patients show a wide variation depending on these various factors. Modern medical therapy has influenced to varying degrees the survival of some of these patients. All studies of medically treated patients, however, show a direct correlation between the number of vessels involved and the long-term survival rate (Fig. 15-1). Left ventricular function also influences survival of patients, as demonstrated in a study in which patients with double vessel disease had a 5-year survival rate of 85 percent when the ejection fraction was normal, 65 percent when the ejection fraction was 31 to 50 percent, and 32 percent when the ejection fraction was below 30 percent.[41]

Randomized trials of medically and surgically treated patients have been difficult and fraught with the problems of selection and crossover. Nonetheless, the Veterans Administration (VA) study demonstrated a clear improvement with surgery for left main disease[9] (Fig. 15-2) and later with surgery for triple vessel disease.[42] Some subsets of double

Figure 15-1 Cleveland Clinic survival curves of medically treated candidates for partial or complete revascularization. LCA = left main coronary artery. *Adapted from Bruschke, AV: Ten year followup of 601 nonsurgical cases of angiographically documented coronary disease. Angiographic correlations. An international symposium "Syllabus" prepared by the Cleveland Clinic Foundation, September 1977. (From Hurst JW (ed):* The Heart (5th ed), *McGraw-Hill, New York, 1982, Fig. 45-30.)*

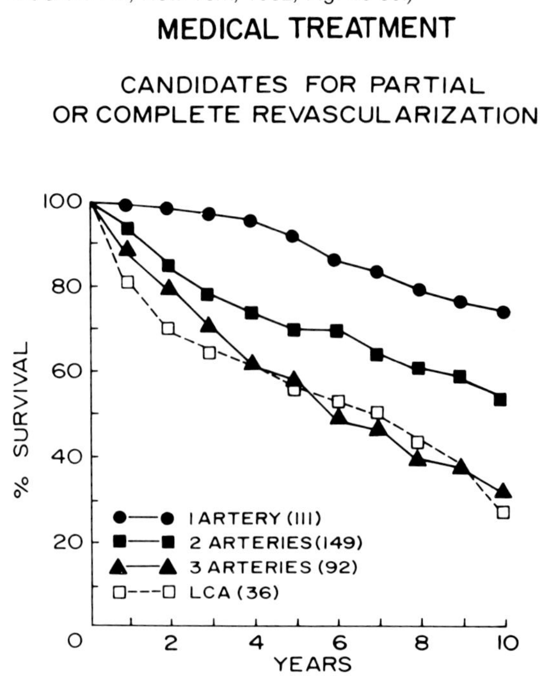

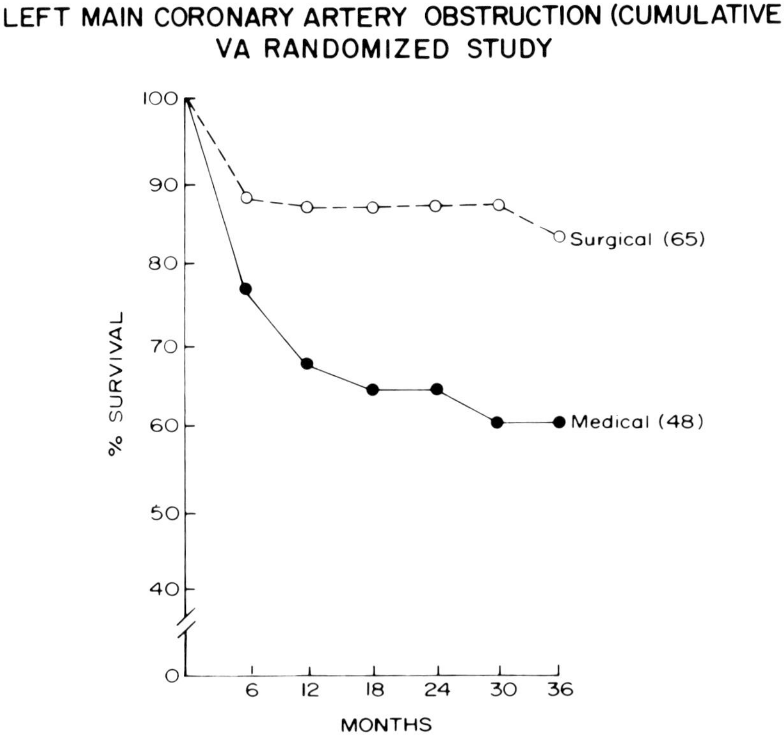

Figure 15-2 Results of the Veterans Administration prospective randomized clinical trial of patients with obstruction of the left main coronary artery.[9] *(From Hurst JW (ed): The Heart (5th ed), McGraw-Hill, New York, Fig. 45-33)*

vessel disease were improved in this study as well as in the European multicenter trial.[19]

A problem in all randomized trials of medical and surgical therapy has been the exclusions allowed. In addition to the VA study, the recently released Coronary Artery Surgery Study (CASS) sponsored by the National Heart, Lung, and Blood Institute (NHLBI)[43] suffered from this problem. Among over 16,000 patients eligible for the study, only 2099 could be randomized because of exclusions such as left main stenosis, unstable angina, class II or III angina, ejection fraction less than 35 percent (only about 15 percent were below 50 percent), age less than 65, other illnesses, etc. Then of the 2099 eligible for randomization, another 1319 were excluded by physician and patient preferences, leaving only 780 patients selected for the study. This represents an average of slightly more than one patient per month selected from each of the 11 participating centers. Such selection results in a low-risk population for medical or surgical therapy.

The other problem with such studies is crossover to surgical therapy. In both the VA and CASS studies, patients with increasing symptoms were, of course, allowed to have surgical therapy in the follow-up period. Using so many exclusions in selecting low-risk patients and then operating on the patients who became worse, it was possible to achieve similar 5-year survival rates in medically and surgically treated groups. The danger is in applying this conclusion to the broad group of patients with coronary disease, patients who have not been through this tight selection process.

Patient survival following PTCA gives few clues as to the overall impact of this procedure on longevity. Those patients selected to date have had largely single vessel coronary artery disease, constituting a subset in which a difference in long-term survival between medical and surgical treatment has been difficult to establish. Since the follow-up of patients treated with PTCA is short and the application of further revascularization treatments is always possible, it will probably never be possible to identify the survival curve of patients undergoing a single PTCA procedure. Among the first 600 patients undergoing PTCA at Emory University Hospital, there have been six late deaths.[44]

Hospital Mortality, Morbidity, and Risks Surgical techniques and anesthetic management have improved the survival of patients undergoing coronary artery bypass surgery. At Emory University Hospital, the operative mortality rate declined from 4 percent in the years 1973 to 1975 to 0.8 percent in the years 1976 to 1981. In 1980, the operative mortality rate was only 0.4 percent (Fig. 15-3). With the mortality risk below 1 percent, cardiologists become more aggressive in referring patients for bypass surgery. This influences surgical selection from both ends of the spectrum of coronary disease, namely, those patients with only moderate coronary disease who wish improvement in symptoms and are willing to undertake a very small risk, as well as patients with far-advanced coronary disease who can now be brought through coronary bypass surgery in much higher percentages than was formerly the case. The selection of higher risk patients will ultimately moderate these low-mortality-rate statistics.

Hospital mortality rate in the early experience of PTCA as reflected by the National Institutes of Health (NIH) registry was 1 percent. In the 2000 patients undergoing PTCA at Emory University Hospital, the incidence of mortality has been confined to two patients, for a rate of 0.1 percent. Hospital mortality rate is not comparable between coronary bypass surgery and angioplasty, however, because patient selection is entirely different, and the most important moderating factor on hospital mortality in angioplasty patients is the availability of expert coronary bypass surgery in cases of failed angioplasty. At Emory, the 70 patients who have undergone emergency bypass surgery following failed angioplasty have all survived the hospital course.

There is, of course, a certain morbidity from revascularization procedures, including universal chest soreness in those patients undergoing bypass surgery and the continuing problems of the occasional patient who has a cerebrovascular accident, myocardial infarction, or pulmonary complications following cardiopulmonary bypass. The main advantage of PTCA rests in the avoidance of the immediate postoperative discomforts of coronary bypass surgery, and certainly the morbidity in this regard is markedly reduced in those patients suitable for angioplasty. The major risk of angioplasty is the closure of the coronary artery resulting in the need for emergency bypass surgery.

In the small group of post-PTCA patients undergoing emergency bypass surgery, the rate of myocardial infarction, of course, is higher than in patients undergoing elective bypass surgery. When

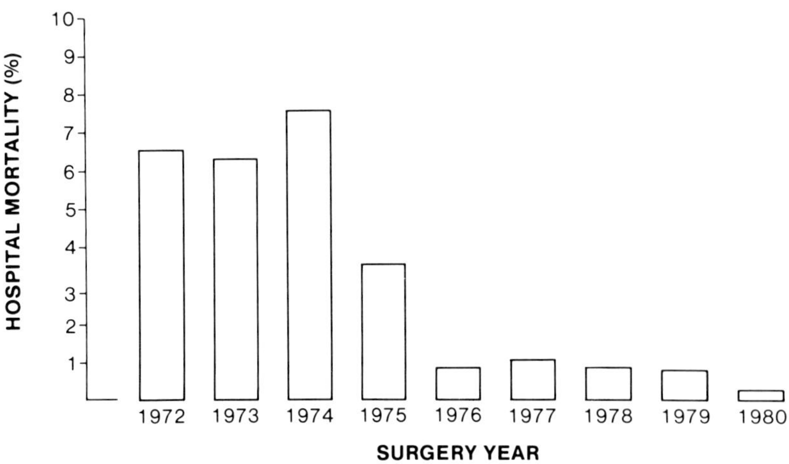

Figure 15-3 Hospital mortality rates for patients undergoing coronary bypass at Emory University Hospital, 1972–1980. Note that the hospital mortality rate during the last year (1980) was about 0.4 percent. *(From Hurst JW (ed): The Heart (5th ed), McGraw-Hill, New York, 1982, Fig. 45-31)*

infarction occurs following angioplasty with emergency surgery or with elective bypass surgery, the extent of infarction appears to be much less than in spontaneously occurring infarction when revascularization is not performed.[45,46]

PROSPECT FOR RELIEF OF ANGINA AND IMPROVED EXERCISE PERFORMANCE

Symptoms

The more severe the patient's symptoms, the greater the likelihood that revascularization procedures will result in improvement. Conversely, in the asymptomatic patient there is no opportunity for relief of symptoms with these procedures. Although the severity of the symptoms may not predict the degree of disease, when considering the relief of symptoms alone, the more one has, the more chance there is for relief. Certainly age and activity level influence these decisions. An older patient who has little need to engage in vigorous physical activity may be satisfied with significantly limiting symptoms whereas a younger patient may be intolerant of such symptoms even if they occur with only moderately heavy exertion.

Revascularization procedures have been effective in relieving angina. Most centers report angina pectoris is relieved in 75 to 95 percent of patients who undergo coronary bypass surgery.[47,48] At Emory University Hospital, the cardiac data bank reveals that of patients surveyed by mail, 91 percent report either angina-free state or marked improvement several years following bypass surgery.[31] The Veterans Administration study of stable angina pectoris showed substantial improvement or no angina in 60 percent of the surgical group as compared with only 16 percent of the medical group 1 year postoperatively.[41] A cooperatively evaluated study of unstable angina pectoris patients which was organized by the National Heart, Lung, and Blood Institute revealed that in the follow-up period of these patients, 45 percent of the medical group developed class III or IV angina compared with only 15 percent of the surgical group.[49]

Symptomatic evaluation of PTCA patients is possible immediately following the procedure and is usually carried out with exercise stress testing. Because of the selection criterion applied to most patients undergoing PTCA, namely, that they have high-grade single vessel disease, a successful procedure is almost always associated with relief of angina pectoris and improved exercise performance.[50]

Objective Evidence of Ischemia

Unstable angina patients are not usually suitable candidates for exercise stress testing; however, in the more stable patients, those with positive exercise ECG testing, thallium myocardial perfusion scanning, and blood pool imaging with exercise have a greater chance for symptomatic improvement than those patients who do not have such objective evidence of ischemia.

Anatomic Factors

The pathoanatomy of the coronary arteries is certainly the critical factor in determining whether patients should undergo revascularization procedures. As has already been indicated, the number of vessels involved and the location of the lesions determines in some part the prognosis of the patient. Anatomic factors which are critical in making the decision for or against revascularization include the location of the lesions, the severity of the lesions, the completeness or incompleteness of the occlusion, the amount of myocardium served by the stenotic vessels, the presence or absence of collateral circulation to the segments distal to the occlusions, the presence or absence of additional stenotic lesions in those vessels supplying collaterals, and the morphology of the lesions themselves.

Predicting the Amount of Myocardium at Risk

The goal of myocardial revascularization is to return as much viable myocardium to a normal perfusion as is possible. Considering the above-mentioned factors, a decision can be made as to whether this can be met adequately with surgery or angioplasty or whether such improvement is actually impossible by either means. The location of the lesion determines in many respects the amount of myocardium that is perfused. Obstruction of the left main artery usually affects up to 75 percent or more of the left ventricular myocardium, while proximal anterior descending stenosis may affect 40 to 50 percent.[66] More distal lesions in each artery affect a smaller percentage of the myocardium. The severity of the lesion determines whether the lesion is hemodynamically significant. If greater than 50 percent of the diameter is involved, then the potential for decreased perfusion with exercise exists. A 50 percent diameter lesion, however, in no way produces the ischemic insult of a 90 percent lesion. When arteries are blocked completely, the most severe interruption in flow occurs, however. One positive factor attends total occlusion. If a vessel is occluded, then one need not worry about the future effects of total occlusion since that event has already taken place and those effects can be readily seen. One would not be equally anxious to bypass a patient with total occlusion of an anterior descending and adequate distal collateral circulation as one would a patient with a 90 percent stenotic anterior descending without evident collaterals.

The amount of myocardium that may be damaged from occlusion of a stenotic artery depends on several factors; however, one of the most important is the distribution of that artery over the myocardium. A coronary artery with a wide distribution may, when occluded, produce a very large infarction, or if collateral circulation develops adequately, may cause little damage. A very tiny coronary segment that serves a small area of myocardium, however, will never result in a large infarction. The presence of collateral vessels does not in itself indicate the lack of myocardial ischemia since collaterals seldom provide adequate perfusion pressure to fully compensate the obstructed vessel. The presence of collaterals is, however, reassuring and is frequently protective from infarction when total occlusion occurs. Again, one would be less anxious to bypass a severely stenotic right coronary artery with a very rich collateral network filling the distal vessel than one would a severely stenotic artery with no evidence of collateral filling.

Finally the morphology of the lesion has assumed increased importance, especially with the advent of PTCA. The morphology may also be important, however, in making decisions for surgery since lesions that exhibit irregular filling defects representing thrombosis or ulcerated plaques may herald acute occlusion of an artery more commonly than lesions with smooth endothelial surfaces. Certainly when considering angioplasty, the morphology of the lesion is critical in determining whether the balloon catheter can be passed beyond the lesion with safety and whether the artery will dilate adequately.

Left Ventricular Function

Patients who have congestive heart failure have little chance for improvement from myocardial revascularization alone. Rarely, in the damaged heart, acute ischemia can precipitate congestive heart failure which will be improved by revascularization of the ischemic segments. These, however, are unusual situations. Also, those patients with mechanical complications of myocardial infarction such as ruptured interventricular septum or papillary muscle or development of ventricular aneurysm can be helped by surgical repair but not by simple revascularization.

Global left ventricular function is an important consideration in the relationship to surgery. If severe left ventricular dysfunction exists, then the operative mortality rate is definitely increased. Most patients with ejection fractions under 20 percent are not good candidates for bypass surgery, although with improved anesthesia techniques some of these patients are brought through surgery and improve symptomatically. Certainly these severely impaired left ventricles should be contraindications in most circumstances to coronary angioplasty as well because further obstruction of coronary segments that may occur as a complication of the angioplasty procedure would reduce the heart's ability to sustain the circulation while moving to emergency bypass surgery. Left ventricular dysfunction is a powerful predictor of survival both in medically and surgically treated patients. At Emory University Hospital, we have been able to demonstrate a marked difference in operative mortality and long-term survival rates in relation to ejection fractions above and below 35 percent (Fig. 15-4).

Left Ventricular Dysfunction in the Setting of Acute Myocardial Infarction in Evolution

Patients in the early stages of acute myocardial infarction have severely impaired left ventricular function which may be partially reversible depending on the promptness with which revascularization is established. The use of intracoronary streptokinase or PTCA or the two in combination or the use of emergency coronary bypass surgery may be effective in salvaging myocardium at risk and restoring left ventricular function partially, as described in Chap. 17.

Graft Patency Following Coronary Artery Bypass Graft Surgery and Restenosis Following PTCA

Bypass graft patency has a direct relationship to symptomatic improvement and long-term survival. The two centers with the largest experience reported early patency rates of 82 and 84 percent.[51,52] The Cleveland Clinic with a large number of patients restudied reported little difference between patency rates of patients restudied at the end of the first year and those studied at the end of the fourth year.[53] The Montreal Heart Institute has conducted a prospective study looking at graft patency at 2 weeks, 1 year, and 3 years postoperatively.[54] The 2-week patency rate was 92 percent, 1 year patency

Figure 15-4 Post–coronary artery bypass graft survival curves for patients with ejection fraction (EFX) above 35 percent and below 35 percent. N = number of patients. *(From Hatcher, CR Jr, Craver, JM, Jones, EL, King, SB III, Hurst, JW: The early and late results of myocardial revascularization, in Hurst, JW (ed): Clinical Essays on the Heart, vol 2, McGraw-Hill, New York, 1984, fig. 4.)*

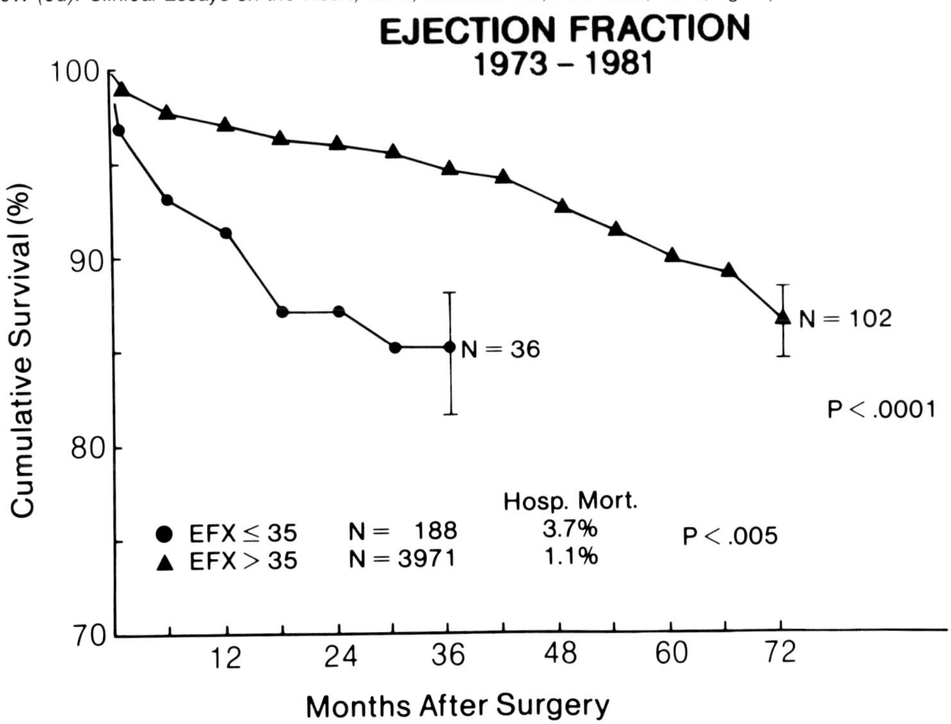

rate 86 percent. Following this first year, the annual rate of attrition was 0.7 percent. Other studies report between 1 and 1.7 percent annual attrition rate for grafts.[55–57] Progression in nongrafted arteries was 9.5 percent in one study.[58] However when these patients were restudied in 6 years, progression was noted in 46 percent of the patients.

Restenosis of dilated coronary arteries following PTCA has been an important consideration. In the first 600 patients undergoing PTCA at Emory University Hospital, the restenosis rate, defined as loss of 50 percent or more of the improvement in diameter stenosis gained at angioplasty, was 33 percent. Several modifications in technique and post-angioplasty management have resulted in an apparent lower restenosis rate in patients undergoing the procedure in the past 2 years. Restenosis of dilated segments in the PTCA population does not have quite the same connotation as the closed vein graft since redilation of a stenosed segment has been associated with a high degree of success and continued patency. In this cohort of 600 patients, continued long-term success was achieved in 78 percent. With increasing use of repeat angioplasty, this long-term benefit will likely rise to near 90 percent. Progression of disease in other arteries will undoubtedly be a feature of patients who have undergone PTCA as it has been in patients undergoing coronary bypass surgery.

LONG-TERM SURVIVAL AFTER CORONARY ARTERY BYPASS GRAFT SURGERY

The Veterans Administration study of left main coronary artery obstruction showed such a dramatic difference in survival rates between the medical and surgical groups that the study was terminated.[9] The randomized European collaborative study of stable angina shows that there is an improved survival rate in the surgical group of patients with left main coronary artery obstruction and triple vessel disease with decreased left ventricular contractility. This study also suggests improved survival rates in patients with double vessel obstruction when one of the lesions involves the proximal anterior descending coronary artery.[59,60] Many of the studies involving triple vessel disease show significant improvement in survival rate in surgically treated cases[10–17] and improvement in double vessel disease patients who are treated surgically when the anterior descending artery is one of the vessels involved.[10,12–17,61] All the patients undergoing coronary bypass surgery at Emory University Hospital have been entered into the cardiac data bank and tabulated for their survival rate in relation to the number of preoperative variables. Factors such as the number of vessels involved, the status of left ventricular function, and the presence or absence of congestive heart failure all influence the survival curves. It is interesting to note, however, that patients with the most severe disease and impaired left ventricular dysfunction have a much improved survival rate when compared to similar patients treated medically before the advent of coronary bypass surgery (Fig. 15-5).

No difference has been documented in the survival rate of patients with single vessel disease treated surgically when compared with those treated medically. Failure to demonstrate this may relate to the longer follow-up needed to demonstrate a high mortality from single vessel disease. During this follow-up period, of course, most patients are undergoing vigorous therapy of various kinds, frequently including bypass surgery as more vessels are involved. Despite this lack of data from randomized trials, we feel that many patients with severe proximal anterior descending lesions which affect large segments of the left ventricular myocardium are at significant jeopardy and should be considered for myocardial revascularization.

Preliminary data from the coronary artery surgery study showed that single vessel disease patients with proximal LAD disease had a 5-year mortality of 32 percent treated medically compared to only 11 percent for all single vessel patients.[67] Proximal LAD disease carries a higher risk than RCA disease[68] or more distal LAD disease.[69]

The presence of proximal LAD disease is also very important in patients with multivessel disease. A recent study by Califf[70] showed a 49 percent 5-

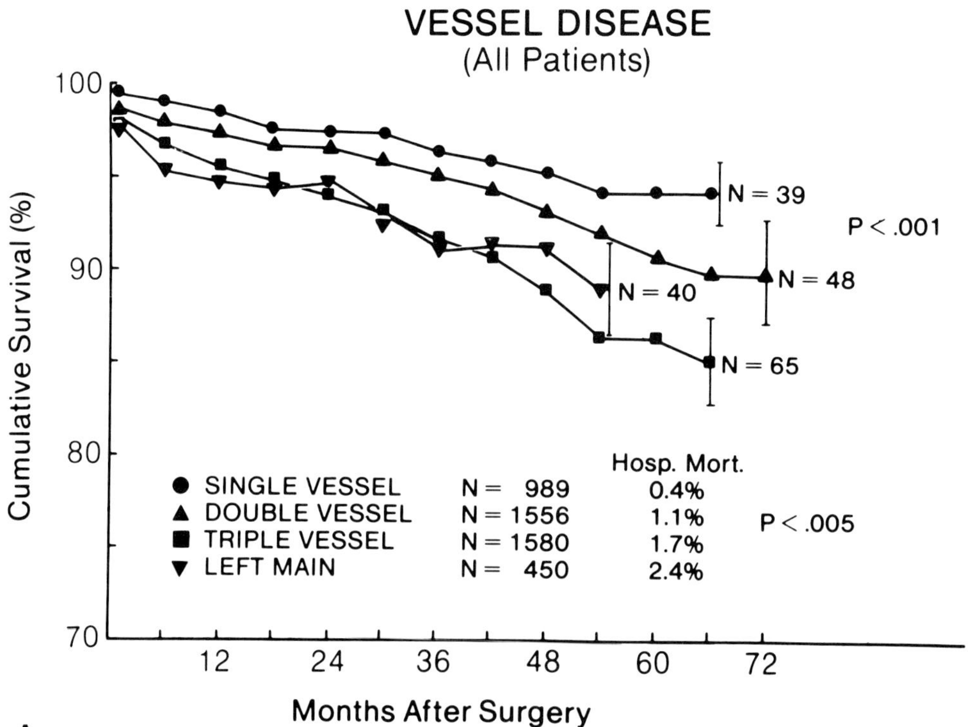

A

Figure 15-5 (*a*) Post–coronary artery bypass graft survival curve for patients according to the extent of their disease. EFX = ejection fraction, N = number of patients. (*b*) Survival curves for those with normal contractility by extent of disease. N = number of patients. (*c*) Survival curves for those with abnormal contractility by the extent of the disease. *(Part* a *from Jones EL, Craver JM, Guyton RA, Bone DK, Hatcher CR Jr: Trends in the treatment of coronary disease today: Selective use of PTCA and bypass surgery. Ann Surg, 197:6, June 1983, fig 3. Parts* b *and* c *from Hatcher, CR Jr, Craver, JM, Jones, EL, King, SB III, Hurst JW: The early and late results of myocardial revascularization in Hurst, JW (ed): Clinical Essays on the Heart, McGraw-Hill, New York, 1984, figs. 1 and 2, respectively.)*

year mortality in patients with proximal LAD and proximal circumflex disease treated without surgery. This was significantly higher than other forms of double or triple vessel disease without proximal LAD involvement.

Noncardiac Determiners of Survival

There are other factors which may influence long-term survival which should be considered when patients are evaluated for coronary revascularization. The potential for survival should certainly be considered in relationship to these other systemic diseases, and the permanent debilitating features of those diseases should be considered in anticipating improvement in symptoms of myocardial ischemia. Neoplastic diseases with palliative or curative potential are not absolute contraindications to either coronary bypass surgery or PTCA. Certainly the palliating effects of PTCA are quite attractive in such patients if that technique is applicable. A number of high-risk patients have had coronary bypass surgery in order to make them candidates for resection of operable pulmonary nodules. Associated vascular lesions must be managed in a way that minimizes the risk to the patient. Significant carotid artery disease is not uncommon in patients undergoing myocardial revascularization.[62,63] At our institution, patients who are severely symptomatic from carotid disease undergo

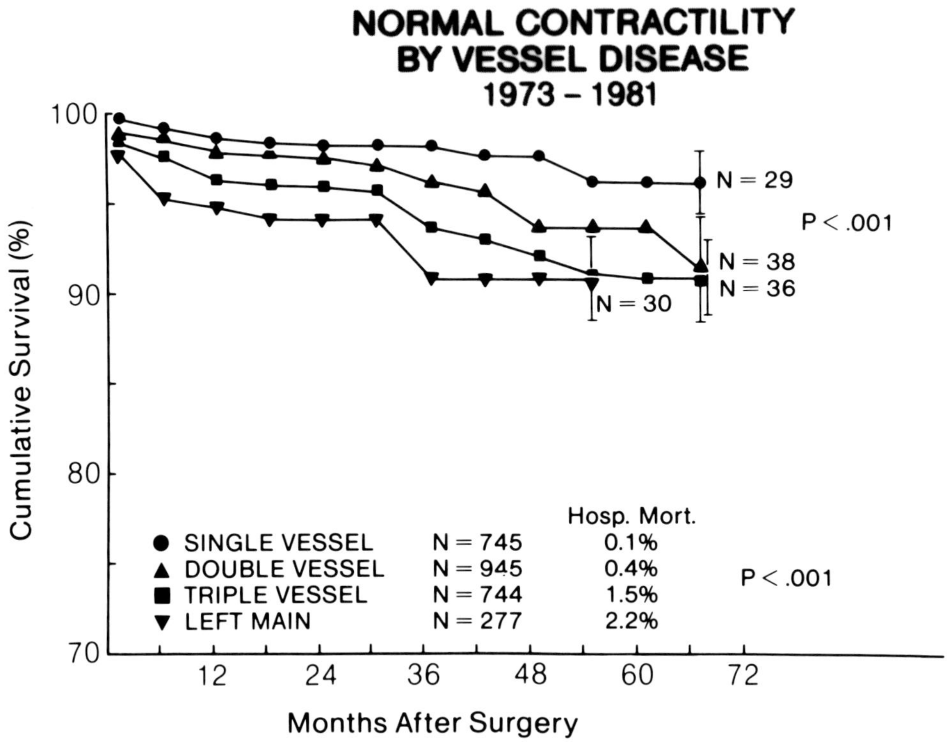

B *(Figure 15-5, continued)*

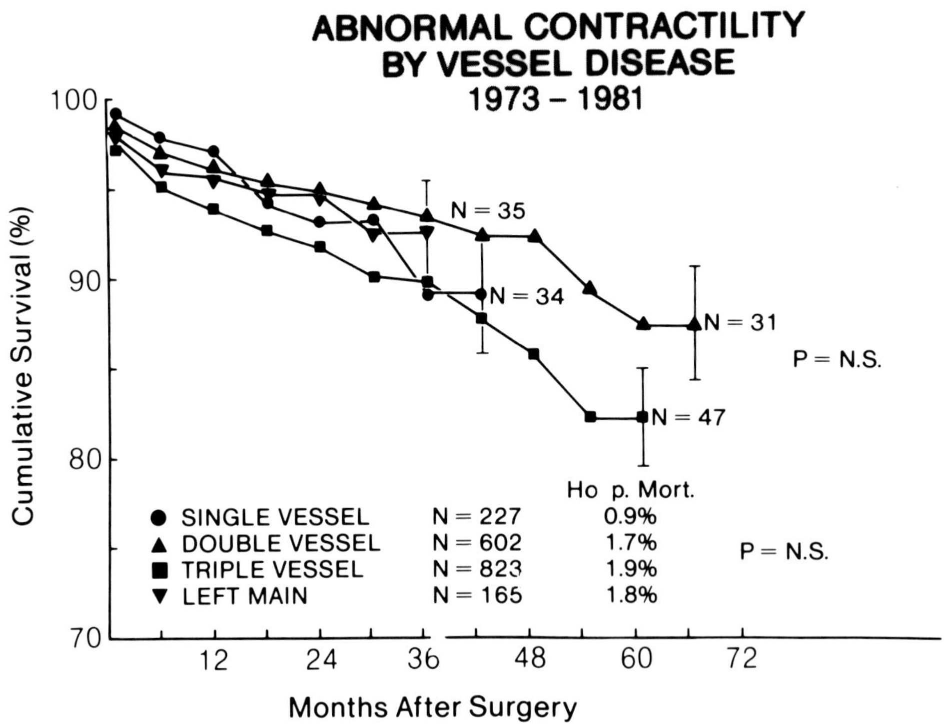

C

carotid surgery first if the cardiac status will tolerate it. If the coronary disease is severe and the carotid disease is less so, then the patient undergoes the coronary bypass surgery and later has the carotid endarterectomy done. When both the carotid artery and the coronary arteries are stenosed in a way that would produce severe insult precluding either surgery alone, then a combined operation attacking both the carotid and the coronary problems is planned.[64]

Coronary bypass surgery to improve angina in a patient with severe peripheral claudication may not result in overall improvement to the patient unless it is possible to attack the peripheral vascular disease as well. If this approach seems impractical because of the location and extent of the peripheral lesions or the patient's age, then there is little reason to perform coronary bypass surgery for improvement of symptomatology in such a limited patient. PTCA may alleviate symptoms of angina in properly selected patients who have a multitude of complicating systemic illnesses which would make them poor candidates for coronary bypass surgery. It must always be kept in mind, however, that PTCA may result in emergency surgery and that must be fully understood prior to application of the technique in such patients.

LIMITATION OF REVASCULARIZATION PROCEDURES

Coronary artery bypass graft surgery is limited by two factors. First, if left ventricular function is so poor as to preclude operative survival, then of course the patient should not undergo surgery. This now applies almost exclusively to those patients in overt congestive heart failure, since when bypassable vessels are present, even those patients with very poor left ventricular function can be brought through the operative procedure. It is true that the long-term outlook for these patients is certainly not as good as for those with adequate left ventricular function, but some of these patients can be helped if they are severely symptomatic. The second reason to deny surgery to an otherwise operative candidate is the condition of the distal coronary vessels. If the disease is diffuse so that the effective placement of bypass grafts is impossible, then the patient should not be offered surgery. With improved surgical experience at placing smaller and smaller grafts, however, the patients falling into this category have decreased in numbers markedly. Still, in order to achieve a significant result from bypass surgery in patients with diffuse multivessel disease, it is necessary to revascularize substantial amounts of myocardium. Patients should not be accepted for surgery if only one small area could be improved when multiple areas are in need of revascularization.

Coronary bypass surgery, of course, requires adequate conduits for constructing the grafts. If patients have been operated on once or twice before, then there may be a problem finding adequate vein material. In our institution, adequate veins have almost always been found, and with the popular use of the internal mammary artery as a conduit, this problem is not a common one. Solving the problem of very poor distal vessels has been approached by endarterectomy in some centers. The results in the right coronary artery have been encouraging; however, left coronary artery endarterectomy has in most hands resulted in a high incidence of anterior myocardial infarction and graft closure. Most surgeons prefer placement of multiple grafts in an artery rather than disrupting the large intimal plaques.

Intraoperative angioplasty has been used in some centers including our own with moderately good result. We have concluded, however, that when multiple grafts can be placed, this is probably superior to performing angioplasty in the operating room to more distal segments of the artery.[65]

Advanced pulmonary disease may make the patient inoperable although superb anesthetic management has improved the chances of patients with moderate pulmonary disease coming through the operative procedure. Sternal infections and systemic infections, of course, would be a contraindication to surgery until those were brought under control.

PTCA is limited by the ability to reach and cross

lesions and by the configuration of the atherosclerotic process itself in terms of how it would respond to an internal expansion of the arterial lumen. The technique is not indicated in totally occluded arteries with one exception. If the arterial anatomy was known by virtue of a recent coronary arteriogram demonstrating subtotal occlusion and then the artery proceeds to total occlusion before the PTCA can be done, then the chance of crossing and dilating that lesion is high. Other chronic total occlusions have such a low success rate that PTCA should not be attempted. In severe multivessel disease, PTCA usually does not have the chance of improving the situation to the same degree as bypass surgery, and therefore the technique should not be chosen. PTCA should not be done in patients with very long diffusely diseased segments, sharp bends preceding the lesion, or bifurcations in the coronary lesion in such a configuration that the side branch would be blocked off. Exceptions to this are small side branches that could be sacrificed with no jeopardy to the patient. PTCA is not recommended in patients with left main coronary stenosis because of the potential for closure of that artery producing massive myocardial damage and death even if emergency surgery is carried out right away.

INDICATIONS FOR CORONARY ARTERY BYPASS GRAFT SURGERY AND PTCA

Before revascularization procedures can be contemplated, it is necessary to have an accurate map of the coronary circulation provided by coronary arteriography. Indications for coronary arteriography have been previously discussed. Selection for further therapy after the coronary arteriogram is performed is based on the patient's symptomatic status, objective evidence of myocardial ischemia, and the anatomic condition of the coronary arteries and the left ventricular function. All these elements are integrated to form a concept of whether the patient will benefit from direct revascularization techniques from the point of view both of improved symptoms and the long-term prognosis.

To alleviate symptoms in symptomatic patients, the first determination to be made is whether the symptoms are indeed the result of the obstructive coronary disease visualized on the arteriogram. This seems obvious; however, many patients have noncardiac chest pain even though some obstructive coronary disease is discovered. These patients have no chance of improvement by coronary bypass surgery and should not be operated on. Sometimes it is difficult to establish this fact but the various noninvasive exercise tests to document myocardial ischemia are most helpful in this regard. Once a determination has been made that symptoms are due to the observed coronary obstructions, the patient's symptoms should be reevaluated. If these symptoms on medical therapy are limiting in a way that is disagreeable to the patient or if the patient's physical activity level is inadequate for his or her needs, then a discussion of revascularization should be carried out. Selection of the type of procedure depends on the location and morphology of the coronary disease. If left ventricular function is adequate to sustain a patient through coronary bypass surgery, then the patient can be evaluated for the prospect of PTCA or coronary artery bypass grafting. Those patients who have discrete, accessible lesions which have a very high chance of responding to PTCA should have that technique recommended to them if experienced operators are available to carry it out. This will be primarily patients with single vessel disease or those who have only a single vessel that can be revascularized by any technique. Some patients with previous total occlusion and obliteration of the distal artery or vessels that are so small that they cannot be bypassed have a severe, high-grade lesion elsewhere that is suitable for angioplasty.

The primary limiting factor in selection for PTCA should be the consideration of what would happen if total occlusion of the vessel occurred during the procedure. If it is felt that a patient would suffer such a hemodynamic insult from closure of the artery attempted that movement to emergency surgery would be jeopardized, then PTCA should not be attempted. In our experience, the number of patients suitable for PTCA at this time represent about 10 to 20 percent of the operative candidates.

Most patients with multivessel involvement should have surgery recommended since this would result in significantly more revascularization than PTCA. Occasional patients have what we call multiple single vessel disease. That is, very discrete, accessible lesions located in more than one artery, usually two, that are exquisitely suitable for PTCA since there is no diffuse disease at all. These patients can have both lesions dilated at the same sitting with a high chance of success.

Most patients with symptomatic coronary disease as described are candidates for coronary bypass surgery, and when adequate revascularization can be performed, the chance of alleviating their symptoms is very high. For prolongation of survival, there is another group of patients who, whether symptomatic or not, should undergo revascularization procedures. These are patients who on coronary arteriography are found to have severe, multivessel obstruction which places them in a high-risk group for long-term complications. We feel the data for the superiority of surgical therapy in improving long-term survival rates is so strong in left main disease and severe triple vessel disease as well as double vessel disease when the proximal anterior descending artery is involved that patients with high-grade lesions in these areas should be recommended for revascularization regardless of the symptomatic status. One should always bear in mind the amount of myocardium in jeopardy when making such decisions since it is possible to have so-called triple vessel disease which may be a rather low-risk proposition with involvement of the distal anterior descending, one marginal branch, and a distal portion of the right coronary artery. These patients are not necessarily in need of urgent coronary bypass surgery; however, those patients with severe proximal obstruction of the artery supplying massive areas of myocardium are.

FOLLOWING MYOCARDIAL INFARCTION

We have previously suggested that patients should undergo cardiac catheterization or at least an objective noninvasive screening procedure following recovery from myocardial infarction. Some of these patients will be asymptomatic and will have high-grade coronary disease identified on the catheterization. Selection for surgery in these patients depends on the finding of high-grade obstructive disease in areas of viable myocardium in addition to the area that was infarcted. There is no opportunity to improve symptoms, of course, in these patients who have none following coronary bypass surgery; therefore it is imperative to make sure that the obstructive disease remote from the myocardial infarction is of such a nature that longevity will be jeopardized unless myocardial revascularization is done. Unfortunately at this time, this is a decision that must be made without adequate hard evidence from randomized clinical trials. Nevertheless, there are certainly patients who have suffered a myocardial infarction who are at great jeopardy of additional infarctions based on the coronary anatomy that is seen. Objective testing for ischemia by exercise ECG or radionuclear means may help identify patients at greatest risk.

Sometimes it is necessary to perform bypass surgery and PTCA in the same patient perhaps more than once over the course of the disease. Since coronary disease is progressive, it is unlikely that either procedure will result in permanent alleviation of the ischemic process if the patient lives long enough. It may therefore be in the best interest of the patient to perform coronary bypass surgery for severe multivessel disease, yet if graft occlusion occurs or progression of disease occurs in unbypassed arteries, then PTCA may be beneficial at that time. On the other hand, patients with high-grade single vessel disease may undergo PTCA and yet if more severe multivessel disease developed in later years, then coronary bypass surgery could be performed in that same patient. In the future undoubtedly other methods of myocardial revascularization will be developed to attack the supply side of coronary artery disease. Until the root causes of the atherosclerotic process can be discovered and controlled, it will be necessary to apply these revascularization procedures in order to enable the patient to enjoy a more fruitful and longer life.

REFERENCES

1 Willius FA, Dry TJ: *A History of the Heart and Circulation*. Saunders, Philadelphia, 1948, p 110.

2 Ibid, p 234.

3 Ibid, p 255.

4 Beck CS: Coronary artery disease: A report to William Harvey 300 years later. Am J Cardiol, 1(1):38, 1958.

5 Vineberg A, Walker J: Six months' to six years' experience with coronary artery insufficiency treated by internal mammary artery implantation. Am Heart J, 54:851, 1957.

6 Favaloro RG: Saphenous vein graft in the surgical treatment of coronary artery disease: Operative technique. J Thorac Cardiovasc Surg, 58:178, 1969.

7 Johnson WD, Flemma RJ, Lepley T Jr, et al: Extended treatment of severe coronary artery disease: A total surgical approach. Ann Surg, 170:460, 1969.

8 Dotter CT, Judkins MF: Transluminal treatment of atherosclerotic obstruction, description of a new technique and preliminary report of its application. Circulation, 30:654–670, 1964.

9 Takaro T, Hultgren HN, Lipton MJ, Detre KM, et al: The VA Cooperative randomized study of surgery for coronary arterial occlusive disease: II. Subgroup with significant left main lesions. Circulation, 54(suppl 3):107, 1975.

10 Hurst JW, King SB III: The prolongation of life by coronary bypass surgery: The Emory University Hospital experience, in Hurst JW (ed): *Update II: The Heart*. McGraw-Hill, New York, 1980, p 141.

11 Rackley CE: Prolongation of life after coronary artery bypass surgery at the University of Alabama Medical Center, in Hurst JW (ed): *Update II: The Heart*. McGraw-Hill, New York, 1980, p 151.

12 Greene DG, Bunnell IL, Arani DT, et al: Preservation of the myocardium by coronary bypass surgery: The effect on survival, in Hurst JW (ed): *Update II: The Heart*. McGraw-Hill, New York, 1980, p 159.

13 Hall RJ, Mathur VS, Garcia E, DeCastro CM: The prolongation of life by coronary bypass surgery: The effect on survival, in Hurst JW (ed): *Update II: The Heart*. McGraw-Hill, New York, 1980, p 175.

14 Gunnar RM, Loeb HS, Palac R, Pifarre R: Improved survival in patients with chronic angina pectoris treated surgically: Report of a randomized prospective study of aortocoronary bypass from Hines, Illinois, in Hurst JW (ed): *Update II: The Heart*. McGraw-Hill, New York, 1980, p 205.

15 Lawrie GM, Morris GC Jr: Improved survival after coronary bypass: A long-term perspective from Baylor College of Medicine, in Hurst JW (ed), *Update II: The Heart*. McGraw-Hill, New York, 1980, p 221.

16 Hammermeister KE, DeRouen TA, Dodge HT: Survival analyses in medically and surgically treated patients with coronary disease: A critical review and experience in Seattle Heart Watch, a nonrandomized series, in Hurst JW (ed): *Update II: The Heart*. McGraw-Hill, New York, 1980, p 239.

17 Proudfit WL: The prolongation of life by coronary bypass surgery: Experience at the Cleveland Clinic, in Hurst JW (ed): *Update II: The Heart*. McGraw-Hill, New York, 1980, p 255.

18 Loop FD, Sheldon WC, Lytle BW, Cosgrove DM, Proudfit WL: The efficacy of coronary artery surgery. Am Heart J, 101(1):86, 1981.

19 European Coronary Surgery Study Group: Long-term results of prospective randomized study of coronary artery bypass surgery in stable angina pectoris. Lancet, 2:1173, 1982.

20 Lichtlen P, Mocetti T, Halter J, et al: Postoperative evaluation of myocardial blood flow in aorto-to-coronary artery vein bypass grafting using xenon-residue detection technique. Circulation, 46:445, 1972.

21 Ormond J, Platt M, Mills L, et al: Thallium 201 scintigraphy and exercise testing in evaluating patients prior to and after coronary bypass surgery. Circulation, 56(suppl 3):131, 1977.

22 Marco JD: Myocardial perfusion following bypass surgery, in Hurst JW (ed): *Update II: The Heart*. McGraw-Hill, New York, 1980, p 13.

23 Furuse A, Klopp EH, Brawley RK, Gott VL: Hemodynamics of aorto-to-coronary artery bypass. Ann Thorac Surg, 14:282, 1972.

24 Kent KM, Borer JS, Green MV, et al: Effects of coronary artery bypass on global and regional left ventricular function during exercise. N Engl J Med, 298:1434, 1978.

25 Tyras DH, Admad N, Kaiser GC, et al: Ventricular function and the native coronary circulation five years after myocardial revascularization. Ann Thorac Surg, 27:547, 1979.

26 Bates ER, Vogel RA, LeFree MT, et al: The chronic coronary flow reserve provided by saphenous vein

bypass grafts as determined by digital coronary radiography. Accepted by Am Heart J (in press).

27 Meier B, Gruentzig AR, Siegenthaler WE, Schlumpf M: Long-term exercise performance after percutaneous transluminal coronary angioplasty and coronary artery bypass grafting. Circulation, 68:796–802. 1983.

28 Hirzel HO, Nuesch K, Gruentzig AR, Horst W, Krayenbuehl HP: Thallium 201 exercise scintigraphy after percutaneous transluminal angioplasty of coronary artery stenosis. Med Clin North Am, 64:163–176, 1980.

29 Peterson R, King SB III, Fajman W, Douglas JS Jr, Jones R: Relationship of coronary artery stenosis and gradient to exercise-induced ischemia. J Am Coll Cardiol I(2):673, 1983 (abstract).

30 Aueron F, Gruentzig A, Vogel RA, King SB, Douglas J, Meier B, et al: Effects of successful percutaneous transluminal coronary angioplasty (PTCA) on acute and chronic coronary flow reserve. Circulation, 68:4, October 1983 (abstract).

31 King SB III, Hurst JW: The relief of angina pectoris by coronary bypass surgery, in Hurst JW (ed): *Update II: The Heart*. McGraw-Hill, New York, 1980, p 71.

32 Oberman A, Wayne JB, Kouchoukos NT, Charles ED, Russell RO Jr, Rogers WL: Employment status after coronary artery bypass surgery. Circulation, 65(suppl II):II-115, 1982.

33 Hammermeister KE, DeRouen TA, English MT, Dodge HT: Effect of surgical versus medical therapy on return to work in patients with coronary artery disease. Am J Cardiol, 44:105, 1979.

34 Benesch L, Neuhaus KL, Rivas-Martin J, Loogen F: Clinical results and return to work after coronary heart surgery, in Roskamm H, Schmuziger M (ed): *Coronary Heart Surgery*. Springer-Verlag, New York, 1979, pp 379–384.

35 David P: Contributing factors preventing return to work of cardiac surgery patients. Cleve Clin Q, 45:177, 1978.

36 Symmes JC, Lenkei SCM, Berman ND: Influence of aortocoronary bypass surgery on employment. Can Med Assoc J, 118:268, 1978.

37 Anderson AJ, Barboriak JJ, Hoffmann RG, Mullen DC: Retention or resumption of employment after aortocoronary bypass operations. JAMA, 243:543, 1980.

38 Almeida D, Bradford JM, Wenger NK, King SB III, Hurst JW: Return to work after coronary bypass surgery. Circulation, 68(suppl II):II-205–II–213, September 1983.

39 Kannel WB, Feinleib M: Natural history of angina pectoris in the Framingham Study: Prognosis and survival. Am J Cardiol, 29:154, 1972.

40 Gazes PC, Mobley EM, Farris MH Jr, et al: Preinfarction (unstable) angina: A prospective study. Ten year follow up. Circulation, 48:331, 1973.

41 Hammermeister KE, DeRouen TA, Dodge HT: Variables predictive of survival in patients with coronary disease: Selection by univariate and multivariate analyses from the clinical, electrocardiographic, exercise, arteriographic, and quantitative angiographic evaluations. Circulation, 59:421, 1979.

42 Read RC, Murphy ML, Hultgren HN, et al: Survival of men treated for chronic stable angina pectoris: A cooperative randomized study. J Thorac Cardiovasc Surg, 75:1, 1978.

43 Coronary Artery Surgery Study (CASS): A randomized trial of coronary artery bypass surgery. Survival data. Circulation, 68(5):939–950, November 1983.

44 Meier B, King SB III, Gruentzig AR, Douglas JS, Hollman J, et al: Repeat coronary angioplasty. J Am Coll Cardiol, September 1984 (in press).

45 Mason DT, Amsterdam EA, DeMaria AN, et al: The prevention of myocardial infarction by coronary bypass surgery, in Hurst JW (ed): *Update II: The Heart*. McGraw-Hill, New York, 1980, p 103.

46 Libow M, Cooke D, King SB III, Gruentzig AR, Douglas JS Jr, et al: Left ventricular function after unsuccessful angioplasty and emergency coronary bypass surgery (submitted to American College of Cardiology annual meeting).

47 Hultgren H, the VA Study participants: VA Cooperative Study of Stable Angina: Comparison of medical versus surgical treatment upon symptoms. Circulation, 58:II-151, 1978 (abstract).

48 Frick MH, Harjola PT, Valle M: Persistence of improved exercise tolerance and degree of revascularization after coronary bypass surgery: A prospective randomized study. Clin Cardiol, 2:81, 1979.

49 Russell RO, Resnekov L, Wolf M, et al: Unstable angina pectoris: National cooperative study group to compare surgical and medical therapy. In-hospital experience and initial follow-up results in patients with one, two, and three vessel disease. Am J Cardiol, 42:839, 1978.

50 Gruentzig AR: Transluminal dilatation of coronary artery stenosis. Lancet, 1:263, 1978.
51 Sheldon WC, Loop FD: Direct myocardial revascularization—1976: Progress report on the Cleveland Clinic experience, Cleve Clin Q 43(3):97, Fall 1976.
52 Walker JA, Friedberg HD, Flemma RJ, Johnson WD: Determinants of angiographic patency of aortocoronary vein bypass grafts. Circulation, 45, 46(suppl I):86, 1972.
53 Sheldon WC: Factors influencing patency of coronary bypass grafts: The first decade of bypass graft surgery for coronary artery disease. An international symposium "Syllabus" prepared by the Cleveland Clinic Foundation, September 1977, p 77.
54 Campeau L, Crochet D, Lesperance J, Bourassa MG, Grondin CM: Postoperative changes in aortocoronary saphenous vein grafts revisited: Angiographic studies at two weeks and at one year in two series of consecutive patients. Circulation, 52:369, 1975.
55 Campeau L, Lesperance J, Corbara F, Hermann J, Grondin CM, Bourassa MG: Aortocoronary saphenous vein bypass graft changes 5 to 7 years after surgery. Circulation, 58(suppl I):170, 1978.
56 Kouchoukas NT, Karp RB, Oberman A, Russell RO Jr, Alison HW, Holt JH Jr: Long-term patency of saphenous veins for coronary bypass grafting. Circulation, 58(suppl I):96, 1978.
57 Lawrie GM, Lie JT, Morris GC Jr, Beazley JL: Vein graft patency and intimal proliferation after aortocoronary bypass: Early and long-term angiopathologic correlations. Am J Cardiol, 38:856, 1976.
58 Bourassa MG, Lesperance J, Corbara F, Saltiel J, Campeau L: Progression of obstructive coronary artery disease 5 to 7 years after aortocoronary bypass surgery. Circulation, 58(suppl I):100, 1978.
59 European Coronary Surgery Study Group: Long term results of prospective randomized study of coronary artery bypass surgery in stable angina pectoris. Lancet, 2:1173–1180, 1982.
60 Special report: National Institutes of Health Concensus-Development Conference Statement: Coronary-artery bypass surgery: Scientific and clinical aspects. N Engl J Med, 304(11):680, 1981.
61 Loop FD, Sheldon WC, Lytle BW, Cosgrove DM, Proudfit WL: The efficacy of coronary artery surgery. Am Heart J, 101(1):86, 1981.
62 Barnes RW, Marszalek PB, Rittgers SE: Asymptomatic carotid disease in preoperative patients. Stroke,II:VII-8, 136, 1980.
63 Mehigan JT, et al: A planned approach to coexistent cerebrovascular disease in coronary artery bypass candidates. Arch Surg, 112:1403, 1977.
64 Jones EL: Combined carotid and coronary surgery—When is it necessary? J Cardiovasc Med, 8(6):676–680. June 1983, p 676–680.
65 Jones EL, King SB III: Intraoperative angioplasty in the treatment of coronary artery disease. J Am Coll Cardiol, 1(3):970–971, March 1983 (editorial).
66 Edwards WD, Tajik AJ, Seward JB: Standardized nomenclature and anatomic basis for regional tomographic analysis of the heart. Mayo Clin Proc, 56:479–497, 1981.
67 Mock MB, Ringquist I, Fischer L, et al: The survival of nonoperated patients with ischemic heart disease: The CASS experience. Am J Cardiol, 49:1007, 1982 (abstract).
68 Califf RM, Tomabechi Y, Lee KL: Outcome in one vessel coronary artery disease. Circulation, 67:283–290, 1983.
69 Brooks N, Cattell M, Jennings K, et al: Isolated disease of left anterior descending coronary artery: Angiographic and clinical study of 218 patients. Br. Heart J, 47:1189–1196, 1982.
70 Califf RM, Conley MJ, Bechar VS: Left main equivalent coronary disease: Its clinical presentation and prognostic significance with non-surgical therapy. Am J Cardiol (in press).

Chapter 16

Thrombolytic Therapy

Douglas C. Morris, M.D.

Any discussion of intracoronary thrombolysis and its applicability in clinical practice must first attempt to resolve three disputable issues. These issues are as follows: (1) Is coronary thrombosis the cause of or the sequela of a myocardial infarction? (2) Is there a lytic agent or agents available capable of lysing this thrombus? (3) Can this lytic process by completed rapidly enough to preserve ischemic myocardium?

Thrombolytic therapy is predicated upon the premise that coronary thrombosis is the cause of myocardial infarction. Just such an assumption led to the recognition for years of *coronary thrombosis* as a clinicopathological entity and an accepted diagnosis for acute myocardial necrosis secondary to ischemia. While in recent years this previously accepted premise has been seriously questioned,[1] there exists a substantial body of data which supports the classic concept of the primary role of thrombosis in the pathogenesis of transmural myocardial infarction.

Table 16-1 lists the pathological studies and Table 16-2 lists the angiographic studies of patients with acute transmural myocardial infarction. The statistically close association of thrombotic arterial occlusion and acute myocardial infarction in most of these studies would suggest a causal relationship. Secondly, the consistent topographical relation between the thrombus and the infarcted tissue in the pathological studies supports this contention. Since the thrombi consistently occurred proximally in the arteries subtending the infarcted tissue, a relationship must be assumed. It would seem that a secondary relationship between the thrombus and the infarction would result in a more haphazard distribution of the occlusions around the periphery and within the confines of the infarcted tissue.[2] Acceptance of the premise that transmural myo-

Table 16-1 Coronary Thrombosis in Transmural Infarction—Pathological Studies

Investigator	Prevalence of thrombus, %	Spatial relations
Chapman	91	Thrombus occurs proximal to infarct in artery supplying infarcted tissue.
Erhardt	100	Thrombus occurs in artery supplying infarcted tissue.
Roberts	54	Site of necrosis corresponds with artery containing thrombus.
Schwartz	86	Most thrombi proximal and anatomically subtend infarct.
Sinapius	97	Constant relation exists between thrombus and infarcted tissue.
Spain	90	Infarcts are associated with arterial thrombus.

cardial infarctions are generally preceded by the formation of a thrombus at the site of a previously established atherosclerotic lesion does not require rejection of the following: Many ischemic events terminating in sudden death are not initiated by an acute thrombus[2]; thrombotic occlusion can occur without infarction in the presence of adequate collateral circulation[8]; and subendocardial infarctions can develop in the absence of coronary occlusion.[9]

The second issue to resolve is whether there are lytic agents available which are capable of lysing thrombi. The mechanism of action of the two currently available lytic agents, streptokinase and urokinase, is portrayed in Fig. 16-1. It is worth noting the slight difference in the manner in which the direct-acting urokinase and the indirect-acting streptokinase enter the fibrinolytic cascade. The efficacy of either of these agents in thrombolysis is irrefutable. The data supporting this efficacy extends from the original studies of lysis of artificially produced thrombi in arteries of dogs[10] and veins of rabbits[11] to more recent work on pulmonary emboli[12] and deep venous thrombosis[13] in human beings. Furthermore, there is nothing about the composition of a coronary thrombus which would render it uniquely refractory to thrombolysis. Dis-

Table 16-2 Coronary Thrombosis in Transmural Infarction—Angiographic Studies

Investigator	Number of patients	Time of study, hours after infarct	Prevalence of total occlusion of artery, %
DeWood[2]	126	4	87
Rentrop[3]	29	15	69
Lee[4]	26	7	85
Reduto[5]	37	18	81
Cowley[6]	11	6	91
Morris	28	5	93

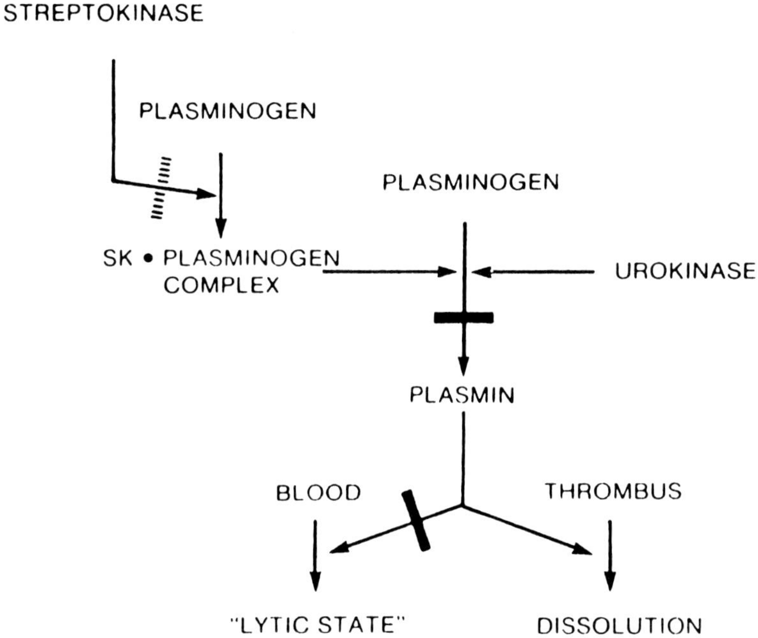

Figure 16-1 Fibrinolytic cascade depicting the point of entry of streptokinase and urokinase.

tally, the thrombus is more likely to be composed of platelets or fibrin or both (white thrombus), whereas proximally it consists of erthrocytes, lesser quantities of fibrin, few platelets, and some leukocytes (red thrombus).

The final premise which must be accepted in order to adopt the application of intracoronary thrombolysis is that the entire process can be completed rapidly enough to preserve a significant portion of the ischemic myocardium. In this regard, data from canine models must be reviewed. Temporary coronary artery occlusion studies, employing a variety of models and techniques, have generally supported the idea that salvageable myocardium is present for 2 to 3 hours after coronary occlusion. On the other hand, permanent occlusion of the vessel for 24 or more hours causes necrosis which is essentially transmural. These observations indicate that not all cells in the ischemic myocardium die simultaneously and that myocardial tissue is available for salvage for a period of hours. Reimer et al. demonstrated by temporary left circumflex coronary artery occlusion in anesthetized open chest dogs that 55 percent of the myocardium at risk of ischemia remained viable after only 40 minutes of occlusion compared with 33 percent in a group of dogs checked after 3 hours of occlusion and 16 percent in a group with 6 hours of occlusion[14] (Fig. 16-2). Their study also established that the progression of necrosis was from the subendocardial myocardial region outward.[14]

Most studies confirming the beneficial effect of coronary artery reperfusion have been performed on anesthesized animals.[15,16] Baughman and associates, however, using conscious dogs found that myocardial infarction size tended to be diminished by reperfusion but that the effect was not statistically significant unless dogs with very small infarcts were excluded.[17] These investigators contended that the inability to reach statistical significance in their study was due to the large variability in infarct size in the animals with permanent coronary occlusion. Other investigators have not observed beneficial effects of reperfusion even 1 to 3 hours after coronary artery occlusion.[18,19] A possible explanation for the lack of improvement in some of these studies is the observation that the recovery of reperfused myocardium is significantly

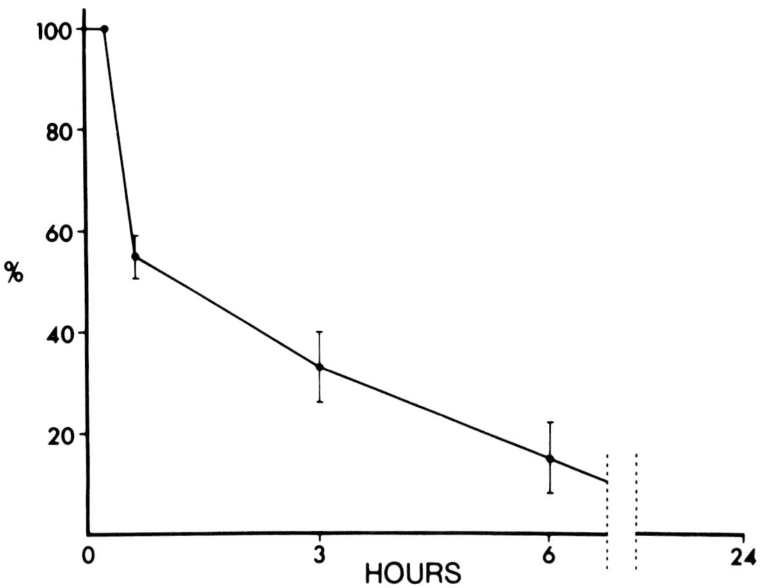

Figure 16-2 This graph depicts the percentage of myocardium which remains viable (ordinate) over time following occlusion of a coronary artery (abscissa). (*From Reimer et al[14]; reprinted with permission of the authors and the American Heart Association.*)

greater at 7 to 14 days following reperfusion than immediately after reperfusion.[20,21]

The other question which has arisen with regard to reperfusion is whether the intramyocardial hemorrhage which often accompanies reperfusion is associated with extension of necrosis. The study of Higginson and associates seems to allay this concern.[22] These investigators demonstrated that hemorrhage during reperfusion was confined to the myocardium which was previously necrotic.

The majority of investigations, therefore, suggest that the very early initiation of thrombolytic therapy after the onset of a myocardial infarction is theoretically justified.

HISTORY OF THROMBOLYTIC THERAPY IN MYOCARDIAL INFARCTION

The first investigation of the use of thrombolytic therapy in the treatment of acute myocardial infarction was made by Anthony Fletcher and associates in 1959.[23] These investigators infused streptokinase intravenously over 30 hours into 22 patients with acute myocardial infarction. The infusion began 5 to 16 hours after the onset of the infarction. The absence of unusual events during the follow-up of the survivors convinced the investigators that streptokinase had no deleterious effects. Secondly, the investigators surmised that in vivo thrombolysis was produced because two of their three immediate deaths had no coronary thrombus and the electrocardiograms in four of their fourteen 6-month survivors were normal.[23]

One year later Boucek and Murphy reported on their technique of segmental perfusion of the coronary arteries with fibrinolysin.[24] In their technique the investigators perfused the occluded coronary artery through a side-hole catheter positioned in the appropriate sinus of Valsalva so that the coronary ostium was in juxtaposition with the catheter orifice. The perfusion was delivered only during the middle and last third of diastole, which had been previously determined in canine models as the critical period of coronary flow. This technique was applied in eight patients without significant complications. A reluctance by the investigators, however, to inject radiopaque material prevented them from providing conclusive evidence of thrombolysis.

These observations coupled with the findings by Nydick and associates in 1961 that lysis of an experimentally induced coronary thrombus caused a reduction in infarct size[25] formed the foundation for subsequent clinical studies of thrombolytic therapy of myocardial infarction. Subsequent studies did not follow immediately primarily because of the significant pyrogenicity of the initial preparations of streptokinase. Secondly, it took the advent of coronary arteriography and its application in acute ischemic events to confirm the causative role of coronary thrombosis in acute myocardial infarction.

The first large clinical evaluation of the systemic infusion of streptokinase in the treatment of myocardial infarction was reported in 1979. This controlled, randomized, multicenter study demonstrated a significant reduction in the 6-month overall mortality rate (15.6 versus 30.6 percent) in the streptokinase group.[26] Rentrop spearheaded the initial clinical studies of intracoronary thrombolysis, and the first large clinical study of this technique was reported by his group in 1981.[4]

CLINICAL RESULTS

Table 16-3 lists the studies which have evaluated the efficacy of intracoronary thrombolysis. While the reported percentage of successful thrombolysis varies between 67 and 95 percent, a reasonable expectation of success would seem to be in the range of 60 to 75 percent. It must also be recognized that an acute restoration of coronary flow does not ensure permanency of this flow.[32] In fact, the 22 percent acute reocclusion rate in our series and the 17.6 percent in the study of Gold and associates[31] points to the high frequency of immediate reocclusion. The angiographic reocclusion rate when evaluated at least 1 week after thrombolysis varies between 5 and 25 percent.[4,5,27] These angiographic results do not accurately reflect the reinfarction rate, probably because of the development of improved collateral circulation in some patients preventing reinfarction upon reocclusion.[7] Conversely, a clinical diagnosis of postthrombolytic reinfarction is often difficult in the setting of an already altered electrocardiographic pattern and frequently still elevated serum enzyme levels. Consequently, some cases of reinfarction may go undiagnosed.

The success of thrombolysis seems to be related both to the duration of chest pain prior to streptokinase infusion and to the coronary artery involved. Both the length of infusion necessary to produce lysis and the likelihood of lysis vary with the duration of symptoms. Lee and associates reported a 75 percent reperfusion rate in patients receiving streptokinase within 5 hours of the onset of chest pain versus 50 percent in those treated at 5 to 7 hours after onset of symptoms and 17 percent when treated beyond 7 hours.[5] Rutsch and his collaborators noted the lysis occurred within 23 minutes if the thrombus was less than 2 hours old versus 43 minutes if the thrombus was older than 4 hours.[33] Successful recanalization of the left an-

Table 16-3 Results of Thrombolysis

Study	Number of patients	Successful lysis, %	Angiographic reocclusion, %	Reopening interval, min
Ganz[26]	20	95	8.3*	21 (average)
Cowley[7]	10	70	25	24 ± 7
Rentrop[4]	29	76	5.2	15–90
Lee[5]	22	82	16	—
Reduto[6]	30	67	—	24 ± 13
Mathey[27]	41	72	20	29 ± 15
Anderson[30]	24	79	—	30 ± 22.7
Khaja[31]	20	60	—	—
Gold[32]	40	85	31	24 ± 17
Kennedy[33]	134	65	—	—
Morris	37	73	26	39 (average)

*Clinical reocclusion; no angiographic restudy performed.

terior descending artery and the right coronary artery requires a briefer infusion time than the recanalization of circumflex coronary artery[33] and is more likely to be successful.[34] Another factor which is not adequately defined in most studies is the number of patients with subtotal occlusions versus total occlusions. The larger the proportion of patients with subtotal occlusion in the study, the higher will be the success rate.

While the importance of expeditious initiation of thrombolysis seems to be confirmed, the optimal total dose and the ideal rate of administration of streptokinase remains undefined. The total doses employed have ranged between 220,000 and 500,000 IU while the rate of administration has ranged between 1000 and 5000 IU/min. Some investigators have initiated streptokinase administration with a 10,000- to 20,000-IU bolus of the lytic agent.[4,6] There is no data to support an improved efficacy of thrombolysis by using this initial bolus. With the exception of Ganz et al.,[27] who observed that patency of the artery was achieved faster with an infusion rate of 4000 IU, an infusion rate of 2000 IU/min has appeared adequate. The use of a subselective infusion technique (a small catheter extended down to the thrombus), at least in canine models, offers some advantage over infusion from a catheter further removed from the thrombus.[35] Reocclusion of a coronary artery does seem to occur more often in those patients who are not adequately anticoagulated following successful thrombolysis. Reocclusion also occurs more often in the left circumflex artery than in either of the other two major arteries.[34] Ganz and associates suggested that infusion of the thrombolytic agent for at least 60 minutes following reperfusion was necessary to prevent early rethrombosis.[27] Our data suggests that in those patients who demonstrate rapid passage of contrast medium past the residual obstruction following reperfusion, continued infusion of the thrombolytic agent is not required.

The average infusion time required to establish patency is approximately 30 minutes. A continuation of infusion beyond 60 minutes is difficult to justify because of the reduced likelihood of reestablishing permanent patency and the reduced likelihood of preserving muscle after this interval of time. Clearly the percentage of patients who will have coronary flow reestablished can be increased by prolonged continuation of streptokinase infusion; however, patency will likely be gained at the expense of producing a systemic lytic state, and there will be little chance of preserving a significant amount of myocardium. Preservation of myocardium is the goal of the efforts at thrombolysis, while reestablishing coronary flow is only the means to this end.

Attempts to measure the degree of myocardial preservation by thrombolysis primarily rest upon follow-up evaluation of the left ventricular ejection fraction. The chronic improvement in the ejection fraction has generally been 9 to 10 percent with a range of 6 to 10 percent (Table 16-4).[4–7,28] It does seem that in many patients at least a week passes before this improvement in contractility becomes evident. Reduto et al., for example, noted no significant change in left ventricular performance from immediately before infusion to immediately after

Table 16-4 Improvement in Left Ventricular Function

	Ejection fraction, %		
Study	Prior to thrombolysis, %	Following thrombolysis, %	Change, %
Cowley[7]	42 ± 5	52 ± 5	(10)
Rentrop[4]	50.5 ± 12	56.6 ± 12.4	(6)
Lee[5]	46	56	(10)
Reduto[6]	46 ± 15	55 ± 10	(9)
Mathey[27]	37 ± 5	47 ± 4	(10)

infusion, but found a 9 percent increase in the ejection fraction at a mean of 10 days after infusion.[6] With a few exceptions, our experience has been similar with a preinfusion ejection fraction of 50 percent, an immediate postinfusion value of 52 percent, and at 10 days after infusion a value of 58 percent. Other studies, however, have noted an immediate improvement in ventricular function.[36] Any immediate improvement in ejection fraction can be attributed, at least in part, to the afterload reduction produced by the administration of streptokinase.

In considering the improvement in ventricular function, we must be cognizant of the fact that there is an anticipated variability in left ventricular ejection fraction of 5 percent or less in patients with depressed contractility (ejection fraction less than 55 percent) and of as high as 12 percent in patients with normal contractility.[32] Furthermore, spontaneous changes in left ventricular ejection fraction from a 32 percent increase to 14 percent decrease have been noted during the first 24 hours of a transmural infarction.[38] Contrary to these results, studies of thrombolytic therapy have shown that only 33 percent of patients with nonreperfused coronary arteries demonstrated sequential improvement in left ventricular contractility as compared with 79 percent of patients with reperfused coronary arteries.[39] Pathological studies and intraoperative inspection also add some validity to the studies demonstrating improved left ventricular contractility following thrombolysis. Intraoperative myocardial biopsy specimens obtained from the center of reperfused tissue in three patients revealed the bulk of tissue was preserved. In two patients the necrosis was subendocardial, and in the third the necrosis was in scattered, nonconfluent areas.[36] Furthermore, cardiovascular surgeons are generally impressed that even akinetic left ventricular segments which have had a restoration of their blood flow demonstrate an absence of epicardial evidence of infarction. Also, a study of coronary artery reperfusion at 1 and 3 hours after occlusion in conscious dogs could not demonstrate a beneficial effect on infarct size but did reveal a striking beneficial effect on survival.[17] Finally, the surgical experiences of Berg et al. suggest an improved hospital and first year survival rate and decreased morbidity rate (lesser prevalence of ventricular septal rupture, ventricular aneurysm, and papillary muscle rupture) in patients receiving myocardial perfusion by coronary artery bypass grafting within 6 hours of the start of chest pain as compared to the general and local medical experience.[40] The patients did not receive thrombolysis prior to surgery.

Another important beneficial effect of thrombolysis is the immediate relief of chest pain due to an alleviation of myocardial ischemia. With a few exceptions, the patients experience prompt relief of chest pain concordant with reestablishment of coronary blood flow. This temporal relation is so striking that it makes for convincing evidence that persistent pain associated with an acute myocardial infarction reflects ongoing ischemia of viable myocardium. Furthermore, a recurrence of pain is generally indicative of reocclusion of the previously occluded coronary artery.

Coronary thrombolysis is usually accompanied by electrocardiographic changes. Usually the ST-segment elevation noted at the initiation of thrombolytic therapy is markedly reduced and often returns to the baseline. Figure 16-3 demonstrates a common electrocardiographic sequence during thrombolysis. Reperfusion dramatically accelerates the electrocardiographic evolution of an acute myocardial infarction. The rapid sequence of electrocardiographic changes concordant with thrombolysis indicates that the absence of "pathological" Q waves at the onset does not imply the absence of irreversible ischemic injury. The evolutionary changes also serve as a reminder that thrombolysis is intended to reduce infarct size and not prevent an infarction.

Figure 16-4 demonstrates the typical patterns for total serum creatine phosphokinase and the MB band for patients with successful reperfusion as compared with controls and those who did not achieve thrombolysis. Typically, the peak creatine phosphokinase level is higher and occurs sooner following reperfusion. The peak serum creatine

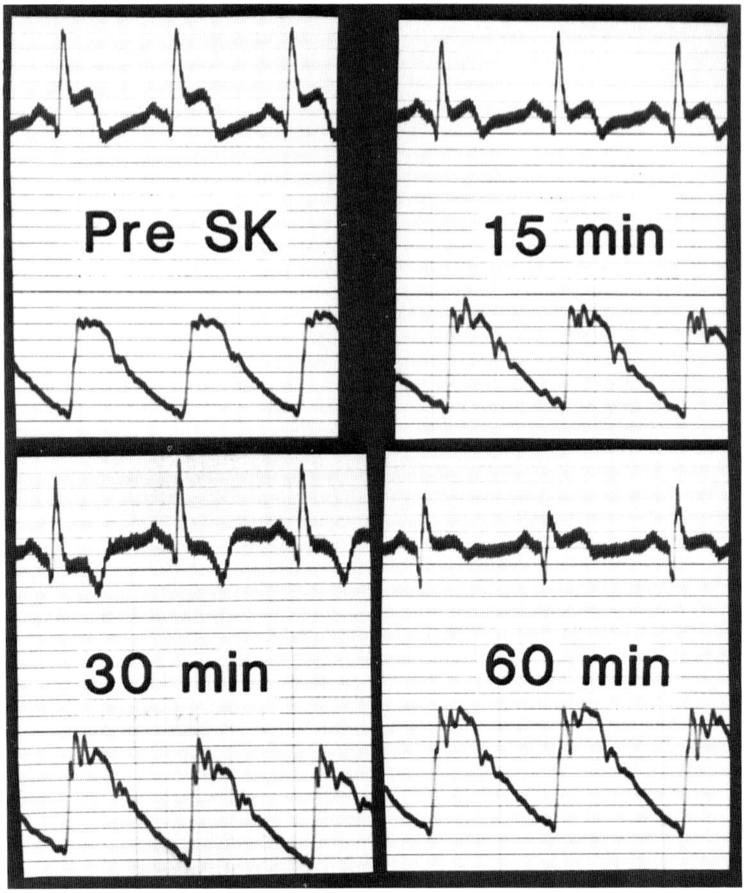

Figure 16-3 Electrocardiographic evolution of an acute inferior myocardial infarction occurring over the 60 minutes of intracoronary streptokinase infusion with reperfusion achieved. Pre SK = prestreptokinase.

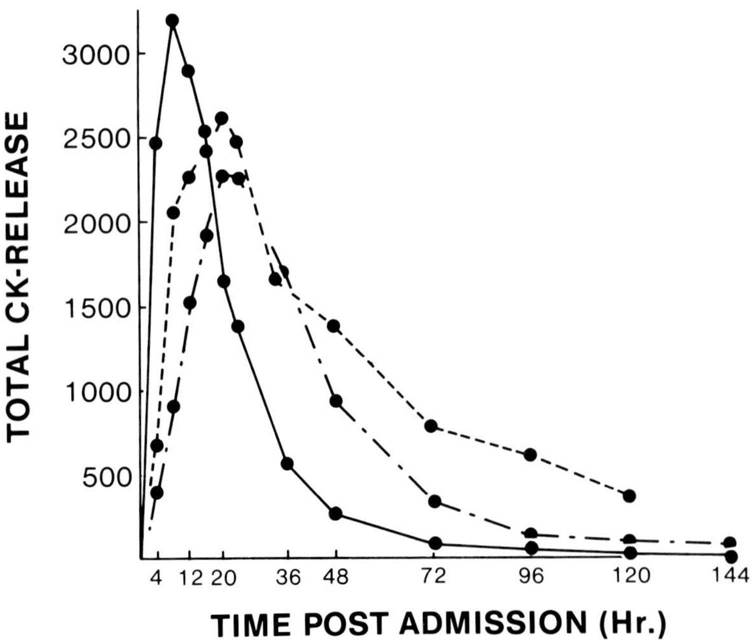

Figure 16-4 Creatine kinase (CK) release following acute myocardial infarction in patients with thrombolysis (————), in patients receiving streptokinase who did not achieve thrombolysis (—·—·—), and in patients not receiving streptokinase (– – – – – –).

phosphokinase was 2879 units occurring at 8 hours after the onset of the infarction as compared to a peak of 2621 occurring at 20 hours in the control group. It is assumed that creatine phosphokinase washout after coronary artery reperfusion contributes significantly to the amount of the enzyme released from the infarcted myocardium. Vatner and associates demonstrated that the total amount of creatine phosphokinase measured in the serum following reperfusion is nearly twice as high per gram of necrotic myocardium as it would be without reperfusion.[41]

CONTRAINDICATIONS AND ADVERSE EFFECTS

Patients with bleeding disorders or contraindications to anticoagulation, those with recent intracerebral or spinal surgery, and patients who have undergone extensive resuscitative efforts should not have thrombolytic therapy.

A possible adverse effect of coronary thrombolysis is the so-called reperfusion arrhythmia. The arrhythmia is generally ventricular extrasystoles, but may be ventricular tachycardia or ventricular fibrillation. Immediate cardioversion is usually followed by sustained stability of the cardiac rhythm. Since the frequency of ventricular fibrillation has been rather low in our experience (1 out of 30), we do not feel compelled to use prophylactic lidocaine infusion during thrombolysis.

The most common adverse effect of streptokinase is hemorrhage. While intracoronary infusion of streptokinase has been purported to produce local thrombolysis without systemic lysis, this is generally not the case. In fact, preliminary data suggests that successful coronary thrombolysis correlates with production of a systemic lytic effect.[39] Major bleeding (defined as that necessitating blood transfusion) has been significantly associated with a fibrinogen concentration below 100 mg/dL. With few exceptions, our patients demonstrated fibrinogen levels in this range following our customary dose of 240,000 to 300,000 units of streptokinase. Strict avoidance of venous or arterial punctures, limiting movement of the patient, and keeping the femoral artery puncture site plugged with a catheter introducer sheath during the first 12 hours after thrombolysis has kept our bleeding complications low. Our only problems with hemorrhage have been persistent bleeding at a puncture site following early removal of a sheath and hematemesis. Other studies have also found these to be the most frequent bleeding problems.[35]

Another possible occurrence which must be considered as an adverse effect of thrombolysis is reinfarction secondary to reocclusion of a coronary artery. This untoward event occurring in as many as 17 percent of the patients[34] is accompanied by chest discomfort and may be accompanied by life-threatening arrhythmias.

POSTREPERFUSION THERAPY

Following completion of thrombolysis, the patient has generally been left with a coronary artery narrowed by the atherogenic process to at least 50 percent of the luminal diameter. Rutsch and his collaborators found only 24 percent of their patients had a residual stenosis which was less severe.[33] Figures 16-5 and 16-6 are examples of the variability of residual stenosis following streptokinase, and Fig. 16-7 is a sequential example taken every 15 minutes of the gradual resolution of a thrombus. In those patients with severe obstructive lesions remaining after thrombolysis, further intervention must be considered. In the only study examining the posthospitalization results of patients undergoing thrombolysis 70 percent of the patients having coronary bypass or coronary angioplasty remained free of chest pain and reinfarction compared to 57 percent of those treated medically.[42] While these results favor surgical intervention, they are not impressive enough to compel a physician to proceed to surgery in those patients who are suboptimal surgical candidates because of poor distal vessels or very little viable myocardium remaining in jeopardy of ischemia. Wisdom would seem to dictate that the physician should substantiate how much myocardium has been

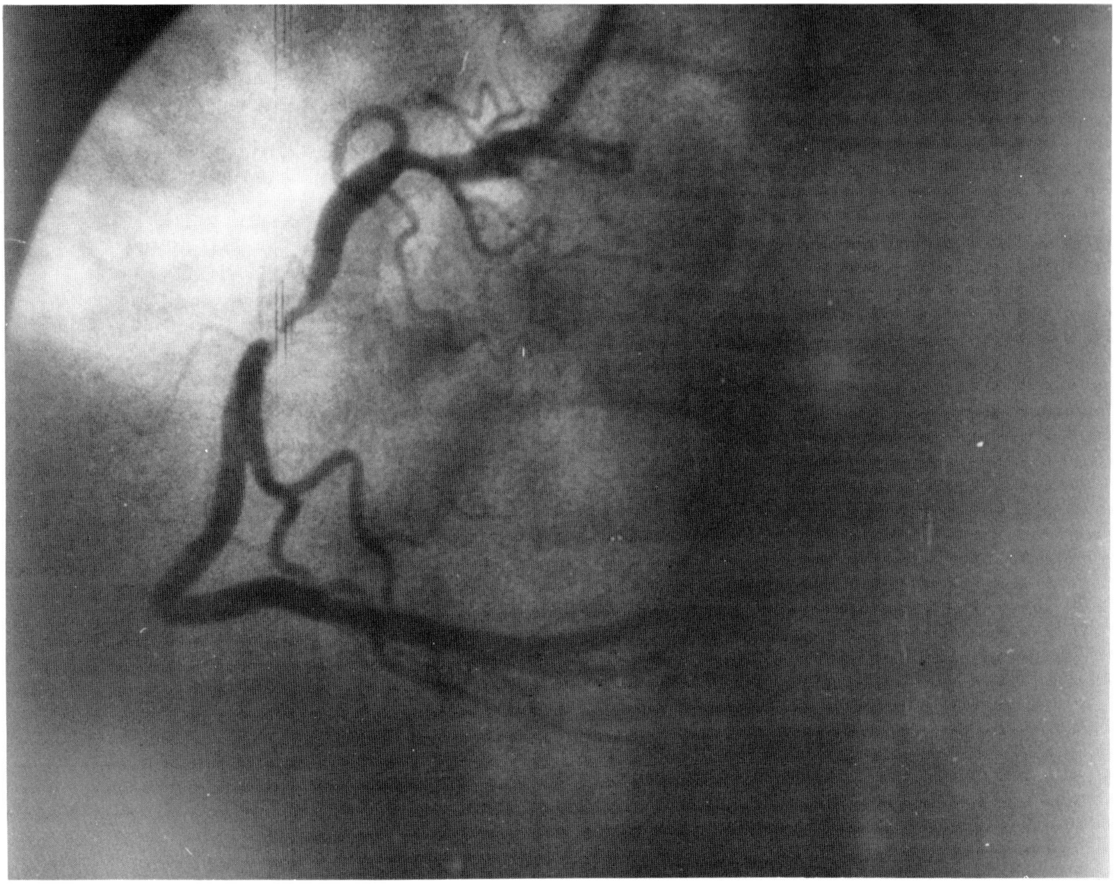

Figure 16-5 Right coronary artery demonstrating severe residual obstruction following thrombolysis. The majority of our patients have had similar significant obstructions.

preserved before recommending further intervention. In our experience an evaluation of left ventricular function by radionuclide ventriculography and of myocardial perfusion by thallium-201 scintigraphy is the best means of assessing the amount of preserved myocardium. Data on the group of patients followed who were on medical therapy revealed that 71 percent of those patients receiving warfarin had no chest pain or reinfarction as compared to only 44 percent of those not receiving warfarin or antiplatelet agents.[42] These results suggest anticoagulation should be part of the therapy in those patients treated medically.

When surgery or angioplasty has appeared indicated because of the presence of a significant residual coronary obstruction following thrombolysis, our practice has been to maintain anticoagulation with heparin and wait 1 to 3 days before proceeding with that more definitive therapy. Our inclination to wait has been based upon the following: a reluctance to proceed to coronary artery bypass grafting until we have documented viable myocardium in the reperfused region, a concern that angioplasty immediately following reperfusion is less successful than that performed several days later after the obstructive lesion has stabilized, and

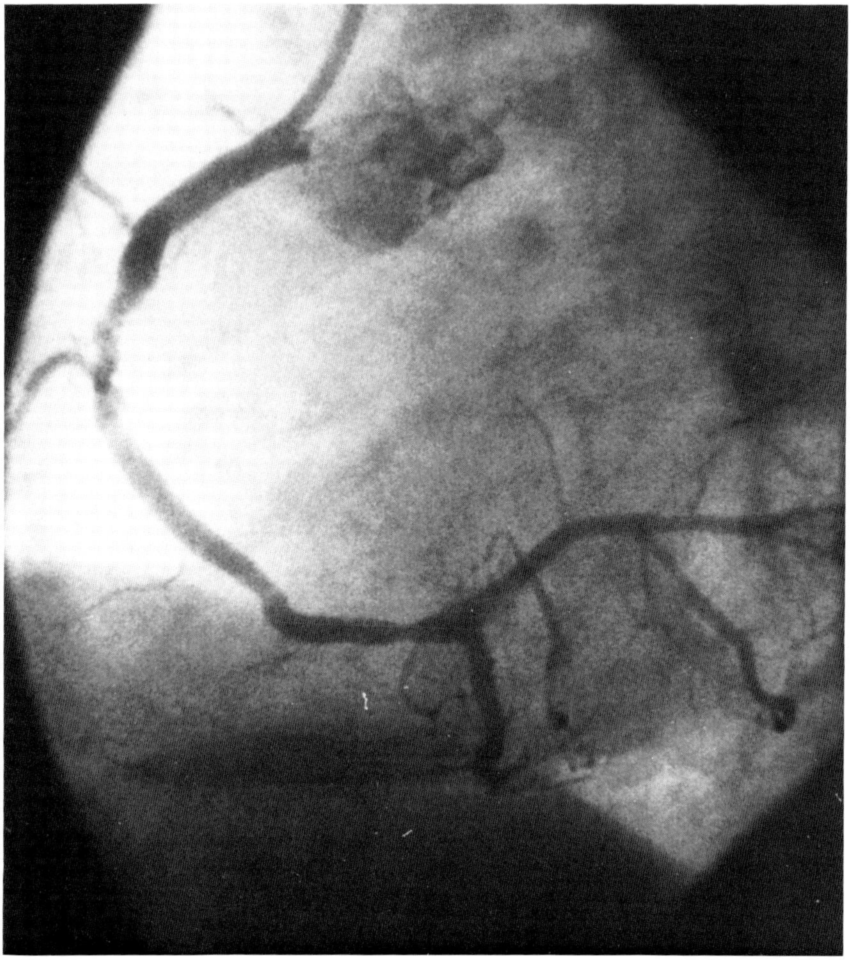

Figure 16-6 Right coronary artery demonstrating mild residual obstruction following thrombolysis. It is unusual to have obstructions of this severity following thrombolysis.

a concern that the bleeding problems arising from operating upon a defibrinogenated patient would be significant. In the limited number of patients we have sent to surgery immediately following attempts at thrombolysis, however, no significant bleeding problems have been encountered. Our results are supported by those of Becker and associates, who found no increase in the risk of bleeding in patients undergoing coronary artery bypass grafting within 24 hours after intracoronary thrombolysis.[43]

Other investigators have advocated early angioplasty because of the threat of early reclosure. We certainly would not hold to our waiting period if the residual lesion was so severe that resting coronary blood flow was reduced.

TECHNIQUE

The most critical factor in successful thrombolytic therapy is time. Successful thrombolysis can only be achieved by a team of persons well-versed in

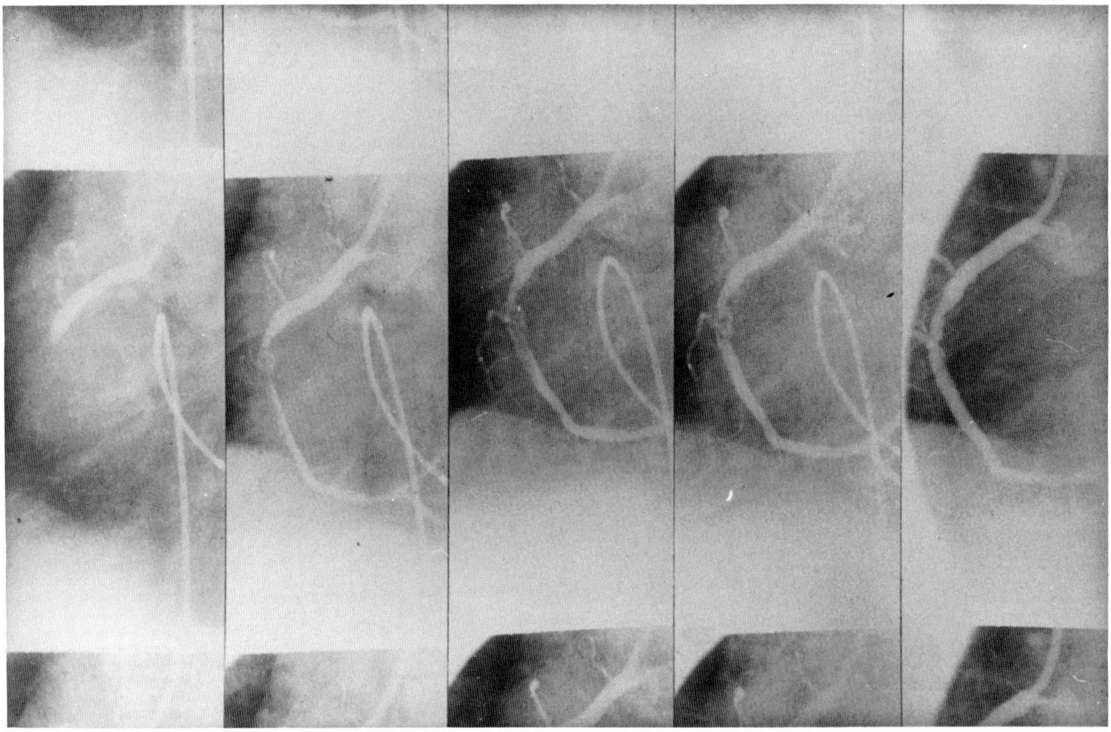

Figure 16-7 Sequential arteriograms of right coronary artery taken at 15-minute intervals during streptokinase infusion.

all details of the procedure and assigned specific responsiblities.

Although bradyarrhythmias have not been encountered in our experience, reports of such with inferior infarctions[39] argues for introduction of a transvenous pacemaker in these cases. Development of cardiogenic shock in two patients with occlusion of a left anterior descending artery prior to any of its branches convinced us to initiate aortic counterpulsation in these patients. Aortic counterpulsation also seems advisable in those patients with an initial left ventricular end-diastolic pressure greater than 30 mmHg.

Once the coronary catheter has been introduced, heparin should be administered (preferably through the catheter) to prevent thrombus formation on the catheter, which will likely remain in the systemic circulation for over an hour; 10,000 units of heparin are administered initially with another 5000 units administered at the end of each hour the catheter remains in the patient.

In addition, systemic administration of steroids prior to streptokinase infusion seems wise. The steroids are given to prevent an allergic reaction to streptokinase which was noted in 5.5 percent of the patients receiving streptokinase in the Urokinase-Streptokinase Embolism Trial.[44] The initial study of thrombolysis by Fletcher, Alkjaersig, and Sherry suggested that steroid administration would also reduce the rate and degree of whole blood fibrinolysis and restrain the development of plasma antithrombin activity.[23]

If the subselective infusion technique (which seems preferable) is to be used, a time limit should be placed on one's efforts to properly position the inner catheter. The inner catheter is a no. 3 or no. 4 French tubing with end and/or side holes which can be extended through the angiographic catheter to the site of the thrombus. If the inner catheter cannot be extended to the site of the thrombus, the angiographer should attempt to position its tip distal to any major branches extending from the occluded artery. The use of a no. 3 or no. 4 French infusion catheter in a high-flow no. 8 French or a no. 9 French angiographic catheter allows for the simultaneous monitoring of systemic pressure through the outer catheter and infusion through the inner catheter.

Remembering that time is of the essence, a more rapidly instituted infusion by the selective technique is preferable to a laborious and time-consuming attempt to achieve a subselective infusion.

Once coronary arteriography confirming coronary artery occlusion is completed, nitroglycerin is usually administered into the coronary artery in doses of 200 to 500 μg. In our experience and that of others,[5] the administration of nitroglycerin (with rare exception) produces no sustained angiographic coronary patency or relief of myocardial ischemic pain. Nevertheless, unless the patient is hypotensive, the adverse affects of the drug are minimal and the time spent administering it is brief. Again, remember the admonition about time and by no means delay administration of the streptokinase because of a problem with the nitroglycerin.

During the administration of streptokinase the arterial pressure should be monitored either through the catheter positioned in the coronary ostium (if the subselective technique is used) or by a catheter positioned in another artery. We believe injections of contrast medium into the occluded artery every 15 minutes during streptokinase administration is beneficial both as a means of monitoring the efficacy of therapy and perhaps as a means of hastening the response to the lytic agent. It has appeared that many of our patients first manifested the electrocardiographic changes characteristic of reperfusion at the instant the contrast medium was injected. Perhaps the force of the injection breaks up the thrombus which has been partially lysed.

The streptokinase should be administered in doses of 2000 to 4000 units per minute diluted in a 1- to 8-mL volume. Although the number of patients studied with a large infusion is too small to make us certain, it does seem that our success with thrombolysis has been greater infusing the same amount of streptokinase in 8 mL diluent per minute than in 1 mL. It also seems that no strong arguments can be made for the initial bolus of 10,000 to 20,000 units of streptokinase. Once patency has been established, a continuation of streptokinase infusion for another 30 minutes should be considered. A continuation of streptokinase infusion for over 60 minutes in the face of continued coronary artery occlusion cannot be endorsed on the basis of the Emory experience. In our experience, coronary arteries reperfused after 1 hour of perfusion have either reoccluded or not been associated with salvageable myocardium. Anticoagulation, first with intravenous heparin and later with oral warfarin, is indicated in any patient in whom thrombolysis is successful, and surgery or angioplasty is not applied.

It is advisable to leave the arterial catheter introducer in place for 12 hours following thrombolysis unless evidence of ischemia distal to the insertion site develops.

PRESENT ROLE OF THROMBOLYSIS

The data accumulated to date on thrombolysis still poses more questions than solutions. We can strongly advocate its use only with the availability of a cardiac catheterization laboratory team who are experienced in the use of thrombolysis and can apply this technique immediately. Furthermore, we would offer thrombolytic therapy to any patient who could have the intracoronary infusion begun within 3 hours of the onset of chest pain. The available data are insufficient to extend these recommendations to other patients.

Current investigation with recombinant tissue type plasminogen activator holds promise of a more dependable lytic agent devoid of the threat of systemic lysis. Perhaps the greatest role of streptokinase in coronary thrombolysis will be that of a forerunner for these later generation thrombolytic agents. Its use has established that myocardial preservation by coronary reperfusion is possible in the clinical setting.

Physicians considering the implementation of this technique must be cognizant of the following:

1 The technique requires a full cardiac catheterization team with members skilled in defibrillation, cardiopulmonary resuscitation, and treatment of pulmonary edema and shock. This would seem to be self-evident, but there is a tendency on off-hours to use a "skeleton crew."

2 The patient who seems very stable during the initial minutes of an infarction may not be so once the endogenous stores of catecholamines are depleted. Nothing is more frightening than to have a patient who was normotensive in the emergency room be discovered to be hypotensive when the catheter is inserted into the arterial system 30 to 60 minutes later. While the evidence may be strong that your procedure did not hasten the demise of a patient, you will have your doubts and probably so will the patient's family.

3 Once the coronary artery flow is reestablished, the patient must be considered to be very unstable due to possibility of reocclusion and hemorrhage and must be dealt with accordingly.

4 This procedure probably as much as any in cardiology causes the physician to experience the ecstasy of victory and the agony of defeat.

REFERENCES

1 Roberts WC, Buja LM: Frequency and significance of coronary arterial thrombi and other observations in fatal acute myocardial infarction: A study of 107 necropsy patients. Am J Med, 52:425–443, 1972.

2 Chandler AB, Chapman I, Erhardt LR, Roberts WC, Schwartz CJ, Sinapius D, Spain DM, Sherry S, Ness PM, Simon TL: Coronary thrombosis in myocardial infarction: Report of a workshop on the role of coronary thrombosis in the pathogenesis of acute myocardial infarction. Am J Cardiol, 34:823–832, 1974.

3 DeWood MA, Spores J, Notske R, Mouser LT, Burroughs R, Golden MS, Lang HT: Prevalence of total coronary occlusion during the early hours of transmural myocardial infarction. N Engl J Med, 303:897–902, 1980.

4 Rentrop P, Blaske H, Karsch KR, Kaiser H, Kostering H, Leitz K: Selective intracoronary thrombolysis in acute myocardial infarction and unstable angina pectoris. Circulation, 63:307–317, 1981.

5 Lee G, Amsterdam EA, Low R, Joye JA, Kimchi A, DeMaria AN, Mason DT: Efficacy of percutaneous transluminal coronary recanalization utilizing streptokinase thrombolysis in patients with acute myocardial infarction. Am Heart J, 102:1159–1167, 1981.

6 Reduto LA, Freund GC, Gaeta JM, Smalling RW, Lewis B, Gould KL: Coronary artery reperfusion in acute myocardial infarction: Beneficial effects of intracoronary streptokinase on left ventricular salvage and performance. Am Heart J, 102:1168–1177, 1981.

7 Cowley MJ, Hastillo A, Vetrovec GW, Hess ML: Effects of intracoronary streptokinase in acute myocardial infarction. Am Heart J, 102:1149–1158, 1981.

8 Blumgart HL, Zoll PM, Wessler S: Angina pectoris: Clinical pathologic study of 177 cases. Trans Assoc Am Physicians, 63:262–267, 1950.

9 Friedberg CK, Horn H: Acute myocardial infarction not due to coronary artery occlusion. JAMA, 112:1675–1679, 1939.

10 Sherry S, Titchner A, Gottesman L, Wasserman P, Troll W: The enzymatic dissolution of experimental arterial thrombi in the dog by trypsin, chymotrypsin and plasminogen activators. J Clin Invest, 33:1303–1313, 1954.

11 Johnson AJ, Tillet WS: The lysis in rabbits of intravascular blood clots by the streptococcal fibrinolytic system. J Exp Med, 95:449–463, 1952.

12 Genton E: Thrombolytic therapy of pulmonary thrombolism. Prog Cardiovasc Dis, 21:333–341, 1979.

13 Marder VJ: Guidelines for thrombolytic therapy of deep-vein thrombosis. Prog Cardiovasc Dis, 21:327–332, 1979.

14 Reimer KA, Lowe JE, Rosmussen MM, Jennings RB: The wavefront phenomenon of ischemic cell death: (1) Myocardial infarct size vs. duration of coronary occlusion in dogs. Circulation, 56:786–793, 1977.

15 Maroko PR, Libby P, Ginks WR, Bloor CM, Shell WE, Sobel BE, Ross J Jr: Coronary artery reperfusion: (1) Early effects on local myocardial function and the extent of myocardial necrosis. J Clin Invest, 51:2710–2716, 1972.

16 Ginks WR, Sybers HD, Maroko PR, Covell JW, Sobel BE, Ross J Jr: Coronary artery reperfusion: (II) Reduction of myocardial infarct size at one week after the coronary occlusion. J Clin Invest, 51:2717–2723, 1972.

17 Baughman KL, Maroko PR, Vatner SF: Effects of coronary artery reperfusion on myocardial infarct size and survival in conscious dogs. Circulation, 63:317–322, 1981.

18 Lang TW, Corday E, Gold H, Meerbaum S, Rabins S, Costantini C, Hirose S, Osher J, Rosen V: Consequences of reperfusion after coronary occlusion. Am J Cardiol, 33:69–81, 1974.

19 Banka VS, Chaddo KD, Helfant RH: Limitations of myocardial revascularization in restoration of regional contraction abnormalities produced by coronary occlusion. Am J Cardiol, 34:164–170, 1974.

20 Puri PS: Contractile and biochemical effects of coronary reperfusion after extended periods of coronary occlusion. Am J Cardiol, 36:244–251, 1975.

21 Costantini C, Corday E, Lang TW, Meerbaum S, Brasch J, Kaplan L, Rubins S, Gold H, Osher J: Revascularization after three hours of coronary arterial occlusion: Effects on regional cardiac metabolic function and infarct size. Am J Cardiol, 36:368–384, 1975.

22 Higginson LAJ, White F, Heggtveit HA, Sanders TM, Bloor CM, Covell JW: Determinants of myocardial hemorrhage after coronary reperfusion in the anesthetized dog. Circulation, 65:62–69, 1982.

23 Fletcher AP, Alkjaersig N, Sherry S: The maintenance of a sustained thrombolytic state in man: I. Induction and effects. J Clin Invest, 38:1111–1121, 1959.

24 Boucek RJ, Murphy WP: Segmental perfusion of the coronary arteries with fibrinolysis in man following a myocardial infarction. Am J Cardiol, 6:525–533, 1960.

25 Nydick I, Ruegsegger P, Boriner C: Salvage of heart muscle by fibrinolytic therapy after experimental coronary occlusion. Am Heart J, 61:93–100, 1961.

26 European Cooperative Study Group for Streptokinase Treatment in Acute Myocardial Infarction: Streptokinase in acute myocardial infarction. N Engl J Med, 301:797–802, 1979.

27 Ganz W, Buchbinder N, Marcus H, Mondkar A, Maddahi J, Charuzi Y, O'Conner L, Shell W, Fishbein MC, Kass R, Muujamoto A, Swan HJC: Intracoronary thrombolysis in evolving myocardial infarction. Am Heart J, 101:4–13. 1981.

28 Mathey DG, Kuck K-H, Tilsner V, Krebber H-J, Bleifield W: Nonsurgical coronary artery recanalization in acute transmural myocardial infarction. Circulation, 63:489–497, 1981.

29 Anderson JL, Marshall HW, Bray BE, Lutz JR, Frederick PR, Yanowitz FG, Datz FL, Klausner SC, Hagan AD: A randomized trial of intracoronary streptokinase in the treatment of acute myocardial infarction. N Engl J Med, 308:1312–1318, 1983.

30 Khaja F, Walton JA, Brymer JF, Lo E, Osterberger L, O'Neill WW, Colper HT, Weiss R, Lee T, Kurian T, Goldberg AD, Pitt B, Goldstein S: Intracoronary fibrinolytic therapy in acute myocardial infarction: Report of a prospective randomized trial. N Engl J Med, 309:1305, 1311, 1983.

31 Gold HK, Leinback RC, Palacios IF, Yasuda T, Block PC, Buckley MJ, Akins CW, Daggett WM, Austen WG: Coronary reocclusion after selective administration of streptokinase. Circulation, 68(suppl I):I-50–I-54, 1983.

32 Kennedy JW, Ritchie JL, Davis KB, Fritz JK: The Western Washington streptokinase in acute myocardial infarction randomized trial. Circulation, 68(suppl III):III-23, 1983.

33 Rutsch W, Schartt M, Mathey D, Kuck K, Merx W, Dorr R, Rentrop P, Blanke H: Percutaneous transluminal coronary recanalization: Procedure, results, and acute complications. Am Heart J, 102:1178–1181, 1981.

34 Merx W, Dorr R, Rentrop P, Blanke H, Karsch KR, Mathey DG, Kremer P, Rutsch W, Schmutzler H: Evaluation of the effectiveness of intracoronary streptokinase infusion in acute myocardial infarction: Postprocedure management and hospital course in 204 patients. Am Heart J, 102:1181–1187, 1981.

35 Kanmatsuse K, Lando U, Mercier JC, Fishbein MC, Swan HJC, Ganz W: Rapid lysis of coronary thrombi by local application of fibrinolysis. Circulation, 59(suppl II):II-216, 1979.

36 Rentrop KP, Blanke H, Karsch KR: Effects of nonsurgical coronary reperfusion on the left ventricle in human subjects compared with conventional treatment: Study of 18 patients with acute myocardial infarction treated with intracoronary infusion of streptokinase. Am J Cardiol, 49:1–8, 1982.

37 Wackers FJ, Berger HJ, Johnstone DE, Goldman L, Reduto LA, Langou RA, Gottschalk A, Zaret BL:

Multiple gated cardiac blood pool imaging for left ventricular ejection fraction: Validation of the technique and assessment of variability. Am J Cardiol, 43:1159–1166, 1979.

38 Wackers FJ, Berger HJ, Weinberg MA, Zaret BL: Spontaneous changes in left ventricular function over the first 24 hours of acute myocardial infarction: Implications for evaluating early therapeutic interventions. Circulation, 66:748–754, 1982.

39 Weinstein J: Treatment of myocardial infarction with intraocoronary streptokinase: Efficacy and safety data from 209 United States cases in the Hoeckst-Roussel registry. Am Heart J, 104:894–898, 1982.

40 Berg R Jr, Selinger SL, Leonard JJ, Grunwald RP, O'Grady WP: Immediate coronary artery bypass for acute evolving mycardial infarction. J Thorac Cardiovasc Surg, 81:493–497, 1981.

41 Vatner SF, Baig H, Manders WT, Marako PR: Effects of coronary artery reperfusion on myocardial infarct size calculated from creatine kinase. J Clin Invest, 61:1048–1056, 1978.

42 Lee G, Low RI, Takeda P, Joe P, DeMaria AN, Amsterdam EA, Lui H, Dietrich P, Lee K, Mason DT: Importance of follow-up medical and surgical approaches to prevent reinfarction, reocclusion, and recurrent angina following intracoronary thrombolysis with streptokinase in acute myocardial infarction. Am Heart J, 104:921–924, 1982.

43 Becker H, Schroder C, Mathey D, Krebber H-J, Tilsner V, Bleifeld W: Coronary artery bypass grafting within 24 hours after intracoronary thrombolysis—risk of bleeding. Circulation, 68(suppl III):III-115, 1983.

44 Urokinase-Streptokinase Embolism Trial: Phase 2 results. JAMA, 229:1606–1613, 1974.

Chapter 17

Percutaneous Transluminal Coronary Angioplasty

Spencer B. King III, M.D.
John S. Douglas, Jr., M.D.
Andreas R. Gruentzig, M.D.

HISTORICAL BACKGROUND

In 1964, Dotter and Judkins[1] performed the first intraluminal angioplasty using a coaxial double-catheter system to stretch the lumen of femoral arteries. The technique did not receive wide acceptance in the United States but was developed further by Porstmann[2] and Zeitler,[3] who utilized a caged distensible balloon for peripheral artery dilation. The technique was modified by Gruentzig, who developed a cylindrical balloon for use in peripheral arterial angioplasty.[4] The balloon was miniaturized by Gruentzig, who applied the technique in coronary arteries first in 1977.[5] This technique has subsequently spread worldwide. Our group at Emory University has performed over 3000 percutaneous transluminal coronary angioplasties (PTCA) as the technique has been refined and improved.

MECHANISM OF INCREASING FLOW

Flow restriction is produced by a severe reduction in the size of the lumen of the coronary artery. PTCA increases the lumen by radial expansion. Since the balloon is nondistensible, it can be inflated only to the constructed size of the balloon. Further attempts to force fluid into the balloon result in increased pressure but no significant increase in its diameter. This radial pressure results in expansion of the lumen by several mechanisms. The atherosclerotic plaque is composed of various elements. Some are of soft lipid composition and may be flattened. Others are quite hard and will not change their shape; therefore compacting is not a reasonable explanation for improvement in that aspect. The internal circumference of the intima is small and must be increased by stretching and splitting. Fissures extend well into the plaque and sometimes into the media of the artery (Fig. 17-1). The media and adventitia faced with the inflating balloon in the artery will expand, resulting in an increased diameter of the outer dimension of the vessel. These mechanisms: flattening of the plaque, splitting of the intima and plaque, and dilation of the artery take place to varying degrees depending on the composition of the atherosclerotic plaque. Soft lesions with extensive lipid infiltration respond by being flattened, while older, hard, or calcified plaques are opened largely by splitting.

METHODOLOGY OF PTCA

The original balloon designed by Gruentzig is fixed to a double-lumen catheter.[5] One lumen terminates in end holes distal to the balloon and is used for measurement of pressure and for contrast medium injection. The other lumen is connected to the balloon for inflation and deflation. The short segment of safety J-guidewire is fixed to the distal end of the catheter to facilitate safe passage of stenotic lesions (Fig. 17-2). This balloon catheter is delivered into the coronary artery through a thin-walled Teflon-coated guiding catheter. After positioning the guiding catheter in the coronary artery, the balloon catheter is advanced down the vessel to the stenotic area. The balloon is then advanced so that the safety guidewire at the tip enters the lesion. When the side holes cross the stenosis, the pressure monitored through the lumen falls. By measuring the proximal pressure through the guiding catheter, the gradient across the lesion can be defined (Fig. 17-3). Radiopaque markers inside the balloon segment of the artery facilitate positioning across the lesion. Distal contrast medium injections ensure

Figure 17-1 Postmortem artery which has been dilated. Note the deep fissuring and splitting of the atherosclerotic plaque.

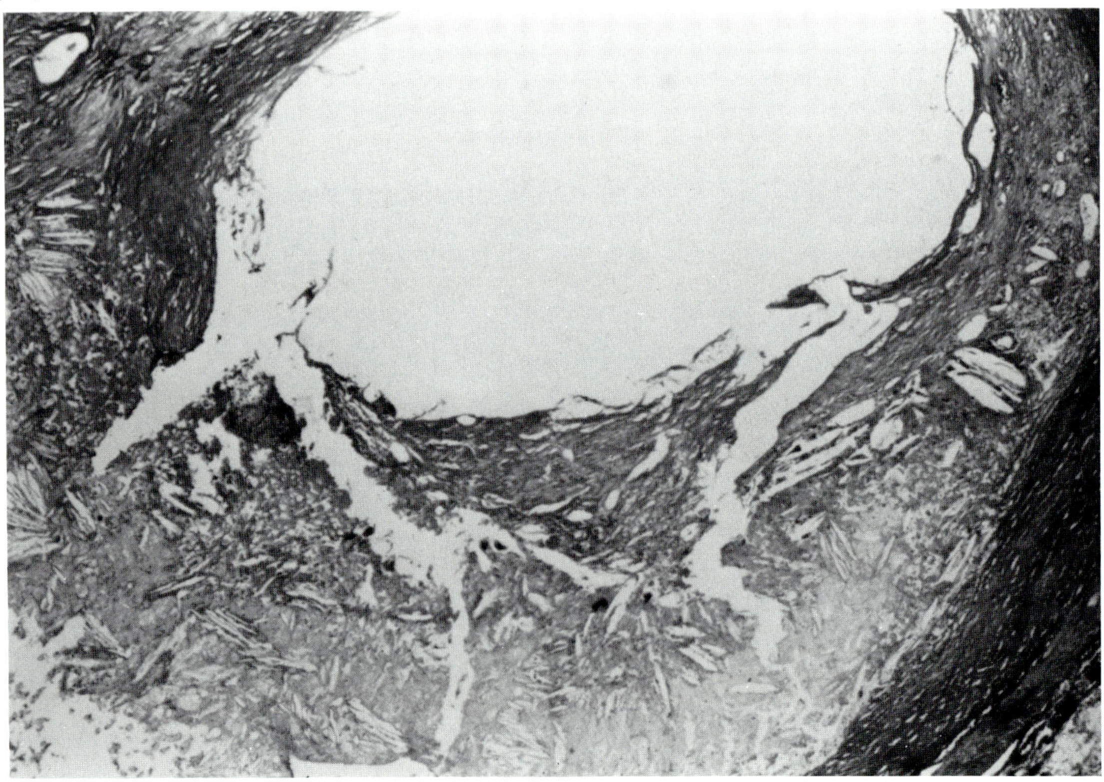

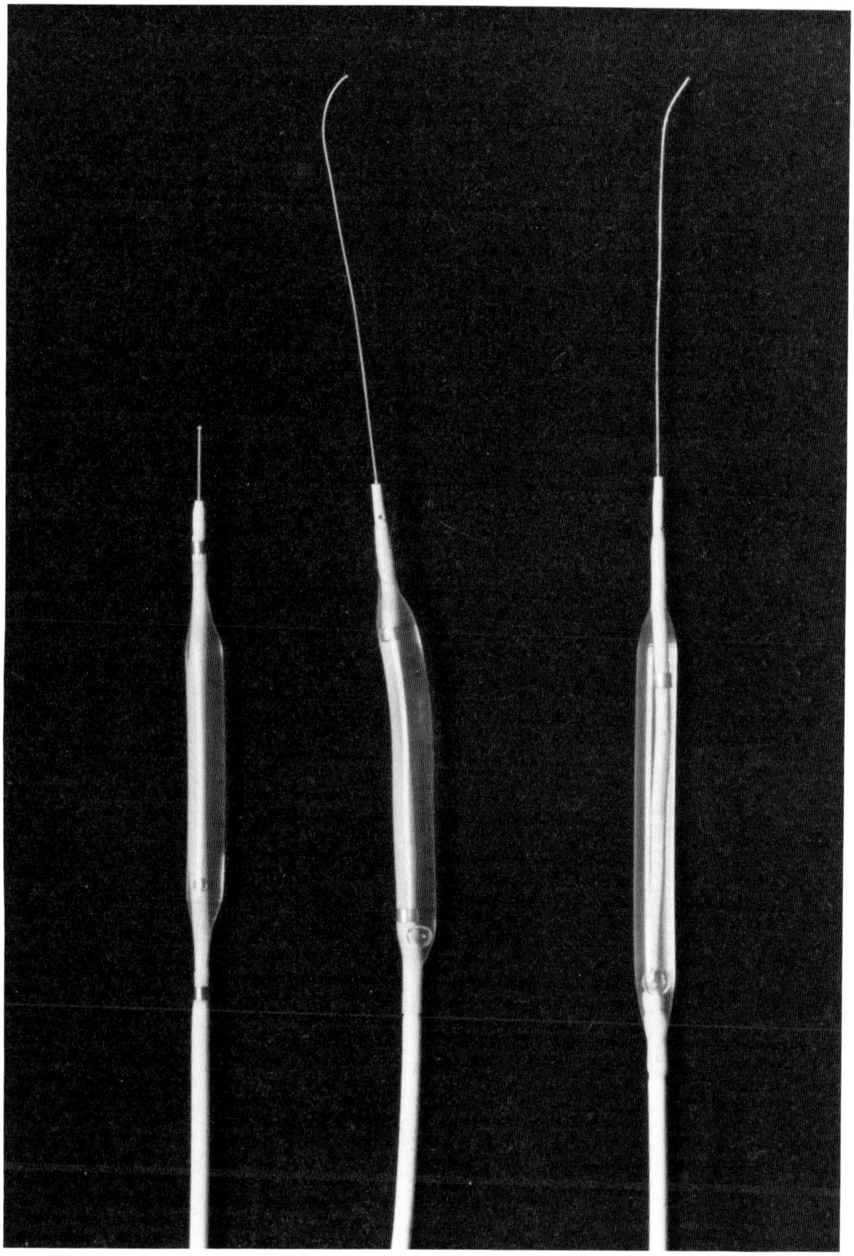

Figure 17-2 *Left:* Original Gruentzig balloon catheter with fixed safety guidewire at the tip and distal side holes for pressure measurement. *Middle:* Steerable catheter system with a central lumen for passage of the guidewire, dye injection, and pressure measurements. *Right:* New low-profile steerable system for utilizing a smaller deflectable guidewire (0.014 inch) and a smaller catheter silhouette for passing severely stenotic lesions.

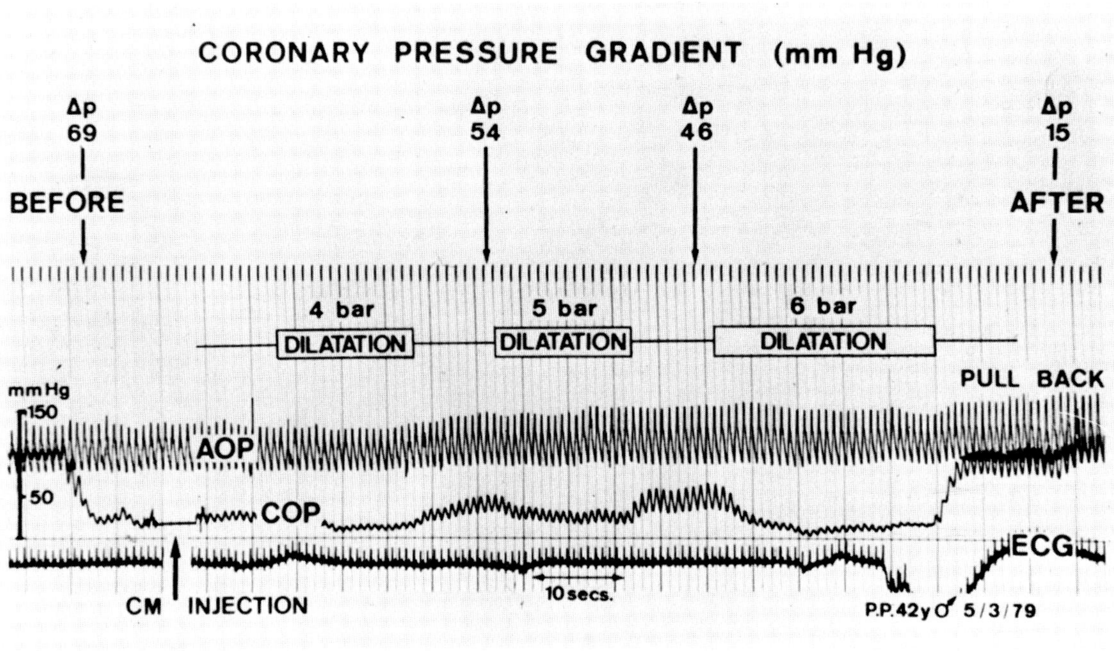

A

Figure 17-3 (*a*) Simultaneous pressure measurements from the guiding catheter, reflecting aortic pressure (AOP), and the tip of the balloon catheter, reflecting distal coronary pressure (COP). Note: with repeated dilatations there is a rise in distal coronary pressure until a final pressure gradient of 15 mmHg is reached. (*From Gruentzig AR: Percutaneous transluminal coronary angioplasty, in Hurst JW (ed):* The Heart (5th ed). *McGraw Hill, New York, 1982, fig 105-4.*) (*b*) Graph of the pressure gradient across the coronary artery stenosis during repeated coronary inflations and deflations. (*From Aueron FM, Gruentzig AR: Percutaneous transluminal coronary angioplasty: Indications and current status. Primary Cardiol, 10(6):97, June 1984.*)

proper location of the tip and provide a check on the presence or absence of antegrade flow. Control of the procedure is by evaluation of the residual pressure gradient after inflation and deflation of the balloon and by visual observation of the lesion by proximal contrast medium injections through the guiding catheter.

Although this catheter was used in the early development of the technique, it has some disadvantages: (1) lesions accessible to the catheter are limited to those proximal in the anterior descending, right, or circumflex arteries and without difficult turns or side branches preceding the lesion, since little can be done to direct the tip of the balloon catheter; (2) crossing complex and eccentric lesions with the relatively stiff-tipped guidewire sometimes leads to disruption of the plaque and dissection of the artery; (3) evaluation of the final result depends on a proximal coronary orifice injection with the balloon in place, which may result in poor visualization; and (4) if the balloon is pulled back across a dilated segment, it is usually unwise to recross the lesion because of the risk of dissection.

In order to address these problems, a catheter with a central lumen housing a movable, steerable guidewire system was developed (Fig. 17-4).[6] Placement of the catheter is again by a guiding catheter. The guidewire is a .016-inch safety guidewire with a flexible tip which has a gentle curve on the distal 3 to 4 mm. This wire is attached to a long segment of hypotubing. By turning the proximal end of the hypotubing, the guidewire's distal tip can be deflected. When this wire is placed 10 to 12 cm outside the balloon catheter, the distal wire deforms easily upon meeting an obstruction, thereby providing an element of safety. The balloon catheter is advanced through the guiding catheter while an assistant rotates the wire tip. By de-

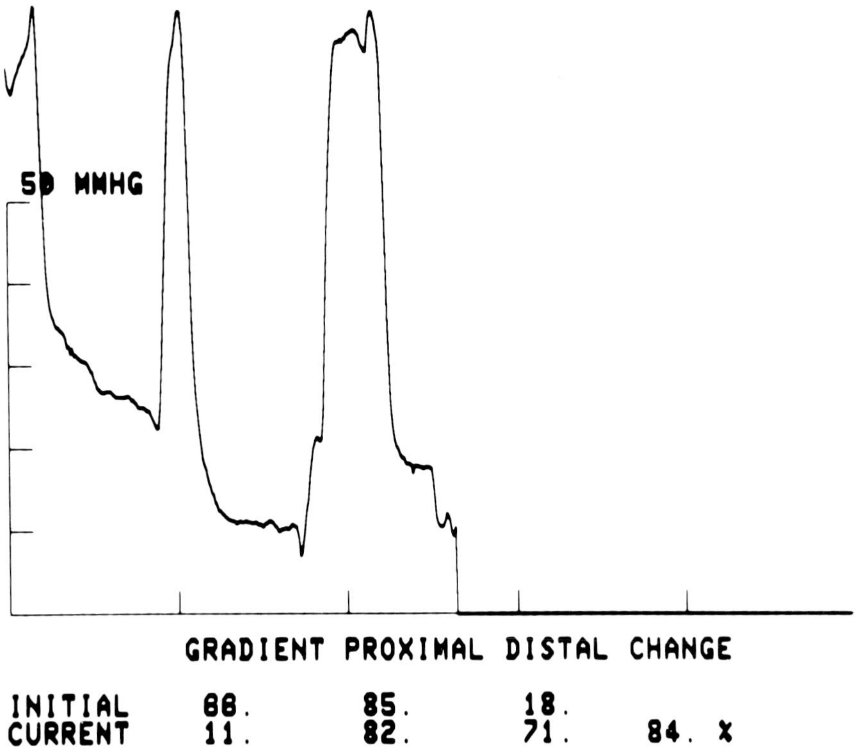

B *(Figure 17-3, continued)*

Figure 17-4 Schematic diagram of steerable catheter system. Note that rotation of the proximal portion of the wire will rotate the distal tip. (*From Aueron FM, Gruentzig AR: Percutaneous transluminal coronary angioplasty: Indications and current status. Primary Cardiol, 10(6):91, June 1984.*)

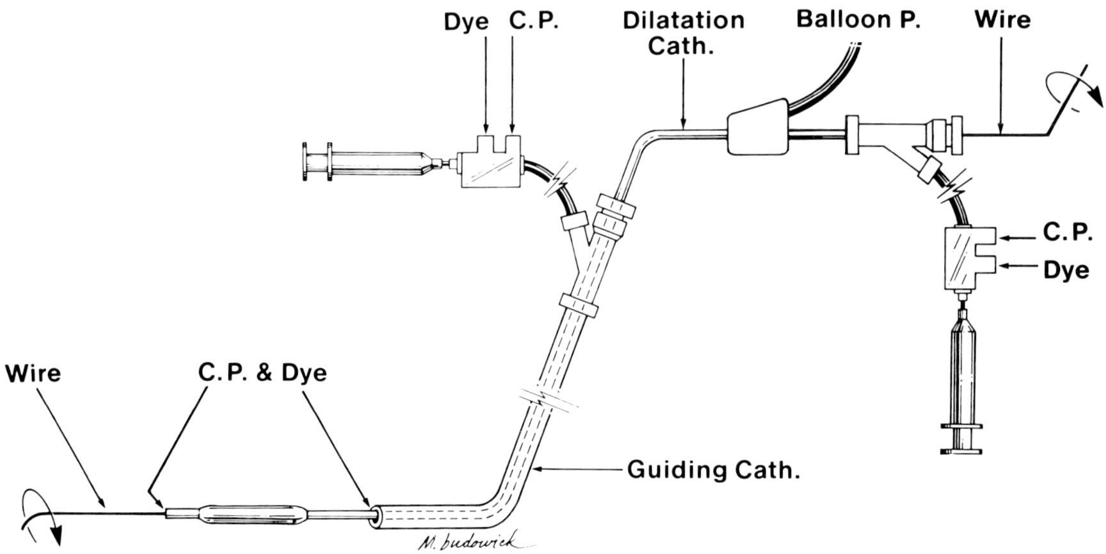

flecting this tip, the operator can bring the wire away from side branches, around curves, and far distal in the arteries to reach lesions which were previously inaccessible (Fig. 17-5).

Eccentric lesions can be safely entered by turning the tip directly into the residual lumen. Observation of the densely radiopaque wire will quickly show if the tip is trapped on an irregular plaque or side branch, in which case the tip will begin to buckle indicating that it should be pulled back and another position tried until the tip slides through the stenosis.

Once the tip passes the lesion, confirmation of the position is made by proximal contrast medium injections using multiple views to ensure that the guidewire is in the distal vessel. The steerable potential of the wire is also useful in avoiding side branches beyond the lesion as the wire is advanced deep into the distal coronary artery. This is important because the stiffer, more proximal part of the wire will now act as a stint over which the balloon catheter can be advanced.

While the assistant pulls back on the guidewire, holding the tip in a stable position, the balloon catheter is advanced until the lesion has been crossed. Confirmation of the position can be made by proximal injections through the guide catheter or by distal injections through the balloon catheter. Ra-

Figure 17-5 (*a*) Stenotic lesion of the left anterior descending artery. (*b*) Steerable guidewire entering the artery. (*c*) Steerable wire pointing toward the diagonal branch. (*d*) Steerable wire rotated into the anterior descending branch. (*e*) Appearance of the artery following angioplasty.

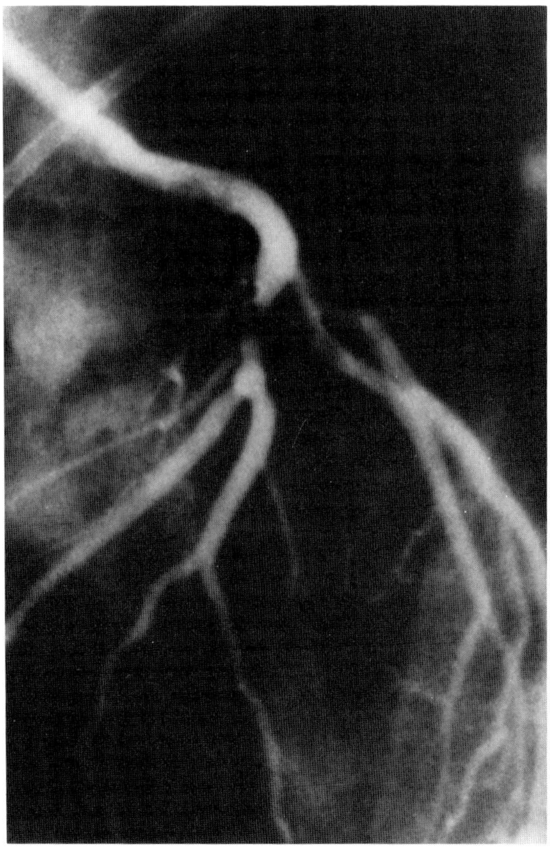

A

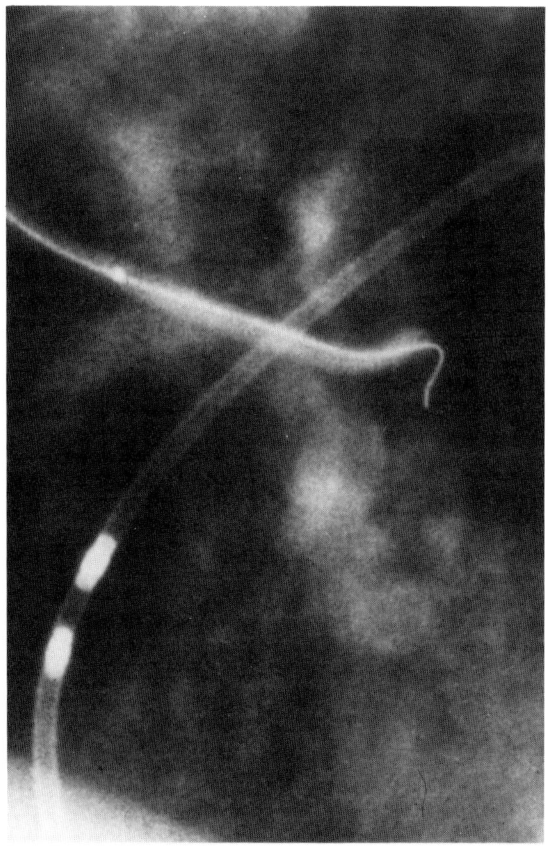

B

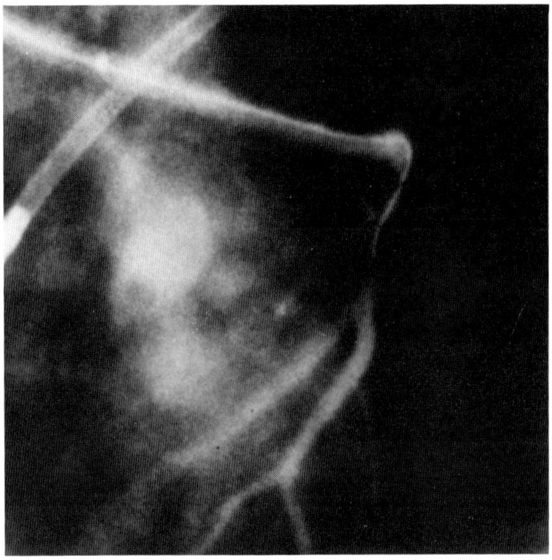

C

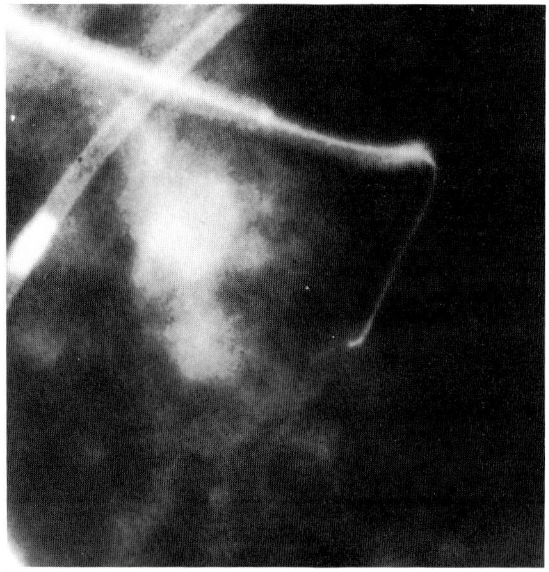

D

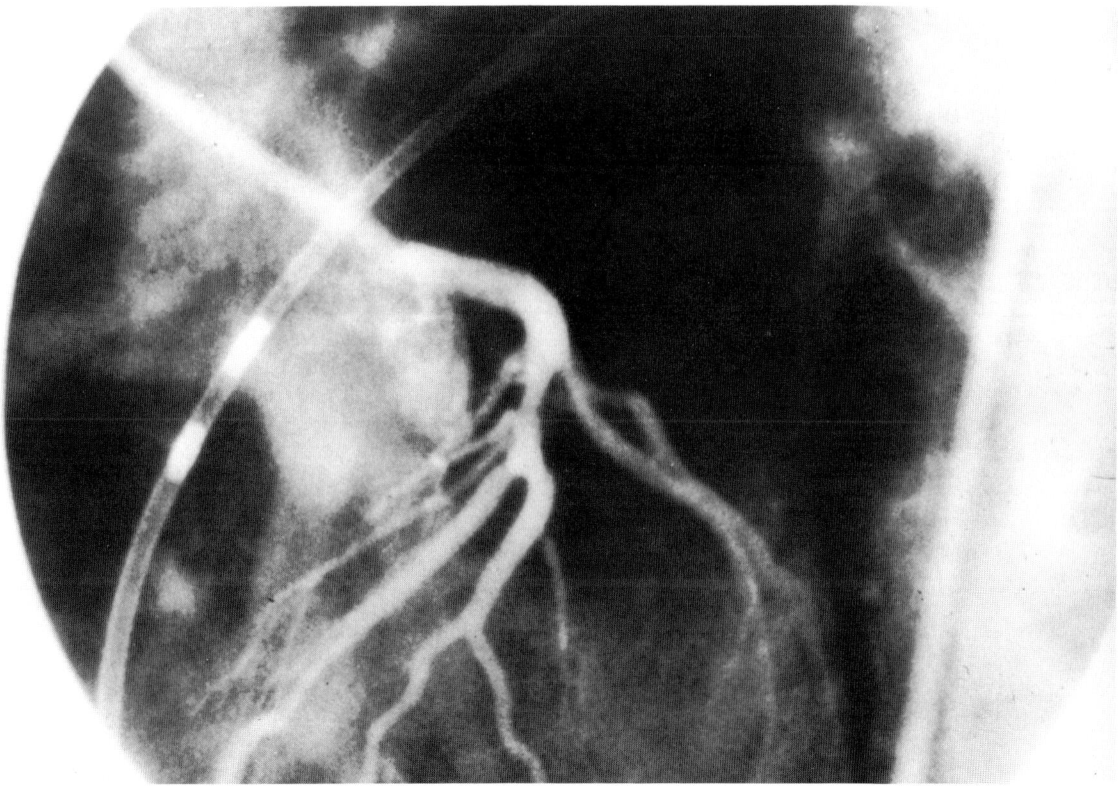

E

diopaque markers within the balloon portion of the catheter aid in proper positioning.

Following several inflations and deflations when the gradient is felt to be at its minimum, the final result can be evaluated angiographically. The balloon is withdrawn across the lesion while the guidewire is advanced so as to keep it far distal to the dilated segment. Injection through the guiding catheter and balloon catheter will show the angiographic result. If the result is unsatisfactory or if dissection or other filling defects obscure the lesion, then the balloon catheter can safely be passed back across the lesion over the guidewire, which has been left in place. If a larger balloon is required to improve the result, then the balloon can be placed distal to the lesion and a long exchange wire inserted into the distal coronary artery. By removing the original balloon and replacing it with a larger balloon over the exchange wire, one can safely recross the lesion. This ability to recross the lesion safely is a major advantage of the guidewire systems.

TECHNIQUE OF PTCA

Patients who are selected for the procedure are admitted to the hospital the day before for the purposes of being educated about the procedure, furnishing any points of history, physical examination, or laboratory data which may point to complicating conditions, and being prepared for the possibility of emergency surgery, and in order that the proper premedications can be administered.[7]

Aspirin is begun the day before the procedure. Some patients also receive dipyridamole; however, it has not been yet established that Persantine adds to the long-term success of PTCA. The patient is kept NPO (nothing by mouth) after midnight the night before the angioplasty if the procedure is to be done in the morning, but if the patient is scheduled for later in the day, then clear liquids are continued to avoid dehydration.

Upon entering the laboratory, patients who give a history of contrast medium allergy are pretreated with diphenhydramine 50 mg and hydrocortisone 100 mg intravenously. Aspirin 5 grains by mouth and nifedipine 10 mg sublingual are given. Low-molecular-weight dextran is infused at 100 mL/h during the procedure and afterward until 500 mL has been given. The vein is punctured for placement of a pacing catheter in the right ventricle. When the artery has been punctured and the guiding catheter has been inserted, 10,000 units of heparin are given intravenously. If the procedure lasts more than 1 hour, an additional 5000 units of heparin are administered.

The guiding catheters for femoral PTCA are of three general configurations: the Judkins shapes, Amplatz shapes, and multipurpose shapes (Figs. 17-6 and 17-7). The Judkins left catheter is commonly used for the left anterior descending (LAD), the Judkins right catheter for the right coronary artery (RCA), the Amplatz for the circumflex and some right coronary arteries, and the multipurpose catheter or an overbent version of it for the vein grafts and some right coronary lesions. The purpose of the guiding catheter is not only to direct the balloon catheter into the diseased coronary artery but also to provide a launching pad or backup platform for exerting some pressure on the balloon catheter to force it through very tight stenoses.

LAD LESIONS

The left Judkins catheter of no. 8 or 9 French size is usually selected. The catheter is inserted through a long femoral sheath over a large safety J-spring guidewire. After the guiding catheter has been positioned in the left main coronary artery, the balloon catheter with the protruding guidewire preceding its tip by 10 to 12 cm is inserted and advanced. If the wire does not enter the LAD, then it is likely that the tip of the guiding catheter is not pointing toward the LAD.

When the tip of the Judkins catheter is in the left coronary orifice, counterclockwise rotation of the catheter will direct the tip in an anterior direction due to the fulcrum effect on the tip in the left orifice (Fig. 17-8). Advancing the catheter slightly will direct the tip more superior and anterior (Fig. 17-9). When the left coronary artery is viewed in

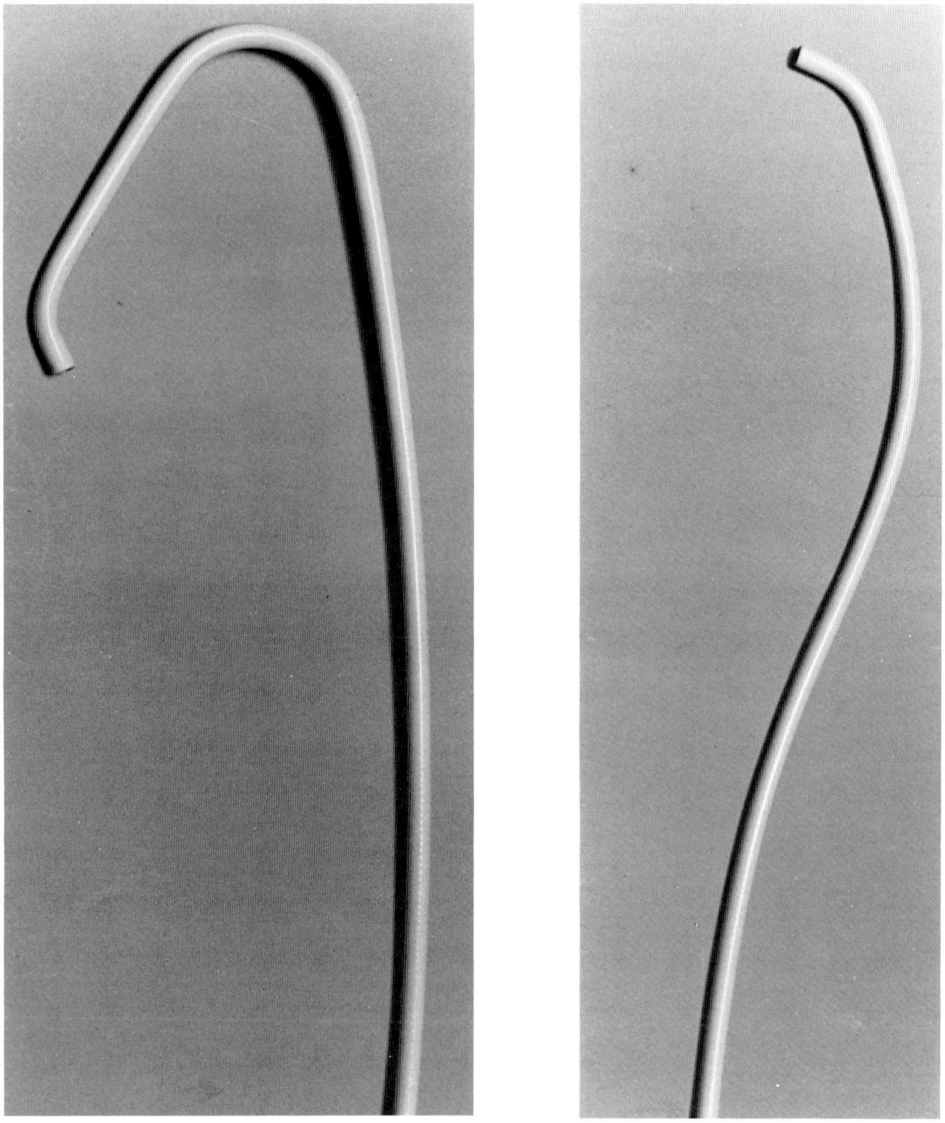

A B

Figure 17-6 (*a*) Left Judkins guiding catheter. (*b*) Right Judkins guiding catheter.

the left anterior oblique (LAO) caudal view, the anterior descending is seen to arise superior with the circumflex artery traveling in an inferior or caudal direction. This view is often helpful in gaining the concept of the direction needed for the tip of the guiding catheter.

A combination of the two maneuvers, i.e., counterclockwise rotation and advancing, results in the tip of the catheter pointing superior and anterior toward the orifice of the anterior descending coronary. Selection of a somewhat undersized Judkins catheter will cause the secondary curve of the cath-

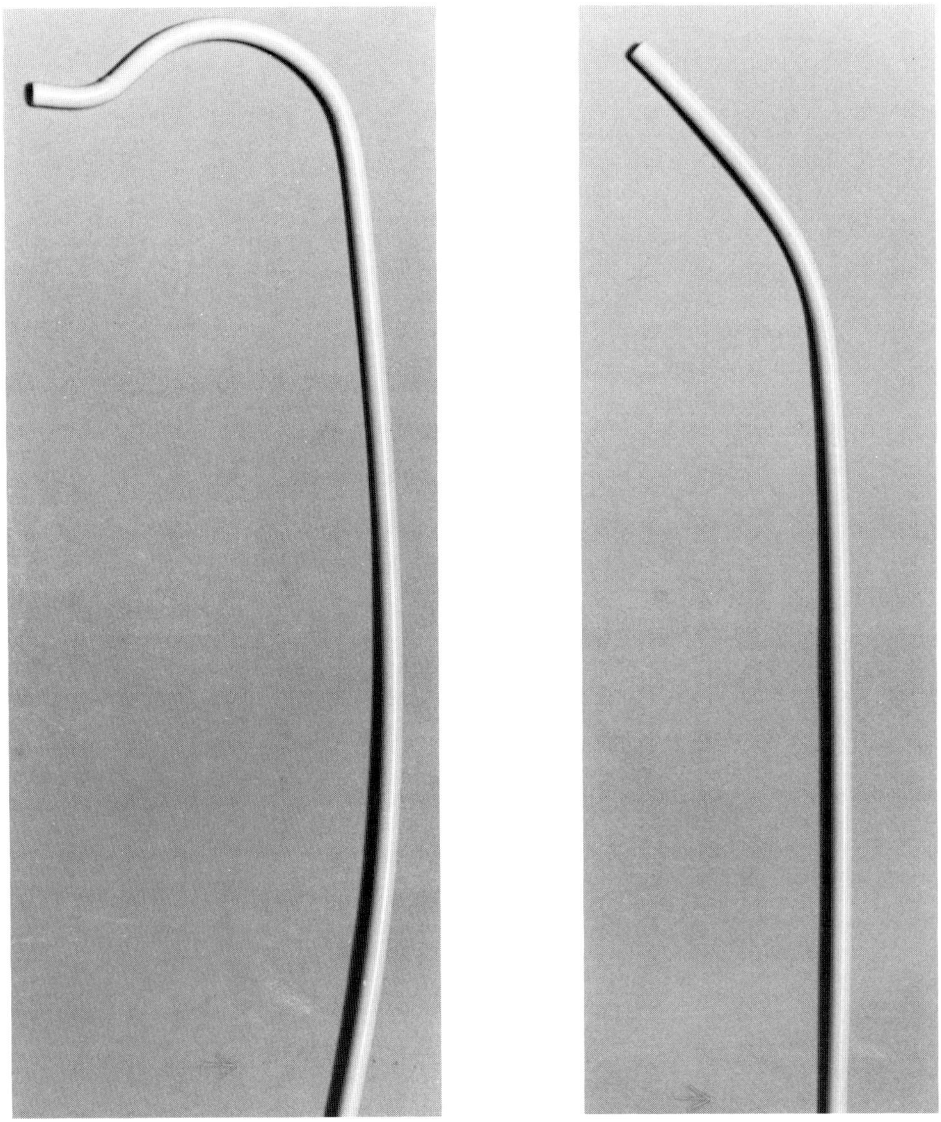

A B

Figure 17-7 (*a*) Amplatz guiding catheter. (*b*) Multipurpose guiding catheter.

eter to pass across the aorta in a horizontal fashion so that the tip of the catheter will be aimed upward when the catheter is advanced. Any placement of the catheter tip deep in the left main poses a potential hazard, but if gentle pressure is used and *no* advancing against resistance or in an area of disease is performed, then complications can be minimized.

If the LAD takes off at a sharp angle from the left main or if the left main is very long so that the guiding catheter cannot aim at the LAD, then most of the maneuvers to enter the LAD must be accomplished with the guidewire. A single curve on the tip will direct the wire in the same direction as the final curve on the Judkins catheter, namely superior and anterior toward the LAD. A long curve on the distal 1 cm of the catheter will usually ensure that the wire enters the LAD, but this severe curve will be a disadvantage in crossing the lesion or placing the catheter distal in the artery. It is therefore preferable to use as little distal curve as needed to enter the LAD so that all the potential for guiding the wire down the vessel and through the stenosis is retained. Often the LAO caudal view will give the best visualization of the separation of the LAD and circumflex and intermediate branches, especially in horizontal hearts. If the left main has a downward direction, as in vertical hearts, then the LAO cranial view will show the division of the left main to best advantage.

The lesion is approached with the guidewire by advancing the catheter and wire as a unit. In the U.S. Catheter Inc. (USCI) system, this gives the best feel and control. In the Advanced Catheter Systems (ACS) catheter, the wire is often advanced independently since it slides a bit easier in that catheter. Steering the tip of the wire is done by the operator or an assistant. It is important to turn the tip back and forth rather than in one direction continuously since a trapped tip of the coiled guidewire could potentially unravel if constantly turned in the direction opposite the coils of the J-guidewire. If the tip is moving in an undesired direction, then slight withdrawal and rotation of the tip will point it in the correct way. Once the wire is safely down the LAD near the apex, the balloon catheter is advanced over it until it crosses the lesion while the assistant pulls back on the guidewire to maintain the tip in a fixed position in the distal coronary.

If resistance is encountered at the lesion, gentle pressure on the balloon catheter will often cause it to cross. If the lesion is too tight or hard, the balloon tip will not cross, and the guiding catheter will begin to back out of the coronary orifice. This is usually solved by obtaining better backup from the guiding catheter by placing the long segment between the primary and secondary curves directly across the root of the aorta so that the catheter rests against the opposite wall of the aorta. This is accomplished by entering the left main artery deeper with the tip of the guiding catheter which, if the left main is free of disease, is safe since the guiding catheter is being stinted over the balloon catheter. To accomplish this maneuver, the operator pulls back slightly on the balloon catheter while advancing the guiding catheter over it to enter the left main and brings the heel of the guiding catheter against the opposite wall of the aorta. In this backup power position, the balloon catheter can be advanced safely over the guidewire, thereby crossing most lesions (Fig. 17-10). Once the lesion is crossed, the guide catheter is pulled back to a free position in the left main orifice and pressure is checked to ensure no damping of the proximal guiding catheter.

If the stenosis is still too tight to cross, a new low-profile catheter must be selected. There are several catheters being developed which present a very low profile to the lesion while sliding through but will still inflate to 3-mm diameter or more.

Our experience indicates that at present when all movable guidewire systems fail to cross a hard lesion, then the standard G20-20 Gruentzig balloon will slip across. The safety of the movable guidewire system must be sacrificed at that point, and the decision to use the G20-20 rests with the operator and that operator's experience. Future catheters with movable guidewires will be sufficiently small to cross virtually all lesions which can be crossed with the guidewire.

The critical point to be remembered in crossing a very hard and stenotic lesion is to identify whether the resistance felt is due to the tight stenosis itself impeding the larger balloon or because one is caught in a side branch or against an eccentric plaque. The steerable guidewire systems almost always ensure that one is in the proper lumen, thereby allowing safe application of moderate force to the balloon catheter to cross the lesion.

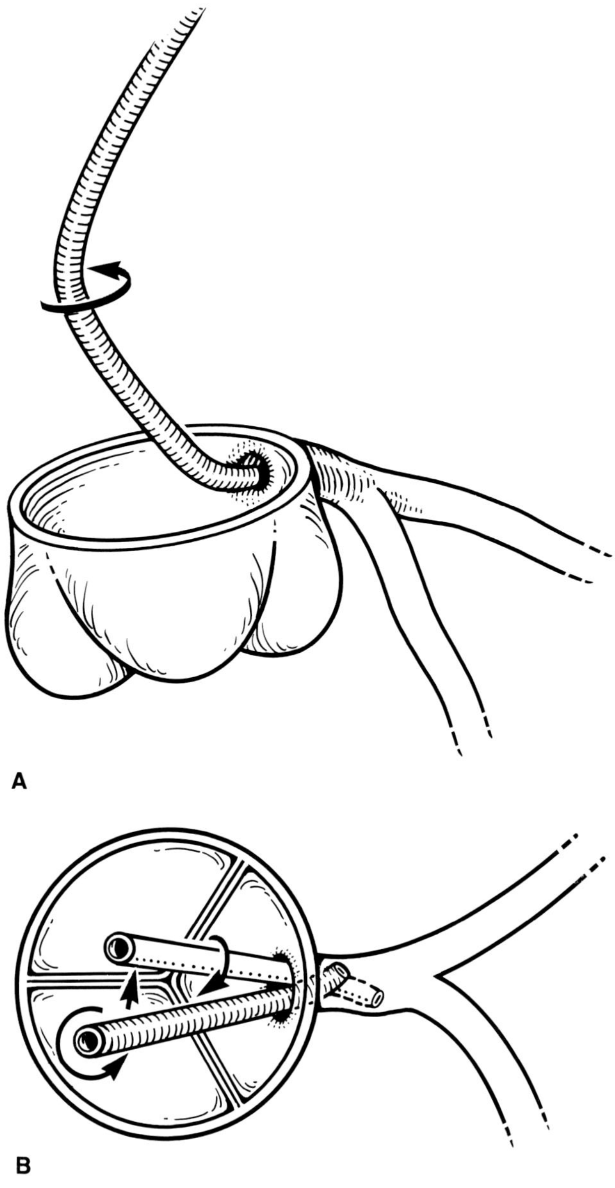

Figure 17-8 (*a*) Left guiding catheter in the left coronary orifice. Counterclockwise rotation brings the heel of the catheter posterior. (*b*) The tip of the catheter is therefore thrust anterior.

THE CIRCUMFLEX ARTERY

Entering the circumflex presents the opposite problem from entering the LAD. The artery takes off from the left main in a posterior and inferior direction. Judkins catheters may allow entry, but if so, it will be an oversized Judkins so that the heel of the catheter rides high on the ascending aorta causing the tip to be in a neutral or downward direction. If the lesion is not too tight so that a strong backup position for the guide catheter is not needed, then the Judkins left coronary catheter is satisfactory. If, however, backup is needed to cross the lesion, then the Amplatz catheter is superior.

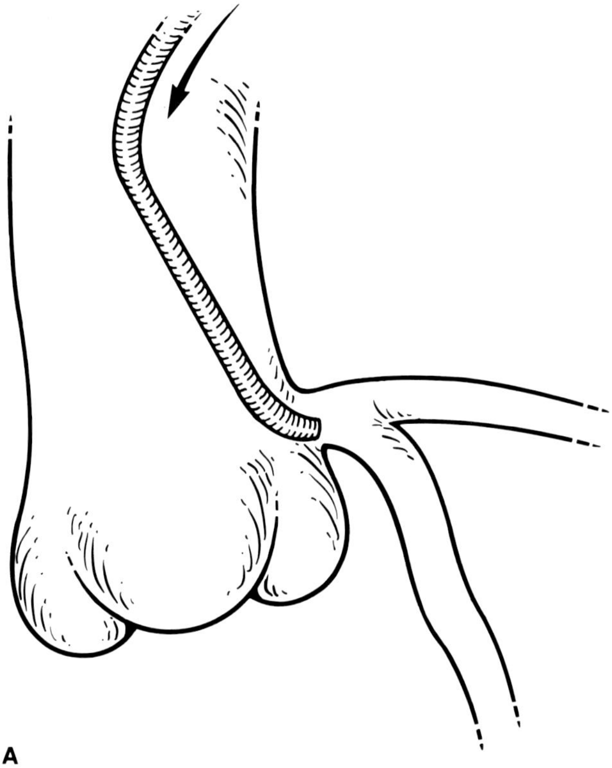

A

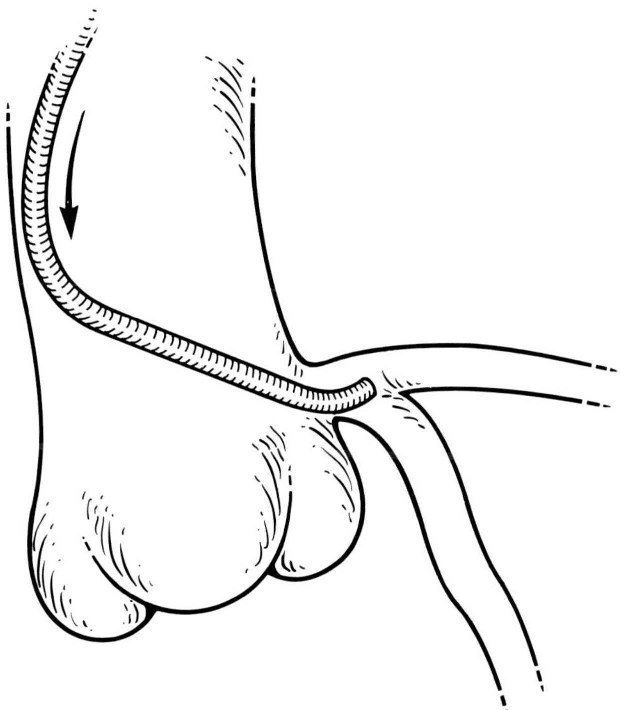

B

Figure 17-9 (*a*) Left Judkins guiding catheter in the left orifice pointed toward the circumflex. (*b*) Advancing the catheter forces the tip into the left main artery and directs it more superiorly toward the anterior descending coronary.

The Amplatz has the advantage of having its tip directed downward in the left main towards the circumflex. In this position, the big curve of the catheter rests in the aortic root against the opposite wall, providing the backup needed (Fig. 17-11). The one disadvantage of the Amplatz is the occasional difficulty in removing it from the left coronary orifice. The catheter should not be removed quickly since there is a chance of injury to the left main if the tip is too well engaged. In this case, the catheter can be removed by advancing the shaft until the tip prolapses out of the orifice down into the aortic cusp and then rotation of the catheter will bring the tip away from the orifice for removal.

If the left main artery is long, the guidewire again may be needed to enter the circumflex artery. A single turn at the end of the wire will direct the tip inferior with the Amplatz catheter, since the terminal curve of the Amplatz is downward (Fig. 17-12). If the Judkins catheter is used, the superior orientation of the final curve will carry a single curve wire upward and toward the LAD. Therefore a double-S type of curve is needed for the circumflex. This type of curve will turn the wire over and point the tip toward the circumflex (Fig. 17-13).

When using the USCI steerable wire, one again wants as straight a wire as possible after entering the diseased artery so that the steerable features can be maintained. If significant shaping of wires has occurred, it may be necessary to advance the balloon catheter into the diseased coronary prior to crossing the lesion and then exchange the shaped wire for a straighter wire in order to continue down the artery. This is the common practice when using the ACS guidewire systems.

THE RIGHT CORONARY ARTERY

The Judkins right catheter will seat in almost all right coronary arteries. If the right coronary has a horizontal, downgoing or slightly upward-directed proximal segment, then the right Judkins is usually the first catheter chosen (Fig. 17-14). The size of the right coronary orifice is occasionally a problem as the tip of the guiding catheter is larger than the diagnostic catheter and may wedge in the orifice. A no. 8 French guiding catheter is less likely to wedge but also has somewhat less backup potential than the no. 9 French for crossing severe lesions. Careful positioning in the ostium can usually solve this wedging problem. Catheters are now being developed with side holes which can be wedged

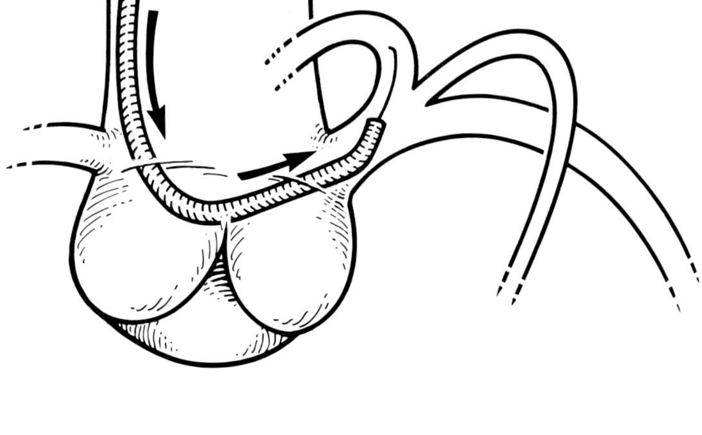

Figure 17-10 Left anterior oblique caudal view showing the left Judkins catheter in a transverse position across the aortic root with its tip directed superiorly toward the left anterior descending artery.

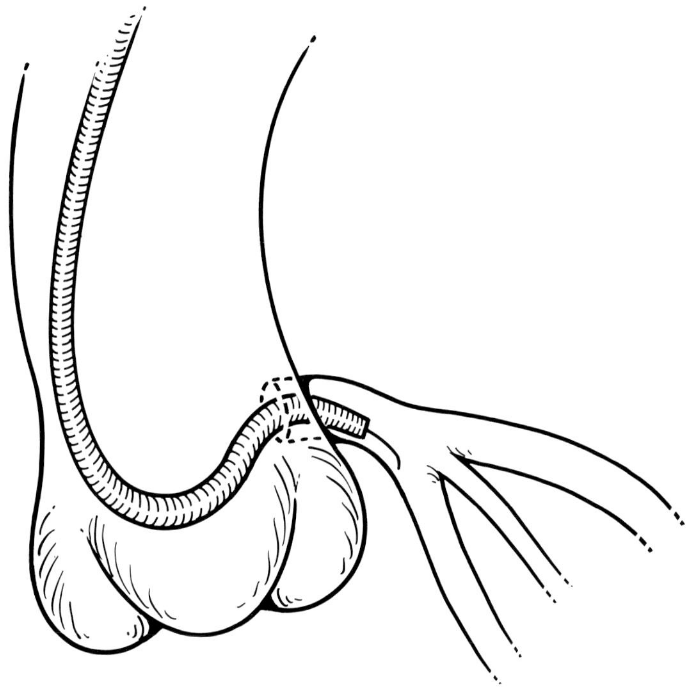

Figure 17-11 Right anterior oblique view with the Amplatz catheter deflecting its tip inferiorly toward the circumflex coronary artery.

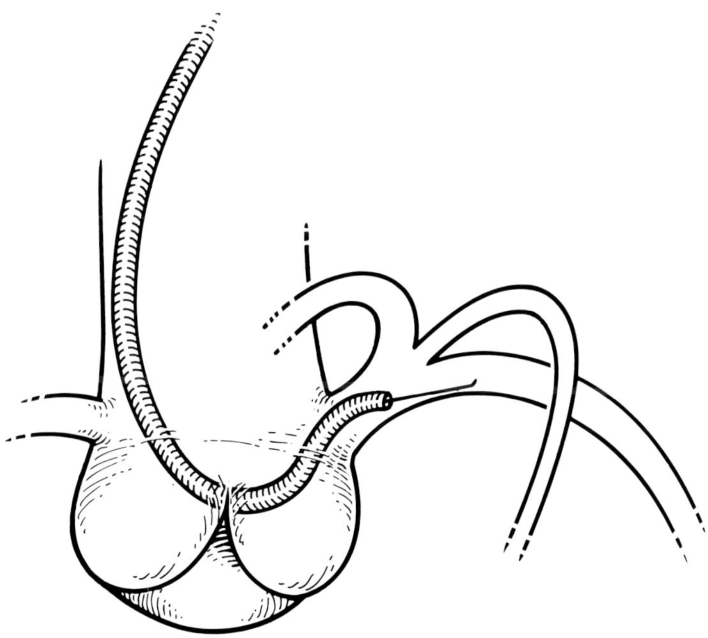

Figure 17-12 Left anterior oblique caudal view of the left coronary artery with a straight guidewire deflected toward the circumflex coronary artery.

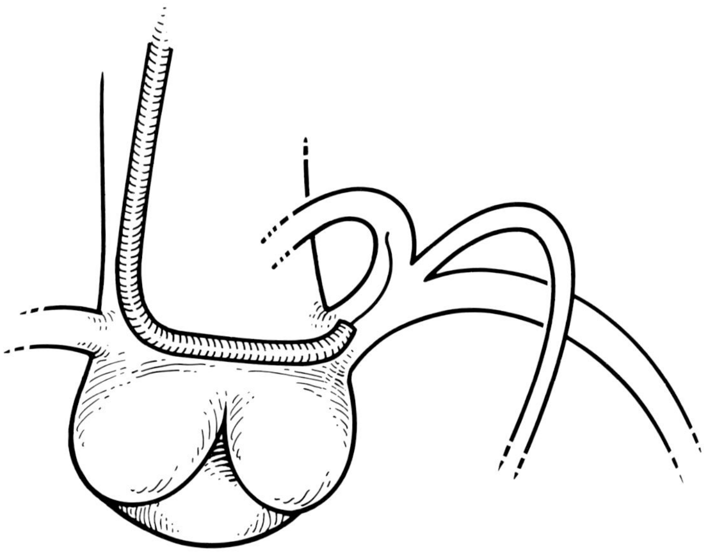

A

Figure 17-13 Left anterior oblique caudal views: (*a*) Single-curved guidewire exiting from Judkins catheter points with the terminal curve of the catheter upward toward the anterior descending coronary. (*b*) Single-curved guidewire exiting from Amplatz catheter points downward toward the circumflex coronary artery. (*c*) Double- or S-curved guidewire exiting from Judkins catheter points away from the terminal curve of the catheter downward toward the circumflex coronary artery.

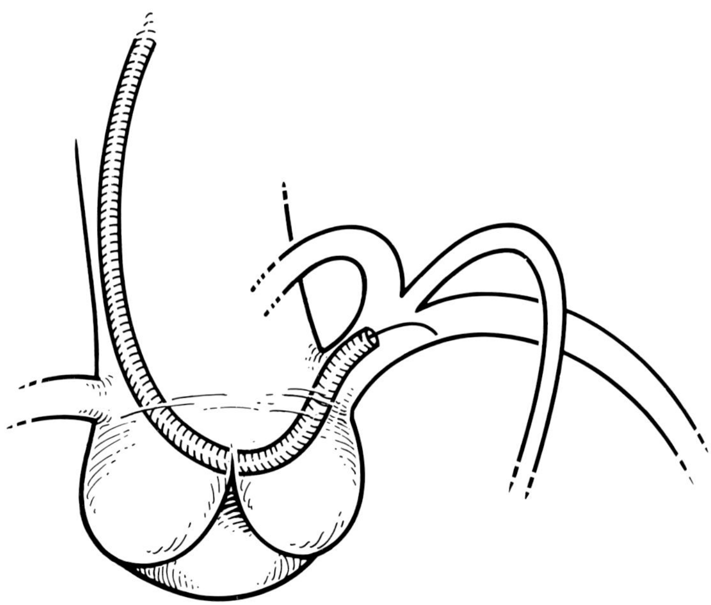

B

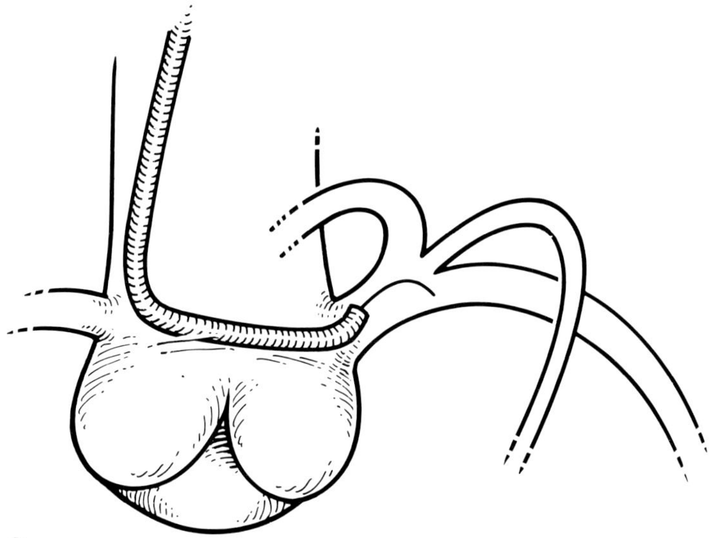

C

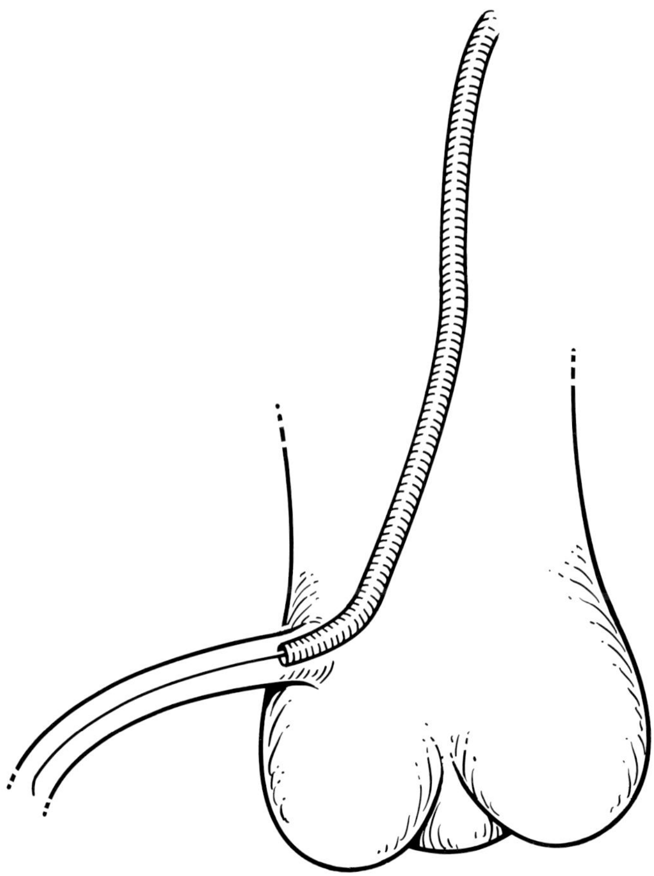

Figure 17-14 Left anterior oblique view showing Judkins shaped right guiding catheter entering the right coronary orifice.

into a difficult right coronary orifice and yet allow antegrade flow through the holes and out the distal opening in the catheter so that perfusion can be maintained despite a wedge position. This flow can be maintained with the guidewire down the right coronary artery but is partially lost once the balloon catheter is advanced into the artery. Still, this produces a solution for the tight right coronary orifice in some cases.

Another problem with the right coronary artery is proximal tortuosity, especially if the proximal right coronary artery starts upward and then turns 180° to travel downward in the atrioventricular groove. This shepherd's crook configuration may make right coronary artery angioplasty impossible. Using a modified Amplatz or multipurpose catheter with an upward crook, one can enter the proximal right coronary artery to the top of the shepherd's crook and provide adequate backup for crossing relatively tight lesions (Fig. 17-15). The multipurpose catheters are also helpful in some right coronary arteries when the proximal segment is downgoing. If the lesion is very tight or distal, the backup provided by the right Judkins catheter may be inadequate. In this case, a straighter catheter such as the multipurpose can be inserted into the right coronary artery for 2 to 3 cm, thereby providing a good backup platform for the balloon catheter to cross tight stenoses.

VEIN GRAFTS

Saphenous vein grafts arise from the anterior portion of the aorta and may travel in a downward, horizontal, or superior direction. The Judkins right coronary catheters are good for angiograms of vein grafts but provide inadequate backup for angioplasty. The multipurpose catheter, as is or with a 90° or greater curve (Fig. 17-16), will enter the graft orifice and with further advancing will be positioned with the heel of the catheter lying in the opposite wall of the aorta so as to provide excellent

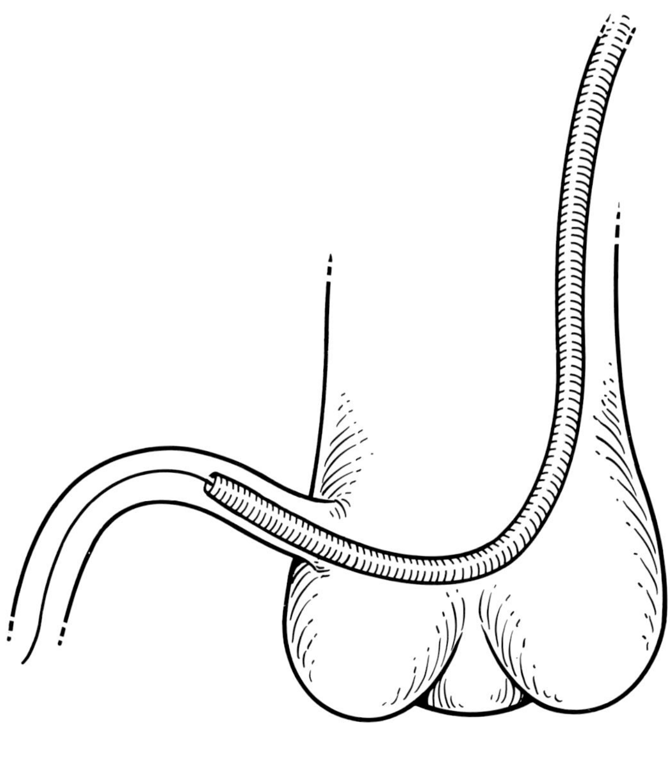

Figure 17-15 Left anterior oblique view showing multipurpose guiding catheter entering an upgoing right coronary artery in order to provide better backup for balloon crossing of the lesion.

backup. Often the tip can be advanced 1 to 3 cm into the graft to provide even better backup position if needed.

The guiding catheter selected for each artery will be determined by the operator's experience. Each has advantages and disadvantages and potential complications which must be avoided.

Following angioplasty, patients are maintained on aspirin 325 mg daily. Trials are currently underway to evaluate the effect of the addition of dipyridamole to aspirin and on the effect of calcium antagonists in conjunction with aspirin. A previous trial comparing warfarin anticoagulation with aspirin therapy showed that the Coumadin was not superior to aspirin in preventing restenosis; therefore, Coumadin anticoagulation has been discontinued.[8]

COMPLICATIONS

Complications of PTCA include all complications of cardiac catheterization itself, including thromboembolic events, arterial dissection, bleeding, and thrombosis of the entry site.[9] Certain complications, however, are more unique to angioplasty. Because of the controlled injury aspects of angioplasty, there is the threat of coronary occlusion due to dissection or expanding intramural hematoma or spasm. If in the process of dilating an artery total occlusion occurs, one must make a judgment about whether to attempt to reopen the vessel. If occlusion occurs with the wire still in place across the lesion, then there is access to the distal artery and the balloon catheter can easily be passed across the lesion and the vessel redilated. Management of this complication usually is best approached by dilating the artery multiple times with long inflations at moderate pressures in an attempt to reattach the intimal surface so that the lumen is maintained. When these attempts fail and the artery continues to reclose, emergency surgery is required.[10] In the process of preparing for surgery, it is often possible to maintain antegrade flow by periodic inflations and deflations with the balloon still in place across the lesion. If acute ischemia cannot be eliminated

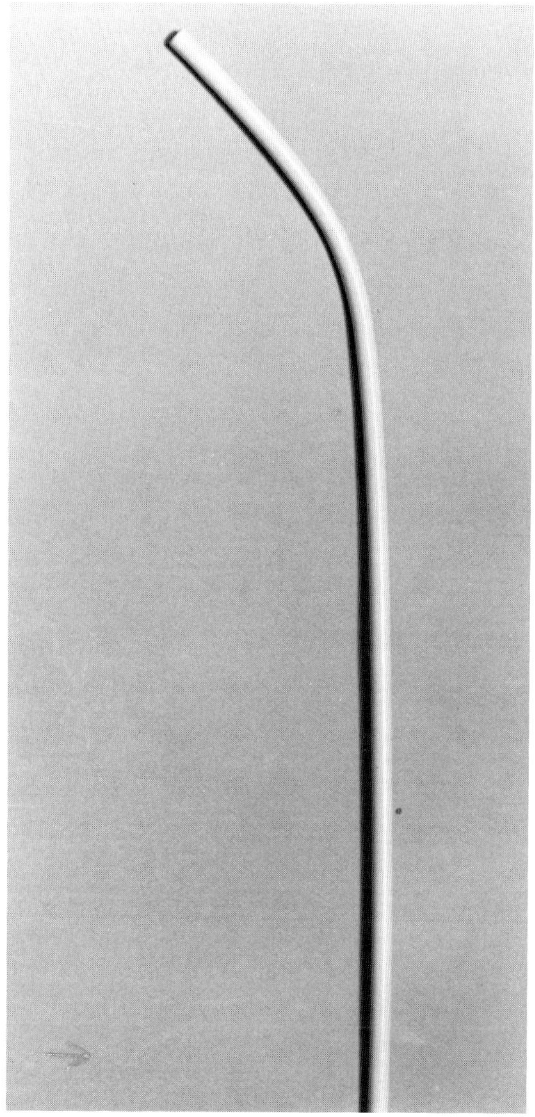

A

Figure 17-16 (*a*) Multipurpose guiding catheter. (*b*) Multipurpose guiding catheter heated and bent to a 90° curve.

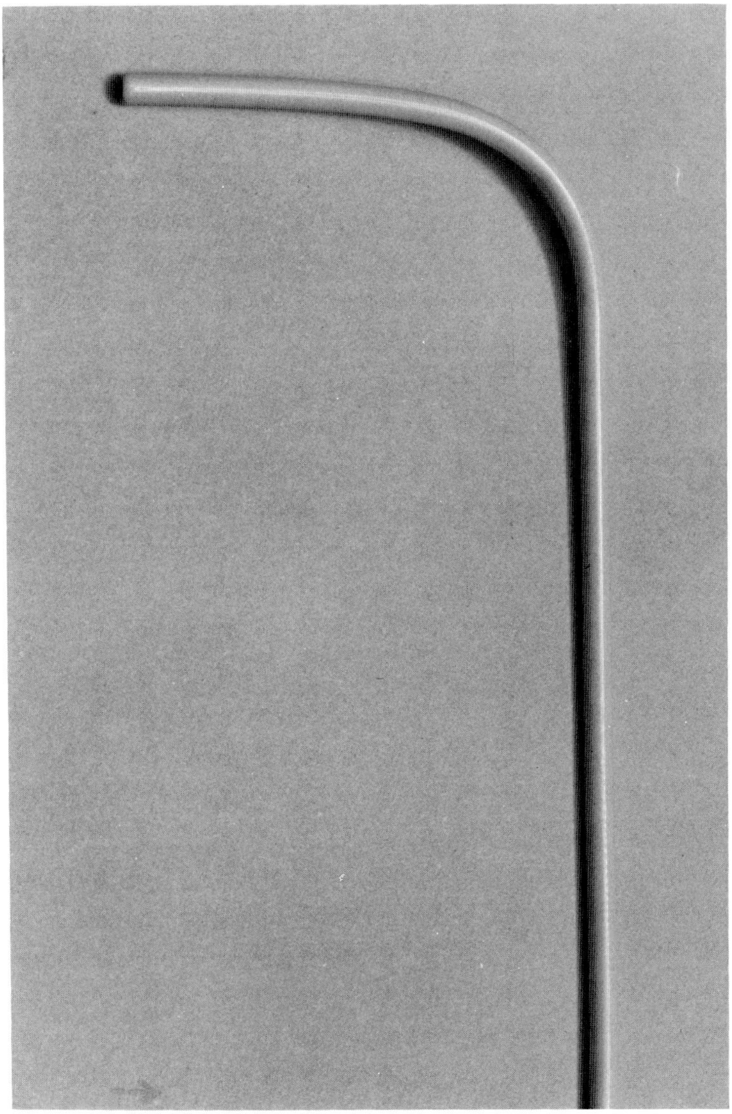

B *(Figure 17-16, continued)*

by that technique, then it is possible to perfuse oxygenated blood from the contralateral femoral artery through the balloon catheter and down the distal vessel. The amount of blood that can be infused is quite limited; however, frequently the pain and ST-segment elevation can be eliminated by this technique while preparing for surgery.

When large areas of myocardium are in jeopardy so that there is hemodynamic instability or there is any delay in moving directly to the operating room, insertion of the intraaortic balloon pump by the percutaneous method will minimize left ventricular work and maximize diastolic coronary filling. We find that the use of the intraaortic balloon pump has been beneficial in reducing the extent of myocardial infarction secondary to acute coronary occlusion and emergency bypass surgery.

If the balloon catheter and guidewire have both

been removed from the artery prior to an acute occlusion, then recrossing of the artery depends on the judgment of the operator based on the anatomy of the artery and the possibilities of opening it.[11] Attempts at opening the artery should be made immediately while making preparations for emergency surgery if the attempts should fail. The patient should not be delayed unduly from receiving emergency bypass surgery by these attempts. In our experience, approximately 50 percent of acute occlusions occurring following angioplasty can be reopened by a second angioplasty without need of moving to the operating room. Similar caution should be exercised when crossing the lesion so as not to create a dissection which may propagate distally and make insertion of distal grafts more difficult.[12]

Some have recommended the use of streptokinase for acutely occluded coronary artery following angioplasty. We have not had extensive experience with this technique, preferring to open the artery mechanically if possible. Occlusions occurring several hours after angioplasty, particularly if these happen at times when mobilization of the laboratory team may take 1 hour or longer, may be properly approached by the use of intravenous streptokinase while making preparations to attempt to recross the vessel if streptokinase attempts are unsuccessful. One must remember, however, that the use of streptokinase will complicate emergency bypass surgery if that is required.

Pericardial tamponade is a serious complication and in our experience has been limited to a few cases of pacemaker wire perforation of the right ventricle. Great care should be exercised in placing pacing catheters in heparinized patients, and one should be alert to the possibility of right ventricular perforation.

Other complications include bleeding from the femoral puncture site, including hematoma formation and retroperitoneal bleeding. Occasionally retroperitoneal bleeding is very insidious and is only picked up by the finding of a decreased hematocrit the day following angioplasty. Usually no further therapy is indicated, but occasionally transfusion is required. Ventricular arrhythmias secondary to coronary occlusion and reperfusion following transient occlusion are more common with angioplasty than with catheterization. All personnel must be well-trained in application of electrical countershock and emergency infusion of lidocaine and other antiarrhythmic drugs. Bradyarrhythmias are usually managed with the prophylactic right ventricular pacemaker, which is inserted prior to the angioplasty procedure.

CONTRAINDICATIONS

Contraindications are based on two factors: (1) the patient's safety, and (2) the chance of success of the angioplasty. First, patients who have left main stenosis should not undergo coronary angioplasty because of the risk of occlusion and the subsequent involvement of massive amounts of left ventricular myocardium should occlusion occur. It should be pointed out that even with emergency surgery immediately available, loss of a very large portion of the left ventricular blood supply may cause profound hypotension and pulmonary edema due to severe generalized left ventricular dysfunction which may jeopardize the patient's survival while moving on to emergency bypass surgery. Even if all vessels are adequately bypassed, it is difficult to resuscitate the patient following an acute total left main occlusion.

Other anatomic situations which carry a high risk include those in which a substantial portion of the left ventricular myocardium has suffered a previous infarction and the artery to undergo angioplasty perfuses a large portion of the remaining myocardium. An example would be total right coronary occlusion with an akinetic inferior wall and a tight stenosis in the proximal LAD. Whereas the chance of success may be in the 95 percent range, if occlusive dissection occurs, a very large segment of the left ventricular myocardium will be affected by this insult. We have found these patients are very unstable, and movement to emergency surgery poses a difficult technical problem.

Contraindications related to the anatomy of the coronary stenoses are becoming less as improved catheter systems are developed which provide accessibility to move difficult and more distal lesions.

Selection for single vessel angioplasty has been dependent on the symptomatic setting, objective evidence of ischemia, and anatomically suitable lesions. A successful angioplasty applied in single vessel disease essentially corrects the entire ischemic insult to the left ventricle and can be easily assessed both subjectively and objectively.

MULTIVESSEL PTCA

As one moves toward multivessel angioplasty, things become a bit more complex. The criteria for multivessel angioplasty are the same as for single vessel, namely, symptomatic status which would require some reperfusion therapy, objective evidence of ischemia, and good possibilities of angioplasty success. Factors to be considered should again be the safety of the patient, the chance of success with angioplasty, and the chance of producing equally satisfactory results as far as myocardial revascularization is concerned when angioplasty is compared to coronary bypass surgery (Fig. 17-17).

SAFETY

If an artery is to be dilated, one should always consider the consequences if the artery became totally occluded. In multivessel angioplasty, the chance of total occlusion must be added to the other, previous insults to the left ventricle. If there has already been occlusion of a vessel with myocardial infarction in a site remote from the angioplasty, then the combined insult of that infarcted area and the area of ischemia resultant from a potential total occlusion of the vessel being dilated must be kept in mind. If that total area exceeds 50 percent of the left ventricular myocardium, then there is the likelihood that severe hemodynamic insult will occur which may make a movement to bypass surgery unsafe for the patient. If, on the other hand, two or three vessels are stenosed and ideally suited for angioplasty, then each vessel can be done with the expectation that if sudden occlusion occurs, there will be adequate remaining perfusion through the other two vessels to maintain left ventricular performance, and safe movement to bypass surgery

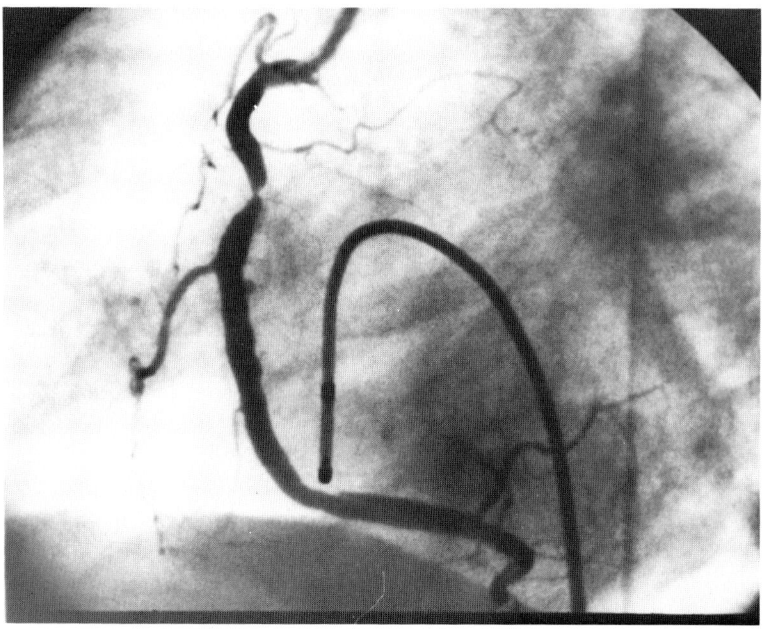

A

Figure 17-17 Double vessel angioplasty. (*a*) Right coronary stenosis, left anterior oblique view. (*b*) After PTCA. (*c*) Circumflex stenosis, right anterior oblique view. (*d*) After PTCA.

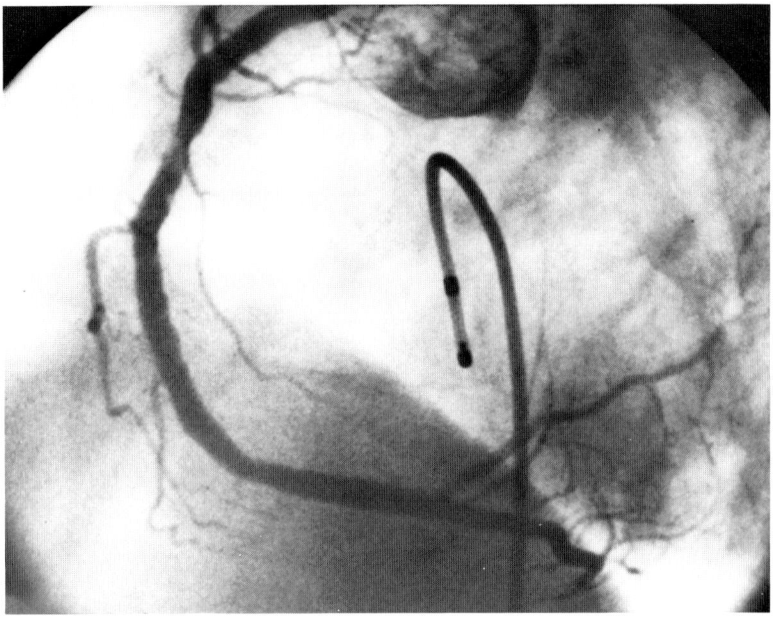

B

(Figure 17-17, continued)

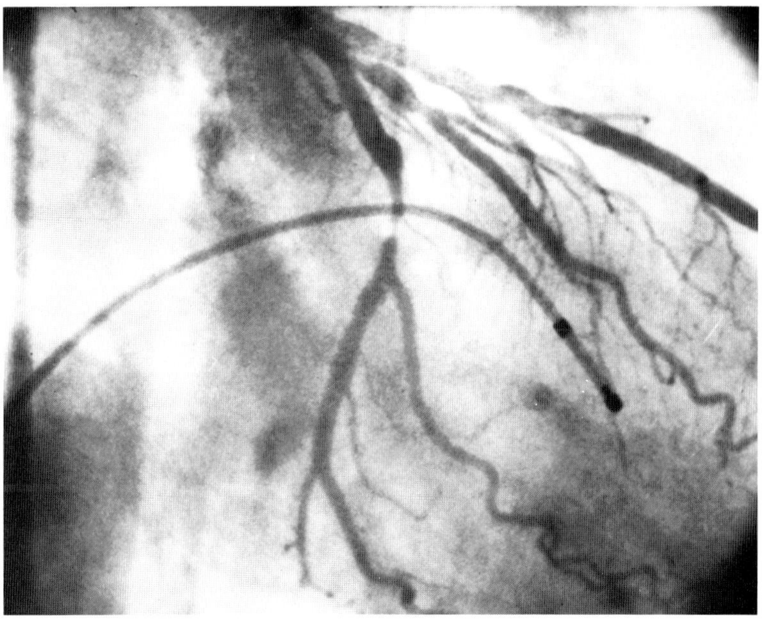

C

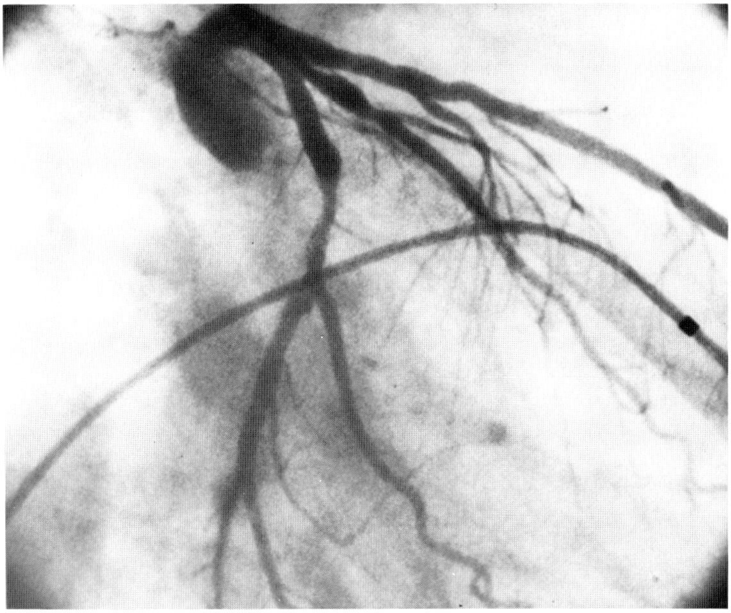

D *(Figure 17-17, continued)*

can be accomplished. The most severe lesion is usually approached first.

CHANCE OF SUCCESS

Patients should be selected for multivessel angioplasty who have uniquely suited discrete stenoses in multiple vessels, rather than those patients with diffuse disease. If such multiple discrete stenoses are present, then one can predict a high chance of success in dilating all lesions. If the chance of success of the angioplasty with all lesions falls to an unacceptable level, then angioplasty should not be attempted.

CHANCE OF RIVALING SURGICAL SUCCESS

If angioplasty would result in opening one or two arteries in multivessel disease, yet bypass surgery would be possible to three, four, or five vessels, then bypass surgery is a better choice in most cases. An example would be a patient with a totally occluded circumflex marginal and diagonal branch who had an LAD suitable for angioplasty. Whereas angioplasty would open the LAD, it would leave the circumflex marginal and diagonal branches unrevascularized, thereby leaving a site for ischemia, perhaps not solving the patient's problem. If those two totally occluded vessels were suitable for bypass surgery, then triple bypass might be a superior solution to angioplasty.

Obviously there are exceptions to these relative contraindications, and some patients who are poor surgical candidates should be considered for angioplasty. There will be, however, increasing pressure to do angioplasty in highly dangerous circumstances because of the high risk of bypass surgery as well. Such pressures should be resisted if the patient's safety is jeopardized by such a decision.

RESULTS

Evaluation of the results of percutaneous transluminal coronary angioplasty have included (1) symptomatic relief; (2) reversal of ECG changes during exercise[13] and positive radionuclear examinations[14,15]; and (3) improvement of the angiographic appearance of the artery. At present, over 3000 coronary angioplasties have been performed by our group; 194 of these procedures were done in Zurich and the remainder at Emory University Hospital in Atlanta. The Atlanta experience demonstrated an improvement in success rate from 81 percent in the first 200 cases to 93 percent in the last 1000 cases. Primary success is defined as the reduction in luminal diameter stenosis of at least 20 percent and has been achieved in over 90 percent of the Emory series. Emergency bypass surgery has been reduced from over 5 percent in the first 400 cases to under 2 percent in the last 1000 cases. These emergency operations have been performed by our surgical teams, which are available throughout the period when angioplasty is being performed. Of the patients in the series, 1.6 percent have suffered acute myocardial infarctions as a result of acute coronary occlusion. However, prompt surgical intervention has resulted in no infarction or in small infarctions as documented by radionuclear ventriculograms in the majority of patients with acute occlusion although a few patients have suffered large transmural infarctions.[12]

RECURRENCE AND REPEAT ANGIOPLASTY

The first 600 patients undergoing angioplasty at Emory University Hospital were followed prospectively for recurrence and late complications. Over 99 percent of the successfully dilated patients have now been followed, and 76 percent have had repeat angiograms. Primary success occurred in 85 percent of these patients, and 89 percent of them have been followed prospectively.[16]

Angiographic recurrence was defined as the loss of 50 percent or more of the initial diameter gain with angioplasty. Repeat angiographic studies have been somewhat biased toward those patients with recurrent symptoms. The recurrence rate in this early series was 33 percent. Changes in methodology since then include longer and higher pressure inflations and anticoagulation with aspirin in all cases, and the addition of dipyridamole or nifedipine in many of the others. These techniques may have resulted in a somewhat lower recurrence rate than in the early experience. Of the variables influencing recurrence, it was found that males had a higher recurrence rate than females, and the right coronary artery showed a lower recurrence rate when compared to the anterior descending coronary artery. Patients who have recurrence can undergo a second angioplasty.

Of the 171 patients with documented recurrences, 95 percent had repeat angioplasty; 92 of the 95 attempts were successful, and the complication rates were lower than in the initial angioplasty series. Following a second angioplasty, recurrence has been documented in 26 percent. Utilizing these figures for initial success plus success following repeat angioplasty, we found a greater than 78 percent chance of continued long-term success if repeat angioplasty is utilized in those cases in which it is needed.

Recurrent stenosis has not been well-studied pathologically; however, a few specimens which have been studied during the recurrence phase of angioplasty show a homogeneous smooth muscle cell proliferation in the intima of the artery. The pathology of this recurrence and methods to prevent it remain the most important aspect of angioplasty research at the present time.

ANGIOPLASTY FOLLOWING CORONARY BYPASS SURGERY

Patients who have undergone angioplasty following bypass surgery make up a very satisfying group in whom repeat bypass surgery has been largely avoided. The distinct advantage of angioplasty in this setting is the avoidance of increased risk of a reoperation while the option to have surgery at a later time remains, should new problems occur. Of concern, however, is the potential risk of emergency reoperation if angioplasty is complicated by vessel closure. Results from the National Heart, Lung, and Blood Institute PTCA Registry suggest a significantly higher risk exists when angioplasty is attempted in postoperative patients.[17,18] In our previously reported experience with 122 angioplasty procedures in postoperative patients, primary success was achieved in 88 percent, 2 percent required emergency reoperation, and there were no

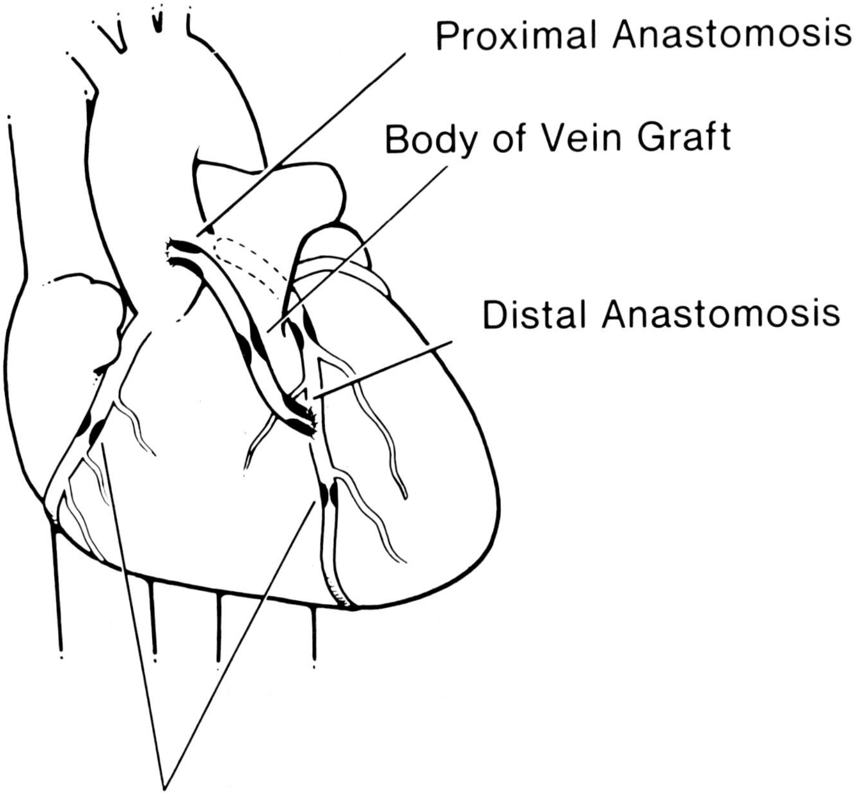

Figure 17-18 Sites of angioplasty in post–coronary bypass patients.

deaths related to the procedure.[19] At last follow-up, 76 percent of patients had persisting benefit from the angioplasty. Angioplasty is needed to correct stenoses which develop in saphenous vein grafts or in native coronary arteries when graft closure occurs or new disease develops (Fig. 17-18). The results of angioplasty are highly influenced by the location of the stenosis attempted. Best results occur with dilation of the distal saphenous vein anastomosis. In 34 patients with stenosis at this site, 94 percent had a successful angioplasty, only 12 percent developed restenosis, and the second angioplasty was successful in all patients attempted with no restenosis. This excellent result makes angioplasty the treatment of choice for stenosis at the junction of the saphenous vein and coronary artery.

Fifty-nine patients required angioplasty of the native coronary artery; roughly half for lesions present at the time of surgery and the remainder because of new atherosclerotic lesions developing postoperatively. Successful angioplasty was obtained in 83 percent of patients, and 2 percent required emergency surgery. There were no other significant complications of the procedure. Only 14 percent of patients followed over 6 months had evidence of restenosis, and at last follow-up, 46 of 59 patients (78 percent) had continued success from their angioplasty. These favorable results lead us to frequently attempt angioplasty of native coronary arteries in postoperative patients when the anatomy is favorable and the risk is not excessive. When stenosis occurs in the midportion of a saphenous vein graft or in the proximal anastomosis (aorta-to–saphenous vein graft junction), it is frequently possible to dilate the lesion successfully, but recurrence is common. Atherosclerotic lesions in vein grafts are notoriously friable, and we have limited our attempts at angioplasty to discrete, focal, hourglass-shaped lesions, avoiding eccentric, irregular, or long vein graft stenoses. In one patient with an eccentric vein graft atheroma, distal embolization of the entire plaque resulted in an inferior infarction. Because of the higher risk of embolization and a restenosis rate that probably exceeds 50 percent, there is not great enthusiasm for angioplasty of mid vein graft stenoses, although carefully selected patients are still attempted. Distal embolization has not occurred with angioplasty of the proximal saphenous vein graft anastomosis, but the restenosis rate at this site also exceeds 50 percent in our experience. The ability to perform coronary angioplasty in postoperative patients has altered our management somewhat, leading us in the direction of early coronary arteriography in order that high-grade stenotic segments amenable to angioplasty can be detected before there is progression of stenosis to total vessel occlusion.

INDICATIONS

Although indications have been covered more thoroughly in the previous chapter, our current indications for coronary angioplasty include (1) demonstrated ischemia in symptomatic patients who would otherwise be candidates for coronary bypass surgery; (2) anatomic suitability of lesions for angioplasty; (3) unacceptable symptoms or unacceptable side effects from medication in patients who also have suitable lesions for angioplasty and who would otherwise not be considered for elective coronary bypass surgery; (4) symptoms occurring in patients who have had coronary bypass surgery who have suitable anatomic lesions. In practice, over 75 percent of our patients remain in the category of single vessel disease whereas the multivessel-diseased patients selected meet the criteria of (1) a high chance of primary success; (2) the ability to survive to emergency bypass surgery should the artery dilated occlude; and (3) an anticipated final result of angioplasty equivalent to that of multivessel bypass surgery. There is a need to compare the long-term results of angioplasty in multivessel disease to the results of coronary bypass surgery. Our prediction is that certain subsets of patients with multivessel disease may benefit over the years from coronary angioplasty and coronary bypass surgery each applied at the proper point in their disease process.

REFERENCES

1 Dotter CT, Judkins MP: Transluminal treatment of arteriosclerotic obstruction: Description of the technique and a preliminary report of its application. Circulation, 30:654, 1964.

2 Porstmann W: Ein Neuer Korsett-Ballonkatheter Fur Transluminalen Rekanalisation Nach Dotter Unter Besonderer Berucksichtigung Von Obliterationen An Den Beckenarterien. Radiol Diagn (Berl), 14:239, 1973.

3 Zeitler E, Schmidtke J, Schoop W: Die Perkutane Behandlung von Arteriellen Durchblutuengasstorungen der Extremiaten mit Katheter. Vasa, 2:401, 1973.

4 Gruentzig AR: Die Perkutane Rekanalisation Chronischer Arterieller Verschlusse (Dotter-Prinzip) mit Einem Doppellumigen Dilatationskatheter. Roefo, 124:80, 1976.

5 Gruentzig AR, Senning A, Siegenthaler WE: Nonoperative dilatation of coronary artery stenosis. N Engl J Med, 301:61, 1979.

6 Gruentzig AR, Hollman J: Improved primary success rate in transluminal coronary angioplasty using a steerable guidewire system. Circulation, 66(suppl II):II–330, 1982 (abstract).

7 King SB, Gruentzig AR, Douglas JS: Coronary angioplasty: Current status and techniques. Cardiovas Pulm, June–July 1983.

8 Thornton MA, Gruentzig AR, Holman J: Coumadin or aspirin after coronary angioplasty? J Am Coll Cardiol, 1(2):725, 1983.

9 Dorros G, Cowley MJ, Simpson J, Bentivoglio LG, Block PC, Bourassa M, et al: Percutaneous transluminal coronary angioplasty: Report of complications from the National Heart, Lung, and Blood Institute PTCA Registry. Circulation, 67:723–729, 1983.

10 Murphy D, Craver J, Jones E, Gruentzig AR, King SB, Hatcher C: Surgical revascularization following unsuccessful percutaneous transluminal coronary angioplasty. J Thorac Cardiovasc Surg, 84:342–348, 1982.

11 Holman J, Gruentzig AR, Douglas JS, King SB, Ischinger T, Meier B: Acute occlusion after percutaneous transluminal coronary angioplasty—a new approach. Circulation, 68:725–732, 1983.

12 Libow M, Cooke D, King SB, Gruentzig AR, Douglas JS et al: Left ventricular function after unsuccessful angioplasty and emergency coronary bypass surgery (submitted to Am Coll Cardiol Annual Meeting).

13 Meier B, Gruentzig AR, Siegenthaler WE, Schlumpf M: Long-term exercise performance after percutaneous transluminal coronary angioplasty and coronary artery bypass grafting. Circulation, 68:796, 1983.

14 Hirzel H, Nuesch K, Gruentzig AR, Luetolf U: Short and long-term changes in myocardial perfusion after percutaneous transluminal coronary angioplasty assessed by thallium-201 scintigraphy. Circulation, 63:1001–1007, 1981.

15 Peterson RJ, King SB, Fajman WA, Douglas JS, Jones RH: Relationship of coronary artery stenosis and gradient to exercise-induced ischemia. J Am Coll Cardiol, I:673, 1983.

16 Meier B, King SB, Gruentzig AR, Douglas JS, et al: Repeat coronary angioplasty. J Am Coll Cardiol (in press).

17 Kent KM, Bentivoglio LG, Block PC, et al: Percutaneous transluminal coronary angioplasty: Report from the Registry of the National Heart, Lung, and Blood Institute. Am J Cardiol, 49:2011–2020, 1982.

18 Mock MB, Kent KM, Bentivoglio LG: The National Heart, Lung and Blood Institute Percutaneous Transluminal Coronary Angioplasty Registry: The first 1116 cases, in Kaltenback M, Gruentzig AR, Rentrop K, Bussmann WD (eds): *Transluminal Coronary Angioplasty and Intracoronary Thrombolysis: Coronary Heart Disease IV*. Springer-Verlag, Berlin, Heidelberg, New York, 1982, pp 11–19.

19 Douglas J, Gruentzig AR, King SB, et al: Percutaneous transluminal coronary angioplasty in patients with prior coronary bypass surgery. J Am Coll Cardiol, 2:745–754, 1983.

Index